Statistical Methods in Radiation Physics

Statistical Methods in Radiation Physics

Editor:

Olga Moreira, Ph.D.

ArclerPress

www.arclerpress.com

Statistical Methods in Radiation Physics

Editor: Olga Moreira, Ph.D.

708 3rd Avenue, 6th Floor
New York
NY 10017
United States of America
www.arclerpress.com

ISBN: 978-1-68094-437-2

Library of Congress Control Number: 2016951134

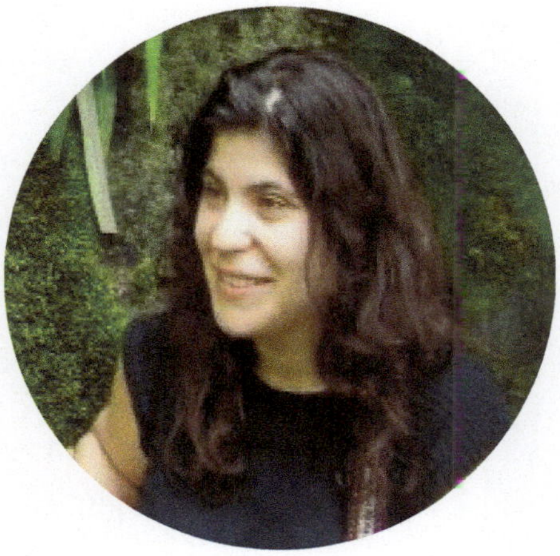

About the Editor

Olga Moreira, Ph.D.

Olga Moreira obtained her Ph.D. in Astrophysics from the University of Liege (Belgium) in 2010, her BSc. in Physics and Applied Mathematics from the University of Porto (Portugal). Her post-graduate travels and international collaborations with the European Space Agency (ESA) and European Southern Observatory (ESO) led to great personal and professional growth as a scientist. Currently, she is working as an independent researcher, technical writer, and editor in the fields of Mathematics, Physics, Astronomy and Astrophysics.

Contents

List of Contributors ..... *xi*

Preface ..... *xv*

Introduction ..... *xvii*

Section I: Radioactive Decay and Radionuclides concentration

Chapter 1 The Uncertainty of the Half-Life 3

1. Introduction 3
2. Applications of Half-Lives 4
3. Measurement of Short Half-Lives 6
4. Measurement of Intermediate Half-Lives 10
5. Measurement of Long Half-Lives 14

Conclusions 15

References 15

Chapter 2 Fundamental Uncertainty Equations for Nuclear Dating Applied to the 140ba-140la and 227th-223ra Chronometers 19

1. Introduction 19
2. Basic Equations 20
3. Uncertainty Propagation 22
4. Procedure for Chronometry 23
5. 140ba-140la Clock 23

Conclusions 31

Acknowledgement 31

Annex a Full Uncertainty Propagation 31

References 33

Chapter 3 Evaluating Summarised Radionuclide Concentration Ratio Datasets for Wildlife 35

1. Introduction 35
2. Methods 38
3. Results and Discussion 39

Conclusions 46

Acknowledgements 46

References 49

Chapter 4 Soil Gas Radon Assessment and Development of a Radon Risk Map 53

1. Introduction 53
2. Geological Setting 54
3. Instruments and Methods 56
4. Results and Discussion 58

Conclusions 63

Footnotes 63

Acknowledgments 63

References 63

Chapter 5 Development of a Neural Network Approach to Characterise 226ra Contamination at Legacy Sites Using Gamma-Ray Spectra Taken from Boreholes 67

1. Introduction 67

2. Materials and Methods ... 70
3. Results and Discussion ... 74
Conclusions ... 77
Acknowledgements ... 78
References ... 78

Section II: Dosimetry and Radiation-Induced Therapy

Chapter 6 Radiological Dose Reconstruction ... 83
1. Results ... 84
2. Discussion ... 89
3. Methods ... 91
Acknowledgements ... 93
References ... 93

Chapter 7 Bayesian Model Selection Validates a Biokinetic Model for Zirconium Processing ... 95
1. Background ... 95
2. Methods ... 96
3. Results And Discussion ... 100
Conclusions ... 104
Acknowledgements ... 104
References ... 104

Chapter 8 Space Radiation Risks for Astronauts ... 107
1. Introduction ... 107
2. Methods ... 108
3. Results ... 110
4. Discussion ... 116
Conclusions ... 119
Acknowledgments ... 119
Author Contributions ... 119
References ... 119

Chapter 9 The Perils of Adapting to Dose Errors in Radiation Therapy ... 123
1. Introduction ... 123
2. Method ... 124
3. Results ... 126
4. Theoretical Insight Into Daily Dose Performance ... 131
Conclusions ... 131
Acknowledgments ... 132
Author Contributions ... 132
References ... 132

Chapter 10 Cell to Cell Variability of Radiation-Induced Foci ... 135
1. Introduction ... 135
2. Materials and Methods ... 135
3. Results ... 137
4. Discussion ... 143
Acknowledgments ... 146
Author Contributions ... 146
References ... 146

Chapter 11 **Electromagnetic Thermography Nondestructive Evaluation: Physics-Based Modeling and Pattern Mining.......... 149**
1. Introduction 149
2. Method 150
3. Results 156
4. Discussion 159
Acknowledgements 159
References 159

Chapter 12 **Radiation Induced Chromatin Conformation Changes Analysed by Fluorescent Localization Microscopy, Statistical Physics, and Graph Theory 161**
1. Introduction 161
2. Materials And Methods 162
3. Results 165
4. Discussion 171
Acknowledgments 172
Author Contributions 172
References 172

Chapter 13 **Therapeutic Application of CCK2R-Targeting Pp-F11 .... 177**
1. Background 177
2. Methods 178
3. Results 182
4. Discussion 187
Conclusions 188
Authors' Contributions 188
Acknowledgements 188
References 188

Chapter 14 **Early Reduction in Tumour [18f] Fluorothymidine (FLT) Uptake In Patients with Non-Small Cell Lung Cancer (NSCLC) Treated with Radiotherapy Alone 191**
1. Introduction 191
2. Materials And Methods 192
3. Results 195
4. Discussion 198
Acknowledgments 200
References 200

Section III: Solar Radiation

Chapter 15 **Measurement Biases Explain Discrepancies Between the Observed and Simulated Decadal Variability of Surface Incident Solar Radiation 205**
1. Introduction 205
2. Results 205
3. Discussion 210
4. Methods 210
Acknowledgements 211
References 211

Chapter 16 **Monthly-Averaged Hourly Solar Diffuse Radiation Models for World-Wide Locations 215**
1. Introduction 215

Conclusions 222
Authors' Contributions 222
References 222

Chapter 17 **Evaluation of Radiometric and Atmospheric Correction Algorithms for Aboveground Forest Biomass Estimation Using Landsat 5 Tm Data 223**
1. Introduction 223
2. Materials and Methods 224
3. Results 228
4. Discussion 232
Conclusions 233
Acknowledgments 233
Author Contributions 233
References 233

Chapter 18 **A Bayesian Method for Short-Term Probabilistic Forecasting of Photovoltaic Generation in Smart Grid Operation and Control 237**
1. Introduction 237
2. Probabilistic Forecasting Method Based on the Bayesian Approach 238
3. Probabilistic Forecasting of the Photovoltaic Generation 239
4. Experimental Section 242
Conclusions 245
Acknowledgements 245
References 245

Index 247

List of Contributors

S Pommé
European Commission, Joint Research Centre, Institute for Reference Materials and Measurements, Retieseweg 111, B-2440 Geel, Belgium

S.M. Collins
National Physical Laboratory, Hampton Road, Teddington, Middlesex TW11 OLW, UK

A. Harms
National Physical Laboratory, Hampton Road, Teddington, Middlesex TW11 OLW, UK

S.M. Jerome
National Physical Laboratory, Hampton Road, Teddington, Middlesex TW11 OLW, UK

M.D. Wood
School of Environment and Life Sciences, University of Salford, Manchester M5 4WT, UK

N.A. Beresford
NERC Centre for Ecology & Hydrology, Bailrigg, Lancaster LA1 4AP, UK

B.J. Howard
NERC Centre for Ecology & Hydrology, Bailrigg, Lancaster LA1 4AP, UK

D. Copplestone
Biological and Environmental Sciences, School of Natural Sciences, University of Stirling, Stirling FK9 4LA, UK

G. Cinelli
European Commission, Joint Research Centre (JRC), Institute for Transuranium Elements (ITU), Via E Fermi 2749, 21027 Ispra, Italy

L. Tositti
Department of Biological, Geological and Environmental Sciences – Section of Geology, Alma Mater Studiorum University of Bologna, Piazza di Porta San Donato 1, 40126 Bologna, Italy

B. Capaccioni
Department of Chemistry «Giacomo Ciamician», Alma Mater Studiorum University of Bologna, Via Selmi 2, 40126 Bologna, Italy

E. Brattich
Department of Biological, Geological and Environmental Sciences – Section of Geology, Alma Mater Studiorum University of Bologna, Piazza di Porta San Donato 1, 40126 Bologna, Italy
Department of Chemistry «Giacomo Ciamician», Alma Mater Studiorum University of Bologna, Via Selmi 2, 40126 Bologna, Italy

D. Mostacci
Laboratory of Nuclear Engineering, Via dei Colli 16, 40136 Bologna, Italy

Adam Varley
Department of Biological and Environmental Sciences, University of Stirling, Stirling FK9 4LA, UK

Andrew Tyler
Department of Biological and Environmental Sciences, University of Stirling, Stirling FK9 4LA, UK

Leslie Smith
Department of Computing Science and Mathematics, University of Stirling, Stirling FK9 4LA, UK

Paul Dale
Scottish Environmental Protection Agency, Radioactive Substances, Strathallan House, Castle Business Park, Stirling FK9 4TZ, UK

Jacqueline Garnier-Laplace
Institut de Radioprotection et de Sûreté Nucléaire, Pôle Radioprotection, Environnement, Déchets, Crise, PRP-ENV/SERIS, Cadarache, Bâtiment 159, BP3, F-13115 Saint Paul lez Durance Cedex, France.

Karine Beaugelin-Seiller
Institut de Radioprotection et de Sûreté Nucléaire, Pôle Radioprotection, Environnement, Déchets, Crise, PRP-ENV/SERIS, Cadarache, Bâtiment 159, BP3, F-13115 Saint Paul lez Durance Cedex, France.

Claire Della-Vedova
Institut de Radioprotection et de Sûreté Nucléaire, Pôle Radioprotection, Environnement, Déchets, Crise, PRP-ENV/SERIS, Cadarache, Bâtiment 159, BP3, F-13115 Saint Paul lez Durance Cedex, France.

Jean-Michel Métivier
Institut de Radioprotection et de Sûreté Nucléaire, Pôle Radioprotection, Environnement, Déchets, Crise, PRP-ENV/SERIS, Cadarache, Bâtiment 159, BP3, F-13115 Saint Paul lez Durance Cedex, France.

Christian Ritz
Department of Nutrition, Exercise and Sports Faculty of Science, University of Copenhagen, Rolighedsvej 26 DK-1958 Frederiksberg C, Denmark.

Timothy A. Mousseau
Department of Biological Sciences, University of South Carolina, Columbia, SC 29208, USA.

Anders Pape Møller
Laboratoire d'Ecologie, Systématique et Evolution, CNRS UMR 8079, Université Paris-Sud, Bâtiment 362, F-91405 Orsay Cedex, France.

Daniel Schmidl
Institute of Bioinformatics and Systems Biology, Helmholtz Zentrum Munchen German Research Center for Environmental Health, Neuherberg, Germany.
Institute for Mathematical Sciences, Technische Universitat¨ Munchen, Garching, Germany.

Sabine Hug
Institute of Bioinformatics and Systems Biology, Helmholtz Zentrum Munchen German Research Center for Environmental Health, Neuherberg, Germany.
Institute for Mathematical Sciences, Technische Universitat¨ Munchen, Garching, Germany.

Wei Bo Li
Research Unit Medical Radiation Physics and Diagnostics, Helmholtz Zentrum Munchen German Research Center for Environmental Health, Neuherberg, Germany.

Matthias B Greiter
Research Unit Medical Radiation Physics and Diagnostics, Helmholtz Zentrum Munchen German Research Center for Environmental Health, Neuherberg, Germany.

Fabian J Theis
Institute of Bioinformatics and Systems Biology, Helmholtz Zentrum Munchen German Research Center for Environmental Health, Neuherberg, Germany.
Institute for Mathematical Sciences, Technische Universitat¨ Munchen, Garching, Germany.

Francis A. Cucinotta
Department of Health Physics and Diagnostic Sciences, University of Nevada Las Vegas, Las Vegas, Nevada, United States of America

Velibor V. Mišić
Operations Research Center, Massachusetts Institute of Technology, Cambridge, Massachusetts, United States of America

Timothy C. Y. Chan
Department of Mechanical and Industrial Engineering, University of Toronto, Toronto, Ontario, Canada

Gaëtan Gruel
Department of Human Health Radiation Protection, Institut de Radioprotection et de Sûreté Nucléaire (IRSN), Fontenay aux Roses, France

Carmen Villagrasa
Department of Human Health Radiation Protection, Institut de Radioprotection et de Sûreté Nucléaire (IRSN), Fontenay aux Roses, France

Pascale Voisin
Department of Human Health Radiation Protection, Institut de Radioprotection et de Sûreté Nucléaire (IRSN), Fontenay aux Roses, France

Isabelle Clairand
Department of Human Health Radiation Protection, Institut de Radioprotection et de Sûreté Nucléaire (IRSN), Fontenay aux Roses, France

Marc Benderitter
Department of Human Health Radiation Protection, Institut de Radioprotection et de Sûreté Nucléaire (IRSN), Fontenay aux Roses, France

Jean-François Bottollier-Depois
Department of Human Health Radiation Protection, Institut de Radioprotection et de Sûreté Nucléaire (IRSN), Fontenay aux Roses, France

Joan Francesc Barquinero
Department of Human Health Radiation Protection, Institut de Radioprotection et de Sûreté Nucléaire (IRSN), Fontenay aux Roses, France

Bin Gao
School of Automation, University of Electronic Science and Technology of China, 610054, Chengdu, China.

Wai Lok Woo
School of Electrical and Electronic Engineering, Newcastle University, NE1 7RU, England, United Kingdom.

Gui Yun Tian
School of Automation, University of Electronic Science and Technology of China, 610054, Chengdu, China.
School of Electrical and Electronic Engineering, Newcastle University, NE1 7RU, England, United Kingdom.

Yang Zhang
Institute for Theoretical Physics, Heidelberg University, Philosophenweg 19, 69120, Heidelberg, Germany

Gabriell Máté
Institute for Theoretical Physics, Heidelberg University, Philosophenweg 19, 69120, Heidelberg, Germany

Patrick Müller
Kirchhoff-Institute for Physics, Heidelberg University, Im Neuenheimer Feld 227, 69120, Heidelberg, Germany

Sabina Hillebrandt
Kirchhoff-Institute for Physics, Heidelberg University, Im Neuenheimer Feld 227, 69120, Heidelberg, Germany

Matthias Krufczik
Kirchhoff-Institute for Physics, Heidelberg University, Im Neuenheimer Feld 227, 69120, Heidelberg, Germany

Margund Bach
Kirchhoff-Institute for Physics, Heidelberg University, Im Neuenheimer Feld 227, 69120, Heidelberg, Germany

Rainer Kaufmann
Kirchhoff-Institute for Physics, Heidelberg University, Im Neuenheimer Feld 227, 69120, Heidelberg, Germany

Michael Hausmann
Kirchhoff-Institute for Physics, Heidelberg University, Im Neuenheimer Feld 227, 69120, Heidelberg, Germany

Dieter W. Heermann
Institute for Theoretical Physics, Heidelberg University, Philosophenweg 19, 69120, Heidelberg, Germany

Mark W. Konijnenberg
Department of Nuclear Medicine, Erasmus MC, PO Box 2040, 3000, CA Rotterdam, The Netherlands.

Wout A. P. Breeman
Department of Nuclear Medicine, Erasmus MC, PO Box 2040, 3000, CA Rotterdam, The Netherlands.

Erik de Blois
Department of Nuclear Medicine, Erasmus MC, PO Box 2040, 3000, CA Rotterdam, The Netherlands.

Ho Sze Chan
Department of Nuclear Medicine, Erasmus MC, PO Box 2040, 3000, CA Rotterdam, The Netherlands.

Otto C. Boerman
Department of Nuclear Medicine, Radboud University Medical Center, 6525, GA Nijmegen, The Netherlands.

Peter Laverman
Department of Nuclear Medicine, Radboud University Medical Center, 6525, GA Nijmegen, The Netherlands.

Petra Kolenc-Peitl
Department of Nuclear Medicine, University Medical Centre Ljubljana, SI-1525 Ljubljana, Slovenia.

Marleen Melis
Department of Nuclear Medicine, Erasmus MC, PO Box 2040, 3000, CA Rotterdam, The Netherlands.

Marion de Jong
Department of Nuclear Medicine, Erasmus MC, PO Box 2040, 3000, CA Rotterdam, The Netherlands.
Department of Radiology, Erasmus MC, 3000, CA Rotterdam, The Netherlands.

Ioannis Trigonis
Institute of Population Health, Wolfson Molecular Imaging Centre, Manchester Academic Health Sciences Centre, The University of Manchester, Manchester M20 3LJ, UK

Pek Keng Koh
Manchester Cancer Research Centre, Manchester Academic Health Sciences Centre, The University of Manchester, Manchester M20 4BX, UK

Ben Taylor
The Christie NHS Foundation Trust, Wilmslow Road, Manchester M20 4BX, UK

Mahbubunnabi Tamal
Institute of Population Health, Wolfson Molecular Imaging Centre, Manchester Academic Health Sciences Centre, The University of Manchester, Manchester M20 3LJ, UK

David Ryder
The Christie NHS Foundation Trust, Wilmslow Road, Manchester M20 4BX, UK

Mark Earl
The Christie NHS Foundation Trust, Wilmslow Road, Manchester M20 4BX, UK

Jose Anton-Rodriguez
Institute of Population Health, Wolfson Molecular Imaging Centre, Manchester Academic Health Sciences Centre, The University of Manchester, Manchester M20 3LJ, UK

Kate Haslett
Manchester Cancer Research Centre, Manchester Academic Health Sciences Centre, The University of Manchester, Manchester M20 4BX, UK
The Christie NHS Foundation Trust, Wilmslow Road, Manchester M20 4BX, UK

Helen Young
AstraZeneca Pharmaceuticals, Alderley Park, Macclesfield SK10 4TG, UK

Corinne Faivre-Finn
Manchester Cancer Research Centre, Manchester Academic Health Sciences Centre, The University of Manchester, Manchester M20 4BX, UK
The Christie NHS Foundation Trust, Wilmslow Road, Manchester M20 4BX, UK

Fiona Blackhall
Manchester Cancer Research Centre, Manchester Academic Health Sciences Centre, The University of Manchester, Manchester M20 4BX, UK
The Christie NHS Foundation Trust, Wilmslow Road, Manchester M20 4BX, UK

Alan Jackson
Institute of Population Health, Wolfson Molecular Imaging Centre, Manchester Academic Health Sciences Centre, The University of Manchester, Manchester M20 3LJ, UK

Marie-Claude Asselin
Institute of Population Health, Wolfson Molecular Imaging Centre, Manchester Academic Health Sciences Centre, The University of Manchester, Manchester M20 3LJ, UK

Kaicun Wang
State Key Laboratory of Earth Surface Processes and Resource Ecology, College of Global Change and Earth System Science, Beijing Normal University, Beijing, 100875, China.

T. Muneer
Edinburgh Napier University, Edinburgh, UK.

EJ Gago
University of Granada, Granada, Spain.

S. Etxebarria
University of Granada, Granada, Spain.

Pablito M. López-Serrano
Doctorado en Ciencias Agropecuarias y Forestales, DICAF, Universidad Juárez del Estado de Durango, Boulevard del Guadiana 501, Ciudad Universitaria, Torre de Investigación, 34120 Durango, Dgo, Mexico

José J. Corral-Rivas
Instituto de Silvicultura e Industria de la Madera, Universidad Juárez del Estado de Durango, Boulevard del Guadiana 501, Ciudad Universitaria, Torre de Investigación, 34120 Durango, Dgo, Mexico

Ramón A. Díaz-Varela
Departamento de Botánica–GI-1908-BIOAPLIC, Universidad de Santiago de Compostela, Escuela Politécnica Superior, 27002 Lugo, Spain

Juan G. Álvarez-González
Departamento de Ingeniería Agroforestal, Universidad de Santiago de Compostela, Escuela Politécnica Superior, 27002 Lugo, Spain

Carlos A. López-Sánchez
Instituto de Silvicultura e Industria de la Madera, Universidad Juárez del Estado de Durango, Boulevard del Guadiana 501, Ciudad Universitaria, Torre de Investigación, 34120 Durango, Dgo, Mexico

Antonio Bracale
Department for Technologies, University Parthenope of Napoli, Centro Direzionale di Napoli, Is. C4, 80143 Napoli, Italy

Pierluigi Caramia
Department for Technologies, University Parthenope of Napoli, Centro Direzionale di Napoli, Is. C4, 80143 Napoli, Italy

Guido Carpinelli
Department of Electrical Engineering and of Information Technologies, University Federico II of Napoli, via Claudio 21, 80125 Napoli, Italy

Anna Rita Di Fazio
Department of Electrical and Information Engineering, University of Cassino and Southern Lazio, via Di Biasio 43, 03042 Cassino, Italy

Gabriella Ferruzzi
Department of Economical-Management Engineering, University Federico II of Napoli, Piazzale V. Tecchio 80, 80125 Napoli, Italy

Preface

Statistics plays a vital role in every fields of human activity. Statistics has important role in determining the existing position of per capita income, unemployment, population growth rate, housing, schooling medical facilities etc…in a country. The application of statistical methods to physics is essential. Whenever we perform an experiment and want to interpret the collected data, we need statistical tools. The accuracy of measurements is limited by the precision of the equipment which we use, and thus the results emerge from a random process. In many cases also the processes under investigation are of stochastic nature, i.e. not predictable with arbitrary precision, such that we are forced to present the results in form of estimates with error intervals. Estimates accompanied by an uncertainty interval allow us to test scientific hypotheses and by averaging the results of different experiments to improve continuously the accuracy. It is by this procedure that a constant progress in experimental sciences and their applications was made possible.

Statistical Methods in Radiation Physics is a collection of contemporary research articles which outline different techniques and methods used in the analysis of radioactive decay, dosimetry, radiation therapy and incident solar radiation data. It is an edited book with a particular emphasis on statistical solutions to problems in the aforementioned research areas. It is mainly addressed to researchers, advanced undergraduate and graduate students in the Natural and Life Sciences. This book consists of 20 chapters, which offer an overview of the statistical methods applied to radiation physics problems, organized into three sections. First section is focused on the measurements and estimate of radionuclides half-life, decay curves, and concentration ratios. It discusses the uncertainty propagation for nuclear dating, activity of radiation sources, contamination and risk maps. It includes methods such as time-interval distribution analysis, maximum likelihood ratio statistic (MLE) for Poisson distributions, log-normal distribution and bimodal distributions fitting, Monte Carlo simulations, and Neural Network training procedure. Second section addresses radiation exposure and protection as well as radiation-induced therapy problems and solutions. It includes techniques based on Bayesian statistics, adaptive robust optimization models, convolution method, radial pair correlation function, graph theory, physics-mathematical pattern modeling and mining. Third section is focused of on surface incident solar radiation modelling. Statistical models included are regression analysis, Analysis of Variance (ANOVA) and Bayesian inference.

Editor
Olga Moreira, Ph.D.

INTRODUCTION

Physics is the scientific study of matter and energy, and their interaction. Energy, such as light, heat or sound, which is emitted from one source, travels through space or material, and then is absorbed by another object, is defined as radiation. Radiation physics is the branch of physics that studies the effects of radiation on matter. This field has been instrumental in providing improved manufacturing processes, nuclear energy, and advanced medical diagnostic and treatment options.

The types of radiation studied by physicists include alpha, beta, and gamma rays, neutrons and x-rays. Alphas are particles containing two protons and two elections which are emitted from the nucleus of an atom. Betas are high speed particles which appear identical to electrons. Neutrons are the neutral particles within the nucleus of all cells. Gamma rays are emitted by the nucleus, and x-rays are a result of energy changes in the nucleus.

X-ray technology is one of the most familiar applications of radiation physics, and has several manufacturing applications. For example, the automobile industry uses high energy x-rays to evaluate engine performance. X-ray microscopes are used to inspect stents and catheters during the production process, and x-ray thickness gauges measure the chemical composition of metal alloys. X-ray radiography is even used by archaeologists to examine ancient artifacts.

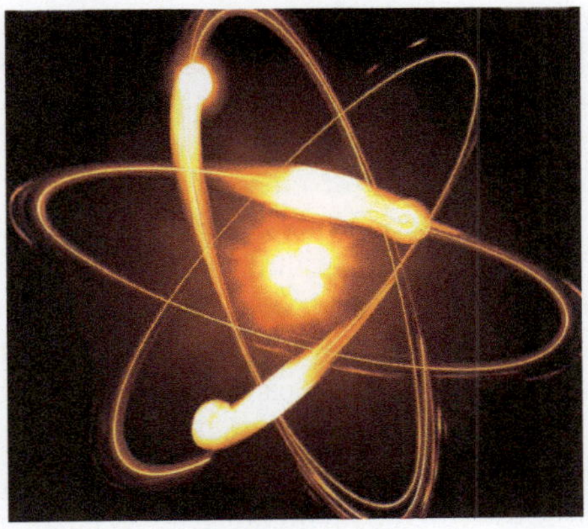

The oil industry has employed radiation physics applications in the treatment and production of petroleum. Oil companies use a radiation process called radiation thermal cracking (RTC) during the production of crude oil, fuel oil, tar and the treatment of the waste byproducts of oil extraction. RTC has a higher production rate, lower cost, and much lower energy consumption than tradition methods. Radiation treatment of oil contaminants provides greater environmental protection than other methods.

Nuclear energy is a growing field which is based on applied radiation physics. Through a process known as nuclear fission, energy is extracted from atoms during controlled nuclear reactions. While the United States produces the largest quantity of nuclear power, France produces the highest percentage of its nation's electrical supply through nuclear reactors.

The field which has benefited the most from radiation physics, however, is medicine. Through the application of physics, scientists have developed methods of using ionizing radiation for diagnosing and treating medical conditions. This includes not only the traditional forms of x-rays, but also ultrasound, magnetic resonance imaging (MRI) and nuclear medicine.

The majority of nuclear medicine involves imaging and employs computers, sensors and radioactive materials called radiopharmaceuticals. X-rays, the oldest form of imaging, uses high frequency light rays to construct images. Gamma rays have even higher frequencies, and are used in nuclear imaging. Positron emission tomography (PET) and single photon emission computer tomography (SPECT) are two of the most widely used pieces of nuclear imaging equipment.

The most common use of radiation therapy is the, for treatment of cancerous tumors. This usually involves depositing high energy x-rays into the cancer cells. The radiation is absorbed by the cell, causing it to die. Radiation is generally delivered to the tumor through an external source. The challenge for medical physicists is to direct the radiation in such a way that the minimum number of healthy cells are destroyed.

Radiation brachytherapy involves the internal application of radiation materials. In this treatment, radioactive "seeds" are implanted near the tumor. The release of radiation is slow, and the distance between the seeds and tumor is short enough that the radiation exposure to healthy cells is limited.

The benefits of radiation physics cross several disciplines and industries. Concerns over potential depletion of fossil fuels make the development of nuclear energy an on-going priority in many nations. The field of nuclear medicine is exploding, with new tests and treatments being developed rapidly, making radiation physics a discipline that will continue to grow.

The Statistical Nature of Radiation, Emission, and Interaction

The statistics, with emphasis on its role in radiation physics, measurements, and radiation protection. That this subject is essential for understanding in these areas stems directly from the statistical nature of the submicroscopic, atomic world, as we briefly discuss in the next section. The principal aspects of atomic physics with which we shall be concerned are radioactive decay, radiation transport, and radiation interaction. Knowledge of these phenomena is necessary for success in many practical applications, which include dose assessment, shielding design, and the interpretation of instrument readings. Statistical topics will be further developed for establishing criteria to measure and characterize radioactive decay, assigning confidence limits for measured quantities, and formulating statistical measures of performance and compliance with regulations. An introduction to biological dose–response relations and to modeling the biological effects of radiation will also be included.

Classical and Modern Physics – Determinism and Probabilities

A principal objective of physical science is to discover laws and regularities that provide a quantitative description of nature as verified by observation. A desirable and useful outcome to be derived from such laws is the ability to make valid predictions of future conditions from a knowledge of the present state of a system. Newtons classical laws of motion, for example, determine completely the future motion of a system of objects if their positions and velocities at some instant of time and the forces acting between them are known. On the scale of the very large, the motion of the planets and moons can thus be calculated forward (and backward) in time, so that eclipses and other astronomical phenomena can be predicted with great accuracy. On the scale of everyday common life, Newtons laws describe all manner of diverse experience involving motion and statics. However, in the early twentieth century, the seemingly inviolate tenets of traditional physics were found to fail on the small scale of atoms. In place of a deterministic world of classical physics, it was discovered that atoms and radiation are governed by definite, but statistical, laws of quantum physics. Given the present state of an atomic system, one can predict its future, but only in statistical terms. What is the probability that a radioactive sample will undergo a certain number of disintegrations in the next minute? What is the probability that a given 100-keV gamma photon will penetrate a 0.5-cm layer of soft tissue? According to modern quantum theory, these questions can be answered as fully as possible only by giving the complete set of probabilities for obtaining any possible result of a measurement or observation. By the close of the nineteenth century, the classical laws of mechanics, electromagnetism, thermodynamics, and gravitation were firmly established in physics. There were, however, some outstanding problems – evidence that all was not quite right. Two examples illustrate the growing difficulties. First, in the so-called ultraviolet catastrophe, classical physics incorrectly predicted the distribution of wavelengths in the spectrum of electromagnetic radiation emitted from hot bodies, such as the sun. Second, sensitive measurements of the relative speed of light in different directions on earth – expected to reveal the magnitude of the velocity of the earth through space – gave a null result (no difference!). Planck found that the first problem could be resolved by proposing a nonclassical, quantum hypothesis related to the emission and absorption of radiation by matter. The now famous quantum of action$^{h=6.6261 \times 10^{-34}\,\mathrm{J\,s}}$, was thus introduced into physics. The second dilemma was resolved by Einstein in 1905 with the revolutionary special theory of relativity. He postulated that the speed of light has the same numerical value for all observers in uniform translational motion with respect to one another, a situation wholly in conflict with velocity addition in Newtonian mechanics. Special relativity further predicts that energy and mass are equivalent and that the speed of light in a vacuum is the upper limit for the speed that any object can have. The classical concepts of absolute space and absolute time, which had been accepted as axiomatic tenets for Newtons laws of motion, were found to be untenable experimentally.

Statistics of Radiation Events

Photons in an x-ray beam and those emitted from a radioactive source are random events with respect to both time and location. The random emission of photons with respect to time makes it somewhat difficult to get a precise measurement of radioactivity. The random distribution of photons with respect to location within an image area is the major source of visual noise in both x-ray and radionuclide imaging. This is because the random distribution produces a fluctuation in the number of photons emitted from one time interval to another or from one area in an image to another. If the photons from a radioactive sample or in a small area of an image are counted for several consecutive time intervals, the number of counts recorded will be different for each, as illustrated below. This natural variation with time introduces an error in the measurement of activity that is generally referred to as the statistical counting error. The variation or random distribution of photons from one area of an image to another is visible as image noise.

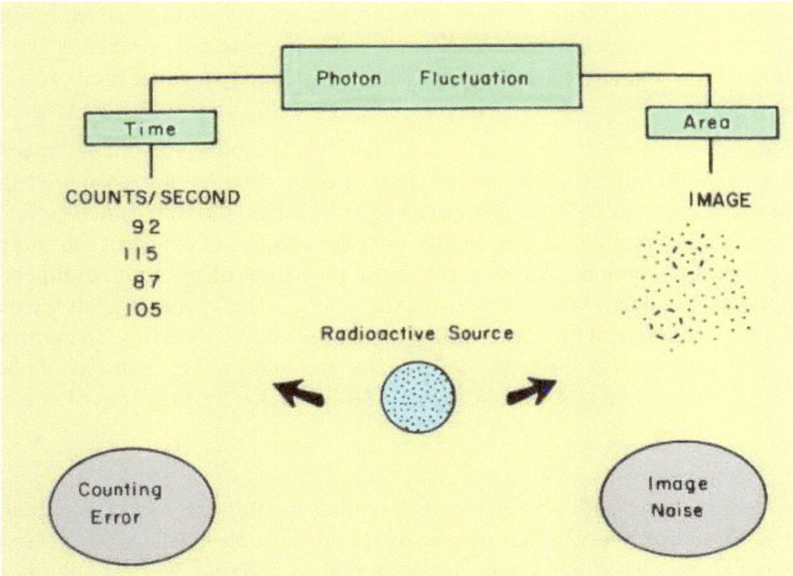

Statistical Photon Fluctuation: As a Source of Counting Error and Image Noise.

The random emission of photons with respect to location, or area, produces image noise. The presence of this spatial noise within an image decreases the ability to see and detect low-contrast objects.

Ionizing Radiation

Radiation with sufficiently high energy can ionize atoms; that is to say it can knock electrons off atoms and create ions. Ionization occurs when an electron is stripped (or "knocked out") from an electron shell of the atom, which leaves the atom with a net positive charge. Because living cells and, more importantly, the DNA in those cells can be damaged by this ionization, exposure to ionizing radiation is considered to increase the risk of cancer. Thus "ionizing radiation" is somewhat artificially separated from particle radiation and electromagnetic radiation, simply due to its great potential for biological damage. While an individual cell is made of trillions of atoms, only a small fraction of those will be ionized at low to moderate radiation powers. The probability of ionizing radiation causing cancer is dependent upon the absorbed dose of the radiation, and is a function of the damaging tendency of the type of radiation (equivalent dose) and the sensitivity of the irradiated organism or tissue (effective dose).

If the source of the ionizing radiation is a radioactive material or a nuclear process such as fission or fusion, there is particle radiation to consider. Particle radiation is subatomic particles accelerated to relativistic speeds by nuclear reactions. Because of their momenta they are quite capable of knocking out electrons and ionizing materials, but since most have an electrical charge, they don't have the penetrating power of ionizing radiation. The exception is neutron particles; see below. There are several different kinds of these particles, but the majority are alpha particles, beta particles, neutrons, and protons. Roughly speaking, photons and particles with energies above about 10 electron volts (eV) are ionizing (some authorities use 33 eV, the ionization energy for water). Particle radiation from radioactive material or cosmic rays almost invariably carries enough energy to be ionizing.

Much ionizing radiation originates from radioactive materials and space (cosmic rays), and as such is naturally present in the environment, since most rock and soil has small concentrations of radioactive materials. The radiation is invisible and not directly detectable by human senses; as a result, instruments such as Geiger counters are usually required to detect its presence. In some cases, it may lead to secondary emission of visible light upon its interaction with matter, as in the case of Cherenkov radiation and radio-luminescence.

Ionizing radiation has many practical uses in medicine, research and construction, but presents a health hazard if used improperly. Exposure to radiation causes damage to living tissue; high doses result in Acute radiation syndrome (ARS), with skin burns, hair loss, internal organ failure and death, while any dose may result in an increased chance of cancer and genetic damage; a particular form of cancer, thyroid cancer, often occurs when nuclear weapons and reactors are the radiation source because of the biological proclivities of the radioactive iodine fission product, iodine-131. However, calculating the exact risk and chance of cancer forming in cells caused by ionizing radiation is still not well understood and currently estimates are loosely determined by population based on data from the atomic bombing in Japan and from reactor accident follow-up, such as with the Chernobyl disaster. The International Commission on Radiological Protection states that "The Commission is aware of uncertainties and lack of precision of the models and parameter values", "Collective effective dose is not intended as a tool for epidemiological risk assessment, and it is inappropriate to use it in risk projections" and "in particular, the calculation of the number of cancer deaths based on collective effective doses from trivial individual doses should be avoided.

Ultraviolet radiation

Ultraviolet, of wavelengths from 10 nm to 125 nm, ionizes air molecules, causing it to be strongly absorbed by air and by ozone (O_3) in particular. Ionizing UV therefore does not penetrate Earth's atmosphere to a significant degree, and is sometimes referred to as vacuum ultraviolet. Although present in space, this part of the UV spectrum is not of biological importance, because it does not reach living organisms on Earth.

There is a zone of the atmosphere in which ozone absorbs some 98% of non-ionizing but dangerous UV-C and UV-B. This so-called ozone layer, starts at about 20 miles (32 km) and extends upward. Some of the ultraviolet spectrum that does reach the ground (the part that begins above energies of 3.1 eV, a wavelength less than 400 nm) is non-ionizing, but is still biologically hazardous due to the ability of single photons of this energy to cause electronic excitation in biological molecules, and thus damage them by means of unwanted reactions. An example is the formation of pyrimidine dimers in DNA, which begins at wavelengths below 365 nm (3.4 eV), which is well below ionization energy. This property gives the ultraviolet spectrum some of the dangers of ionizing radiation in biological systems without actual ionization occurring. In contrast, visible light and longer-wavelength electromagnetic radiation, such as infrared, microwaves, and radio waves, consists of photons with too little energy to cause damaging molecular excitation, and thus this radiation is far less hazardous per unit of energy.

Gamma radiation

Gamma (γ) radiation consists of photons with a wavelength less than $3x10^{-11}$ meters (greater than 1019 Hz and 41.4 keV). Gamma radiation emission is a nuclear process that occurs to rid an unstable nucleus of excess energy after most nuclear reactions. Both alpha and beta particles have an electric charge and mass, and thus are quite likely to interact with other atoms in their path. Gamma radiation, however, is composed of photons, which have neither mass nor electric charge and, as a result, penetrates much further through matter than either alpha or beta radiation.

Gamma rays can be stopped by a sufficiently thick or dense layer of material, where the stopping power of the material per given area depends mostly (but not entirely) on the total mass along the path of the radiation, regardless of whether the material is of high or low density. However, as is the case with X-rays, materials with high atomic number such as lead or depleted uranium add a modest (typically 20% to 30%) amount of stopping power over an equal mass of less dense and lower atomic weight materials (such as water or concrete). The atmosphere absorbs all gamma rays approaching Earth from space. Even air is capable of absorbing gamma rays, halving the energy of such waves by passing through, on the average, 500 ft (150 m).

Alpha radiation

Alpha particles are helium-4 nuclei (two protons and two neutrons). They interact with matter strongly due to their charges and combined mass, and at their usual velocities only penetrate a few centimeters of air, or a few millimeters of low density material (such as the thin mica material which is specially placed in some Geiger counter tubes to allow alpha particles in). This means that alpha particles from ordinary alpha decay do not penetrate the outer layers of dead skin cells and cause no damage to the live tissues below. Some very high energy alpha particles compose about 10% of cosmic rays, and these are capable of penetrating the body and even thin metal plates. However, they are of danger only to astronauts, since they are deflected by the Earth's magnetic field and then stopped by its atmosphere.

Alpha radiation is dangerous when alpha-emitting radioisotopes are ingested or inhaled (breathed or swallowed). This brings the radioisotope close enough to sensitive live tissue for the alpha radiation to damage cells. Per unit of energy, alpha particles are at least 20 times more effective at cell-damage as gamma rays and X-rays. See relative biological effectiveness for a discussion of this. Examples of highly poisonous alpha-emitters are all isotopes of radium, radon, and polonium, due to the amount of decay that occur in these short half-life materials.

Neutron radiation

Neutrons are categorized according to their speed/energy. Neutron radiation consists of free neutrons. These neutrons may be emitted during either spontaneous or induced nuclear fission. Neutrons are rare radiation particles; they are produced in large numbers only where chain reaction fission or fusion reactions are active; this happens for about 10 microseconds in a thermonuclear explosion, or continuously inside an operating nuclear reactor; production of the neutrons stops almost immediately in the reactor when it goes non-critical.

Neutrons are the only type of ionizing radiation that can make other objects, or material, radioactive. This process, called neutron activation, is the primary method used to produce radioactive sources for use in medical, academic, and industrial applications. Even comparatively low speed thermal neutrons cause neutron activation (in fact, they cause it more efficiently). Neutrons do not ionize atoms in the same way that charged particles such as protons and electrons do (by the excitation of an electron), because neutrons have no charge. It is through their absorption by nuclei which then become unstable that they cause ionization. Hence, neutrons are said to be "indirectly ionizing." Even neutrons without significant kinetic energy are indirectly ionizing, and are thus a significant radiation hazard. Not all materials are capable of neutron activation; in water, for example, the most common isotopes of both types' atoms present (hydrogen and oxygen) capture neutrons and become heavier but remain stable forms of those atoms. Only the absorption of more than one neutron, a statistically rare occurrence, can activate a hydrogen atom, while oxygen requires two additional absorptions. Thus water is only very weakly capable of activation. The sodium in salt (as in sea water), on the other hand, need only absorb a single neutron to become Na-24, a very intense source of beta decay, with half-life of 15 hours.

In addition, high-energy (high-speed) neutrons have the ability to directly ionize atoms. One mechanism by which high energy neutrons ionize atoms is to strike the nucleus of an atom and knock the atom out of a molecule, leaving one or more electrons behind as the chemical bond is broken. This leads to production of chemical free radicals. In addition, very high energy neutrons can cause ionizing radiation by "neutron spallation" or knockout, wherein neutrons cause emission of high-energy protons from atomic nuclei (especially hydrogen nuclei) on impact. The last process imparts most of the neutron's energy to the proton, much like one billiard ball striking another. The charged protons, and other products from such reactions are directly ionizing.

High-energy neutrons are very penetrating and can travel great distances in air (hundreds or even thousands of meters) and moderate distances (several meters) in common solids. They typically require hydrogen rich shielding, such as concrete or water, to block them within distances of less than a meter. A common source of neutron radiation occurs inside a nuclear reactor, where a meters-thick water layer is used as effective shielding.

What does a Radiation Physicist do?

A radiation physicist ensures the safety and proper operation of medical devices that use radiation sources. Professionals typically work in hospitals, oncology centers, universities, and specialty medical centers that provide radiology equipment to diagnose and treat different conditions. A medical radiation physicist makes frequent rounds in a facility to monitor radiation levels, determine whether or not patients or medical professionals are at risk of exposure, and establish effective safety procedures.

Many machines and pieces of equipment in hospitals rely on radiation sources to operate properly. Testing equipment such as X-ray machines and computerized tomography devices, and cancer treatment equipment like linear particle accelerators, emit radiation that can be potentially harmful or fatal if administered incorrectly. It is the job of a skilled radiation physicist to make sure that such equipment is operating properly and that patients, doctors, and others are not overexposed to harmful radiation. An expert uses sophisticated testing equipment to monitor emissions and recommend safe doses for patients.

A radiation physicist may also research and analyze the effects of radiation from certain medical devices, and make policy recommendations on how to improve their effectiveness and safety. Physicists are frequently held responsible for ensuring that a hospital is in compliance with federal and local regulations regarding radiation exposure, preventative measures, emergency procedures, and safety equipment. A professional may also lead training courses or seminars for other medical professionals to explain safe operating procedures of potentially hazardous devices.

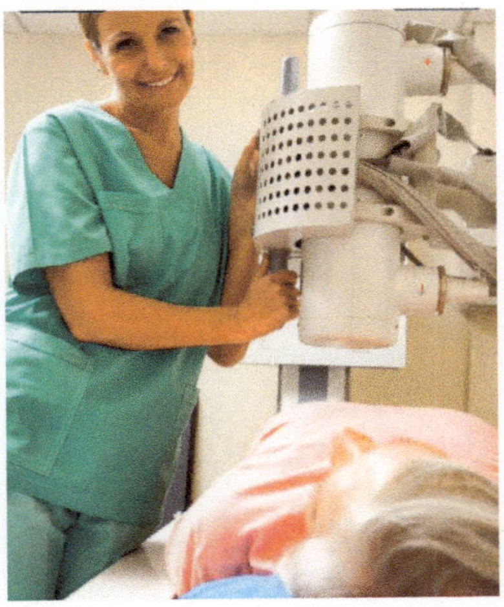

The requirements to become a radiation physicist vary by location and employer, though most professionals hold at least bachelor's degrees in medical physics, radiation biology, or similar disciplines. After receiving degrees, most new physicists must work as technicians or assistants to established professionals in the field for a period of up to two years, gaining hands-on experience and becoming more familiar with the practical aspects of the job. Many countries require a prospective radiation physicist to gain certification by logging a set number of practical training and passing a written examination. In the United States, certification is offered through the American Board of Health Physics.

Continuing education is usually considered very important for a practicing medical radiation physicist. Professionals frequently attend refresher courses and seminars to make sure they stay up-to-date on the latest radiation research and equipment technology. With continuing education, time, and proven skills, radiation physicists may be are able to advance to supervisory positions within a hospital. Some experienced physicists decide to work in private or university laboratories, conducting independent research studies on different aspects of radiation and medical treatment.

SECTION I - RADIOACTIVE DECAY AND RADIONUCLIDES CONCENTRATION

CHAPTER 1

THE UNCERTAINTY OF THE HALF-LIFE

S. Pommé

Keywords: Uncertainty, half-life, radioactivity

INTRODUCTION

The exponential decay of radionuclides as a function of time is a cornerstone of nuclear physics and radionuclide metrology. Since its discovery in 1903 by Rutherford and Suddy [1], it has been confirmed in numerous measurements of radioactive decay (see e.g. in [2]). Theoretical derivations of the exponential law can be achieved from probabilistic and quantum-mechanical points of view [3]. Both approaches imply that spontaneous nuclear transitions occur with a constant rate coefficient λ. At the level of single atoms, it is a stochastic process in which the survival time in a time period t is given by $e^{-\lambda t}$. For a set of atoms, the number of surviving and decayed atoms are ruled by a binomial distribution which, in the limit of a large number of atoms, $N >> 1$, and short time period, $\lambda t << 1$, reduces to a Poisson process.

Whereas decay constants for spontaneous nuclear decay are considered invariable in time and space, there is an area of research that explores possible violations of the exponential decay law. The quantum-mechanical theory is based on certain assumptions valid for intermediate values of λt, which may be violated for extreme cases of $\lambda t >> 1$ and $\lambda t << 1$ [2–6]. There is experimental evidence of changes in radioactive decay constants in cases where the nuclear decay is coupled to the atomic environment, i.e. decays that proceed through electron capture or internal conversion [3]. In recent years, controversy arose due to claims that half-lives are affected by temperature, conductivity of the hosting material, solar proximity or neutrino flux, which were subsequently refuted by others (see [7–12]).

At the heart of this controversy are the metrological difficulties inherent to the measurement of half-lives. When based on repeated measurements of activity, the half-life result is strongly influenced by instabilities in the measurement conditions [13–15]. From a metrological point of view it is obvious that instruments, electronics, geometry and background may vary due to external influences such as temperature, pressure, humidity and natural or man-made sources of radioactivity. Claims of non-constancy of half-lives on the basis of deviations from an exponential decay curve can only be considered when these instrumental effects have been fully compensated and/or accounted for in the uncertainty budget.

Therein lies the problem with half-life measurements: they are undeservedly perceived as easy and the experimental uncertainties are often underestimated, sometimes by an order of magnitude [14,15]. Consequently, nuclear data evaluators are frequently confronted with the problem of deriving a recommended value for half-lives from a discrepant set of data. Evaluations show that, for the majority of the radionuclides, the spread of experimentally determined half-life values is larger than expected from the claimed accuracies [16]. The published data not being completely reliable, one has to use alternative methods to obtain a mean and associated uncertainty value. The power-moderated mean applied by the Consultative Committee for Ionizing Radiation, CCRI(II), in key comparisons is a recommendable tool for that purpose [17, 18].

The situation is often aggravated by experimenters providing insufficient detail on how the half-life and its uncertainty were determined. A more comprehensive reporting

Citation: S Pommé (2015), The uncertainty of the half-life, Metrologia, 52, S51–S65. DOI:10.1088/0026-1394/52/3/S51.

style, which provides traceability for all major aspects of the measurement that may influence the result and tools that allows assessing the quality of the data, is recommended [15]. With time, one can expect evaluators to disregard published decay data lacking a sufficient level of traceability when a growing number of well-documented experiments become available in the literature.

It is of interest to the user community that the quality of decay data, and half-lives in particular, be improved [19, 20]. Whether the applications are situated in the field of nuclear medicine, power generation, nuclear forensics, radioactive waste management, analytical techniques, astrophysics, geochronology, basic nuclear research or detector calibration using reference sources, there is generally a half-life correction factor involved for rescaling measured activities to a reference time. This paper addresses some issues from the viewpoints of the user community and of the decay data provider. It discusses the propagation of the uncertainty of the half-life in activity measurements and the difficulties with providing an uncertainty budget when measuring half-lives.

APPLICATIONS OF HALF-LIVES

Rescaling of Activity

As the activity in a radioactive sample changes with time, it is appropriate to associate a measured activity with a reference time t_0, which does not necessarily coincide with the start or stop time of measurement (t_1, t_2). Rescaling of a measured amount of decays N of a radionuclide with decay constant λ involves correction factors for decay between the reference time and the start of the measurement $t_d = t_1 - t_0$ and during the measurement $t_m = t_2 - t_1$.

$$A(t_0) = \frac{N}{t_\mathrm{m}} \mathrm{e}^{\lambda t_\mathrm{d}} \frac{\lambda t_\mathrm{m}}{(1 - \mathrm{e}^{-\lambda t_\mathrm{m}})} \tag{1}$$

The counting factor, $C = (1 - \mathrm{e}^{-\lambda t_\mathrm{m}})/\lambda t_\mathrm{m}$, accounts for decay during the measurement and is significant (>x%) only if t_m is not negligibly small compared to the half-life $T_{1/2}$ = ln2/λ or, using a first order series expansion $C = 1 - \lambda t_\mathrm{m}/2 + O(\lambda^2 t_\mathrm{m}^2)$, if $t_\mathrm{m}/T_{1/2} > 2/\ln 2x\% \approx 3x\%$.

The standard uncertainty of the half-life, $\sigma_{T_{1/2}}$, propagates through the decay correction factors as follows

$$\begin{aligned}
\left(\frac{\sigma_A}{A}\right)^2 &= \left(\frac{\partial A}{\partial \lambda}\right)^2 \left(\frac{\lambda}{A}\right)^2 \left(\frac{\sigma_\lambda}{\lambda}\right)^2 \\
&= \left(\lambda t_\mathrm{d} + 1 - \frac{\lambda t_\mathrm{m}}{\mathrm{e}^{\lambda t_\mathrm{m}} - 1}\right)^2 \left(\frac{\sigma_\lambda}{\lambda}\right)^2 \\
&= \left(\lambda t_\mathrm{d} + \lambda t_\mathrm{m} - \frac{1 - C}{C}\right)^2 \left(\frac{\sigma_{T_{1/2}}}{T_{1/2}}\right)^2 \\
&= \left(\lambda t_\mathrm{d} + \frac{\lambda t_\mathrm{m}}{2} + O(\lambda^2 t_\mathrm{m}^2)\right)^2 \left(\frac{\sigma_{T_{1/2}}}{T_{1/2}}\right)^2
\end{aligned} \tag{2}$$

The uncertainty on the corrected activity increases linearly in time (via t_d and t_m, if $t_m < T_{1/2}$) and the propagation factor is significant for time periods of comparable magnitude as the half-life. With every 0.1% uncertainty on the half-life, the uncertainty of the activity increases by 0.07% per half-life.

Routine laboratories calibrate their activity detectors by means of secondary standards; calibrated sources with traceable activities of certain radionuclides. These standards are kept and reused for a practical period of time. Consider for example 10 year-old ^{22}Na (2.6029 (8) a), ^{54}Mn (312.13 (3) d), ^{55}Fe (2.747 (8) a), ^{57}Co (271.80 (5) d), ^{65}Zn (244.01 (9) d), ^{109}Cd (461.4 (12) d), ^{124}Sb (60.208 (11) d) and ^{134}Cs (2.0644 (14) a [21]) sources being used for calibration in an x- and γ -ray spectrometry laboratory. The standard uncertainty on the calibration factor due to uncertainty on the half-life is then respectively 0.08% (^{22}Na), 0.08% (^{54}Mn), 0.7% (^{55}Fe), 0.17% (^{57}Co), 0.4% (^{65}Zn), 1.4% (^{109}Cd), 0.8% (^{124}Sb) and 0.23% (^{134}Cs), which is significant for some of these nuclides. Larger errors can occur for radionuclides with shorter or less reliably known half-life.

More intricate rescaling is applied in the field of neutron activation analysis, where the link between elemental concentrations and measured activity of decay products is established through complex activation and decay formulas obtained as solutions of sets of linear first-order differential equations [22]. They typically contain a saturation factor $S = (1 - \mathrm{e}^{-\lambda t_\mathrm{irr}})$ for the activation during a period t_{irr}, a decay factor $D = \mathrm{e}^{-\lambda t_\mathrm{d}}$ and a counting factor C as above. The relative uncertainty of a measured count rate via such factors SDC is

$$\begin{aligned}
\left(\frac{\sigma_\mathrm{SDC}}{SDC}\right)^2 &= \left(\frac{\lambda}{S}\frac{\partial S}{\partial \lambda} + \frac{\lambda}{D}\frac{\partial D}{\partial \lambda} + \frac{\lambda}{C}\frac{\partial C}{\partial \lambda}\right)^2 \left(\frac{\sigma_\lambda}{\lambda}\right)^2 \\
&= \left(\lambda\left(t_\mathrm{d} + t_\mathrm{m} - t_\mathrm{irr}\frac{1 - S}{S}\right) - \frac{1 - C}{C}\right)^2 \left(\frac{\sigma_{T_{1/2}}}{T_{1/2}}\right)^2 \\
&= \left(\lambda\left(t_\mathrm{d} + \frac{t_\mathrm{m}}{2} + \frac{t_\mathrm{irr}}{2}\right) - 1 + O(\lambda^2 t_\mathrm{irr}^2) + O(\lambda^2 t_\mathrm{m}^2)\right)^2 \left(\frac{\sigma_{T_{1/2}}}{T_{1/2}}\right)^2
\end{aligned} \tag{3}$$

Assuming that the time periods involved—t_{irr}, t_d and t_m—are of similar magnitude, the propagation factor is about 1 for long-lived nuclides ($\lambda t \ll 1$, $\lambda t_{irr}(1 - S)/S \approx 1$, $C \approx 1$) and $\lambda t_d + 1$ for extremely short-lived nuclides ($\lambda t \gg 1$, $\lambda t_{irr}(1 - S)/S \approx 0$, $\lambda t_m - (1 - C)/C \approx 1$). For intermediate half-lives ($\lambda t \approx 0.1$–1), the propagation factor can be <1 or even cancel out completely, because the activation and decay terms have opposite signs.

Radiometric Dating

Radiometric dating methods are based on the exponential decay law describing the decreasing number of radioactive atoms in a material, and/or the related ingrowth of daughter nuclides [23]. One way of age dating is based on known atomic concentrations P(t) of the parent nuclide at different times, via

$$\mathrm{Age} = t = \frac{1}{\lambda}\ln\left[\frac{P(0)}{P(t)}\right] \tag{4}$$

A typical example is ^{14}C dating (5700 (30) a).

If the daughter atoms are stable and their initial concentration is zero, D(0) = 0, the sum of parent and daughter concentrations is constant, D(t) = P(0) − P(t) or P(0) = P(t) + D(t), and the age can be obtained from

$$\text{Age} = \frac{1}{\lambda}\ln\left[1 + \frac{D(t)}{P(t)}\right] \tag{5}$$

This scheme can be used in uranium-lead dating for systems that remained closed and with both decay routes $^{238}U/^{206}Pb$ and $^{235}U/^{207}Pb$ yielding concordant ages.

Corrections are required if $D(0) \neq 0$ or if the concentrations have varied in the sample through physicochemical processes. Isochron dating methods use the concentration S of a stable isotope of the daughter element as a reference. Since $(P(0) + D(0))/S = (P(t) + D(t))/S$, the relative concentration of the daughter isotopes $D(t)/S$ is the sum of the initial isotopic ratio $D(0)/S$ and a fraction originating from the decay of the parent nuclide:

$$\frac{D(t)}{S} = \frac{P(t)}{S}[e^{\lambda t} - 1] + \frac{D(0)}{S} \tag{6}$$

As $P(t)/S$ can vary freely within material samples of the same age, a consistent set of data is characterised by a linear relationship, called isochron. The age follows from the slope $(e^{\lambda t} - 1)$

$$\text{Age} = \frac{1}{\lambda}\ln\left[1 + \frac{\Delta(D(t)/S)}{\Delta(P(t)/S)}\right] \tag{7}$$

This procedure is routinely used in rubidium-strontium dating, in which the parent ^{87}Rb and daughter ^{87}Sr are compared to stable ^{86}Sr. Ratios are used instead of absolute concentrations because they are conveniently measured with mass spectrometers. Another application is dating 'young' groundwater, i.e. assessing when it became isolated from the atmosphere, through the decay of tritium ^{3}H to the rare stable daughter ^{3}He.

The isochron method can also be applied in uranium-lead dating, using ^{204}Pb as the non-radiogenic isotope. Combining the isochron equations for the $^{238}U/^{206}Pb$ and $^{235}U/^{207}Pb$ systems, one can derive the mathematical basis of 'lead-lead dating' based merely on measurement of the lead isotopic ratios $R_{6,4}(t) = {}^{206}Pb/^{204}Pb$ and $R_{7,4}(t) = {}^{207}Pb/^{204}Pb$

$$\frac{R_{7,4}(t) - R_{7,4}(0)}{R_{6,4}(t) - R_{6,4}(0)} = \frac{1}{137.88}\left(\frac{e^{\lambda_{235}t} - 1}{e^{\lambda_{238}t} - 1}\right) \tag{8}$$

where the factor of 137.88 is the present-day $^{238}U/^{235}U$ ratio. The initial Pb isotopic ratios (extracted from meteorites) and age of the system are the two factors determining the present day Pb isotopic ratios. In a closed system, equation (7) represents a linear relationship in which the slope depends on the age. The age of Earth, 4.54 (5) 10^9 a, was thus obtained (see e.g. [24]).

The dating equations (4), (5) and (7) are linearly proportional to the half-life of the parent (and equation (8) roughly on a ratio of half-lives), which means that the relative uncertainty of the half-life constitutes an upper limit to the attainable accuracy on the age. For several applications, this has become the bottleneck [25].

Another dating technique, ^{210}Pb sediment radiochronology [26], is frequently applied to reconstruct past environmental conditions of ecosystems. In systems that have been closed for a sufficiently long time (>150 a), the supported ^{210}Pb is in equilibrium with its parent radionuclide ^{226}Ra. Due to various transport processes, e.g. exhalation of ^{222}Rn and subsequent deposition of daughter products, excessor unsupported ^{210}Pb can accumulate in bottom sediments. The amount of excess ^{210}Pb in various layers of a sediment core is an indicator of the accumulation rate. For this technique, the uncertainty on the half-life is of minor importance compared to the modelling issues and the measurement uncertainty on the difference between ^{210}Pb and $^{226}Ra/^{214}Pb$ activities.

Nuclear forensics

Radioactive disequilibrium between parent and daughter arises when both are separated by physicochemical processes, e.g. by applying radiochemical separation techniques. Following this separation, the daughter starts to grow in again. Information on the time of separation may be obtained from measuring the ratio of parent to daughter atoms. This property is applied in nuclear forensics, aiming at fingerprinting of nuclear materials [23, 27, 28]. The relative amounts of parent and decay products can be used to identify the age and source of the material. Nuclides of interest are actinides (Th, U, Np, Pu, Am) with potential applications in improvised nuclear devices or other nuclides that can be applied in radiological dispersion devices (Co, Sr, Cs). A sample consisting of mixed U-Pu isotopes provides as many as a dozen chronometers, including $^{234}U/^{230}Th$, $^{235}U/^{231}Pa$, $^{238}Pu/^{234}U$, $^{239}Pu/^{235}U$, $^{240}Pu/^{236}U$ and $^{241}Pu/^{241}Am$. The time scale of interest is in the 1–50 year range, which is much shorter than in geology. Age dating of U is more difficult than Pu dating, because their long half-lives lead to minute amounts of ingrowing daughter nuclides. Besides the quality of the separation, the current uncertainties on the relevant half-lives are a major limiting factor on the attainable accuracy.

Parent and daughter both being unstable, the ratio of their atom concentrations at a time t after complete separation ($D(0) = 0$) is calculated from [29]

$$R(t) = \frac{D(t)}{P(t)} = \frac{\lambda_P}{\lambda_D - \lambda_P}(1 - e^{-(\lambda_D - \lambda_P)t}) \tag{9}$$

and the 'age' t is solved from

$$\text{Age} = \frac{1}{\lambda_P - \lambda_D}\ln\left(1 - \frac{D(t)}{P(t)}\frac{\lambda_D - \lambda_P}{\lambda_P}\right) \tag{10}$$

Linear propagation of uncertainty on the atom ratio R(t) and the half-lives λ_P and λ_D results to [29]

$$\left(\frac{\sigma_t}{t}\right)^2 = \left(\frac{\lambda_D}{\lambda_P - \lambda_D}\left(\frac{T}{t} - \frac{\lambda_P}{\lambda_D}\right)\right)^2\left(\frac{\sigma_{\lambda_P}}{\lambda_P}\right)^2 + \left(\frac{-\lambda_D}{\lambda_P - \lambda_D}\left(\frac{T}{t} - 1\right)\right)^2\left(\frac{\sigma_{\lambda_D}}{\lambda_D}\right)^2 + \left(\frac{T}{t}\right)^2\left(\frac{\sigma_R}{R}\right)^2 \tag{11}$$

in which the variable T is defined through

$$\frac{T}{t} = \frac{e^{(\lambda_D - \lambda_P)t} - 1}{(\lambda_D - \lambda_P)t} \tag{12}$$

For material with a relatively young age compared to the half-lives involved, $\lambda_P t << 1$ and $\lambda_D t << 1$, the propagation factors for λ_P and R are unity, while the factor for λ_D is insignificantly small. Consequently, age determinations based on atom ratios are more sensitive to the parent half-life than to the daughter half-life. This is compatible with the fact that R(t) $\approx \lambda_P t$ for small values of t, i.e. linear with λ_P and independent of λ_D.

Only for old material, $|\lambda_D - \lambda_P|t >> 1$, does the uncertainty propagation of the daughter half-life become important, but under these conditions, the over-all accuracy of the method is relatively poor as the propagation factors increase almost exponentially with $\lambda_D t$.

Similar equations can be derived for cases in which the activity ratio R_A of parent and daughter nuclide is measured instead of the atom ratio, with a subtle change in a multiplication factor

$$\text{Age} = \frac{1}{\lambda_P - \lambda_D}\ln\left(1 - \frac{A_D(t)}{A_P(t)}\frac{\lambda_D - \lambda_P}{\lambda_D}\right) \tag{13}$$

The uncertainty propagation of the concentration ratio $R_A(t)$ and the half-lives λ_P and λ_D to the age is given by [29]

$$\left(\frac{\sigma_t}{t}\right)^2 = \left(\frac{\lambda_P}{\lambda_P - \lambda_D}\left(\frac{T}{t} - 1\right)\right)^2\left(\frac{\sigma_{\lambda_P}}{\lambda_P}\right)^2 + \left(\frac{-\lambda_P}{\lambda_P - \lambda_D}\left(\frac{T}{t} - \frac{\lambda_D}{\lambda_P}\right)\right)^2\left(\frac{\sigma_{\lambda_D}}{\lambda_D}\right)^2 + \left(\frac{T}{t}\right)^2\left(\frac{\sigma_{R_A}}{R_A}\right)^2 \tag{14}$$

For material with a young age compared to the half-lives involved, $\lambda_P t << 1$ and $\lambda_D t << 1$, the propagation factors for λ_D and R_A are unity, while the factor for λ_P is insignificantly small. Consequently, age determinations based on activity ratios are more sensitive to the daughter half-life than to the parent half-life, which is the opposite of the effect noticed for atom ratios (equation (11)).

Activity ratio measurements enhance the signal of the short-lived nuclide, and may be a good alternative to atom ratio measurements in cases where the atom concentration of the short-lived nuclide is particularly low. The relative uncertainty of the half-lives of the parent (via R) or the daughter nuclide (via R_A) is of equal importance as the relative uncertainty of the measured ratio (Ror R_A). In order to achieve a time resolution of 50 d (k = 1) over a period of 1–50 years, the half-life uncertainties need to be lower than 0.25%, which has not yet been achieved for several important nuclides.

Dating of a nuclear event

The principles of radiometric dating can also be applied to fission products created in a nuclear explosion. Radionuclides may attach to aerosols or be released as noble gases and get collected in air samplers at a remote location. One can distinguish isobaric and non-isobaric clocks [30]. Non-isobaric clocks start from theoretical (cumulative) fission yields for the calculation of initial activity ratios and use the current activity ratio of fission products with different half-lives to estimate the time elapsed since the nuclear event. Isobaric clocks are based on parent–daughter pairs of which the daughter nuclide is not directly produced in the fission reaction. The equations are the same as the equations (9)–(14) applied in nuclear forensics. For example, they are directly applicable to the ^{140}Ba-^{140}La clock [31], based on progeny of the short-lived noble gas ^{140}Xe (13.6 s). The aerosol-bound ^{95}Zr-^{95}Nb chronometer is another important clock that requires a more elaborate mathematical treatment due the presence of meta-stable ^{95m}Nb in the decay scheme [32]. Specific equations for time-zero and uncertainty calculation are available to perform bias-free ^{95}Zr-^{95}Nb dating of a nuclear event over a time range of more than a year [33].

Nuclear medicine

Radionuclides introduced as nuclear medicine into the human body deliver a dose that depends on their effective half-life $T_{eff} = \ln2/\lambda_{eff}$, a combination of radioactive decay and biological excretion:

$$\lambda_{\text{eff}} = \lambda + \lambda_{\text{bio}} \tag{15}$$

Starting from an initial activity A, the accumulated dose is proportional to the number of atoms that decay in the body:

$$\text{dose} \propto \int_0^{T\to\infty} Ae^{-\lambda_{\text{eff}}t} = \lim_{T\to\infty}\frac{A}{\lambda_{\text{eff}}}\left(1 - e^{-\lambda_{\text{eff}}T}\right) \tag{16}$$

The relative uncertainty of the effective half-life propagates linearly to the dose. The biological half-life cannot be determined as precisely as the physical half-life, and the dominance of either rate differs from one radionuclide to another. For many long-lived nuclides, such as ^{3}H, ^{14}C, ^{22}Na, ^{36}Cl,^{60}Co, ^{137}Cs and ^{235}U, the much shorter biological half-life (10–70 d) is dominant [34]. The inverse is true for short-lived nuclides, such as ^{32}P, ^{59}Fe, ^{99m}Tc, ^{123,131}I, ^{140}Ba and ^{198}Au. The latter are the only cases in which the dose calculation depends significantly on the accuracy of the physical half-life. The bone seekers ^{90}Sr, ^{226}Ra and ^{239}Pu have extremely long effective half-lives (18–197 a [34]), which reduces their uncertainty propagation towards the accumulated dose during a person's lifetime.

MEASUREMENT OF SHORT HALF-LIVES

Half-lives of excited nuclear states, giving access to transition probabilities, provide direct insight into the structure of the nucleus and offer one of the most stringent tests of nuclear models. Different measurement techniques are applied to cover half-life ranges between picoseconds and seconds.

Picoseconds–Nanoseconds

Short lifetimes of excited nuclear levels ranging between about 1 ps to several ns have been measured by the Recoil Distance Doppler-Shift (RDDS) method [35, 36] for a large variety of nuclei all over the nuclear chart. In this method, nuclei produced by a beam-induced nuclear reaction in a thin target are allowed to fly freely in vacuum over variable distances from the target to a stopper ('plunger'). Gamma-spectroscopy measurements are performed with a single off-axis HPGe detector, preferably at extreme forward or backward angles, or by a cluster of detectors arranged at the same polar angle to increase sensitivity. Gamma rays emitted in flight are distinguished from those emitted after the nucleus has come to rest in the stopper, due to their Doppler shift. The mean life of a given level (and the accumulated time delay from higher lying states that feed it) can be deduced from the relative intensities of the shifted and unshifted peaks at different target-to-stopper distances.

In principle all the effects which should be considered when applying the RDDS method were known right from the beginning when the method was developed, but from time to time some of these effects were underestimated or invalid assumptions were made. In some cases the reasons for failures could be identified later but for other cases the situation remained unclear. Typical sources of uncertainty mentioned in the review paper by Dewald et al [35] are:

- Fit of decay curve: the decay curve comprises of a single exponential if only one excited level is involved, but usually a more complex level-feeding scheme needs to be solved with many free parameters, such as level lifetimes, branching ratios and initial populations. Assumptions have to be made for time behaviour of side-feeding, i.e. level feeding for which no discrete transitions are observed. Advanced code was developed to deal with the complexity of the non-linear fitting problem, but in many cases the solution is not unique. In general, the function to be fitted is not exactly known since the feeding states are not completely known.
- Distances and solid angles: the standard method relies on absolute distances, incl. the position of the plunger. Solid angle effects show up in the shifted peak when the target–stopper distance becomes comparable to the stopper–detector distance. In this case, only the unshifted component is analysed or a fixed stopper and moving target is used instead.
- Detector efficiencies: the shifted and unshifted peaks are registered with different detector efficiencies, depending also on the angle of observation with respect to the recoil velocity.
- Relativistic effects: high recoil velocities affect the lifetime of the excited nuclear state (time dilation), the emission angle (aberration) and the solid angle (Lorentz boost).
- Line shapes: knowledge of the line shapes of the shifted and unshifted peaks is needed when both are not well separated. The recoil velocity distribution is significantly broadened and asymmetric due to the finite target thickness. Moreover, the faster recoils reach the stopper in a shorter time and therefore contribute less to the area of the flight peak. Also during slowing-down time in the stopper, the ion velocity changes magnitude and direction, leading to a tailed γ-line shape that prevents determination of comparably small lifetimes.
- Deorientation: the angular distribution of the γ-ray emissions becomes more and more isotropic with increasing flight time, due to a decay of the spin orientation during the relaxation period. Even though this effect has been known for a long time, it was often underestimated, resulting in wrong half-lives. The error may reach 20% when using only the unshifted peak or 6% when using both.

These problems stimulated efforts to improve the technique with respect to higher reliability and to make it more transparent so that the presence of possible systematic errors is revealed more easily. Some of these improvements are [35, 36]:

- γ–γ coincidence measurements: by gating on specific feeding transitions, the problem of side-feeding and unknown feeding intensities and times can be circumvented. The drawback is the need for longer beam time and many Ge-detectors. Gating as a means of reducing background is beneficial to the statistical precision only if it improves the peak-to-background ratio by a large factor.
- The differential decay curve method and new alternatives: powerful new analysis techniques help solve problems of the standard method, relying more on experimentally accessible data, requiring only relative flight times/target-to-stopper distances and taking into account the angular and velocity spread of recoiling nuclei due to energy loss and multiple scattering in the target.

Nanoseconds–Microseconds

Nano- and microsecond nuclear states are mostly measured electronically in delayed coincidence experiments or alternatively by time interval analysis.

Delayed Coincidence Counting

The radiation yielding the state of interest is detected to provide a start pulse for an electronic clock, and the radiation by which the state decays is detected in the same or another device to provide a stop pulse. The half-life is derived from the analysis of the time difference between both signals. Using ultrafast scintillators (plastic scintillator, $LaBr_3$(Ce), BaF_2), the applicability range of the method has been extended down to picoseconds [37]. Also states of tens of milliseconds (or even seconds) are within reach, provided that the count rate is sufficiently low. Conventional experimental set-ups contain electronic modules, such as delay line amplifiers, timing single channel analysers (TSCA), time-to-amplitude converters (TAC) and multi-channel analysers (ADC), but they can also be replaced by programmable processors (FPGA) or software performing off-line data analysis of digitally acquired data saved in list files [38].

Common features of the delayed coincidence method are that time differences are stored in a spectrum, that the decay constant is derived from the slope of an exponential function fitted to a part of the spectrum and that account has to be taken for data not due to the intended parent–daughter pairs. Random coincidences may be recorded due to background signals, decays from other states or closely spaced but unrelated parent and daughter events. The first two interferences can be significantly reduced if the experiment allows for energy selectivity, e.g. by selecting peaks in γ- or α-spectra, and the third by keeping the count rate well below the decay constant. By means of energy selection, multiple half-lives can be derived from one experiment.

There exist different variants of how the data are recorded, each requiring a specific mathematical basis for the functional shape of the time spectrum. Two options are discussed below, based on different manners to collect and interpret time differences.

Single Delayed Coincidence

In a classical set-up, a timer is started whenever a parent decay is detected and stopped when a daughter decay is detected. Then the system is made sensitive again for parent decays. In doing so, all the parent events arriving before the first daughter event are ignored. In this type of experiment, the time spectrum theoretically takes the following shape: [39]

$$N(t)\cdot \mathrm{d}t = A \cdot \mathrm{e}^{-(R_2+\lambda)t}\mathrm{d}t + B \cdot \mathrm{e}^{-R_2 t}\mathrm{d}t \quad (17)$$

in which A and B are multiplication factors related to efficiency and count rate, λ is the decay constant of the state of interest and R_2 is the count rate of the daughter decay. If the count rate R_2 is kept small ($R_2 << \lambda$), this formula can be approximated by:

$$N(t)\cdot \mathrm{d}t = [A \cdot \mathrm{e}^{-\lambda t} + B] \cdot \mathrm{d}t \quad (18)$$

which is commonly used for the determination of a half-life from experimental data.

Multiple Delayed Coincidences

If the activity of the source is high – i.e. R_2 is not negligible compared to λ – the true parent–daughter decays are being interfered by uncorrelated events, leading to a distortion of the single-coincidence time spectrum. In that case, systematic errors are to be expected from using equation (18). This can be solved by means of an alternative time analysing circuit in which a parent decay starts the timer and not a single but multiple delayed coincidences are added to the time spectrum, one time value for every recorded daughter decay over a long period of time [40]. Theoretical analysis [39] predicts that time spectra obtained by this approach are represented by the sum of a constant term and an exponential function with the time constant of the radioactive decay of the daughter, exactly as in equation (18). Using multiple delayed coincidences eliminates the spectral distortion effect, but at the price of an increased number of random coincidences.

Time-interval Distribution Analysis Method

Time-interval distribution analysis is a well-established method for measuring the activity of radiation sources [41–43]. For a simple decay, the probability density of the time interval between two successive disintegrations is given by the formula:

$$P(t)\,\mathrm{d}t = \lambda N \mathrm{e}^{-\lambda N t}\mathrm{d}t \quad (19)$$

in which λN denotes the activity of the source. This formula can also be applied to a good approximation in short time intervals for a mixture of long-lived radionuclides – decaying independently or in radioactive equilibrium in a decay chain – but is incorrect if the decay chain also contains short-lived members. Lindeman and Rosen [42] deduced the general formula for the time-interval distribution of decays from a long-lived parent in equilibrium with n – 1 short-lived daughters. For a large number of parent atoms N_1, the probability of a given time interval between two successive disintegrations is given by:

$$P(t) = \frac{1}{n}\mathrm{e}^{-\lambda_1 N_1 t - \sum_i N_i(1-e^{-\lambda_i t})}\left[\lambda_1 N_1\left(1 + \sum_i \mathrm{e}^{-\lambda_i t}\right)^2 + \sum_i \lambda_i \mathrm{e}^{-\lambda_i t}\right] \quad (20)$$

It shows that, at low time intervals, the shape of the curve has a term that depends not on the activity of the daughter nuclide, but on its half-life. The time-interval spectrum is obtained by binning the time differences between all events. It is possible to focus on one of the transitions separately by selecting regions in the energy spectrum mainly belonging to the parent-daughter sequence of interest. The resulting curves have the characteristics of equation (20) applied to a single daughter nuclide (i = 2), but need the inclusion of a weighting factor C to balance both parts of the curve:

$$P(t) = \frac{1}{2}\mathrm{e}^{-\lambda_1 N_1 t - N_2(1-\mathrm{e}^{-\lambda_2 t})}\left[\lambda_1 N_1 (1 + \mathrm{e}^{-\lambda_2 t})^2 + C\lambda_2 \mathrm{e}^{-\lambda_2 t}\right] \quad (21)$$

in which C is included as a free parameter in the fit. For a source in equilibrium, the number of short-lived daughter atoms $N_2 = N_1 \lambda_1/\lambda_2$ will be low compared to N_1 and thus the second term in the first exponential is small. Time-interval distribution analysis yields comparable results to the delayed coincidence method [38, 43].

Data Analysis

The half-life of the nuclide is usually derived from a least-squares fit of an exponential function to the measured time spectra. However, some complications have to be taken into account. Least squares fitting procedures imply the assignment of proper weighting factors to the stochastically distributed data involved. In the case of a Poisson distribution, the obvious choice of setting the weighting factor equal to the inverse of the measured value is prone to bias towards low values. Alternatively, using the inverse of the fitted value may turn out to be biased towards higher values, depending on the procedure followed. Additional problems arise when also the possibility of zero counts has to be taken into account. An overview of the problems and possible solutions can be found in [44, 45] and references therein.

In fact, it is possible to perform unbiased least-squares fitting with Pearson's chi-square i.e. using the fitted value Y as weighting factor,

$$\chi_P^2 = \sum_{i=1}^{n} \frac{(y_i - Y)^2}{Y} \quad (22)$$

on condition that the weighting factor is kept fixed during each iteration of the fit. After each optimisation, it is set equal to the fit value Y obtained in the last iteration and a new fit is performed until convergence is reached [45]. There exist alternative estimators that allow using existing software for least-squares in a less biased way, with a minimal adaptation to the procedure. For example, one can minimise [45]

$$T^2 = \sum_{i=1}^{n} \frac{(y_i - Y - 0.5)^2}{Y} \tag{23}$$

freely without the need for an iterative procedure, and obtain an unbiased result if the data are not too close to zero.

A recommended solution to the problem of bias is to replace the χ^2 estimator by a maximum likelihood ratio statistic (MLE) for Poisson distributions [44]:

$$\chi_\lambda^2 = 2\sum_{i=1}^{n}\left[Y - y_i - y_i \ln\left(\frac{Y}{y_i}\right)\right] \tag{24}$$

in which y_i is the observed number of events in time bin i, Y is the fitted value and the last term is set equal to zero for $y_i = 0$.

To decay curves with a (quasi) purely exponential shape, another excellent method to derive an unbiased value for the decay constant is applying 'moment analysis'. It is known that the 'first moment' (i.e. the expectation value for the decay time t) and the 'second central moment' of the exponential distribution are equal to λ^{-1} and λ^{-2}, respectively. If the moment analysis of the decay curve is restricted to a time interval (t_1,t_2), the following relationship can be derived between the half-life and the first moment [45]:

$$T_{1/2} = \ln(2)\left(\mu_1(t_1, t_2) - t_1 + C_1\right) \tag{25}$$

and with the second central moment [45]:

$$T_{1/2} = \ln(2)\left(\mu_2'(t_1, t_2) + C_2\right)^{1/2} \tag{26}$$

in which the correction factors C_i are calculated from:

$$C_i = \frac{(t_2 - t_1)^i e^{-\lambda(t_2 - t_1)}}{(1 - e^{-\lambda(t_2 - t_1)})^i} \qquad i = 1, 2 \tag{27}$$

The statistical uncertainty associated with equation (25) is:

$$\frac{\sigma(T_{1/2})}{T_{1/2}} = \frac{\sigma(\lambda)}{\lambda} = 1/\sqrt{N_{(t_1,t_2)}(1 - \lambda^2 C_2)} \tag{28}$$

in which $N_{(t_1,t_2)}$ represents the number of events observed within the time interval (t_1,t_2). The relative uncertainty associated with $T_{1/2}$ of equation (26) is about a factor $\sqrt{2}$ higher, i.e. proportional to $\sqrt{2/N_{(t_1,t_2)}}$. Equation (26) confirms the observation by others [46, 47] that the best attainable precision on a decay constant is equal to $1/\sqrt{N}$.

The first moment, which is not a central moment, is sensitive to the time value assigned to each time bin. The data being distributed into time bins of equal duration Δt, the weighted mean time value of the first time bin, going from $t = 0$ to Δt, is calculated from:

$$\langle t \rangle = \frac{1}{\lambda} + \frac{\Delta t}{1 - e^{\lambda \Delta t}} \tag{29}$$

The time values for the other bins are found by adding to equation (29) a multiple of Δt. Central moments are insensitive to a linear translation of the time origin. Moment analysis should be performed only in a region (t_1,t_2) of the spectrum in which the random coincidence part (B in equation (18)) or contributions of other nuclides with a significantly shorter or longer half-life are negligible.

Uncertainties

The time spectrum is the convolution of the prompt peak (the width of which shows the variation in the timing between truly coincident events) and the slope generated by the lifetime of the nuclear level. For relatively long half-lives, the width of the prompt peak is negligibly small and the half-life is extracted from a fit to the exponential slope. If the half-life is short compared to the time resolution of the detection system, the time spectrum resembles the prompt peak of which the centroid has been displaced. The lifetime can be extracted from this shift [37]. The 'shift' method is less precise than the 'slope' method.

Typical uncertainty components are:

- Time resolution: indicates the lowest time difference that a coincidence set-up is able to determine. It is represented by the FWHM of the prompt time spectrum, which is generally a Gaussian distribution obtained by measuring simultaneous events in the two timing branches. Contributors to the FWHM are variances due to scintillator, photomultiplier and time pickoff.
- Time jitter in a scintillator is proportional to the figure of merit $\eta \propto \sqrt{\tau_f / N_f}$, in which τ_f and N_f are the intrinsic decay time and light yield of the scintillator, respectively. Photomultipliers are matched to the scintillator for maximum spectral response at the required wave length, large quantum efficiency, short rise time, transit time and transit-time spread. The development of ultrafast scintillators and multipliers have contributed most to improving the sensitivity of the fast timing technique down to the picosecond region.
- Walk, drift: whereas jitter is caused by noise and statistical fluctuations of the signals, walk stems from differences in pulse shape and amplitude and drift relates to aging and temperature variations. These effects are considerably reduced by using constant fraction discrimination, resulting in a bipolar pulse of which the zero crossing is nearly independent of pulse height. This results in more precise time pickoff.
- Counting statistics: statistical precision lowers the uncertainty on either the centroid shift or the slope of the time distribution. Ideally the best attainable precision is $1/\sqrt{N}$.
- Secondary effects: systematic errors due to difference in the traveling time of particles and photons from source to detector as well as spatial distribution of interactions within the detector, ambiguity in the separation of parent and daughter radiation, scattering of radiation between detectors, spurious shifts due to changing counting rates, time calibration and its linearity, different signal velocities in cables, interfering signals from other transitions, etc.
- Data analysis: the theoretical model of the time distribution analysis has to match with the electronic scheme by which the data were collected. Parent-

daughter transitions should be correctly separated from random coincidences and interfering signals, while influences from the latter need to be accounted for in the uncertainty. For example, one can quantify the sensitivity of the decay constant to an error on B in equation (18) by fitting a hypothetical λ for B ± σ(B). In spectra with low counting statistics and long slopes, the least-squares analysis underestimates the lifetime and proper fitting should be based on Poisson statistics [37].

MEASUREMENT OF INTERMEDIATE HALF-LIVES

Decay Curve

Many radionuclides with practical implications and applications have half-lives varying between seconds and about 100 years. This is a range of half-lives that can be measured directly by repeated activity measurements of a source. The simplicity of the measurement principle has incited many authors to publish thus obtained half-life data, unsuspecting of hidden processes that inflate the measurement errors far beyond their uncertainty estimates. A common scenario is that an exponential decay curve is fitted to various activity values measured as a function of time and that the uncertainty on the decay constant is obtained from the least-squares minimisation algorithm. This procedure is often faulty [48], as real measurement data may deviate in a subtle but systematic way from the theoretically assumed decay curve. The fitted decay constant is the value leading to the smallest residuals, which explains why an erroneous result seldom raises suspicion in the mind of the experimenter [14, 15]. Also other methods can be applied to extract the half-life from the data, such as moment analysis (section 3.2.3) and statistical sampling [14, 49], but they are equally sensitive to systematic errors.

The sum of an exponential function superposed on a constant background is often assumed to model the temporal dependence of the measured activity:

$$\widehat{A}(t) = A_0 \cdot e^{-\lambda t} + B \tag{30}$$

The fitted value of the parameter λ is believed to be the most probably value of the decay constant and the uncertainty is derived from the covariance matrix provided by the fitting algorithm, which implicitly assumes that the measurement data rigorously follow the prescribed decay function, the residuals being purely stochastic. In reality, there is a less than perfectly linear relationship between the activity and the measured signal (count rate or current) in a detector. Various processes make measurement data deviate from the ideal decay curve, long-term instabilities being at the same time the most influential but least visible sources of error. Due to differences in uncertainty propagation, it is convenient to subdivide these process according to the frequency at which they occur [14, 15]:

- High-frequency deviations: these sources of uncertainties occur at a rate that is higher than or comparable to the measurement duration of one data point. A typical example would be counting statistics: Poisson processes are characterised by an exponential distribution of the interval times between successive events. By extending the measurement, one improves the statistical uncertainty on the actual count rate. Also ultra-high frequency instabilities, such as e.g. electronic noise, are included in this category. They are partly cancelled, though, by the ‹integrating› effect of the duration of the measurement. Normal statistical treatments (including least squares fitting) apply because of the preservation of randomness of the data.
- Medium-frequency deviations: these instabilities show up (at least partly) as a trend in the residuals and can also be identified by means of an autocorrelation plot [14]. They include the so-called ‹seasonal effects› (e.g. day-night effects or changes with the seasons of the year), but also other variations occurring at a rate that can be observed over the measurement campaign. Their effect on the fitted half-life is greatly underestimated if treated as just a random residual. Moreover, a fit tends to minimise the residuals and partly covers up the true size of the medium frequency effects. Typical examples are the activity interference by radioactive impurities, reproducibility of the source-detector geometry, noticeable changes in the detector efficiency (e.g. through temperature, pressure, humidity, electronic flaws, scale changes in an electrometer) and modelling errors (e.g. neglecting a decay correction during measurement when progressively adjusting the measurement duration with time, inadequate separation between photopeak and underlying Compton continuum by gamma-ray spectrometry).
- Low-frequency deviations: these sources of uncertainties occur at a rate that is lower than or comparable to the duration of the whole measurement campaign. They remain practically invisible in the residuals, as the fit will compensate for this trend, hence erase it erroneously. Common problems in this range are a non-linear detector response to activity (charge recombination in ionisation chamber, discharge of a capacitor, non-linearity in an electrometer, pile-up and dead time in counter), systematic errors in the background subtraction, under- or over-compensation of count loss by live-time systems (double count loss through summing-out of piled-up events, hidden dead time due to unexpected behaviour of detector and electronic modules, pulse undershoot and overshoot, cascade effects of pile-up and dead time, effect of variation of dead time during measurement of short-lived nuclides), long-term drift of the counting efficiency and source degradation (e.g. oxidation of the source, mechanical wear, precipitation of active material in a solution).

In figure 1, hypothetical residuals of a fitted decay curve to data with high, medium and low frequency instabilities are shown. The dark dots represent the deviations of the data from the ‹true› decay curve, the light circles show the deviations of the data from the fitted decay curve and the solid curve is the difference between the fitted and true decay curve. The observer that performs the fit perceives only the light points. Considering that a slope equal to zero corresponds to the true half-life, the medium and low frequency deviations in figure 1 lead to a biased result. As the residuals give insufficient indication of these errors, one has to evaluate an exhaustive list of potential uncertainty components and combine them in a squared sum in the uncertainty budget.

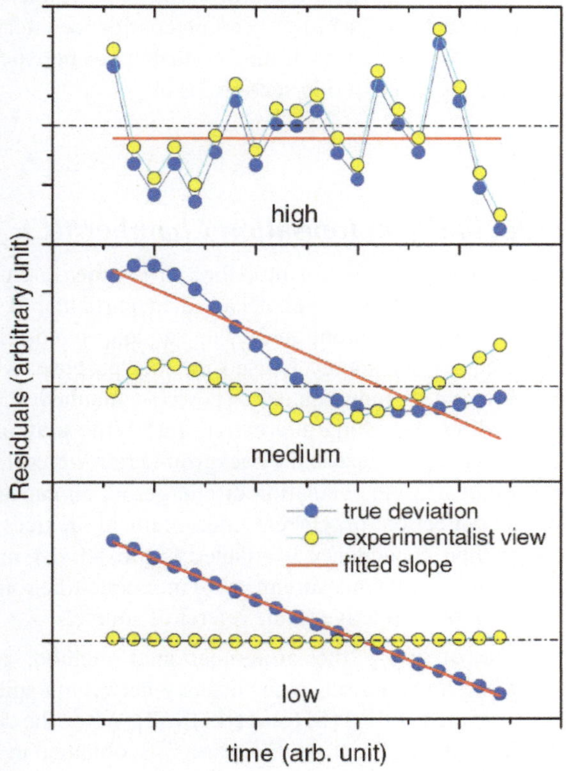

Figure 1. True (dark dots) and perceived (light dots) residuals from a fit of a decay curve through hypothetical data affected by high (top), medium (middle) and low (bottom) frequency instabilities. Systematic deviations are not fully observed by the experimentalist, as the fit tends to minimise them.

Impact of Systematic Errors

In a simplified scheme, the decay constant in equation (30) can be determined from two activity measurements of a source: A_0 at t = 0 and A at time t. Generally, corrections have to be made to transform the measured signals Â into the activity A of the radionuclide, which can be represented by a subtraction of a value B (e.g. background signals) and multiplication by a factor f (e.g. dead-time correction). The estimated value of the decay constant is

$$\hat{\lambda} = \frac{1}{\hat{t}}\ln\left(\frac{\widehat{A_0}}{\widehat{A}}\right)$$

$$= \frac{1}{\hat{t}}\left[\ln\left(\frac{A_0 f_0 + B - \widehat{B_0}}{Af + B - \widehat{B}}\right)\right]$$

$$\approx \frac{1}{t}\left[\ln\left(\frac{A_0}{A}\right) + \ln\left(\frac{f_0}{f}\right) + \ln\left(1 + \frac{\Delta B}{A}\right)\right] \quad (31)$$

Errors ΔB and Δf in the corrections propagate into an error in the decay constant:

$$\frac{\hat{\lambda} - \lambda}{\lambda} \approx \frac{1}{\lambda t}\left[\left(\frac{\Delta f}{f}\right)_0 - \left(\frac{\Delta f}{f}\right) + \left(\frac{\Delta B}{A}\right) - \left(\frac{\Delta B}{A}\right)_0\right] \quad (32)$$

Some conclusions can be derived from equation (32):

- Assuming the errors to be constant, the uncertainty on the half-life is inversely proportional with time via the factor 1/λt. Consequently, in order to reduce the uncertainty by a factor of two, one needs to double the decay time. This entails a linear relationship on a log-log scale, therefore less and less is gained by continuing the experiment at great length. Moreover, the gain in accuracy can be counteracted by a long-term increase of ΔB/A and Δf/f with time.
- A systematic relative error $\Delta f/f = (\Delta f/f)_0$ does not alter the half-life result; e.g. there is no need to determine the detection efficiency of the detector, as long as it is constant in time. On the other hand, a systematic error in the characteristic dead time leads to non-constant relative error in the count-loss correction factor. Some authors, even in recent publications, make the error of emphasising efficiency calibration over linearity checks.
- The impact of systematic errors ΔB in background (or impurity) subtraction are dependent on their size relative to the net signal A. Energy-selectivity is a useful tool to separate the source activity from interfering signals and to be insensitive to variations in threshold settings and instrumental noise. Therefore it is easier to measure half-lives through (high-energy) gamma rays and alpha particles than through (low-energy) x-ray, electron and beta emissions. The latter decay types are more sensitive to medium-frequency instabilities, which explains the speculations about the non-constancy of half-lives involved in, e.g. electron capture decay.
- The ideal time interval for a measurement campaign is typically chosen in function of non-linearity effects at the start (e.g. dead-time, short-lived impurities) and poor signal quality at the end (e.g. counting statistics, background subtraction, long-lived impurities, instability).

Uncertainty Propagation

The uncertainty propagation formula for a half-life $T_{1/2}$ = T ln2/lnR determined from the activity ratio $R = A/A_0$ at time t = 0 and t = T is

$$\frac{\sigma(T_{1/2})}{T_{1/2}} = \frac{1}{\ln R}\frac{\sigma(R)}{R} = \frac{1}{\lambda T}\sqrt{\frac{\sigma^2(A_0)}{A_0^2} + \frac{\sigma^2(A)}{A^2}} \quad (33)$$

In practice, measurements are repeated at regular time intervals during a measurement campaign over a time interval [0,T], with the intention to reduce the uncertainty on the half-life. Assuming a hypothetical situation in which the relative uncertainty on the activity measurement σ(A)/A is identical for each data point, the uncertainty propagation can be calculated from [50]:

$$\frac{\sigma_{T_{1/2}}}{T_{1/2}} \approx \frac{2}{\lambda T}\sqrt{\frac{3(n-1)}{n(n+1)}}\frac{\sigma_A}{A} \quad (34)$$

The formula implicitly assumes that the data are independent; therefore, it is applicable only to statistical (short-term) variations and not to auto-correlated (medium and long-term) variations. When performing three measurements, the middle data point neither affects the half-life nor its uncertainty. It makes a fitted decay curve shift as a whole in the vertical direction, but does not alter its slope.

A similar approximating formula was derived independently [14, 15] from the assumption that the relative impact of a measurement on the fitted half-life is proportional to the time difference with the middle of the campaign, i.e. ~|t − T/2|/(T/2). Under the aforementioned conditions, and data points being spread somewhat evenly in time over the period T, the uncertainty on $T_{1/2}$ is approximated by:

$$\frac{\sigma(T_{1/2})}{T_{1/2}} \approx \frac{2}{\lambda T}\left(\sum_{i=1}^{n}\left|\frac{2t_i}{T}-1\right|\right)^{-1/2}\frac{\sigma(A)}{A} \quad (35)$$

and the reduction factor (for n > 2) is roughly equal to

$$\sqrt{\sum_{i=1}^{n}\left|\frac{2t_i}{T}-1\right|} = \sqrt{\sum_{i=0}^{n-1}\left|\frac{2i}{n-1}-1\right|} \approx \sqrt{\frac{n+1}{2}} \quad (36)$$

resulting in

$$\frac{\sigma(T_{1/2})}{T_{1/2}} \approx \frac{2}{\lambda T}\sqrt{\frac{2}{n+1}}\frac{\sigma(A)}{A} \quad (37)$$

Using equations (34) or (37), an evaluator as well as an experimenter can make a quick estimate of the contribution of, e.g. counting statistics to the half-life if three variables are available: the number of activity measurements, n, the duration of the campaign, T, and a measure of the uncertainty for a typical activity measurement, σ(A). Equation (34) is probably more rigorous for large n, but the difference is less than 20% and significant only in the rare case that high-frequency uncertainty components are dominant. If an uncertainty component σ(A)/A is not constant with time, an average is taken of its value at time t = 0 and t = T.

It is important to apply independent uncertainty propagation according to the 'frequency' of the uncertainty components. When pertaining to medium and low-frequency instabilities, the parametern in equations (34) and (37) receives a new meaning. For (cyclic) medium-frequency components, the value of n is set equal to the number of periods covered by the measurement campaign. In the case of, e.g. yearly repeating effects, n would correspond to the number of years covered. For low-frequency effects, the value n = 1 is always selected and the propagation factor is 2/λT. For example, a hypothetical 1% change in detection efficiency during the measurement campaign leads to an average uncertainty at t = 0 and t = T of < σ(A)/A > = (0% + 1%)/2 = 0.5% and is propagated to an uncertainty of $\sigma(T_{1/2})/T_{1/2}$ = 1%/ λT, in agreement with equation (33).

Whereas two activity measurements in principle suffice for a half-life determination, repeated measurements have the advantage of reducing the propagation of random uncertainties, as well as allowing quantification of medium frequency components if they are not insignificant compared to the random variations. For this purpose, it is important to measure with good statistical precision. As time progresses, the main weight of the uncertainty budget typically shifts from random variations to cyclic instabilities and systematic errors [14]. The latter are the most difficult to quantify, so the most precise half-lives have the most uncertain confidence intervals. Also the analysis method itself may contribute to unexpected errors, as already discussed in section 3.2.3.

Examples

Reproducibility in Ionisation Chamber (IC)

Ionisation chambers are well-suited for half-life measurements because of their stability over decades, in particular if that stability is regularly monitored with a long-lived check source. Often a ^{226}Ra source is used for that purpose, which requires care that its radon daughter is well-contained; ^{166m}Ho is considered an interesting alternative. Instability may occur if, e.g. the chamber leaks gas, the background rate varies due to external sources, radon emanation discharges an air capacitor, the charge collection or current measurement devices are replaced or their capacitance is adapted to the activity range. For this reason, current measurements of mononuclidic sources are often performed relative to the reference source.

In spite of using the aforementioned method, there appeared to be a mysterious inconsistency between a suite of half-lives obtained at PTB [51] and NIST [52]. While the decay curves of, e.g. ^{60}Co, ^{133}Ba, ^{137}Cs, ^{152}Eu and ^{207}Bi obtained in both laboratories looked exponential, they had different slopes. The explanation was eventually found in a gradual slippage of the positioning ring that determines the height of the sample in the re-entrant tube of the NIST ionisation chamber during 35 years of use [53, 54]. This unaccounted-for height change caused a change in the detector response on the order of 10^{-5} to 10^{-3} per year, depending on the radionuclide. The changes are dependent onγ-ray energy and have particularly affected the half-lives of long-lived nuclides with different IC response than the reference source. The long-term instabilities remained unperceived in the residuals of the fitted decay curves, yet simulations of their influence have led to significant corrections (~1%) and an increase of the uncertainty [53, 54].

Impurity and Background Correction

An ionisation chamber is used to measure a source that is not perfectly mono-nuclidic due to the presence of an impurity, possibly a radionuclide occurring in the same decay chain. Gamma-ray spectrometry may be used to determine the relative activity of both nuclides and to calculate the impurity signal in the IC to be subtracted. Errors in the γ-ray emission probabilities and response of the IC and spectrometer can influence the half-life result. As an alternative, the signals of both nuclides can be fitted simultaneously to the decay curve. Another possible source of error is neglecting the decay rate change during measurements of variable duration, which requires a different correction factor $C_i(t_m) = (1 - e^{-\lambda_i t_m})/\lambda_i t_m$ (see also section 2.1) for the fractions of the signal associated with both decay constants. The following function can be fitted to the measured data (average current over a measurement time interval [55]):

$$I(t, t + t_m) = aC_1(t_m)e^{-\lambda_1 t} + bC_2(t_m)e^{-\lambda_2 t} + B \quad (38)$$

in which a and b are constants and B represents the background signal. For measurements of constant duration t_m in real time, the factors C_i are invariable and can be integrated in the factors a and b. Assuming that these corrections have been taken into account, the activity ratio at two different moments in time $t = t_1$ and $t = t_2$ is calculated from:

$$R = \frac{\widehat{A}\,(t_1)}{\widehat{A}\,(t_2)} = \frac{I(t_1) - \widehat{b}\,e^{-\widehat{\lambda}_2 t_1} - \widehat{B}}{I(t_2) - \widehat{b}\,e^{-\widehat{\lambda}_2 t_2} - \widehat{B}} \quad (39)$$

in which I(t) is measured IC current, $\hat{b}$ is a fitted or calculated impurity signal and $\hat{B}$ is the measured or fitted background signal. The most straightforward way to investigate the uncertainty on the half-life $T_{1/2} = (t_2 - t_1)\ln 2/\ln R$ due to potential errors on background and impurity subtraction is to compare the result of hypothetical half-life calculations using equation (38) with different values of $\hat{B}, \hat{b}$ and $\hat{\lambda}_2$. Alternatively, one can calculate the uncertainty from a first order series expansion [55] and equation (33):

$$\frac{\sigma_R}{R} \approx \frac{1 + \left(\frac{\sigma_b}{a} + \frac{b}{a}\sigma_{\lambda_2} t_1\right) e^{-(\lambda_2 - \lambda_1)t_1} + \frac{\sigma_B}{a} e^{\lambda_1 t_1}}{1 + \left(\frac{\sigma_b}{a} + \frac{b}{a}\sigma_{\lambda_2} t_2\right) e^{-(\lambda_2 - \lambda_1)t_2} + \frac{\sigma_B}{a} e^{\lambda_1 t_2}} - 1 \quad (40)$$

The fitted values of background $\hat{B}$ and impurity signal $\hat{b}$ may be anti-correlated as they compete in describing the part of the decay curve not following the exponential decay of the main nuclide. This should be taken into account when combining the different uncertainty components. It is important to take into account that the number of background counts may show statistical fluctuations higher than expected from a Poisson process. It is good practice to include a fraction of $\hat{B}$ also as a hypothetical systematic uncertainty component, e.g. because the counting conditions for a blank and a source may differ.

The above reasoning and equations (38)–(40) are also formally applicable to the case of a parent and daughter half-life being derived simultaneously from a fit to an ingrowth-and-decay curve obtained with an IC or calorimeter. The resulting half-lives can be highly correlated and their uncertainty underestimated. For example, this could be the case with ^{227}Th where applying a fixed value for the half-life of the ^{223}Ra daughter has led to a significant but questionable reduction of the uncertainty estimate (see discussion in [56]).

Counting with Dead Time and Pileup

The activity is registered as a pulse counting process, as opposed to current measurements in non-selective methods as ionisation chambers and calorimeters. The weakness of counting methods lies in the finite time resolution of the detector and associated pulse processing electronics [57, 58]. The linearity of the detector response is affected by count loss due to pulse pileup and system dead time. This prohibits the use of high amounts of activity at the start and therefore shortens the duration of the measurement campaign, since it is also limited at the end by poor counting statistics and significant background subtraction.

Live-timing techniques can compensate for count loss, by accounting for the characteristic dead timeτ associated with each recorded event. If the dead time is of the extending type, the activity ratio R of the activities A1 and A2 at a time t1 and t2, respectively, is obtained from the measured count rates r1and r2 and an exponential correction factor [57–59] to estimate the true input rates ρ1 and ρ2:

$$R = \frac{\rho_1}{\rho_2} = \frac{r_1}{r_2} e^{(\rho_1 - \rho_2)\tau} \quad (41)$$

The relative error on R produced by applying a slightly incorrect characteristic dead time $\tau + \Delta$ is

$$\frac{\sigma_R}{R} = e^{(\rho_1 - \rho_2)\Delta} - 1 \approx (\rho_1 - \rho_2)\Delta$$

$$\approx \frac{\Delta}{\tau}\left\{\ln\left[\frac{T_R}{T_L}\right]_1 - \ln\left[\frac{T_R}{T_L}\right]_2\right\} \quad (42)$$

in which T_R and T_L represent the system real time and live time, respectively, and the ratio of both corresponds to the dead time correction factor used in the respective measurements. The error grows exponentially with the count rate ρ_1, which overrules the $1/\lambda T$ reduction factor in the uncertainty propagation to $T_{1/2}$ (via equation (33)):

$$\frac{\sigma_{T_{1/2}}}{T_{1/2}} \approx (\rho_2 \tau)\left(\frac{\Delta}{\tau}\right)\frac{e^{\lambda T} - 1}{\lambda T} \quad (43)$$

For a fixed end point of the measurement campaign with count rate ρ_2, the uncertainty due to extending dead time or pileup increases by a factor of 1.5 or more for every half-life that the measurement campaign is started earlier. Therefore, there is no gain in accuracy by increasing the initial activity if dead time or pileup is the main uncertainty component.

In the case of non-extending dead time, the uncertainty on the activity ratio is

$$\frac{\sigma(R)}{R} = \frac{1 + \rho_1\Delta/(1 + \rho_1\tau)}{1 + \rho_2\Delta/(1 + \rho_2\tau)} - 1 \quad (44)$$

and propagates to $T_{1/2}$ via equation (33). Equations (42) and (43) apply by approximation only for moderate count rates, i.e. $\rho_1\tau < 0.2$.

The influence of dead time on the activity measurement is even more complicated for radionuclides with a short half-life, such that the count rate and corresponding dead time varies during one measurement. Mathematical equations are available to convert the integrated count rate to a momentary value [57]. In the field of primary standardisation of activity, counting is usually performed with a single-channel system and an artificial dead time of selectable length and type (extending or non-extending) imposed on every counted event. However, this live-time technique may also suffer from residual cascade effects of pileup with the imposed dead time, a process which can be corrected for through confirmed theoretical models [60, 61].

Time Interval Analysis

A formalism has been developed to replace histogram analysis of the decay curve by time interval analysis of valid events [62, 63]. The events are saved in list mode and subsequently analysed, first by assigning a fixed extendable dead time τ to each event and eliminating all events falling within a dead time period, and second by calculating a likelihood function for each surviving event i from a total ofn:

$$L = \prod_{i=1}^{n} \rho(t_i) \exp(- \int_{t_i - T_L(i)}^{t_i} \rho(t') \, dt') \quad (45)$$

in which $T_L(i)$ is the 'live time' that preceded the event and the count rate is made slightly variable with time (cf non-homogenous Poisson process). Rate-related count loss is mostly compensated for through the imposed extending dead time, but similar issues remain regarding time interval distortions and cascade effects with pulse-pileup [59–61], impurity and background subtraction, etc.

Spectrometric Method

Spectrometric methods have the advantage of energy selectiveness, allowing partial or full discrimination of the interfering signals from other radionuclides, decay progeny and background. High-resolution gamma-ray spectrometry is a popular method that allows simultaneous half-life analyses from a single series of measurements of a mixed source. Typical contributors to uncertainty are pileup, dead time, geometrical changes in source positioning and activity distribution, other instabilities influencing detection efficiency, spectral interference and background signals.

The method can be optimised by measuring in the same spectra also a reference source which is in a firmly fixed position close to or even mixed with the radionuclide of interest [50]. Relative to the latter, the reference nuclide preferably emits non-interfering gammas of comparable energy and is long-lived and/or has a well-known half-life. Its activity should be high enough to ensure good statistically accuracy in each spectrum, yet moderate with respect to its contribution to pileup, dead time and the Compton continuum. The measured quantities are ratios of peak areas from both sources, which are less sensitive to rate-related count loss and detection instabilities.

The peak areas of the reference source typically vary with time due to uncompensated count loss from pileup and geometrical changes. The method assumes that all instabilities affect the source and reference peaks equally if precautions are taken [50]. However, it is still sensitive to imperfect separation of the full-energy peaks from the underlying Compton continuum, in particular if it has a curved shape and a temporal behaviour that reflects the presence of nuclides with other half-lives. The fitted peak areas are always 'contaminated' with a positive or negative number of counts from the continuum of which the relative amount may vary smoothly like a medium-frequency instability.

Mass Spectrometry

The decay of a radionuclide can also be followed with a mass spectrometry technique, by measuring isotopic abundance relative to a stable isotope. An example is the ^{241}Pu half-life measured from isotopic atomic abundance ratios in a homogenised stock of plutonium [64–66]. The same formalism (equations (33)–(37)) can be applied for the uncertainty calculations. In spite of the notoriously low uncertainty achievable with this technique [67], it is not uncommon to find indications of an uncertainty budget being incomplete. The half-life determination of ^{241}Pu is such an example, since a continuation of the experiment revealed discrepant results [65, 66].

MEASUREMENT OF LONG HALF-LIVES

For half-lives longer than hundreds of years it is not feasible to measure accurately the decrease in counting rate over a reasonable length of time. Even with a repeatability of 0.01%, at least a measurement period of 100 years is needed to achieve 0.1% accuracy on a 500 year half-life (equation (34)). In such cases, a measurement of specific activity may be resorted to:

$$\lambda_{A,Z} = \frac{A_{A,Z}}{N_{A,Z}} = \left(\frac{A}{m_{tot}}\right) / \left(\frac{N_A}{M_{A,Z}} \frac{m_{A,Z}}{m_Z} \frac{m_Z}{m_{tot}} m_{tot}\right) \quad (46)$$

in which $A_{A,Z}$ is the activity and $N_{A,Z}$ is the number of atoms of nuclide ^AZ of the measured source,N_A is the Avogadro number, $M_{A,Z}$ is the molar mass of the isotope, m_{tot} is the total source mass andm_Z is the mass of its content of element Z.

The method implies three main stages: absolute measurement of activity concentration [68] in the source material, weighing of the source mass and determination of the isotopic composition. Mass spectrometry is well-suited for the latter, which allows determination of $m_{A,Z}/m_Z$ and correcting the total source activity for decays from other isotopes. A difficulty may arise in the mass determination of the base material if the chemical state of the element is not exactly defined. The composition of uranium oxides, for example, varies with the conditions in which it is produced and stored and therefore the oxygen/uranium ratio may vary. The uranium concentration may be investigated with titrations, coulometry, oxygen analysis or isotope dilution mass spectrometry (IDMS) relative to a pure metallic reference material [69].

The mass determination can be skipped by means of a relative measurement of two (or more) isotopes in one material

$$\lambda_{A,Z} = \frac{A_{A,Z} / A_{A*,Z}}{N_{A,Z} / N_{A*,Z}} \lambda_{A*,Z} \quad (47)$$

in which A* represents the mass number of the other isotope(s). Half-life ratios of Pu and U isotopes can be determined from relative peak areas in alpha spectra of quantified mixtures [70].

For a subset of long-lived nuclides having a short-lived parent, e.g. ^{243}Cm-^{239}Pu, ^{244}Cm-^{240}Pu, ^{249}Cf-^{245}Cm and ^{250}Cf-^{246}Cm, the daughter half-life can be determined relatively to the parent half-life by measuring the ingrowth in an initially pure parent source. The daughter-to-parent activity ratio measured after a decay time by a spectrometric technique is roughly proportional to the ratio of their decay constants [71].

Also the activity measurement can be avoided for nuclides appearing in a parent-daughter relationship in a decay chain in secular equilibrium, the activity ratio being constant in this case. Typical examples are the half-life measurements of ^{234}U and ^{230}Th by mass spectrometry of very old materials [72] using the ^{238}U parent as reference, of which the half-life was determined by alpha counting at a defined solid angle [73]. The uncertainty on $T_{1/2}$(^{238}U) should probably be increased [74], which in turn should be propagated to the daughter nuclides [29].

CONCLUSIONS

A multitude of techniques have been used to measure nuclear half-lives, their applicability very much depending on the order of magnitude of the value itself. The half-life data are essential for our knowledge of nuclear structure and fundamental natural laws and lead the way to applications in radioactivity measurements, dating techniques and dosimetry. Work is still in progress to measure new data and to confirm or improve existing half-life values. Whereas the quality of the published work has generally improved with time regarding accuracy and traceability, there is still room for improvement in accounting for all factors that may influence the measurement result and providing a complete uncertainty assessment. Underestimation of uncertainties is still a problem today, mostly because the random uncertainty component is often reduced to a minimum and systematic errors and their propagation towards the half-life uncertainty are more difficult to quantify. This has its consequences in scientific debate and societal consequences derived from radioactivity-based techniques.

REFERENCES

1. Rutherford E and Soddy F 1903 Radioactive change Phil. Mag. S 6 576–91
2. Norman E B, Gazes S B, Crane S G and Bennett D A 1988 Tests of the exponential Decay law at short and long times Phys. Rev. Lett. 60 2246–9
3. Semkow T M 2007 Exponential Decay law and nuclear statistics Applied Modeling and Computations in Nuclear Science ed T M Semkow et al (Washington, DC: ACS/OUP) pp 42–56
4. Norman E B, Sur B, Lesko K T, Larimer R M, DePaolo D J and Owens T L 1995 An improved test of the exponential decay law Phys. Lett. B 357 521–5
5. The OPAL Collaboration et al 1996 Test of the exponential decay law at short decay times using tau leptons Phys. Lett. B 368 244–50
6. Rothe C, Hintschich S I and Monkman A P 2006 Violation of the exponential-Decay law at long timesPhys. Rev. Lett. 96 163601
7. Krause D E, Rogers B A, Fischbach E, Buncher J B, Ging A, Jenkins J H, Longuski J M, Strange N and Sturrock P A 2012 Searches for solar-influenced radioactive decay anomalities using spacecraft RTGsAstropart. Phys. 36 51–6
8. Semkow T M, Haines D K, Beach S E, Kilpatrick B J, Khan A J and O'Brian K 2009 Oscillations in radioactive exponential decay Phys. Lett. B 675 415–9
9. Pierre S, Cassette P, Loidl M, Branger T, Lacour D, Le Garrérès I and Morelli S 2010 On the variation of the 210Po half-life at low temperature Appl. Radiat. Isot. 68 1467–70
10. Hardy J C, Goodwin J R and Jacob V E 2012 Do radioactive half-lives vary with the Earth-to-Sun distance? Appl. Radiat. Isot. 70 1931–3
11. Kossert K and Nähle O J 2014 Long-term measurements of 36Cl to investigate potential solar influence Astropart. Phys. 55 33–6
12. Meier M M M and Wieler R 2014 No evidence for a decrease of nuclear decay rates with increasing heliocentric distance based on radiochronology of meteorites Astropart. Phys. 55 63–75
13. Siegert H, Schrader H and Schötzig U 1998 Half-life measurements of Europium radionuclides and the long-term stability of detectors Appl. Radiat. Isot. 49 1397–401
14. Pommé S 2007 Problems with the uncertainty budget of half-life measurements Applied Modeling and Computations in Nuclear Science ed T M Semkow et al (Washington, DC: ACS/OUP) 282–92
15. Pommé S, Camps J, Van Ammel R and Paepen J 2008 Protocol for uncertainty assessment of half-lives J. Radioanal. Nucl. Chem. 276 335–9
16. Woods M J and Collins S M 2004 Half-life data—A critical review of TECDOC-619 update Appl. Radiat. Isot. 60 257–62
17. Pommé S 2012 Determination of a Reference Value, Associated Standard Uncertainty and Degrees of Equivalence–for CCRI(II) Key Comparison Data JRC Scientific and Policy Reports, EUR 25355 EN EUR – Scientific and Technical Research series (European Commission) ISSN 1831–9424 (online), ISSN 1018–5593 (print), ISBN 978-92-79-25104-7 doi: 10.2787/61338 2012
18. Pommé S and Keightley J 2014 Determination of a reference value through a power-moderated meanMetrologia 52 S200–12
19. Nichols A L 2006 Nuclear decay data: observations and reflections Appl. Radiat. Isot. 64 1384–91
20. Kellett M 2012 Assessment of actinide decay data evaluations: findings of an IAEA Coordinated Research Project Appl. Radiat. Isot. 70 1919–23
21. DDEP Monographie BIPM-5—Table of Radionuclides www.nucleide.org/DDEP_WG/DDEPdata.htm
22. Pommé S, Hardeman F, Robouch P, Etxebarria N, De Corte F, De Wispelaere A, Van Sluijs R and Simonits A P 1996 General activation and decay formulas and their application in neutron activation analysis with k0 standardization Anal. Chem. 68 4326–34
23. Magil J and Galy J 2005 Radioactivity Radionuclides Radiation (New York: Springer) ISBN: 3-540-21116-0
24. Dalrymple G B 2001 The age of the Earth in the twentieth century: a problem (mostly) solved Special Publications Geolog. Soc. Lond. 190 205–21

25. Begemann F, Ludwig K R, Lugmair G W, Min K, Nyquist E, Patchett P J, Renne P R, Shih C-Y, Villa I M and Walker R J 2001 Call for an improved set of decay constants for geochronological use Geochim. Cosmochim. Acta 65 111–21
26. Sanchez-Cabeza J A and Ruiz-Fernández A C 2012 210Pb sediment radiochronology: an integrated formulation and classification of dating models Geochim. Cosmochim. Acta 82 183–200
27. Mayer K, Wallenius M and Fanhängel T 2007 Nuclear forensic science—From cradle to maturity J. Alloy. Comp. 444–445 50–6
28. Mayer K, Wallenius M and Varga Z 2013 Nuclear forensic science: correlating measurable material parameters to the history of nuclear material Chem. Rev. 113 884–900
29. Pommé S, Jerome S M and Venchiarutti C 2014 Uncertainty propagation in nuclear forensics Appl. Radiat. Isot. 89 58–64
30. Nir-El Y 2004 Dating the age of a nuclear event by gamma spectrometry Appl. Radiat. Isot. 60 197–201
31. Ihantola S, Toivonen H and Moring M 2013 140La/140Ba ratio dating of a nuclear release J. Radioanal. Nucl. Chem. 298 1283–91
32. Harms A, Johansson L and MacMahon D 2009 Decay correction of 95Nb Appl. Radiat. Isot. 67 641–2
33. Pommé S and Collins S 2014 Unbiased equations for 95Zr–95Nb chronometry Appl. Radiat. Isot. 90234–40
34. Tuszynski J A and Dixon J M 2001 Biomedical Applications of Introductory Physics (Hoboken, USA: Wiley) ISBN: ISBN-10: 0471412953 ISBN: ISBN-13: 9780471412953
35. Dewald A, Möller O and Petkov P 2012 Developing the recoil distance Doppler-shift technique towards a versatile tool for lifetime measurements of excited nuclear states Progr. Part. Nucl. Phys. 67 786–839
36. Bizzeti P G and Bizzeti-Sona A M 2014 Integral- and differential-Decay-curve methods for recoil distance measurements of nuclear lifetimes Nucl. Instrum. Methods A 736 179–83
37. Mach H, Gill R L and Moszyński M 1989 A method for picosecond lifetime measurements for neutron-rich nuclei (1) outline of the method Nucl. Instrum. Methods A 280 49–72
38. Suliman G and Pommé S 2012 Measurements of the half-life of 214Po and 218Rn using digital electronics Appl. Radiat. Isot. 70 1907–12
39. Radeloff J, Buttlera N, Kesternich W and Bodenstedt E 1967 Measurement of lifetimes up to one second of isometric nuclear states populated in the decay of radioactive sources Nucl. Instrum. Methods 47 109–15
40. Tove P A 1957 Electronic time analyzer applied to the measurement of the half-lives of metastable nuclear states Nucl. Instrum. Methods 1 95–100
41. Tatcher M and Lindeman H 1968 Measurement of half-lives of isomeric nuclear states by a method of time interval analysis Nucl. Instrum. Methods 61 58–60
42. Lindeman H and Rosen N 1957 A generalization of the Marsden–Barratt law for time-correlated radioactive decay Physica 23 436–40
43. Erlik A, Felsteiner J, Lindeman H and Tatcher M 1971 Lifetime measurements of alpha emitters in the millisecond region Nucl. Instrum. Methods 92 45–9
44. Hauschild T and Jentschel M 2001 Comparison of maximum likelihood estimation and chi-square statistics applied to counting experiments Nucl. Instrum. Methods A 457 384–401
45. Pommé S and Keightley J 2007 Count rate estimation of a Poisson process: unbiased fit versus central moment analysis of time interval spectra In Applied Modeling and Computations in Nuclear Science ed T M Semkow (Washington, DC: ACS/OUP) pp 316–34
46. Maller R A 1979 On the precision of estimation of half life in delayed coincidence experiments Nucl. Instrum. Methods 167 479–81
47. Jaffey A H 1970 Statistical considerations in half-life measurements, I Nucl. Instrum. Methods 81155–63
48. Walz K F, Debertin K and Schrader H 1983 Half-life measurements at the PTB Int. J. Appl. Radiat. Isot.34 1191–9
49. Silverman M 2014 Theory of nuclear half-life determination by statistical sampling Europhys. Lett.105 22001-p1–5
50. Parker J L 1990 Near-optimum procedure for half-life measurement by high resolution gamma-ray spectroscopy Nucl. Instrum. Methods A 286 502–6
51. Schrader H 2004 Half-life measurements with ionization chambers—a study of systematic effects and results Appl. Radiat. Isot. 60 317–23
52. Unterweger M 2002 Half-life measurements at the National Institute of Standards and TechnologyAppl. Radiat. Isot. 56 125–30
53. Fitzgerald R 2012 NIST ionization chamber 'A' sample-height corrections J. Res. Natl. Inst. Stand. Technol. 117 80
54. Unterweger M P and Fitzgerald R 2014 Update of NIST half-life results corrected for ionization chamber source-holder instability Appl. Radiat. Isot. 87 92–4
55. Pommé S, Paepen J, Altzitzoglou T, Van Ammel R and Yeltepe E 2011 Measurement of the 177Lu half-life Appl. Radiat. Isot. 69 1267–73
56. Collins S M, Pommé S G, Jerome S M and Pearce A K 2014 The half-life of 227Th by direct and ingrowth measurements in press
57. Pommé S, Fitzgerald R and Keightley J 2014 Uncertainty of nuclear counting Metrologia 52 S3–17
58. Pommé S 2007 Dead time, pile-up and counting statistics Applied Modeling and Computations in Nuclear Science (ACS Symp. Series vol 945) ed T M Semkow et al (Washington, DC: American Chemical Society) pp 218–33 ISBN: 0-8412-3982-7
59. Pommé S, Denecke B and Alzetta J-P 1999 Influence of pileup rejection on nuclear counting, viewed from the time-domain perspective Nucl. Instrum. Methods A 426 564–82

60. Pommé S 2008 Cascades of pile-up and dead time Appl. Radiat. Isot. 66 941–7

61. Choi H D 2011 Counting statistics modified by two dead times in series Nucl. Eng. Technol. 43 287–300

62. Horvat V and Hardy J C 2013 Time-interval analysis of beta decay Nucl. Instrum. Methods A 713 19–26

63. Fynbo H O U and Riisager K 2014 Extended time-interval analysis Nucl. Instrum. Methods A 735 557–63

64. De Bièvre P and Verbruggen A 1999 A new measurement of the half-life of 241Pu using isotope mass spectrometry Metrologia 36 25–31

65. Wellum R, Verbruggen A and Kessel R 2009 A new evaluation of the half-life of 241Pu J. Anal. At. Spectrom. 24 801–7

66. Croft S, Burr T L and Favalli A 2013 Estimating the half-life of 241Pu and its uncertainty Radiat. Meas.59 94–102

67. Richter S and Goldberg S A 2003 Improved techniques for high accuracy isotope ratio measurements of nuclear materials using thermal ionization mass spectrometry Int. J. Mass Spect. 229 181–97

68. Pommé S 2007 Methods for primary standardization of activity Metrologia 44 S17–26

69. Milton M J T and Wielgosz R I Uncertainty in SI-traceable measurements of amount of substance by isotope dilution mass spectrometry Metrologia 37 199–206

70. Aggarwal S K 2006 Precise and accurate determination of alpha decay half-life of 244Pu by relative activity method using thermal ionization mass spectrometry and alpha spectrometry Radiochim. Acta94 397–401

71. Ahmad I, Kondev F G, Greene J P, Kellet M A and Nichols A L 2007 Measurement of the 240Pu half-life Nucl. Instrum. Methods A 579 458–60

72. Cheng H et al 2013 Improvements in 230Th dating, 230Th and 234U half-life values, and U–Th isotopic measurements by multi-collector inductively coupled plasma mass spectrometry Earth Planet. Sci. Lett. 371–372 82–91

73. Jaffey A H, Flynn K F, Glendenin L E, Bentley W C and Essling A M 1971 Precision Measurement of half-lives and specific activities of 235U and 238U Phys. Rev. C 4 1889–906

74. Schön R, Winkler G and Kutschera W 2004 A critical review of experimental data for the half-lives of the uranium isotopes 238U and 235U Appl. Radiat. Isot. 60 263–73

CHAPTER 2

FUNDAMENTAL UNCERTAINTY EQUATIONS FOR NUCLEAR DATING APPLIED TO THE 140BA-140LA AND 227TH-223RA CHRONOMETERS

S. Pommé, S.M. Collins, A. Harms and S.M. Jerome

Keywords: Nuclear chronometry, Uncertainty, CTBT, Non-proliferation, Geochronology, Nuclear medicine, and Dosimetry

INTRODUCTION

Nuclear chronometry is based on the statistical laws ruling the temporal dependence of the expected number of radioactive atoms in a decay chain, commonly known as the Bateman equations (Bateman, 1910 and Pommé et al., 1996). If the initial conditions of the atom or activity ratios in a closed system are known, the elapsed time since this 'time zero' can be derived from the current atom or activity ratio of a radionuclide and its decay product(s). The most commonly used chronometers are mathematically equivalent to a parent-daughter decay, for which the derivation of the dating equation is straightforward (Nir-El, 2004, Magill and Galy, 2005 and Pommé, 2015).

However, the formulae for the uncertainty propagation were always considered difficult to derive (Harms and Jerome, 2004, Harms et al., 2009, Douysset et al., 2014 and Axelsson and Ringbom, 2014) and therefore sometimes addressed by simulation methods. Uncertainty equations presented by Pan and Ungar (2012) showed a high degree of complexity. Only recently, succinct but rigorous mathematical solutions were published for nuclear dating by atom ratio (mass spectrometry) and activity ratio (nuclear spectrometry) measurements of parent-daughter pairs (Pommé et al., 2014 and Pommé, 2015). In addition, approximating formulae were presented that showed in certain conditions the propagation factors of relative uncertainties on decay constants and measured ratios towards the age can approach unity, but also large or small numbers are possible. Specific unbiased equations have been presented for ^{95}Zr-^{95}Nb chronometry of a nuclear event (Pommé and Collins, 2014). Precise dating in this particular case was complicated by a decay branch passing through a meta-stable state, ^{95m}Nb.

In this work, equations are presented for relatively short-lived parent-daughter pairs and applied to two valuable chronometers: (1) the ^{140}Ba-^{140}La parent-daughter pair, which is a prominent nuclear chronometer used for the dating of nuclear explosions in the frame of the International Monitoring System (IMS) for the verification of the Comprehensive Nuclear Test-Ban Treaty (CTBT), and (2) the ^{227}Th-^{223}Ra pair and their progeny, where ^{227}Th is an α-particle emitter being investigated for targeted radiotherapy of lymphoma cells (Dahle et al., 2009, Heyerdahl et al., 2012 and Bayer, 2014). Age dating of the material is needed for accurate dose administration to the patient, since the ingrowth of the daughter nuclides progressively affects the hospital dose calibrator response.

Due to the relatively short half-lives of the radionuclides involved ($T_{1/2} < 20$ d), the dating formulae need a significant correction for decay during the measurement. The uncertainty propagation of the half-life uncertainties through this correction factor needs to be included within the uncertainty budget. Solutions to this mathematical problem are provided. They are applicable only to activity ratio measurements, not to atom ratio measurements. The effect of using inaccurate decay data is demonstrated for both nuclear chronometers.

The uncertainties within this paper are stated as standard uncertainties or combined standard uncertainties as defined in the Guide to the Expression of Uncertainty in Measurement (GUM) (JCGM, 2008).

Citation: S. Pommé, S.M. Collins, A. Harms, S.M. Jerome, Fundamental uncertainty equations for nuclear dating applied to the 140Ba-140La and 227Th-223Ra chronometers, Journal of Environmental Radioactivity, Volumes 162–163, October 2016, Pages 358-370, ISSN 0265-931X, http://dx.doi.org/10.1016/j.jenvrad.2016.06.013.

BASIC EQUATIONS

Activity Ratio

General solutions to the Bateman equations (Bateman, 1910) are available for subsequent activation and decay in various branching schemes (Pommé et al., 1996). Some simplified initial conditions are applied in the derivation of the basic equations for chronometry: (i) the activation time is assumed to be small (i.e. a delta function), (ii) the initial amounts of parent and daughter nuclides are zero at t < 0 and (iii) the amount of the parent is at its maximum at t = 0, whereas the daughter is only produced through the decay of the parent. The symbols used in this paper are summarised in Table 1.

Table 1. Overview of symbols used in this paper.

Variable		Estimate	
t	Time elapsed since nuclear event	$\hat{t}$	Eq. (9)
$t^{(0)}$	1st order approximation of t	$\hat{t}^{(0)}$	Eq. (10)
$t^{(1)}$	Close approximation of t	$\hat{t}^{(1)}$	Eq. (11)
T	Timing variable for t	$\hat{T}$	Eq. (17)
$T^{(0)}$	Timing variable for $t^{(0)}$	$\hat{T}^{(0)}$	Eq. (18)
$T^{(1)}$	Timing variable for $t^{(1)}$	$\hat{T}^{(1)}$	Similar to Eq. (18)
λ_1	Decay constant of parent	$\hat{\lambda}_1$	Literature
λ_2	Decay constant of daughter	$\hat{\lambda}_2$	Literature
T_1	Half-life of parent	$\hat{T}_1$	Literature
T_2	Half-life of daughter	$\hat{T}_2$	Literature
F	Factor of decay constants	$\hat{F}$	Eq. (4)
$N_1(t)$	Number of parent atoms at time t	$\hat{N}_1(t)$	Eq. (1)
$N_2(t)$	Number of daughter atoms at time t	$\hat{N}_2(t)$	Eq. (2)
$A_1(t)$	Parent activity at time t	$\hat{A}_1(t)$	Eqs. (3) and (8)
$A_2(t)$	Daughter activity at time t	$\hat{A}_2(t)$	Eqs. (3) and (8)
R_A	Activity ratio, A_2/A_1	$\hat{R}_A$	Eqs. (3) and (8)
t_1	Time at start of measurement	$\hat{t}_1$	From clock
t_2	Time at end of measurement	$\hat{t}_2$	From clock
Δt	Duration of measurement	$\hat{t}_2 - \hat{t}_1$	From clock
$I_1(t_1,t_2)$	Parent activity integral in $[t_1,t_2]$	$\hat{I}_1(\hat{t}_1,\hat{t}_2)$	Eqs. (6), (20), (21)
$I_2(t_1,t_2)$	Daughter activity integral in $[t_1,t_2]$	$\hat{I}_2(\hat{t}_1,\hat{t}_2)$	Eqs. (6), (20), (21)
C_i	Counting factor for λ_i and $[t_1,t_2]$	$\hat{C}_i$	Eq. (7)
t_{irr}	Duration of production process	$\hat{t}_{irr}$	From clock
I_γ (x keV)	x keV γ-ray intensity	$\hat{I}_\gamma$	Literature
n_{P+C}	Counts in+underneath γ-ray peak	$\hat{n}_{P+C}$	From spectrum
n_C	Counts underneath γ-ray peak	$\hat{n}_C$	From peak fit
n_B	Background counts in peak	$\hat{n}_B$	Background spectrum
F_{DT}	Dead-time correction factor	$\hat{F}_{DT}$	Real time/live time
ΔF_{DT}	Difference in F_{DT} of γ-rays	$\Delta\hat{F}_{DT}$	Small
ε	Detection efficiency of γ-ray	$\hat{\varepsilon}$	Calibration
$\Delta\varepsilon$	Difference in ε of γ-rays	$\Delta\hat{\varepsilon}$	Calibration
$\sigma(t)$	Standard deviation of t	$u(t)$	Uncertainty evaluation

Denoting the parent and daughter by indices 1 and 2, respectively, one can represent the temporal dependence of the number of atoms by

$$N_1(t) = N_1(0)e^{-\lambda_1 t} \tag{1}$$

$$N_2(t) = N_1(0)\frac{\lambda_1}{\lambda_2-\lambda_1}\left[e^{-\lambda_1 t} - e^{-\lambda_2 t}\right] \tag{2}$$

The temporal dependence of the daughter to parent activity ratio is calculated from:

$$R_A(t) = \frac{A_2(t)}{A_1(t)} = \frac{\lambda_2}{\lambda_1}\frac{N_2(t)}{N_1(t)} = F\left(1 - e^{-(\lambda_2-\lambda_1)t}\right) \tag{3}$$

in which the factor F is defined as

$$F = \frac{\lambda_2}{\lambda_2 - \lambda_1} \tag{4}$$

As a measurement is performed over a finite time interval $[t_1,t_2]$ which may be non-negligible compared to the half-lives involved, one does not obtain a momentary activity ratio but instead a ratio of integrated activities

$$\frac{I_2(t_1,t_2)}{I_1(t_1,t_2)} = F\frac{\left[C_1e^{-\lambda_1 t} - C_2e^{-\lambda_2 t}\right]}{C_1e^{-\lambda_1 t}} \tag{5}$$

in which

$$I_i(t_1,t_2) = \int_{t_1}^{t_2} A_i(t)dt \tag{6}$$

is the integrated activity (or measured amount of decays divided by the measurement time $\Delta t = t_2 - t_1$), and

$$C_i = \frac{1 - e^{-\lambda_i(t_2-t_1)}}{\lambda_i(t_2-t_1)}(i = 1,2) \tag{7}$$

is the counting factor that corrects for decay during the measurement. Even small deviations of C_i from unity create significant differences between I_2/I_1 and A_2/A_1 and eventually lead to erroneous dating results (Harms et al., 2009 and Pommé and Collins, 2014).

The relationship between both quantities is established by

$$\frac{A_2(t_1)}{A_1(t_1)} = \frac{I_2(t_1,t_2)}{I_1(t_1,t_2)}\frac{C_1}{C_2} + F\left[1 - \frac{C_1}{C_2}\right] \tag{8}$$

Time Zero

The activity ratio has been expressed as a function of time in Eq. (3), and this relationship can be inverted to express the elapsed time as a function of the activity ratio:

$$t = \frac{1}{\lambda_1 - \lambda_2}\ln\left(1 - \frac{A_2(t)}{A_1(t)}\frac{1}{F}\right) \tag{9}$$

It is of interest to compare the exact Eq. (9) with two approximate formulae, as they are of use in the uncertainty propagation (see section 3). A first order approximation $t^{(0)}$ of the time t can be obtained by ignoring decay during the measurement, thus using the integrated decay rates $I(t_1,t_2)$ instead of the momentary activities A(t):

$$t^{(0)} = \frac{1}{\lambda_1 - \lambda_2}\ln\left(1 - \frac{I_2(t_1,t_2)}{I_1(t_1,t_2)}\frac{1}{F}\right) \tag{10}$$

The error, $t^{(0)}$–t, induced by the use of Eq. (10) can be shown clearly by deriving a more precise approximation $t^{(1)}$ of Eq. (9) (by introducing Eq. (8) into Eq. (9)):

$$\begin{aligned} t^{(1)} &= \frac{1}{\lambda_1 - \lambda_2}\ln\left(\left[1 - \frac{I_2(t_1,t_2)}{I_1(t_1,t_2)}\frac{1}{F}\right]\frac{C_1}{C_2}\right) \\ &= t^{(0)} + \left(-\frac{1}{2}\Delta t + \frac{1}{24}(\lambda_1 + \lambda_2)\Delta t^2 + \dots\right) \end{aligned} \tag{11}$$

in which a serial expansion of the natural logarithm of the counting factor Ci (i = 1,2) was applied:

$$\ln(C_i) = -\frac{1}{2}\lambda_i\Delta t + \frac{1}{24}(\lambda_1\Delta t)^2 - \frac{1}{2880}(\lambda_1\Delta t)^4 \tag{12}$$

The contribution by the last term in Eq. (12) is relatively small (<1%) on condition that the measurement time Δt is shorter than three times the half-life Ti (or $\lambda i \Delta t < 2.2$). Given that Eq. (11) is accurate under these conditions, it is clear that the approximation $t^{(0)}$overestimates the elapsed time t by about half the duration of the measurement, Δt/2. This means that $t^{(0)}$ roughly refers to the midpoint of the measurement, whereas $t^{(1)}$refers to the start of the measurement due to the application of the decay correction factors.

Time Zero of a 'Long Event'

The basic equations were derived under the assumption that the nuclear event at time zero is negligibly short in time. In reality, one has to consider that the production process of the parent nuclide (and by subsequent decay also the daughter nuclide) occurs over a finite period. Assuming that the parent – but not the daughter – is produced via a nuclear reaction at a constant rate over a time period t_{irr}, the production and ingrowth rates of parent and daughter are ruled by the activation-decay formulae used in activation analysis (Pommé et al., 1996). The activity ratio $A_2(t_{irr})/A_1(t_{irr})$ at the end of the production period is then expressed by:

$$\frac{A_2(t_{irr})}{A_1(t_{irr})} = F\left(1 - \frac{\lambda_1}{\lambda_2}\frac{1 - e^{-\lambda_2 t_{irr}}}{1 - e^{-\lambda_1 t_{irr}}}\right) \tag{13}$$

and the perceived time zero at the end of the irradiation is found by introducing Eq.(13) into Eq. (9):

$$t(0) = \frac{1}{\lambda_1 - \lambda_2} \ln\left(\frac{\lambda_1}{\lambda_2} \frac{1 - e^{-\lambda_2 t_{irr}}}{1 - e^{-\lambda_1 t_{irr}}}\right)$$

$$\approx \left(\frac{t_{\text{irr}}}{2} - \frac{1}{24}(\lambda_1 + \lambda_2)t_{\text{irr}}^2 + \frac{(\lambda_1 + \lambda_2)\left(\lambda_1^2 + \lambda_2^2\right)}{2880} t_{\text{irr}}^4 + \ldots\right) \tag{14}$$

In the case that t_{irr} is relatively small compared to the chronometer half-lives, i.e. ($\lambda_i t_{irr} < 1$), the perceived time zero in Eq. (14) corresponds to the middle of the irradiation period, $t_{irr}/2$. For very long irradiation periods, the parent and daughter activities will approach an equilibrium and the perceived time zero will become independent of the start of the production period, approaching a constant value of

$$t(0) \underset{t_{irr} \to \infty}{\to} \frac{\ln(\lambda_1) - \ln(\lambda_2)}{\lambda_1 - \lambda_2} \tag{15}$$

In the case of the ^{140}Ba-^{140}La clock, time zero in Eq. (15) would refer to 5.65 days before the end of the production period.

UNCERTAINTY PROPAGATION

Basic Propagation Formulae

In recent work, basic formulae have been derived for the uncertainty propagation of nuclear chronometry in the case of a simple parent-daughter decay by means of Eq. (9)(Pommé et al., 2014). The uncertainties on the half-lives and the activity ratio were propagated to the time using the following equations:

$$\left(\frac{\sigma(t)}{t}\right)^2 \approx \left(\frac{\lambda_1}{\lambda_1 - \lambda_2}\left(\frac{T}{t} - 1\right)\right)^2 \left(\frac{\sigma(\lambda_1)}{\lambda_1}\right)^2 + \left(\frac{-\lambda_1}{\lambda_1 - \lambda_2}\left(\frac{T}{t} - \frac{\lambda_2}{\lambda_1}\right)\right)^2 \times \left(\frac{\sigma(\lambda_2)}{\lambda_2}\right)^2 + \left(\frac{T}{t}\right)^2 \left(\frac{\sigma(R_A)}{R_A}\right)^2 \tag{16}$$

in which the variable T is defined as:

$$\frac{T}{t} = \frac{e^{(\lambda_2 - \lambda_1)t} - 1}{(\lambda_2 - \lambda_1)t} \tag{17}$$

The uncertainty propagation factors have also been stated as a series expansion (Pommé et al., 2014). For small values of t, where $|\lambda_2 - \lambda_1| t < 1$, the propagation factors for λ_2 and R_A are close to unity, while the factor for the parent decay constant λ_1 is small; however, the latter gains importance with time and is of comparable magnitude after a single half-life, T_1. The relative uncertainties on the decay constants are equal to (minus) the relative uncertainties on the half-lives, i.e. $\sigma(\lambda)/\lambda = -\sigma(T_{1/2})/T_{1/2}$.

Extended Propagation Formula

The formulae in Eq. (16) are incomplete if there is significant decay during the measurement, i.e. if the measurement time is significantly large compared to the half-lives involved. Then the uncertainty on the half-lives also propagates through the conversion of the counting integrals I_2/I_1 into activities A_2/A_1 via Eq. (8). In Annex A, a full uncertainty propagation is done to take these effects into account. In the following, a shorter and more efficient solution is derived from the approximations in Eqs. (10), (A.1),(A.2), (A.3), (A.4), (A.5), (A.6), (A.7) and (11). For the first order approximation, $t^{(0)}$ in Eq.(10), one can calculate a matching propagation factor, comparable to T/t in Eq. (17):

$$\frac{T^{(0)}}{t^{(0)}} = \frac{e^{(\lambda_2 - \lambda_1)t^{(0)}} - 1}{(\lambda_2 - \lambda_1)t^{(0)}} \tag{18}$$

The same can be done for $t^{(1)}$, which is usually a very accurate approximation of t, and therefore $T^{(1)}/t^{(1)} = T/t$. The uncertainty propagation of the half-lives to $t^{(1)}$, comprises of two components: (i) a term with $t^{(0)}$ for which similar propagation laws hold as in Eq. (16)and (ii) the higher order term(s) derived from $\ln(C1/C2)/(\lambda_1 - \lambda_2)$, which is a polynomial function of the decay constants. The following uncertainty propagation formula can be considered as a more complete version of Eq. (16):

$$\left(\frac{\sigma(t)}{t}\right)^2 \approx \left(\frac{\sigma(t^{(1)})}{t^{(1)}}\right)^2 \approx \left(\frac{-\lambda_1}{\lambda_1 - \lambda_2}\left(\frac{T^{(0)}}{t^{(0)}} - 1\right)\frac{t^{(0)}}{t^{(1)}} - \frac{\lambda_1 \Delta t}{24}\frac{\Delta t}{t^{(1)}}\right)^2 \left(\frac{\sigma(T_1)}{T_1}\right)^2 + \left(\frac{\lambda_1}{\lambda_1 - \lambda_2}\left(\frac{T^{(0)}}{t^{(0)}} - \frac{\lambda_2}{\lambda_1}\right)\frac{t^{(0)}}{t^{(1)}} - \frac{\lambda_2 \Delta t}{24}\frac{\Delta t}{t^{(1)}}\right)^2 \left(\frac{\sigma(T_2)}{T_2}\right)^2 + \left(\frac{T^{(0)}}{t^{(0)}}\frac{t^{(0)}}{t^{(1)}}\right)^2 \left(\frac{\sigma(I_2/I_1)}{I_2/I_1}\right)^2 \tag{19}$$

The validity of these equations has been confirmed numerically for measurements performed with the ^{140}Ba-^{140}La and ^{227}Th-^{223}Ra clocks, and data are provided in sections5 and 6.

PROCEDURE FOR CHRONOMETRY

Measurement

Sampling of material should be done in a way to ensure that the parent and daughter atoms are in a closed system, or both have equal probability of being sampled. The validity of such conditions is implicitly assumed, but not scrutinised in this paper.

The activity measurement consists of γ-ray spectrometry of the sample, e.g. an air filter, and quantifying in the spectrum the peaks of γ-ray emissions from the parent and daughter decays. The integrated activity is estimated from:

$$\widehat{I}_i(t_1,t_2)=\left(\frac{\widehat{n}_{P+C}-\widehat{n}_C}{\widehat{t}_2-\widehat{t}_1}F_{DT}-\frac{\widehat{n}_B}{\widehat{t}_2-\widehat{t}_1}\right)\frac{1}{I_\gamma\varepsilon} \tag{20}$$

in which the net number of counts in a full-energy peak (FEP), n_p, is obtained from a spectral fit that allows subtraction of counts in the spectral continuum underneath the FEP, n_C. It may be necessary to correct for interfering peaks from other radionuclides, especially in the inherently complex γ-ray spectra produced by a mixture of fission products (Pommé et al., 1993). If the background spectrum contains FEPs at the same energy as the chronometer FEPs $(\hat{n}_B \neq 0)$, a background subtraction should be performed on the measured count rate in the FEP. The counts in the FEPs can be considered as statistically uncorrelated (except if the daughter half-life is very short and the detection efficiency very high), but measurement conditions such as detection efficiency (ε) and dead time are highly correlated. The link between theory and measurement is made by the calculation of the integrated activity ratio from the FEP areas:

$$\frac{\widehat{I}_2(t_1,t_2)}{\widehat{I}_1(t_1,t_2)}\approx\frac{\left(\widehat{n}_{P+C}-\widehat{n}_C\right)_2}{\left(\widehat{n}_{P+C}-\widehat{n}_C\right)_1}\frac{I_{\gamma,1}}{I_{\gamma,2}}\left(1+\frac{\Delta\varepsilon}{\varepsilon}\right)\left(1+\frac{\Delta F_{DT}}{F_{DT}}\right) \tag{21}$$

The dead time correction can, in principle, vary among radionuclides with different decay curves if the count rate varies significantly during the measurement, but in common conditions one may assume that $\Delta F_{DT} = 0$. The uncertainty on the FEP detection efficiency ratio is an important systematic component, which is relatively small if the γ-ray emissions by parent and daughter are of similar energy (since the error on the efficiencies of closely spaced γ rays are highly correlated). If the sample is measured close to the detector crystal, also true-coincidence summing effects need to be taken into account.

The measured integrated activity ratio $\hat{I}_2(t_1,t_2)/\hat{I}_1(t_1,t_2)$ is then converted into a momentary activity ratio $\widehat{A_2(t_1)/A_1(t_1)}$, using Eq. (8). This involves the use of accurate values for the parent and daughter half-lives and realistic estimates of their uncertainties, preferably taken from nuclear decay data evaluations provided by the Decay Data Evaluation Project (DDEP, 2004–2015) or the Evaluated Nuclear Structure Data File (ENSDF). The estimated elapsed time $\hat{t}_1$ between the nuclear event and the start of the measurement follows then from Eq. (9). Alternatively, the time $\hat{t}_1$ can be calculated directly from the $\hat{I}_2/\hat{I}_1$ ratio via Eq. (11) for $t^{(1)}$, which comprises of $t^{(0)}$ (Eq. (10)) minus half the measurement time and a small correction term.

Counting Statistics

The uncertainty on the activity ratio R_A is a squared sum of relative uncertainties on the factors I_γ, ε, peak fitting, background subtraction and Poisson distribution of counts. The latter statistical uncertainty will depend on the inverse square root of the number of counts $n_{P,1}$ and $n_{P,2}$ in the parent and daughter FEPs, respectively. The best statistical accuracy can be expected when the count rates in both peaks are similar of size, i.e. when the daughter nuclide has sufficiently grown in and well before the parent nuclide has decayed away.

As long as the Poisson variance is by far the dominant uncertainty component, the accuracy of the nuclear dating can be improved by extending the measurement time: increasing Δt by a factor of 4 reduces the statistical uncertainty by a factor of 2 (when disregarding subtraction of continuum and background signals). However, at the same time the propagation factor increases through $\frac{t^{(0)}}{t^{(1)}}\approx 1+\frac{1}{2}\frac{\Delta t}{t^{(0)}}$. Therefore, no accuracy is gained by continuing a measurement in which the systematic uncertainties (efficiency, intensities, etc.) are larger than the statistical uncertainty. This will be demonstrated in the example in section 5.

^{140}BA-^{140}LA CLOCK

Production through Fission

Asymmetric fission of uranium and plutonium being favoured by nuclear shell effects, the yield of mass A = 140 fragments is relatively high, in particular around nuclear chargeZ = 54 (xenon) (Pommé et al., 1993). The xenon, being a noble gas, can go airborne and facilitate detection of its progeny in remote places (De Geer, 2013 and Ihantola et al., 2013). The A = 140 isobars produced directly in fission are short-lived ($T_{1/2} < 63.7$ s) and the isobaric fission yield accumulates in the longer-lived successor $^{140}_{55}Ba$ ($T_{1/2}$ = 12.753 (4) days (Helmer, 2004a)), its daughter nuclide $^{140}_{57}La$ ($T_{1/2}$ = 1.67858 (21) days (Chechev and Kuzmenko, 2015)) and by further decay in the stable nuclide $^{140}_{58}Ce$. The isobaric decay scheme is presented in Fig. 1. In the case of a nuclear explosion, the initial abundances of ^{140}Ba and ^{140}La are assumed to be zero and the A = 140 isobaric fission yield accumulates in the ^{140}Ba-^{140}La chronometer within a few minutes.

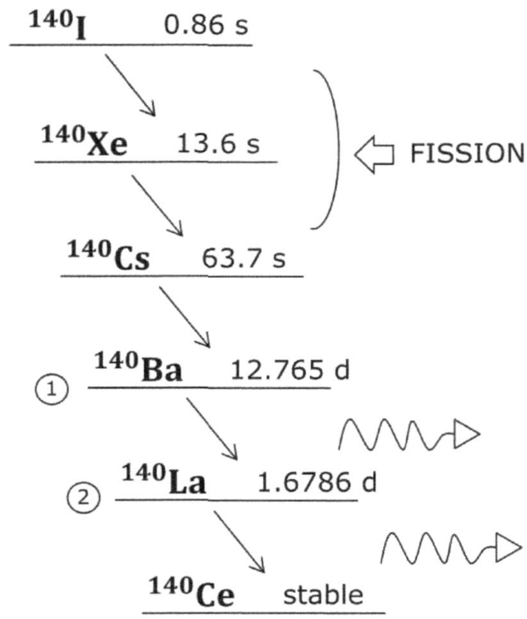

Figure 1. Isobaric decay scheme for mass A = 140 fission fragments and their decay products. The mass yield readily accumulates in the longer-lived isobars (1) ^{140}Ba and (2) ^{140}La and the gamma radiation emitted after their decay is used for chronometry.

In this work, two experiments are discussed in which the ^{140}Ba-^{140}La chronometer is applied to determine the 'age' of fission products produced under controlled conditions at a nuclear facility. Time zero refers to the time when the barium was chemically separated from the target (and the lanthanum daughter). Useful decay data for ^{140}Ba-^{140}La chronometry are summarised in Table 2.

Table 2. Evaluated decay data relevant for chronometry in this work, from three references: (Helmer, 2004a and Helmer, 2004b), (Nica, 2007), and (Chechev and Kuzmenko, 2015)

Variable	DDEP (2004)	ENSDF (2007)	DDEP (2015)
T_1 (^{140}Ba) (days)	12.753 (4)	12.7527 (23)	
I_γ (537.3) (%)	24.39 (22)	24.39 (23)	
T_2 (^{140}La) (days)	1.67850 (17)	1.67855 (12) d	1.67858 (21) d
I_γ (487.0) (%)	46.1 (4)	45.5 (9)	46.1 (5)
I_γ (815.8) (%)	23.72 (12)	23.3 (4)	23.72 (20)
I_γ (1596.2) (%)	95.40 (8)	95.4 (1.4)	95.40 (5)

Experiment 1

Irradiation and Sample Preparation

Experiment 1 refers to a re-analysis of data published by Harms and Jerome (2004). The ^{140}Ba was produced by the neutron irradiation of a >98% enriched ^{235}U target at the Imperial College research reactor, over a period of 18,000 s. The details of the irradiation and chemical separation were described in the original paper. The irradiated material was passed through cation and anion exchange columns and barium was precipitated and redissolved into a solution from which sources for measurement were made. The reference time, corresponding to the last chemical separation, was assigned an uncertainty of 1155 s or 0.013 days.

Chronometry Measurements & Results

The activity ratio was measured at NPL by γ-ray spectrometry with the HPGe detector 'MAGGIE', using the characteristic γ ray emissions following the decay of ^{140}Ba at 537.3 keV (I_γ = 24.39 (22) %) and of ^{140}La at 487.0 keV (I_γ = 46.1 (4) %), 815.8 keV (I_γ = 23.72 (12) %) and 1596.2 keV (I_γ = 95.40 (8) %) (Helmer, 2004a and Helmer, 2004b).

Relevant measurement data are summarised in Table 3. In total 16 γ-ray spectra were collected between 0.09 and 5.8 days after time zero. The duration of the measurements varied between 0.05 and 0.97 days, and the corresponding correction factors (C_1, C_2) for decay during the measurements ranged from 0.9986 to 0.8236. As a result, the integrated activities I significantly differed from the decay-corrected activities A, and so did the approximate time estimate $t_1^{(0)}$ (referring approximately to the midpoint) deviate from the corrected value $t_1^{(1)}$ (referring to the start of the measurement). The agreement between the estimated and real 'time zero' is generally good, the absolute differences are always below 0.4 days, the relative difference generally below 10% and the zeta score mostly between 0 and -2.

Table 3. Measurement results with the ^{140}Ba-^{140}La chronometer, including reference time of production through ingrowth of ^{140}La into chemically separated ^{140}Ba (Experiment 1, by Harms and Jerome (2004)) or directly from an induced fission process (Experiment 2, this work), (i) spectrum number, (ii) elapsed time at start of measurement, (iii) duration of measurement, (iv, v) counting factors correcting for decay during measurement, (vi, vii) measured (integrated) activity, (viii) integrated activity ratio, (ix) momentary activity ratio (x) initial time zero estimate via Eq. (10), (xi) final estimate of time zero via Eq. (9) or Eq. (11), (xii), absolute and (xiii) relative difference between estimated time and reference time, (xiv) uncertainty on calculated time, increased with uncertainty of 0.013 days (#1)/0.012 days (#2) on reference time (xv) zeta score for $\hat{t}_1 - t_1$ calculated as a ratio between columns (xii) and (xiv).

Experiment 1 Separation		t_{ref}	25 April 2002		(10:00)									
(i)	(ii)	(iii)	(iv)	(v)	(vi)	(vii)	(viii)	(ix)	(x)	(xi)	(xii)	(xiii)	(xiv)	(xv)
#	t_1 (days)	t_2-t_1 (days)	C_1 (−)	C_2 (−)	$\hat{I}_1$ (Bq)	$\hat{I}_2$ (Bq)	$\hat{I}_2/\hat{I}_1$ (−)	$\hat{A}_2/\hat{A}_1$ (−)	$\hat{t}_1^{(0)}$ (days)	$\hat{t}_1$ (days)	$\hat{t}_1 - t_1$ (days)	$\frac{\hat{t}_1}{t_1} - 1$ (%)	$u(\hat{t}_1 - t_1)$ (days)	ζ (−)
1	0.0917	0.0528	0.9986	0.9892	125,737	6182	0.0492	0.0387	0.122	0.095	0.004	4.0	0.014	0.3
2	0.1486	0.1020	0.9972	0.9792	124,640	9833	0.0789	0.0592	0.198	0.147	−0.001	−1.0	0.014	−0.1
3	0.2543	0.0575	0.9984	0.9882	124,276	13,517	0.1088	0.0980	0.277	0.248	−0.006	−2.5	0.015	−0.4
4	0.3157	0.0848	0.9977	0.9827	122,853	16,455	0.1339	0.1184	0.345	0.303	−0.013	−4.2	0.015	−0.9
5	0.403	0.8326	0.9777	0.8462	120,500	33,181	0.2754	0.1392	0.762	0.359	−0.043	−10.7	0.023	−1.9
6	1.237	0.1130	0.9969	0.9770	117,847	47,584	0.4038	0.3885	1.204	1.148	−0.089	−7.2	0.034	−2.6
7	1.352	0.8115	0.9784	0.8497	115,760	58,557	0.5058	0.4081	1.613	1.220	−0.131	−9.7	0.048	−2.7
8	2.165	0.2942	0.9920	0.9416	112,190	69,755	0.6218	0.5934	2.165	2.020	−0.145	−6.7	0.070	−2.1
9	2.463	0.7277	0.9805	0.8637	109,418	76,693	0.7009	0.6400	2.616	2.263	−0.200	−8.1	0.092	−2.2
10	3.194	0.3767	0.9898	0.9261	106,804	82,962	0.7768	0.7510	3.130	2.945	−0.250	−7.8	0.123	−2.0
11	3.573	0.7261	0.9805	0.8640	103,559	87,349	0.8435	0.8019	3.677	3.324	−0.250	−7.0	0.161	−1.5
12	4.301	0.3777	0.9898	0.9259	100,482	90,490	0.9006	0.8832	4.248	4.062	−0.239	−5.6	0.211	−1.1
13	4.681	0.7168	0.9808	0.8656	97,887	92,086	0.9407	0.9127	4.735	4.386	−0.295	−6.3	0.263	−1.1
14	5.400	0.1523	0.9959	0.9692	95,235	93,011	0.9766	0.9718	5.255	5.180	−0.221	−4.1	0.328	−0.7
15	5.715	0.1276	0.9965	0.9741	94,916	93,430	0.9843	0.9805	5.381	5.317	−0.398	−7.0	0.346	−1.1
16	5.844	0.9724	0.9740	0.8236	92,253	93,845	1.0173	0.9927	5.992	5.524	−0.320	−5.5	0.445	−0.7
Experiment 2 Irradiation		t_{ref}	6 May 2015		11:50		(11:20–12:20)							
1	5.028	0.0455	0.9988	0.9907	7872	7140	0.9070	0.9050	4.320	4.298	−0.730	−15	0.219	−2.7
2	5.075	0.0551	0.9985	0.9887	9196	8315	0.9042	0.9018	4.289	4.261	−0.814	−16	0.186	−3.4
3	5.195	0.7173	0.9808	0.8655	7477	7226	0.9663	0.9417	5.096	4.747	−0.447	−9	0.164	−1.6
4	5.913	1.0283	0.9726	0.8148	8561	8471	0.9895	0.9581	5.468	4.975	−0.939	−16	0.188	−3.0
5	6.973	1.0222	0.9727	0.8158	6632	7018	1.0582	1.0402	7.005	6.515	−0.458	−7	0.379	−0.8
6	8.192	0.8256	0.9779	0.8474	7644	8159	1.0674	1.0544	7.295	6.895	−1.297	−16	0.397	−2.0
7	9.162	1.0160	0.9729	0.8167	7121	7869	1.1052	1.0963	8.956	8.468	−0.695	8	0.743	−0.6
8	10.522	1.0131	0.9730	0.8172	6716	7460	1.1108	1.1030	9.315	8.828	−1.694	−16	0.841	−1.2
9	11.536	0.7335	0.9803	0.8628	6395	7144	1.1171	1.1123	9.781	9.425	−2.111	−18	1.429	−1.1

The residuals are also presented in Fig. 2, which reveals that the chronometer has a bias towards underestimation of the elapsed time since time zero. Such anomaly may originate from various sources of error, possibly in the detection efficiencies, γ-ray intensities or half-lives. The uncertainty components coming into play in the 16 measurements have been compiled in Table 4. The uncertainty propagation factors of the integrated activity ratio $\hat{I}_2/\hat{I}_1$ and daughter half-life $\hat{T}_2$ are of comparable magnitude, whereas the one for the parent half-life $\hat{T}_1$ is negligibly small. Remarkably, the propagation factors are larger for spectra taken over a longer period of time, such as e.g. #5, 7, 9, 11, 13, and 16. This gave rise to a relatively large uncertainty on the chronometry with these spectra, since the improved statistical precision did not compensate for the inflated systematic uncertainties. This counterintuitive effect follows directly from application of the uncertainty propagation in Eq. (19).

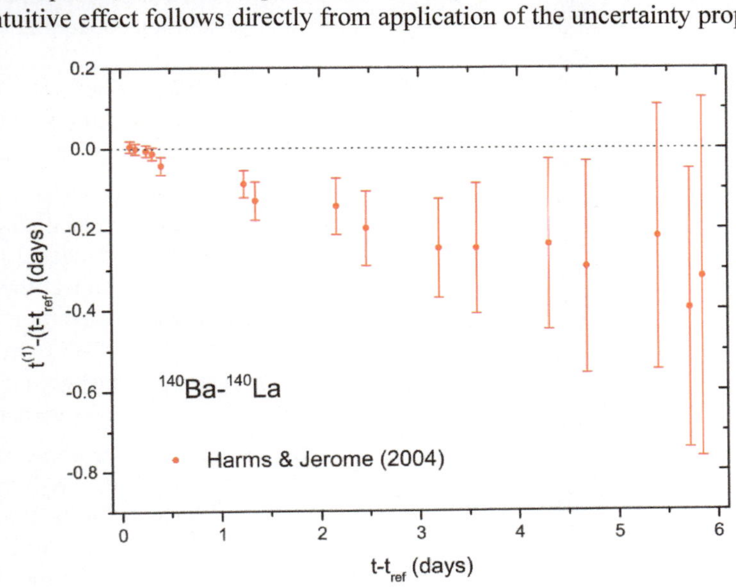

Figure 2. Deviation of the chronometry results from time zero for the ^{140}Ba-^{140}La pair from experiment 1 by Harms and Jerome (2004).

Table 4. Uncertainty components related to the ^{140}Ba-^{140}La chronometry data in Table 2: (i) spectrum number, (ii–iv) uncertainties and propagation factors for the integrated activity ratios and the ^{140}Ba (T_1 = 12.753 (4) days) and ^{140}La (T_2 = 1.67850 (17) days) half-lives towards $\hat{t}_1$, (v) relative uncertainty on the estimated time zero $\hat{t}_1$, (vi) uncertainty on reference time t_1 divided by $\hat{t}_1$, (vii) uncertainty of the residuals $\hat{t}_1 - t$ divided by $\hat{t}_1$. Timing uncertainties on t_1 and t_2 (Δt) were assumed to be negligible.

Uncertainties and propagation factors						
(i)	(ii)	(iii)	(iv)	(v)	(vi)	(vii)
	$\frac{u(\hat{I}_2/\hat{I}_1)}{I_2/I}$	$\frac{u(\hat{T}_1)}{T_1}$	$\frac{u(\hat{T}_2)}{T_2}$		$u(t_1)$	
Exp. 1	2.1%	0.031%	0.010%		1155 s	
Exp. 2	~2%	idem	idem		30 min	
#	$\frac{u(\hat{t}_1)/\hat{t}_1}{u\left(\frac{I_2}{I_1}\right)/\frac{I_2}{I_1}}$	$\frac{u(\hat{t}_1)/\hat{t}_1}{u(\hat{T}_1)/\hat{T}_1}$	$\frac{u(\hat{t}_1)/\hat{t}_1}{u(\hat{T}_2)/\hat{T}_2}$	$\frac{u(\hat{t}_1)}{\hat{t}_1}$	$\frac{u(t_1)}{\hat{t}_1}$	$\frac{u(\hat{t}_1-t_1)}{\hat{t}_1}$
	Eq. (19)	Eq. (19)	Eq. (19)	ii² + iii² + iv²		v² + vi²
	(–)	(–)	(–)	(%)	(%)	(%)
Experiment 1						
1	1.30	0.0042	1.27	2.8	14.0	14.3
2	1.39	0.0072	1.34	2.9	9.1	9.6
3	1.17	0.0086	1.11	2.5	5.4	5.9
4	1.21	0.0111	1.13	2.6	4.4	5.1
5	2.44	0.044	2.04	5.1	3.7	6.3
6	1.31	0.040	1.01	2.8	1.2	3.0
7	1.79	0.070	1.24	3.8	1.1	3.9
8	1.62	0.083	0.99	3.4	0.7	3.5
9	1.92	0.115	1.04	4.0	0.6	4.1
10	1.96	0.136	0.93	4.1	0.5	4.2
11	2.30	0.180	0.92	4.8	0.4	4.9
12	2.46	0.215	0.83	5.2	0.3	5.2
13	2.84	0.266	0.81	6.0	0.3	6.0
14	3.01	0.30	0.71	6.3	0.3	6.3
15	3.09	0.31	0.70	6.5	0.3	6.5
16	3.82	0.41	0.67	8.1	0.2	8.1
Experiment 2						
1	2.406	0.212	0.793	6.2	0.3	6.2
2	2.392	0.210	0.796	5.6	0.3	5.6
3	3.065	0.302	0.770	5.7	0.3	5.7
4	3.423	0.352	0.744	6.4	0.3	6.4
5	4.851	0.572	0.501	9.3	0.2	9.3
6	5.128	0.617	0.440	9.6	0.2	9.6
7	7.843	1.028	0.027	14.6	0.2	14.6
8	8.600	1.143	−0.090	16.0	0.2	16.0
9	9.577	1.294	−0.257	20.9	0.1	20.9

Experiment 2

Irradiation and Sample Preparation

Experiment 2 refers to new work in which ^{140}Ba was produced by proton induced fission in a uranium target, then chemically separated from the target and measured by HPGe γ-ray spectrometry. A target of 1.51 g $^{nat}UO_2$ compacted between an aluminium holder and a 0.025 mm Ti foil was irradiated at the Birmingham University cyclotron. The target was exposed to a beam of 25 MeV protons, with a current of 10 µA, for 50 min. The irradiation was started at 11:30 UTC and stopped at 12:20 UTC on 2015-05-06. The irradiated target of $^{nat}UO_2$ was dissolved in 30 g of 2 M HNO_3, containing 0.01 mg g^{-1} each of strontium, caesium, yttrium, molybdenum and hafnium. A 1 g aliquot of this solution was dispensed to a 2 mL flamed sealed ISO ampoule. The solution was further extracted three times with 40 mL 30% v/v tributyl phosphate (TBP) in n-dodecane to separate the fission products from the uranium. A 1 g aliquot of this final solution was dispensed to a 2 mL flamed sealed ISO ampoule.

Gamma-ray Spectrometry

The HPGe γ-ray spectrometer 'LISA' of NPL was used. It was contained in a lead shield with internal dimensions of 1 m × 1.5 m × 1 m, constructed of 10-cm-thick walls with a cadmium-copper graded lining. The FEP efficiency of this detector had been calibrated for a 1 g solution in a 2 mL ISO ampoule mounted at 20 cm from the detector window using a radionuclide solution containing ^{241}Am, ^{109}Cd, ^{57}Co, ^{139}Ce, ^{51}Cr, ^{113}Sn, ^{85}Sr, ^{137}Cs, ^{54}Mn, ^{88}Y, ^{65}Zn and ^{60}Co, which were traceable to primary standards of activity. The nuclear data used for each radionuclide were derived from the DDEP evaluations (DDEP, 2004–2015).

The detector chain consisted of an analogue CANBERRA AFT Research amplifier, analogue-to-digital converter (ADC) and AIM electronics connected to a PC using CANBERRA GENIE 2000 v2.1c to collect the spectra. The dead time and pulse-pileup were corrected for using the live-time correction/pile-up rejection (LTC/PUR) circuit built into the amplifier-ADC combination. A background spectrum was collected for 200,000 s prior to the measurements.

The two samples were measured for a total of nine times over a campaign of one week, starting five days after the irradiation mid-point, for live times of ~3800 s–86,400 s. The source-detector distance of 20 cm made the effect of true coincidence summing negligible relative to the uncertainties of the measurement, therefore no corrections were applied.

Thirty plus γ ray emitting fission products were present in the samples, with over 300 full energy peaks measured. The collected spectra were therefore complex, with a number of interferences and convolutions of some of the selected ^{140}Ba and ^{140}La FEPs present, thus the peak fits of the spectra were manually verified using interactive peak fitting and adjusted as required. The ^{132}I (812.0 keV) and ^{136}Cs (818.5 keV) FEP were de-convoluted from the 815.8 keV FEP of ^{140}La to determine the net peak area.

Chronometry Results

The mid-point of the irradiation was taken as the reference time for chronometry. The 'time zero' was calculated from the activity of the ^{140}Ba and ^{140}La derived from each spectrum, following the procedure detailed in section 3. The correction factors for count loss through dead time and uncompensated pile-up were of the order of 1.04–1.01 and 1.005–1.0015, respectively. A summary of relevant numbers is included in Table 3 and Table 4, relying on the old DDEP evaluated data from Helmer, 2004a and Helmer, 2004b for direct comparison with experiment 1. In Fig. 3, a combined graph is shown of the residuals of the timing results relative to the reference time obtained in both experiments. An alarming finding is that the chronology in this new experiment is also biased towards an underestimation of the elapsed time. The systematic bias is comparable with experiment 1 around $t - t_0 = 5$ days and grows even further for spectra taken at a later stage. The arithmetic mean of the time zero estimates is 2015-05-07 12:19 UTC ± 0.57 days, which is discrepant from the reference time 2015-05-06 11:50 UTC ± 0.012 days by a day.

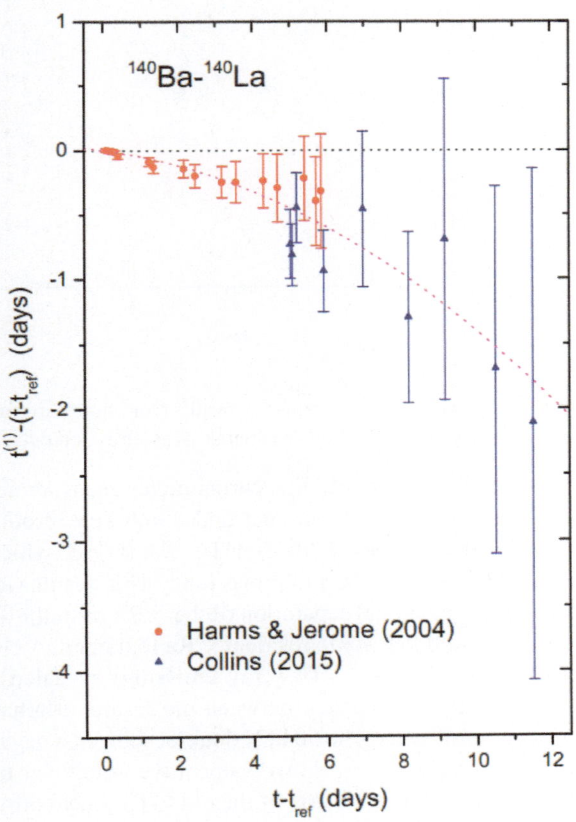

Figure 3. The residuals of ^{140}Ba-^{140}La chronometry results obtained in experiments 1 and 2, using DDEP decay data (Helmer, 2004a and Helmer, 2004b).

Impact of Nuclear Data

The two samples produced similar results, even though the second sample was made after a further chemical separation stage, and so it cannot be excluded that the equilibrium of the ^{140}Ba-^{140}La pair was disrupted during the initial sample preparation stage. As an alternative explanation, one may suspect a bias in the γ-ray intensities. As summarised in Table 2, the DDEP evaluation data of Helmer, 2004a and Helmer, 2004bhave been updated by Chechev and Kuzmenko (2015) with a small effect on the ^{140}La half-life and changes in the uncertainties of the characteristic γ-ray intensities. The most recent ENSDF evaluation (Nica, 2007) has been tried as an alternative to the DDEP reference data: it contains similar half-life values with smaller uncertainties, the same intensity for the main ^{140}Ba line, but lower intensities with higher uncertainties for the^{140}La lines.

Replacing the nuclear data with those from ENSDF, the consistency in the results shows an improvement. In Fig. 4 the new results are compared with those based on the old DDEP data (cf. Table 4). Whereas the uncertainties are higher, the bias is clearly smaller. The average estimate of the time zero is 2015-05-07 03:36 UTC ± 0.41 d, which is still 0.66 days off target. The increase in the uncertainties of the chronometer measurements derived from the ENSDF nuclear data are due to the significantly larger uncertainty determined for the 1596.2 keV emission of the ^{140}La with a value of 1.5% (ENSDF) versus 0.08% (DDEP), as well as for the other γ-rays listed in Table 2.

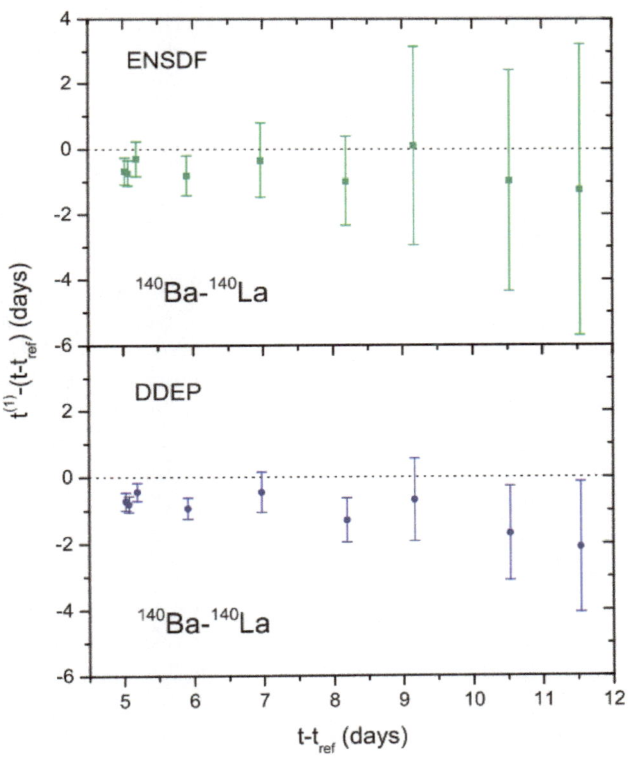

Figure 4. Comparison of the chronometry residuals in experiment 2 when using the ENSDF(2007) and DDEP(2004) data sets in Table 2.

Investigation of the individual chronometry performance of the γ-ray emissions of ^{140}La revealed that the DDEP and ENSDF data provide identical trends for the 1596.2 keV γ-ray, but significantly different ones for the 487.0 keV and 815.8 keV γ-rays. Whereas the trends in the residuals are consistent for all

DDEP data, the ENSDF data lead to opposing trends which explains why its average result is better. The uncertainties on the ENSDF emission probabilities are comparable for the three γ-rays, which gives extra weight to the mutually consistent subset of the 487.0 keV and 815.8 keV results.

In summary, one can conclude that the ENSDF database is inconsistent – and therefore more 'accurate' for the 'wrong' reasons – whereas the DDEP database is consistent but may be inaccurate due to an error in either or both of the γ-ray intensity normalisation factors for ^{140}Ba and ^{140}La decay.

^{227}Th-^{223}Ra CLOCK

The radionuclide ^{227}Th ($T_{1/2}$ = 18.697 days (Collins et al., 2015c)) and several of its daughter nuclides are alpha emitters suitable for application in alpha immunotherapy. Two nuclides in the decay chain, ^{223}Ra ($T_{1/2}$ = 11.4354 days (Collins et al., 2015a)) and ^{221}Pb ($T_{1/2}$ = 36.161 min (Aitken-Smith and Collins, 2016)), have a non-negligibly long half-life which prevents the decay chain from establishing a secular equilibrium when starting from an isolated amount of ^{227}Th. For months, the decay chain acts as a dynamic system in which the combined activity is not an exact integer multiple of the parent activity. The dosimetric impact varies with time, as well as the response of a hospital calibrator to the gradually changing composition of the radionuclide mixture. Precise modelling of these processes through the decay formulae (Pommé et al., 1996) requires knowledge of the decay constants and the effective time zero of chemical separation. A systematic study of the decay characteristics of the ^{227}Th decay series has recently been performed (Collins et al., 2015a, Collins et al., 2015b, Collins et al., 2015c, Collins et al., 2016 and Aitken-Smith and Collins, 2016). Establishment of the effective time zero through ^{227}Th-^{223}Ra chronometry has been tested in the experiment described below.

Sample Preparation

A ^{227}Th solution that had been radiochemically separated from an ^{227}Ac sample was supplied to NPL by Bayer (Norway) as $[^{227}Th(NO_3)_6]^{2-}$ in 8 M HNO_3 at a nominal activity of 70 MBq. A chemical separation was performed to remove residual ^{227}Ac and the ^{227}Th decay progeny, passing the solution through a Bio-Rad AG1-X8(100–200 mesh) anion exchange resin; 2 g of this resin was used as a 50 mm × 7.5 mm column. The chemical separation commenced at 09:00 UTC and completed at 09:38 UTC on 2013-09-17; the mid-point of the separation was at 09:19 UTC.

The column was washed with 3 × 3 mL aliquots of 8 M HNO_3 to remove the decay products and any residual actinium. The ^{227}Th was eluted from the column using 3 × 3 mL aliquots of 2 M HNO_3 and further diluted by the addition of 2 M HNO_3 containing 10 μg g^{-1} Ce^{4+}, added as a proxy carrier for thorium to avoid absorption of the thorium onto the glass container walls. A 1 g aliquot of the solution was dispensed to a 2 mL ISO ampoule, which was flame sealed in order to stop the release of ^{219}Rn, before being measured by HPGe γ-ray spectrometry.

Gamma-ray Spectrometry

The HPGe γ-ray spectrometer 'BART', described in detail by Collins et al. (2015b), was used to perform ^{227}Th-^{223}Ra chronometry of the radiochemical separation. The ^{227}Th/^{223}Ra activity ratios were determined utilising the γ-ray emissions of the 50 keV doublet (comprised of the 49.8 keV and 50.1 keV γ-ray emissions) and 236.0 keV of ^{227}Th and the 154 keV of the ^{223}Ra. The 269.5 keV of ^{223}Ra was not used due to a small interference from the 267 keV from ^{227}Th and the 271.0 keV of ^{219}Rn. The activities for the ^{227}Th and ^{223}Ra were determined using the γ-ray emission probabilities from ENSDF (Browne, 2001) and Collins et al. (2015b), respectively. The half-lives were taken fromCollins et al., 2015a and Collins et al., 2015c.

A series of 56 measurements were made over a period ~105 days, for live times of 3600 and 5000 s. The peaks were manually verified and adjusted where required using interactive peak fitting software, the net peak areas were corrected for any background interferences.

Chronometry Results

The deviation of the measured time zero values from the separation mid-point are presented in Fig. 5. The chronometry performs well throughout the campaign, with the residuals being significantly smaller than the uncertainties. The latter are quite large, due to the considerable uncertainty on the ENSDF decay data (Browne, 2001). Higher precision can be achieved with the recently improved decay data (see section 6.4).

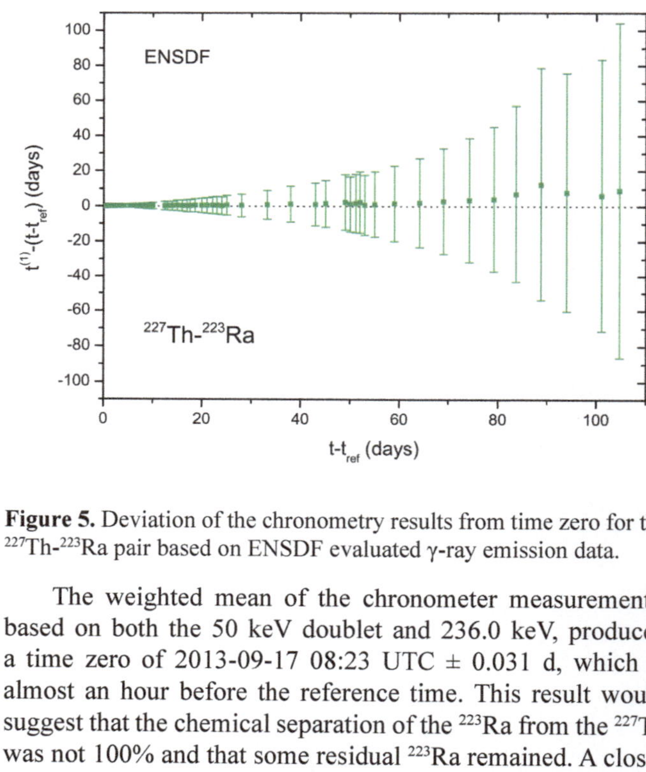

Figure 5. Deviation of the chronometry results from time zero for the ^{227}Th-^{223}Ra pair based on ENSDF evaluated γ-ray emission data.

The weighted mean of the chronometer measurements, based on both the 50 keV doublet and 236.0 keV, produced a time zero of 2013-09-17 08:23 UTC ± 0.031 d, which is almost an hour before the reference time. This result would suggest that the chemical separation of the ^{223}Ra from the ^{227}Th was not 100% and that some residual ^{223}Ra remained. A closer investigation of the two ^{227}Th γ ray emissions revealed that there was a large discrepancy between the results originating from the two emissions. The 50 keV doublet showed a negative trend, while the 236.0 keV showed a positive trend over time. Mainly due to the low precision of the old ^{227}Th γ-ray emission probabilities, it is clear that determining the time zero with any precision becomes impossible after only a few days.

Table 5 provides uncertainty propagation factors of the activity ratio and the half-lives towards the age dating for hypothetical measurements started at time t_1 and continued over a period Δt. The values from the new formulae in Eq.

(19) are compared with those of the solution for long-lived radionuclides in Eq. (16); the magnitude of the propagation factors is visibly enhanced for measurements of relatively long duration. In Fig. 6, propagation factors are shown for hypothetical measurements of 2 days. The factor for I_2/I_1 is always larger than 1, for T_1 it is small at first but rises above 1 after 39 days, whereas for T_2 it changes sign. The difference between Eqs. (16), (A.1), (A.2), (A.3),(A.4), (A.5), (A.6), (A.7) and (19) is visible at all times, particularly in the beginning.

Table 5. Uncertainty propagation for hypothetical ^{227}Th-^{223}Ra chronometry measurements: (i) start time t_1, (ii) measurement duration Δt, (iii,v,vii) rigorous propagation factors calculated from Eq. (19) for I_2/I_1, T_1 and T_2, respectively, (iv,vi,viii) approximate propagation factors from Eq. (16), which is applicable only if measurements are negligibly short compared to half-lives.

Uncertainty propagation factors							
		T_1 T_2	18.697 (7) d 11.4354 (17) d		$u(T_1)/T_1$ $u(T_2)/T_2$		0.037% 0.015%
(i)	(ii)	(iii)	(iv)	(v)	(vi)	(vii)	(viii)
t_1	Δt	$\dfrac{u(\hat{t}_1)/\hat{t}_1}{u\left(\frac{I_2}{I_1}\right)/\frac{I_2}{I_1}}$		$\dfrac{u(\hat{t}_1)/\hat{t}_1}{u(T_1)/T_1}$		$\dfrac{u(\hat{t}_1)/\hat{t}_1}{u(T_2)/T_2}$	
(days)	(days)	Eq. (19) (–)	Eq. (16) (–)	Eq. (19) (–)	Eq. (16) (–)	Eq. (19) (–)	Eq. (16) (–)
2	0.1	1.050	1.024	0.040	0.038	0.985	0.962
2	1	1.285	1.024	0.058	0.038	1.188	0.962
2	2	1.546	1.024	0.081	0.038	1.402	0.962
5	0.1	1.072	1.061	0.098	0.096	0.912	0.904
5	2	1.285	1.061	0.138	0.096	1.056	0.904
5	5	1.616	1.061	0.208	0.096	1.252	0.904
10	1	1.191	1.128	0.222	0.201	0.827	0.799
20	1	1.317	1.277	0.460	0.436	0.564	0.564
40	1	1.693	1.661	1.072	1.041	–0.060	–0.041
40	5	1.819	1.661	1.195	1.041	–0.137	–0.041
40	10	1.972	1.661	1.346	1.041	–0.241	–0.041
50	0.1	1.910	1.907	1.432	1.429	–0.431	–0.429
60	1	2.233	2.199	1.929	1.888	–0.921	–0.888
80	1	3.001	2.960	3.142	3.087	–2.136	–2.087
100	0.1	4.053	4.048	4.807	4.800	–3.807	–3.800
100	1	4.100	4.048	4.875	4.800	–3.870	–3.800
100	10	4.559	4.048	5.530	4.800	–4.488	–3.800

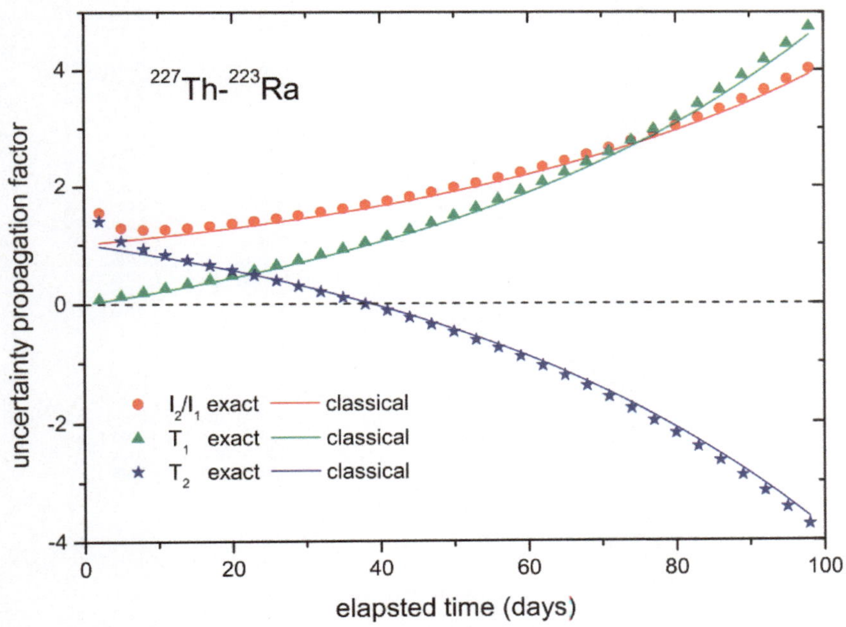

Figure 6. Propagation factors of the activity ratio and the parent and daughter half-lives towards the calculated time zero derived from measurements of 2 days. The exact values from Eq. (19) (symbols) are compared to the approximate values from Eq. (16) (lines).

Impact of Decay Data on Chronometer

The accuracy of ^{227}Th-^{223}Ra chronometry can be drastically improved with the availability of recently determined decay data (Collins et al., 2015a, Collins et al., 2015b,Collins et al., 2015c and Collins et al., 2016). New absolute γ-ray emission probabilities for ^{227}Th have been determined in Collins et al. (2016), which show a significant difference with the values of the 50.1 keV doublet and 236.0 keV emission probabilities, as shown in Table 6. The quoted precision of these emission intensities have been reduced by at least a factor of 10. The time zero of the separation has been re-determined using these new intensity data.

Table 6. Evaluated decay data applied for ^{227}Th-^{223}Ra chronometry in this work, from ENSDF (Browne, 2001) and Collins et al., 2015a, Collins et al., 2015b, Collins et al., 2015c and Collins et al., 2016.

Variable	ENSDF	Collins et al.
T_1 (^{227}Th) (days)	–	18.697 (7)
I_γ (49.8 + 50.1) (%)	8.81 (85)	9.013 (50)
I_γ (236.0) (%)	12.9 (11)	12.578 (64)
T_2 (^{223}Ra) (days)	–	11.4354 (17)
I_γ (154.2) (%)	5.699 (20)	6.02 (3)

In Table 7, an overview is presented of relevant quantities used in this chronometry experiment. The uncertainty contribution of the half-lives is negligible compared to the activity ratio. As shown in Fig. 7, the dating results are consistent and have a much smaller uncertainty compared to Fig. 5. Fig. 8 showing a zoom in over the first 25 days of the campaign, demonstrates a high correlation between the dating results derived from both γ ray emissions combined and separately. The time zero determined from the weighted mean for the 50 keV doublet and 236 keV γ-ray emissions was 08:26 (16) UTC and 08:29 (16) UTC on 2013-09-17, respectively. These are both in agreement with the results derived from the ENSDF data in section 6.3.

Table 7. Measured data from the ingrowth of ^{223}Ra into chemically separated ^{227}Th, including reference time of chemical separation, (i) spectrum number, (ii) elapsed time at start of measurement, (iii) duration of measurement, (iv, v) counting factors correcting for decay during measurement, (vi, vii) measured (integrated) activity, (viii) integrated activity ratio, (ix) momentary activity ratio (x) initial time zero estimate via Eq. (10), (xi) final estimate of time zero via Eq. (9), (xii), absolute and (xiii) relative uncertainty on the measured integrated activity ratio, (xiv) uncertainty on calculated time, increased with uncertainty of 11 min on reference time (xv) zeta score for $\hat{t}_1 - t_1$ calculated as a ratio between columns (xii) and (xiv).

Separation														
		t_{ref} $u(t_{ref})$	17 September 2013 11 min		09:19 0.00764 days		(09:00–09:38)							
(i)	(ii)	(iii)	(iv)	(v)	(vi)	(vii)	(viii)	(ix)	(x)	(xi)	(xii)	(xiii)	(xiv)	(xv)
#	t_1	t_2-t_1	C_1	C_2	$\hat{I}_1$	$\hat{I}_2$	$\hat{I}_2/\hat{I}_1$	$\hat{A}_2/\hat{A}_1$	$\hat{t}_1^{(0)}$	$\hat{t}_1$	$\hat{t}_1-t_1$	$\frac{u(\hat{I}_2/\hat{I}_1)}{\hat{I}_2/\hat{I}}$	$u(\hat{t}_1-t_1)$	ξ
	(days)	(days)	(–)	(–)	(Bq)	(Bq)	(–)	(–)	(days)	(days)	(days)	(%)	(days)	(–)
1	0.282	0.043	0.9992	0.9987	662,024	12,934	0.0195	0.0182	0.324	0.302	0.020	3.6	0.014	1.4
2	0.328	0.043	0.9992	0.9987	660,754	14,944	0.0226	0.0213	0.375	0.353	0.026	3.1	0.014	1.8
3	0.373	0.043	0.9992	0.9987	658,521	17283	0.0262	0.0249	0.435	0.413	0.040	2.5	0.013	3.0
4	0.433	0.043	0.9992	0.9987	656,463	20,332	0.0310	0.0297	0.514	0.492	0.060	2.5	0.015	4.0
5	0.481	0.044	0.9992	0.9987	656,448	21,574	0.0329	0.0316	0.546	0.524	0.043	2.4	0.015	2.8
6	0.525	0.044	0.9992	0.9987	653,323	23,121	0.0354	0.0341	0.588	0.566	0.041	2.3	0.016	2.6
7	0.569	0.044	0.9992	0.9987	652,675	25,697	0.0394	0.0381	0.655	0.633	0.063	6.4	0.043	1.5
8	0.982	0.044	0.9992	0.9987	641,420	39,665	0.0618	0.0606	1.033	1.011	0.029	1.6	0.018	1.6
9	1.030	0.044	0.9992	0.9987	642,321	40,732	0.0634	0.0621	1.059	1.037	0.007	4.6	0.050	0.1
10	1.078	0.194	0.9964	0.9941	639,385	46,092	0.0721	0.0664	1.206	1.109	0.031	1.0	0.015	2.1
11	1.990	0.061	0.9989	0.9982	618,856	74,695	0.1207	0.1189	2.039	2.009	0.019	1.1	0.025	0.8
12	2.069	0.195	0.9964	0.9941	614,809	80,547	0.1310	0.1254	2.218	2.121	0.052	0.9	0.023	2.3
13	2.273	0.061	0.9989	0.9982	612,182	83,335	0.1361	0.1344	2.307	2.277	0.004	1.1	0.027	0.1
14	3.170	0.061	0.9989	0.9982	591,860	110,802	0.1872	0.1855	3.207	3.176	0.006	1.0	0.035	0.2
15	4.060	0.061	0.9989	0.9981	573,168	135,210	0.2359	0.2342	4.082	4.051	−0.008	1.0	0.043	−0.2
16	5.351	0.061	0.9989	0.9981	543,447	169,270	0.3115	0.3098	5.477	5.446	0.095	1.0	0.058	1.6
17	6.160	0.089	0.9984	0.9973	529,866	187,660	0.3542	0.3518	6.286	6.242	0.082	0.9	0.064	1.3
18	7.165	0.124	0.9977	0.9963	507,847	205,341	0.4043	0.4012	7.257	7.195	0.030	0.9	0.073	0.4
19	8.196	0.062	0.9989	0.9981	488,936	222,947	0.4560	0.4544	8.280	8.249	0.053	1.0	0.087	0.6
20	8.983	0.062	0.9989	0.9981	473,748	233,280	0.4924	0.4909	9.016	8.985	0.002	1.0	0.096	0.0
21	10.020	0.062	0.9989	0.9981	455,777	248,771	0.5458	0.5443	10.120	10.089	0.069	1.0	0.109	0.6
22	12.467	0.062	0.9989	0.9981	417,672	274,354	0.6569	0.6555	12.511	12.480	0.013	0.9	0.138	0.1
23	12.959	0.062	0.9989	0.9981	410,574	279,325	0.6803	0.6789	13.034	13.003	0.043	0.9	0.143	0.3
24	13.988	0.062	0.9989	0.9981	394,996	286,114	0.7243	0.7230	14.032	14.001	0.014	0.9	0.156	0.1
25	14.987	0.062	0.9989	0.9981	378,584	293,063	0.7741	0.7728	15.190	15.159	0.172	0.9	0.172	1.0
26	15.989	0.062	0.9989	0.9981	365,403	296,255	0.8108	0.8095	16.064	16.033	0.044	0.9	0.184	0.2
27	16.985	0.062	0.9989	0.9981	353,181	299,818	0.8489	0.8476	16.993	16.962	−0.023	0.9	0.197	−0.1
28	17.592	0.062	0.9989	0.9981	345,572	301,798	0.8733	0.8721	17.598	17.567	−0.025	0.9	0.207	−0.1
29	18.584	0.062	0.9989	0.9981	331,242	304,994	0.9208	0.9196	18.799	18.768	0.184	0.9	0.224	0.8
30	19.871	0.062	0.9989	0.9981	316,113	305,404	0.9661	0.9650	19.980	19.949	0.078	1.0	0.244	0.3
31	20.936	0.062	0.9989	0.9981	304,844	307,469	1.0086	1.0075	21.117	21.086	0.150	1.0	0.260	0.6
32	22.080	0.062	0.9989	0.9981	291,816	307,183	1.0527	1.0516	22.329	22.298	0.218	1.0	0.281	0.8
33	22.987	0.062	0.9989	0.9981	281,235	304,847	1.0840	1.0829	23.212	23.181	0.194	1.0	0.302	0.6
34	23.960	0.062	0.9989	0.9981	272,727	302,347	1.1086	1.1075	23.920	23.889	−0.071	1.0	0.314	−0.2
35	24.995	0.062	0.9989	0.9981	262,570	303,293	1.1551	1.1541	25.288	25.258	0.262	1.0	0.333	0.8
36	27.967	0.061	0.9989	0.9981	234,749	292,273	1.2450	1.2441	28.069	28.038	0.071	1.0	0.385	0.2
37	33.212	0.061	0.9989	0.9982	193,292	271,824	1.4063	1.4054	33.560	33.529	0.318	1.0	0.505	0.6
38	37.954	0.061	0.9989	0.9982	161,549	248,582	1.5387	1.5380	38.670	38.640	0.686	1.0	0.634	1.1
39	43.003	0.060	0.9989	0.9982	135,571	223,369	1.6476	1.6470	43.387	43.357	0.354	1.0	0.759	0.5
40	45.067	0.060	0.9989	0.9982	124,927	212,350	1.6998	1.6992	45.847	45.817	0.750	1.0	0.848	0.9
41	48.993	0.060	0.9989	0.9982	108,008	193,297	1.7897	1.7891	50.450	50.421	1.428	1.1	1.018	1.4
42	49.999	0.060	0.9989	0.9982	104,479	186,960	1.7895	1.7889	50.439	50.409	0.411	1.1	1.021	0.4
43	51.132	0.060	0.9989	0.9982	100,122	181,866	1.8164	1.8159	51.925	51.895	0.763	1.1	1.070	0.7
44	51.997	0.060	0.9989	0.9982	96,948	178,492	1.8411	1.8406	53.329	53.299	1.302	1.1	1.129	1.2
45	52.985	0.060	0.9989	0.9982	93,674	171,751	1.8335	1.8330	52.892	52.862	−0.123	1.1	1.116	−0.1
46	54.997	0.060	0.9989	0.9982	86,577	162,186	1.8733	1.8728	55.237	55.207	0.210	1.1	1.227	0.2
47	58.991	0.059	0.9989	0.9982	75,079	145,687	1.9405	1.9400	59.510	59.481	0.490	1.1	1.431	0.3
48	64.113	0.059	0.9989	0.9982	62,303	125,478	2.0140	2.0136	64.745	64.715	0.603	1.1	1.712	0.4
49	68.995	0.059	0.9989	0.9982	51,654	107,951	2.0899	2.0895	70.921	70.892	1.897	1.2	2.127	0.9
50	74.239	0.059	0.9989	0.9982	42,678	91,854	2.1523	2.1520	76.770	76.741	2.503	1.2	2.645	0.9
51	79.134	0.059	0.9989	0.9982	35,648	77,899	2.1852	2.1850	80.223	80.193	1.059	1.3	2.991	0.4
52	83.612	0.059	0.9989	0.9982	29,766	67,123	2.2550	2.2548	88.608	88.578	4.966	1.5	4.387	1.1
53	88.725	0.058	0.9989	0.9982	24,719	57,166	2.3126	2.3124	97.043	97.014	8.288	1.4	5.152	1.6
54	93.991	0.058	0.9989	0.9982	20,379	47,533	2.3324	2.3323	100.383	100.353	6.363	1.5	5.979	1.1
55	101.076	0.058	0.9989	0.9982	15,757	37,107	2.3550	2.3548	104.531	104.502	3.426	1.6	7.204	0.5
56	104.685	0.058	0.9989	0.9982	13,892	32,505	2.3399	2.3397	101.709	101.680	−3.005	1.7	7.133	−0.4

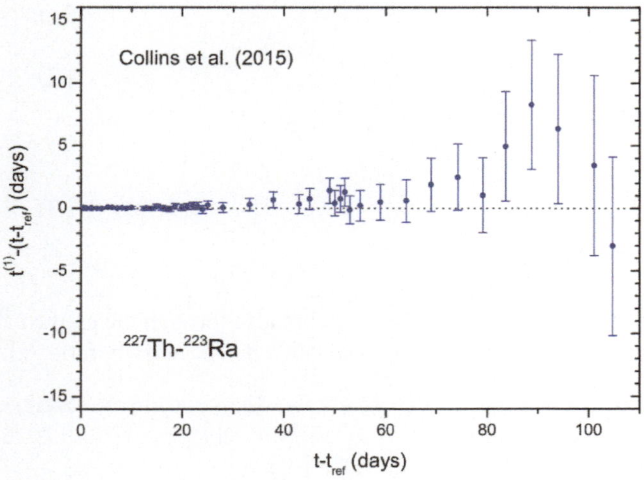

Figure 7. The residuals of ^{227}Th-^{223}Ra chronometry results, using recently determined decay data by Collins et al., 2015b and Collins et al., 2016.

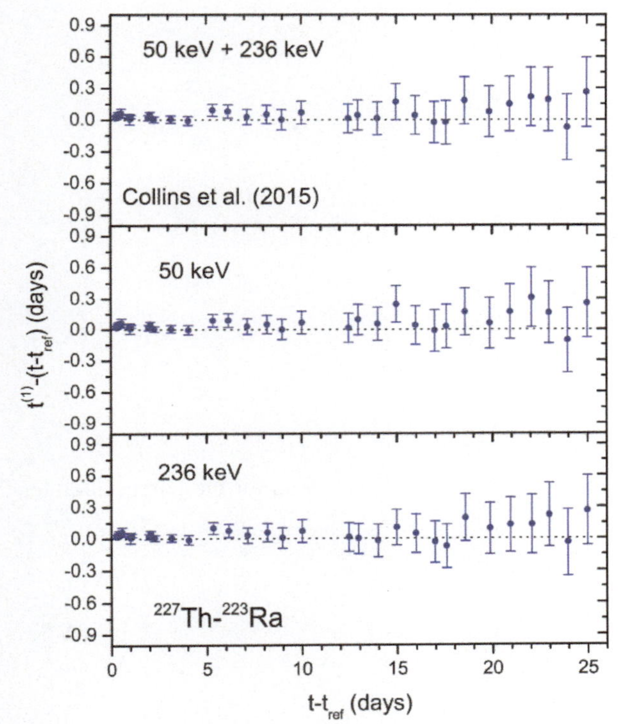

Figure 8. The residuals of ^{227}Th-^{223}Ra chronometry results in the first 25 days, for combined and separate use of the 50 keV and 236 keV peaks.

It is recommended that the accuracy of ^{227}Th-^{223}Ra chronometry is also checked in another laboratory, since the new decay data sets have been determined on the same detector and therefore inconsistencies are unlikely to show up in this context. For completeness, a new ^{227}Th-^{223}Ra chronometry experiment (not described in this paper) has recently been performed at NPL using another HPGe detector, leading to equally consistent results.

CONCLUSIONS

The general uncertainty equations for nuclear dating in Eq. (16) have been amended for the particular case of parent-daughter chronometry involving radionuclides with relatively short half-life. Deriving time zero from the measured count ratios in parent and daughter γ-ray peaks through Eq. (10) leads to a time estimation $t^{(0)}$ which deviates from the true value by about half the measurement time. A more precise approximation $t^{(1)}$ is obtained by including correction factors for decay during measurements, via Eq. (11). The principally correct dating value follows from the ratio of the decay-corrected activities in Eq. (8) implemented in Eq. (9).

In the Annex, a full mathematical derivation of the uncertainty budget for parent-daughter dating has been performed. It includes the propagation of the half-life uncertainties through the conversion formula from count integrals to activity (Eq. (8)). The effect of the latter can be so significant for short-lived radionuclides that the dating uncertainty for a long measurement may be inferior to that of a short one. A simplified but accurate uncertainty formula, Eq. (19), was derived from the approximations $t^{(0)}$ and $t^{(1)}$, which can be considered an amendment to Eq. (16).

The formulae have been successfully applied for dating of an irradiation or chemical purification of a sample, using γ-ray spectra taken of ^{140}La-^{140}Ba and ^{227}Th-^{223}Ra parent-daughter pairs. The accuracy and precision of both chronometers showed heavy dependency on the nuclear decay data set used. Some bias in the results may be caused by incomplete chemical separation or inadvertent disturbance of the chemical composition of the sample.

ACKNOWLEDGEMENT

The authors would like to thank Dr Peter Ivanov for the preparation of the fission product solution used in the ^{140}Ba-^{140}La experiment 2. This work gives indirect support to the research projects MetroERM, 'Metrology for radiological early warning networks in Europe' and MetroNORM, 'Metrology for processing materials with high natural radioactivity', funded by the European Union.

ANNEX A FULL UNCERTAINTY PROPAGATION

In section 3.2, a shortcut solution is presented for the uncertainty propagation of the half-lives T_1, T_2 and the counting integral ratio I_2/I_1. The same numerical results can be obtained from a rigorous uncertainty propagation of the basic dating formulae (Eqs.(8) and (9))). For completeness, the derivation and mathematical result is succinctly presented in this annex.

Uncertainty of Activity Integral

In Eq. (16), the propagation of the uncertainty on A_2/A_1 is correctly taken into account, however it is more convenient to propagate the uncertainty on the ratio of the measured quantities I_2/I_1. Using the partial derivative $\frac{\partial(A_2/A_1)}{\partial(I_2/I_1)} = \frac{C_1}{C_2}$ one readily obtains the following equation:

$$\frac{\sigma(t)}{t} \approx \left(\frac{T}{t}\right)\frac{\sigma(A_2/A_1)}{A_2/A_1} = \left(\frac{T}{t}\frac{C_1}{C_2}\frac{I_2/I_1}{A_2/A_1}\right)\frac{\sigma(I_2/I_1)}{I_2/I_1} \quad \text{(A.1)}$$

Eq. (A.1) is equivalent with the third term of Eq. (19), and therefore the equality of the sensitivity factors holds:

$$\frac{T^{(0)}}{t} = \frac{T}{t}\frac{C_1}{C_2}\frac{I_2/I_1}{A_2/A_1} \tag{A.2}$$

which yields an alternative relationship between the activity ratio and the integral ratio:

$$\frac{A_2/A_1}{I_2/I_1} = \frac{T}{T^{(0)}}\frac{C_1}{C_2} \tag{A.3}$$

Uncertainty of Parent Half-life

The uncertainty of the parent half-life not only propagates through the dating equation (Eq. (9)), but also through the conversion formula of I_2/I_1 to A_2/A_1 (Eq. (8)), and its relative uncertainty propagates with a sensitivity factor of T/t. The activity ratio A_2/A_1 depends onλ_1 through the factors F and C_1:

$$\frac{\partial(A_2/A_1)}{\partial\lambda_1} = \frac{\partial F}{\partial\lambda_1}\left(1-\frac{C_1}{C_2}\right) + \frac{\partial C_1}{\partial\lambda_1}\left(\frac{1}{C_2}\frac{I_2}{I_1} - \frac{F_1}{C_2}\right) \tag{A.4}$$

in which

$$\frac{\partial F}{\partial\lambda_1} = \frac{\lambda_2}{(\lambda_2-\lambda_1)^2}$$

$$\frac{\partial C_1}{\partial\lambda_1} = \frac{e^{-\lambda_1\Delta t}}{\lambda_1} - \frac{1-e^{-\lambda_1\Delta t}}{\lambda_1^2\Delta t} \approx \Delta t\left(-\frac{1}{2}+\frac{\lambda_1\Delta t}{3}\right)$$

The full uncertainty propagation of the parent half-life T_1 to the time t is calculated from

$$\frac{\sigma(t)}{t} \approx \frac{-\sigma(T_1)}{T_1} \times \left\{\frac{\lambda_1}{\lambda_1-\lambda_2}\left(\frac{T}{t}-1\right) + \frac{\lambda_1\lambda_2}{(\lambda_2-\lambda_1)^2}\left(\frac{1-C_1/C_2}{A_2/A_1}\right)\frac{T}{t} + \lambda_1\Delta t\left(-\frac{1}{2}+\frac{\lambda_1\Delta t}{3}\right)\frac{1}{C_1}\left(1-F\frac{A_1}{A_2}\right)\frac{T}{t}\right\} \tag{A.5}$$

The terms in Eq. (A.5) are summed linearly, not quadratically.

Uncertainty of Daughter Half-life

The propagation of the uncertainty on the daughter nuclide half-life is derived in a similar way as for the parent nuclide. The activity ratio A_2/A_1 depends on λ_2 through the factors F and C_2:

$$\frac{\partial(A_2/A_1)}{\partial\lambda_2} = \frac{\partial F}{\partial\lambda_2}\left(1-\frac{C_1}{C_2}\right) + \frac{\partial C_2}{\partial\lambda_2}\left(\frac{-1}{C_2}\left(\frac{I_2}{I_1} - F\frac{C_1}{C_2}\right)\right) \tag{A.6}$$

in which

$$\frac{\partial F}{\partial\lambda_2} = \frac{-\lambda_1}{(\lambda_2-\lambda_1)^2}$$

$$\frac{\partial C_2}{\partial\lambda_2} = \frac{e^{-\lambda_2\Delta t}}{\lambda_2} - \frac{1-e^{-\lambda_2\Delta t}}{\lambda_2^2\Delta t} \approx \Delta t\left(-\frac{1}{2}+\frac{\lambda_2\Delta t}{3}\right)$$

The full uncertainty propagation of the daughter half-life T_2 to the time t is calculated from

$$\frac{\sigma(t)}{t} \approx \frac{\sigma(T_2)}{T_2} \times \left\{\frac{\lambda_2}{\lambda_1-\lambda_2}\left(\frac{T}{t}-\frac{\lambda_2}{\lambda_1}\right) + \frac{\lambda_1\lambda_2}{(\lambda_2-\lambda_1)^2}\left(\frac{1-C_1/C_2}{A_2/A_1}\right)\frac{T}{t} + \lambda_2\Delta t\left(-\frac{1}{2}+\frac{\lambda_2\Delta t}{3}\right)\frac{1}{C_2}\left(1-F\frac{A_1}{A_2}\right)\frac{T}{t}\right\} \tag{A.7}$$

Total Uncertainty

The full uncertainty on t is obtained from the quadratic sum of Eqs. (A.1), (A.5) and (A.7).

REFERENCES

1. Aitken-Smith, P., Collins, S., 2016. Measurement of the 211Pb half-life using recoil atoms from 219Rn decay. Appl. Radiat. Isot. 110, 59–63.
2. Axelsson, A., Ringbom, A., 2014. On the calculation of activity concentrations and nuclide ratios from measurements of atmospheric radioactivity. Appl. Radiat. Isot. 92, 12–17.
3. Bateman, H., 1910. The solution of a system of differential equations, occurring in the theory of radioactive decay. Proc. Camb. Philos. Soc. 15, 423–427.
4. Bayer, 2014. Investor Handout Meet Management in London, p. 28.
5. Browne, E., 2001. Nuclear Data Sheets for A=215, 219, 223, p. 231.
6. Chechev, V., Kuzmenko, N., 2015. Update of $^{140}_{56}$La Evaluation by Helmer (2004b). http://www.nucleide.org/DDEP_WG/DDEPdata.htm.
7. Collins, S.M., Pearce, A.K., Ferreira, K.M., Fenwick, A.J., Regan, P.H., Keithley, J.D., 2015a. Direct measurement of the half-life of 223Ra. Appl. Radiat. Isot. 99, 46–53.
8. Collins, S.M., Pearce, A.K.A.J., Regan, P.H., Keithley, J.D., 2015b. Precise measurements of the absolute g-ray emission probabilities of 223Ra and decay progeny in equilibrium. Appl. Radiat. Isot. 102, 15–28.
9. Collins, S.M., Pearce, A.K.A.J., Regan, P.H., Keithley, J.D., 2015c. The half-life of 227Th by direct and indirect measurements. Appl. Radiat. Isot. 104, 203–211.
10. Collins, S.M., et al., 2016. Standardisation of 227Th and the Precision Measurements of the Absolute g-ray Emissions from its Decay. 2016.
11. Dahle, J., Krogh, C., Melhus, K.B., Borrebaek, J., Larsen, R.H., Kvinnsland, Y., 2009. In vitro cytotoxicity of low-dose-rate radioimmunotherapy by the alphaemitting radioimmunoconjugate Thorium-227-DOTA-rituximab. Int. J. Radiat. Oncol. Biol. Phys. 75, 886–895.
12. DDEP, 2004e2015. Table of Radionuclides, 1–7. Monographie BIPM-5 BIPM, Sevres. http://www.nucleide.org/DDEP_WG/DDEPdata.htm.
13. De Geer, L.-E., 2013. Reinforced evidence of a low-yield nuclear test in North Korea on 11 May 2010. J. Radional. Nucl. Chem. 298, 2075–2083.
14. Douysset, G., Le Petit, G., Gross, P., Jutier, C., 2014. Long-term performances of the 95Zr/95Nb chronometer for nuclear events dating. Appl. Radiat. Isot. 87, 152–156.
15. Harms, A.V., Jerome, S.M., 2004. On the integrated decay and ingrowth equations used in the measurement of radioactive decay families: the general solution. Appl. Radiat. Isot. 61, 367–372.
16. Harms, A., Johansson, L., MacMahon, D., 2009. Decay correction of 95Nb. Appl. Radiat. Isot. 67, 641–643.
17. Helmer, R.G., 2004a. Table of Radionuclides (Vol. 1 e A=1 to 140). $^{140}_{56}$Ba. Monographie BIPM-5. Bureau International des Poids et Mesures, pp. 271–276.
18. Helmer, R.G., 2004b. Table of Radionuclides (Vol. 1 e A=1 to 140). $^{140}_{56}$La. Monographie BIPM-5. Bureau International des Poids et Mesures, pp. 277–285.
19. Heyerdahl, H., Abbas, N., Brevik, E.M., Mollatt, C., Dahle, J., 2012. Fractionated therapy of HER2-expressing breast and ovarian cancer xenografts in mice with targeted alpha emitting 227Th-DOTA-p-benzyl-trastuzumab. PLoS ONE 7 (8), e42345. http://dx.doi.org/10.1371/journal.pone.0042345.
20. Ihantola, S., Toivonen, H., Moring, M., 2013. 140La/140Ba ratio dating of a nuclear release. J. Radional. Nucl. Chem. 298, 1283–1291.
21. JCGM, 2008. Evaluation of measurement data d guide to the expression of uncertainty in measurement. JCGM 100, 2008 (Bureau International des Poids et Mesures).
22. Magill, J., Galy, J., 2005. Radioactivity · Radionuclides · Radiation. Springer-Verlag Berlin Heidelberg and European Communities, Germany.
23. Nica, N., 2007. Nuclear data Sheets for A = 140. Nucl. Data Sheets 108, 1287–1470.
24. Nir-El, Y., 2004. Dating the age of a nuclear event by gamma spectrometry. Appl. Radiat. Isot. 60, 197–201.
25. Pan, P., Ungar, K.R., 2012. Nuclear event zero-time calculation and uncertainty evaluation. J. Env. Rad. 106, 65–72.
26. Pomme, S., 2015. The uncertainty of the half-life. Metrologia 52, S51–eS65.
27. Pomme, S., Collins, S., 2014. Unbiased equations for^{95}Zr-^{95}Nb chronometry. Appl. Radiat. Isot. 90, 234–240.
28. Pomme, S., Jacobs, De Frenne, D., Persyn, K., Govaert, K., Yoneama, M.-L., 1993. Excitation energy dependence of charge odd-even effects in the fission of ^{238}U close to the fission barrier. Nucl. Phys. A560, 689–714.
29. Pomme, S., Hardeman, F., Robouch, P., Etxebarria, N., De Corte, F., De Wispelaere, A., van Sluijs, R., Simonits, A., 1996. General activation and decay formulas and their application in neutron activation analysis with k0 standardization. Anal. Chem. 68, 4326–4334.
30. Pomme, S., Jerome, S.M., Venchiarutti, C., 2014. Uncertainty propagation in nuclear forensics. Appl. Radiat. Isot. 89, 58–64.

CHAPTER 3

EVALUATING SUMMARISED RADIONUCLIDE CONCENTRATION RATIO DATASETS FOR WILDLIFE

M.D. Wood, N.A. Beresford, B.J. Howard, and D. Copplestone

Keywords: Radionuclide transfer, Statistical analysis, Geometric statistic, Lognormal distribution, Environmental assessment, and Model parameter

INTRODUCTION

Concentration ratios ($CR_{wo\text{-}media}$) are equilibrium transfer parameters which are used to predict wildlife transfer in most models that have been developed for assessing the impact of ionising radiation on wildlife under chronic exposure conditions (Beresford et al., 2008a). Also known as the Biological Concentration Factor (BCF), Concentration Factor (CF), Biological Intake Value (B_{iv}), Transfer Factor (TF) or Lumped Parameter, the $CR_{wo\text{-}media}$ is a coefficient which relates the whole-body ($_{wo}$) activity concentration of a radionuclide (R_{act}) in an organism on a fresh mass (fm) basis to the activity concentration of that radionuclide in an environmental medium ($_{media}$). Depending on the environment and radionuclide under consideration, the reference medium may be soil, sediment, water or air. If soil or sediment, the activity concentration in the environmental medium is reported as dry mass (dm).

For terrestrial ecosystems, Beresford et al. (2008b) defined the $CR_{wo\text{-}media}$ value as:

$$CR_{wo-soil} = \frac{R_{act} \text{ in biota whole} - \text{body } (\text{Bq kg}^{-1} \text{ fm})}{R_{act} \text{ in soil } (\text{Bq kg}^{-1} \text{ dm})} \quad (1)$$

with the exception of chronic atmospheric releases of ^3H, ^{14}C, $^{32,33}P$ and ^{35}S, which are defined as:

$$CR_{wo-air} = \frac{R_{act} \text{ in biota whole} - \text{body}(\text{Bq kg}^{-1}\text{fm})}{R_{act} \text{ in air}(\text{Bq m}^{-3})} \quad (2)$$

For aquatic ecosystems, Hosseini et al. (2008) define the $CR_{wo\text{-}media}$ as:

$$CR_{wo-water} = \frac{R_{act} \text{ in biota whole} - \text{body}(\text{Bq kg}^{-1}\text{fm}}{R_{act} \text{ in filtered water}(\text{Bq l}^{-1})} \quad (3)$$

although some models use sediment as the medium for aquatic ecosystems (Copplestone et al., 2013).

Recent work within the International Atomic Energy Agency (IAEA) EMRAS II programme has led to the development of a Wildlife Transfer Database (WTD, http://www.wildlifetransferdatabase.org/), which provides the most comprehensive compilation of $CR_{wo\text{-}media}$ values available to date for both terrestrial and aquatic ecosystems (Copplestone et al., 2013). The $CR_{wo\text{-}media}$ values within the WTD have been calculated from direct measurements of wildlife whole-body activity concentrations and/or from tissue measurements converted to whole-body estimates using conversion factors (e.g.Wood et al., 2010 and Yankovich et al., 2010) if the information is not given in the source paper. The WTD has collated both radioisotope and stable element data for a range of elements that may need to be considered within environmental radiation protection assessments. The WTD has been used to provide summarised $CR_{wo\text{-}media}$ statistics for an IAEA handbook (IAEA, 2013) and an International Commission on Radiological Protection report (ICRP, 2009). Although $CR_{wo\text{-}media}$ values are used widely within all tiers of environmental radiation protection assessments (from initial

Citation: M.D. Wood, N.A. Beresford, B.J. Howard, D. Copplestone, Evaluating summarised radionuclide concentration ratio datasets for wildlife, Journal of Environmental Radioactivity, Volume 126, December 2013, Pages 314-325, ISSN 0265-931X, http://dx.doi.org/10.1016/j.jenvrad.2013.07.022.

screening assessments to detailed assessments involving the use of $CR_{wo\text{-}media}$ value probability density functions), there have been various criticisms of the $CR_{wo\text{-}media}$ value approach.

A criticism of the $CR_{wo\text{-}media}$ approach is the simplistic assumption that all of the complexity associated with radionuclide behaviour within environmental media, the interaction of organisms with these media and subsequent food chain transfer can be appropriately represented by a simple ratio. For instance, the assumption of instantaneous equilibrium between organism and medium is unrealistic (e.g. Mann et al., 2007) and various factors will influence uptake. These factors include physico-chemical influences on uptake (Vives i Batlle, 2012), such as pH, cation exchange capacity, concentrations of chemical analogues and temperature (Jeffree, 1991 and Whicker et al., 1990), heterogeneity of contaminant distribution (Beresford et al., 2005), the effect of seasonal changes in both the endocrine cycle and diet (Scott et al., 1986, Rudge et al., 1993 and Wood et al., 2009a) and organism age (Albrecht et al., 2007, Gochfeld and Burger, 1987 and Sakai et al., 2000), especially for radionuclides with a long biological half-life (ICRP, 2009). Non-linearity of transfer has also been reported for some elements/radionuclides, with different transfer values being calculated for different media concentrations (Tuovinen et al., 2011) although data from sites with high heavy metal concentrations, at which non-linear transfer may be observed, were excluded from the WTD (Copplestone et al., 2013).

As a result of the complex interactions of factors influencing transfer, comparisons between predicted and measured radionuclide activity concentrations in wildlife can vary by several orders of magnitude (e.g. Beresford et al., 2008c, Beresford et al., 2008d,Johansen et al., 2012 and Wood et al., 2009b). Recognising this variability in comparisons between predictions and measurements of whole-body radionuclide activity concentrations and the underlying complexity of radionuclide transfer, the adoption of mechanistic modelling approaches for predicting transfer has been identified in the Strategic Research Agenda developed through the EC Strategy for Allied Radioecology (STAR) project (Hinton et al., 2013; http://www.star-radioecology.org) as a priority for radioecology research over the next 20 years.

Some of the criticisms of using $CR_{wo\text{-}media}$ values to predict transfer are, in part, countered by the lack of available data to parameterise mechanistic models (ICRP, 2009 and Wood et al., 2009b) and the potential to calculate condition-specific $CR_{wo\text{-}media}$ values, such as for different broad soil types as done in human food chain modelling (e.g.IAEA, 2009). Improving the parameter database for mechanistic models is one of the objectives of the forthcoming International Atomic Energy Agency's MOdelling and DAta for Radiological Impact Assessments (MODARIA) programme (http://goto.iaea.org/modaria). However, the extent to which available data can be used to calculate condition-specific $CR_{wo\text{-}media}$ values, such as for ecosystem and organism sub-categories, needs further evaluation.

Recognising both the conflicting viewpoints surrounding the applicability of $CR_{wo\text{-}media}$ values and the significant international effort to develop the WTD, there is a need to critically review the equilibrium transfer parameter approach and to provide some clear guidance on the application of this approach within environmental radiation protection. In this paper, we propose a method for evaluating summarised CR datasets and assess the extent to which terrestrial ecosystem data within the WTD can be disaggregated to produce $CR_{wo\text{-}media}$ values for ecosystem and organism sub-categories (see Tables 1and 2).

Table 1. Terrestrial organism groupings and sub-categories used for collating data within the Wildlife Transfer Database (Copplestone et al., 2013).

Broad group	Available sub-categories
Amphibian	–
Annelid	
Arachnid	–
Arthropod	Arthropod – Carnivorous
	Arthropod – Detritivorous
	Arthropod – Herbivorous
Bird	Bird – Carnivorous
	Bird – Herbivorous
	Bird – Omnivorous
Mollusc – gastropod	–
Grasses and herbs	–
	Grasses
	Herbs[a]
Lichens and Bryophytes	–

Mammal	Mammal – Carnivorous
	Mammal – Herbivorous[b]
	Mammal – Omnivorous
	Mammal – Marsupial[c]
	Mammal – Rangifer spp.
Reptile	–
	Reptile – Carnivorous
	Reptile – Herbivorous
Shrub	–
Tree	–
	Tree – Coniferous
	Tree – Broadleaf

[a]Any non-woody plant which does not fall into one of the other categories.

[b]Excludes Rangifer spp. (reindeer and caribou) in recognition of the high transfer of some elements to this group compared to other mammals.

[c]No distinction made between marsupials based on feeding strategy.

Table 2. Terrestrial ecosystem sub-categories used within the Wildlife Transfer Database (Copplestone et al., 2013); definitions are from (IAEA, 2013).

Ecosystem sub-category	**Definition**
Terrestrial	Generic ecosystem including all terrestrial ecosystem types (excludes terrestrial areas of estuarine systems)
Terrestrial – semi-natural grassland	Includes: mountain and upland grasslands, heath and shrub lands, and some Arctic ecosystems
Terrestrial – forest	Land with tree crown cover of more than 10% over an area of more than 0.5 ha and with trees, which are able to reach a minimum in situ height of 5 m at maturity
Terrestrial – agricultural grassland	Managed grasslands
Terrestrial – coastal sand dunes	Coastal sand dunes (excludes marine organisms)
Terrestrial – wetland	Marsh, fen, peatland (excludes estuarine saltmarshes)

Summarising $CR_{wo\text{-}media}$ values in the WTD

The WTD provides summary tables of $CR_{wo\text{-}media}$ values for organism group and radionuclide combinations across generic ecosystems (terrestrial, freshwater, brackish and marine) (Howard et al., 2013a). Where the number of values across all studies in the whole dataset (N) for a given organism radionuclide combination is greater than 2 and the available $CR_{wo\text{-}media}$ values are all individual values, the summarised data are presented as the arithmetic mean (μ) and standard deviation (σ):

$$\mu = \frac{\sum_{i=1}^{N} x_i}{N} \tag{4}$$

$$\sigma = \sqrt{\frac{\sum_{i=1}^{N} (x_i - \mu)^2}{N-1}} \tag{5}$$

where xi represents each value (x) from 1 to N and all other terms have been defined. The $CR_{wo\text{-}media}$ values are entered into the WTD as either individual values or summarised data: the number of observations in a study (ni)[1], arithmetic mean and standard deviation for individual studies. Therefore weighted arithmetic mean (μw) and associated standard deviation (σw) are calculated using Equations (6) and (7) respectively (Howard et al., 2013a):

$$\mu_W = \frac{\sum_{i=1}^{n} n_i CR_i}{N} \tag{6}$$

$$\sigma_W = \sqrt{\frac{\sum_{i=1}^{n}\left((n_i - 1)\sigma_i^2 + n_i CR_i^2\right) - \frac{\left(\sum_{i=1}^{n} n_i CR_i\right)^2}{N}}{N-1}} \tag{7}$$

where CR_i is the arithmetic mean $CR_{wo\text{-}media}$ value used in the derivation of the summarised data for study i, n is the number of studies and all other terms have been defined. The range (minimum and maximum values) of the weighted dataset is also presented in the WTD. However, because the weighted dataset is derived from a combination of individual values (i.e.

entries where ni = 1) and summarised datasets, the minimum and/or maximum value may be the arithmetic mean of one of the input datasets rather than the overall range derived from all of the underlying data (Copplestone et al., 2013).

$CR_{wo\text{-}media}$ values tend to be lognormally distributed (Beresford et al., 2008a and Brown et al., 2008); transforming $CR_{wo\text{-}media}$ values by taking the natural logarithm (ln) of the individual data values within the distribution produces a dataset with the properties of a normal distribution. Therefore, although summarised $CR_{wo\text{-}media}$ data are generally presented using the arithmetic mean and standard deviation, from a statistical analysis perspective that approach is often incorrect because it implies that the untransformed data follow a normal distribution. The correct approach for describing the central tendency and variability of a lognormally distributed dataset (assuming all entries are individual values) is to calculate the geometric mean (μg) and its associated standard deviation (σg):

$$\mu_g = \sqrt[N]{x_i x_{i+1} \cdots x_N} \tag{8}$$

$$\sigma_g = \exp\left(\sqrt{\frac{\sum_{i=1}^{N}\left(\ln\frac{x_i}{\mu_g}\right)^2}{N}}\right) \tag{9}$$

However, because many of the data inputs into the WTD are of summarised data and the geometric mean and standard deviation are rarely presented in the source references, the above approach to deriving geometric means and standard deviations cannot be applied readily across the whole WTD. As some users may want geometric values, the WTD uses the weighted arithmetic mean and associated standard deviation to estimate weighted geometric means (μgw) and standard deviations (σgw) for the weighted dataset (IAEA, 2013):

$$\mu_{gw} = \exp\left(-0.5\ln\left(\frac{\sigma_w^2 + \mu_w^2}{\mu_w^4}\right)\right) \tag{10}$$

$$\sigma_{gw} = \exp\left(\sqrt{\ln\left(\frac{\sigma_w^2 + \mu_w^2}{\mu_w^2}\right)}\right) \tag{11}$$

There are a number of challenges in summarising data within the WTD:

- Although the WTD presents $CR_{wo\text{-}media}$ values for some organism sub-categories, the decision to present these data was based on the number of values available for each sub-category and the significance of any differences was not considered. Testing the significance of differences between sub-category $CR_{wo\text{-}media}$ values is not straightforward because the datasets used within the WTD include both individual and summarised data.
- As noted previously, the range of $CR_{wo\text{-}media}$ values in the WTD summary tables may be the range of arithmetic means rather than of underlying data. Therefore, users of the WTD are unable to assess the 'true' range of the underlying data, which may be important for screening assessments if the maximum value is used (e.g. USDoE, 2002).
- Some of the data entries within the WTD provide ni and arithmetic mean $CR_{wo\text{-}media}$, but no standard deviation. These data entries were used ni times within the derivation of arithmetic summary statistics in IAEA (2013).
- The estimation of the weighted geometric mean and standard deviation from the weighted arithmetic mean and standard deviation may result in poor estimates of the geometric parameters, especially when the underlying arithmetic data include summarised data where ni > 2 but no standard deviation (σi) is reported. As can be seen in Equations (10) and (11), the calculation of geometric summary statistics utilises the arithmetic standard deviation and this is likely to be underestimated where datasets include entries with ni > 2 but no standard deviation.

To analyse the statistical significance of differences in $CR_{wo\text{-}media}$ values within specific organism and/or ecosystem sub-categories, it is necessary to identify a method that enables such analyses to be performed on weighted datasets, taking into account that the WTD includes summarised data entries with missing arithmetic standard deviation values. The ideal approach would be to access the underlying data for each individual study for which summarised data have been entered into the WTD. However, with more than 520 data sources from the period 1956 to 2010 providing data to the WTD, this approach is impossible. In the subsequent sections we propose and discuss a database reconstruction approach to enable the data to be analysed and more robust summary statistics to be calculated.

METHODS

Database Reconstruction

One option for deriving summary statistics is to use each summarised data line ni times within the analysis, but this creates artificial discrete data clusters within a resulting distribution and does not account for the variation described within the summarised data. An alternative is to treat each summarised data line as ni = 1, but this also 'loses' information on within study variation and omits the weighting of larger studies compared with smaller studies (this is the approach used in the IAEA data collation for human foodstuffs (IAEA, 2009 and IAEA, 2010)). Therefore, a more statistically defensible approach, assuming data are lognormally distributed, is to use the summarised data from each individual study to generate a lognormal distribution and then randomly sample nitimes within that distribution to approximate the underlying dataset that produced the summarised data.

For each individual study for which summarised data are provided, the arithmetic mean ($\mu_{ln}x$) of the natural logarithms of the underlying data values (x) and the corresponding standard deviation ($\sigma_{ln}x$) are derived as:

$$\mu_{\ln x} = \ln\mu_x - \frac{1}{2}\sigma_{\ln x}^2 \tag{12}$$

$$\sigma_{\ln x} = \sqrt{\ln\left(1 + \frac{\sigma_x^2}{\mu_x^2}\right)} \quad (13)$$

Assuming that the distribution of the untransformed data is lognormal, the natural logarithms of the dataset will follow a normal distribution. Therefore, the arithmetic mean of the natural logarithms of the underlying data values and the corresponding standard deviation describe a normal distribution. To sample n_i times within this distribution it is necessary to derive n_i random percentile values and determine the value of lnx at each percentile. These values can then be reverse transformed to the corresponding value of x in the original scale ($\exp^{\ln}x = x$). The random percentile values were derived using the MS Excel™ 2007 random number generator.

Given that the arithmetic mean of the natural logarithms of the underlying data values and the corresponding standard deviation describe a normal distribution, lnx can be standardised to derive the standard normal distribution random variable z, which defines the distance in standard deviation units between lnx and the arithmetic mean of the natural logarithms of variable x:

$$z = \frac{\ln x - \mu_{\ln x}}{\sigma_{\ln x}} \quad (14)$$

Published 'z tables' relate z values to specific probabilities of the standard normal distribution. For example, the probabilities for z values of −2 and +2 are 0.0228 and 0.9772 respectively, so approximately 95% of the values within the standard normal distribution occur within 2 standard deviation units of the arithmetic mean. For the purposes of the analysis presented here, we needed to derive values of lnx for specific percentiles, so Equation (14) was modified to:

$$z_p = \frac{\ln x_p - \mu_{\ln x}}{\sigma_{\ln x}} \quad (15)$$

where z_p is the value of z at probability p, x_p is the value of x at probability p and all other terms have been defined. The ni randomly generated percentiles were converted to probabilities by dividing by 100 and the corresponding z values for each probability obtained from a 'z table', as reproduced in most statistics textbooks. Equation (15) was rearranged to calculate x_p:

$$x_p = \exp(\sigma_{\ln x} z_p + \mu_{\ln x}) \quad (16)$$

The calculated values of x_p for each study from which summarised data had been reported were used to replace the summarised data line for that study within the subsequent data analysis.

For studies reporting $n_i > 2$ and an arithmetic mean but not a standard deviation, we needed to estimate the arithmetic standard deviation. For a given wildlife group-radionuclide combination, the coefficient of variation (CV) was calculated for each study reporting both an arithmetic mean and a standard deviation:

$$\mathrm{CV} = \frac{\sigma_i}{\mu_i} \quad (17)$$

For each radionuclide, the arithmetic mean of the CVs (CV_μ) for the wildlife group was used to estimate the missing arithmetic standard deviation values (σ_i):

$$\sigma_i = \mathrm{CV}_\mu \cdot \mu_i \quad (18)$$

The calculation approach described above was implemented using a purpose-built spreadsheet (available at https://wiki.ceh.ac.uk/x/PgC6Cw). The resultant dataset (referred to hereafter as the reconstructed database or RDB) was used to derive full summary statistics: N, means, standard deviations, minimum, maximum and 95th percentile values. Equations (4), (5), (8) and (9) were used to calculate the arithmetic weighted mean and standard deviation and the geometric mean and standard deviation from the RBD. The min and max values were taken to be the minimum and maximum for each category within the RDB derived by applying Equation (16). Two estimates of 95th percentile were made: (i) from weighted arithmetic mean and standard deviation assuming a lognormal distribution and using Equation (16); and (ii) from weighted geometric mean and standard deviation using the following equation:

$$\mathrm{GM}_{95} = \exp\left(\ln \mu_{gw} + 1.645 \cdot \ln \sigma_{gw}\right) \quad (19)$$

where GM_{95} is the 95th percentile estimated from the geometric summary statistics and 1.645 is the z value for the 95th percentile.

Statistical Approach to Sub-category Comparison

The RDB was used to test for significant differences between sub-categories (wildlife sub-categories, habitats and stable element v's radioisotope) for examples with comparatively large N (N > 40). Minitab v16 was used to analyse the log-transformed data using a General Linear Model with Tukey's pairwise comparisons (see Minitab v16 help file).

RESULTS AND DISCUSSION

Improving WTD Summary Statistics

Table 3 compares the WTD summary statistics presented in IAEA (2013) with those calculated in the present paper using the data within the RDB; although not presented inIAEA (2013), for comparative purposes we have calculated 95th percentiles (as described above) from the IAEA summarised data.

Table 3. Comparison of wildlife group $CR_{wo\text{-}media}$ summary statistics calculated using the IAEA WTD (Howard et al., 2013a) approach and the RDB approach presented in this paper.

Element	Wildlife group	Data source[a]	N (% of studies with $n_i > 2$, but no SD)	Arithmetic mean ± SD	Geometric mean (SD)	Lognorm95[b]	GM95[c]	Range
Am	Mammal[d]	IAEA	139	(3.2 ± 10) E-2	9.8E-3(4.7)	1.2E-1	1.2E-1	2.6E-4–1.7E-1
		RDB	139 (0%)	(4.6 ± 17) E-2	6.2E-3(10.4)	2.0E-1	2.9E-1	5.1E-6–1.7
Cs	Grasses & Herbs	IAEA	2028	1.2 ± 2.6	5.1E-1(3.7)	4.5	4.4	1.9E-3–37
		RDB[e]	2028 (20%)	1.2 ± 2.7	2.3E-1(9.0)	4.4	8.6	2.0E-5–41
Cs	Mammal[d]	IAEA	2463	3.5 ± 8.3	1.3(4.0)	13	13	2.8E-3–140
		RDB[e]	2463 (2%)	3.4 ± 7.8	1.2(5.2)	12	19	1.5E-3–140
Cs	Shrub	IAEA	354	2.3 ± 4.0	1.2(3.3)	8.2	8.0	9.8E-3–16
		RDB[e]	354 (7%)	2.3 ± 4.1	6.5E-1(5.4)	7.9	11	4.9E-3–30
Pb	Annelid	IAEA	647	(5.2 ± 7.5) E-1	2.9E-1(2.9)	1.7	1.7	2.3E-3–2.8
		RDB[e]	647 (50%)	(5.2 ± 7.5) E-1	1.2E-1(7.8)	1.7	3.5	1.1E-3–2.8
Pb	Arthropod	IAEA	561	(4.0 ± 4.7) E-1	2.6E-1(2.5)	1.2	1.2	4.6E-3–1.0
		RDB[e]	561 (64%)	(4.0 ± 4.6) E-1	9.6E-2(7.9)	1.2	2.9	4.6E-3–2.2
Pb	Mammal[d]	IAEA	515	(3.8 ± 3.6) E-2	2.8E-2(2.2)	1.0E-1	1.0E-1	2.7E-4–2.0E-1
		RDB[e]	515 (6%)	(3.8 ± 2.8) E-2	2.6E-2(3.2)	1.0E-1	1.7E-1	7.7E-6–3.3E-1
Pu	Arthropod	IAEA	150	(3.1 ± 4.9) E-2	1.7E-2(3.1)	1.1E-1	1.0E-1	4.2E-4–2.5E-1
		RDB	150 (0%)	(3.0 ± 4.5) E-2	9.7E-3(5.8)	1.0E-1	1.7E-1	2.1E-4–2.5E-1
Pu	Mammal[d]	IAEA	219	(5.0 ± 26) E-2	9.3E-3(6.3)	2.0E-1	1.9E-1	1.6E-4–2.6
		RDB[e]	219 (3%)	(5.4 ± 24) E-2	3.0E-3(8.5)	2.0E-1	1.0E-1	3.7E-5–2.6
Sr	Grasses & Herbs	IAEA	519	(9.8 ± 18) E-1	4.7E-1(3.4)	3.5	3.4	6.7E-3–8.8
		RDB[e]	519 (41%)	(9.8 ± 19) E-1	2.1E-1(6.6)	3.5	4.8	5.7E-4–15
Sr	Shrub	IAEA	307	(4.8 ± 7.8) E-1	2.5E-1(3.1)	1.7	1.6	4.7E-3–6.7
		RDB	307 (0%)	(4.9 ± 7.8) E-1	1.0E-1(9.0)	1.7	3.9	3.8E-4–6.7

[a]IAEA from handbook of radionuclide transfer parameters for wildlife (IAEA, 2013), RDB values estimated from the reconstructed database.

[b]The 95th percentile $CR_{wo\text{-}soil}$ value estimated from the arithmetic mean and standard deviation using Tier 3 of the ERICA Tool and assuming a log-normal distribution.

[c]The 95th percentile $CR_{wo\text{-}soil}$ value calculated from the geometric mean and standard deviation.

[d]Does not include Rangifer spp. (as per IAEA, 2013).

[e]Included data entries where $n_i > 2$ but no SD reported, which required SD values to be generated using the approach described in the text.

There is little difference in the estimates of arithmetic mean, which demonstrates that both the IAEA WTD approach and the approach presented in this paper can be used. The arithmetic standard deviations are generally similar between the two approaches because the missing standard deviation values for data from particular sources were derived from the arithmetic mean of the coefficients of variation for the full dataset. Any differences in arithmetic standard deviation are not consistent, reflecting the random sampling taking place within the distributions for each individual data source and the location of data sources with missing values within the overall data distribution.

The geometric mean as presented by the IAEA is consistently higher than that calculated for the RDB, whilst the geometric standard deviation is consistently lower. IAEA (2013)acknowledges that the geometric mean and associated standard deviation values are approximations as Equations (10) and (11) are dependent upon the distribution of the underlying data. It is evident from the RDB arithmetic mean and standard deviation values presented in Table 3 that, if the approach outlined in IAEA (2013) was used to estimate geometric statistics, the same values as obtained by calculating geometric mean and standard deviation from the full dataset would not be estimated (e.g. Cs transfer to grasses and herbs and Pb transfer to arthropods, where the arithmetic statistics are similar for both IAEA and RDB, but the geometric statistics differ). Whilst IAEA could not assess the distribution of the underlying data, we have investigated the distributions present within each RDB for the various element-organism combinations considered and found that they all tend towards lognormal (e.g. Figs. 1 and 2). For the mammal Am $CR_{wo\text{-}media}$ dataset, the Kolmogorov–Smirnov test (K–S Z = 1.251, $p < 0.1$) indicates that the observed cumulative distribution function (OBD cdf) is not significantly different from the cdf that would be expected (EXP cdf) if the data are lognormal (Fig. 1). For the shrub Cs $CR_{wo\text{-}media}$ data, the Kolmogorov–Smirnov test (K–S Z = 1.455,$p < 0.05$) indicates that the OBD cdf are significantly different from the cdf that would be expected (EXP cdf) if the data are lognormal (Fig. 2). However, Fig. 2 suggests that the data are tending towards lognormal.

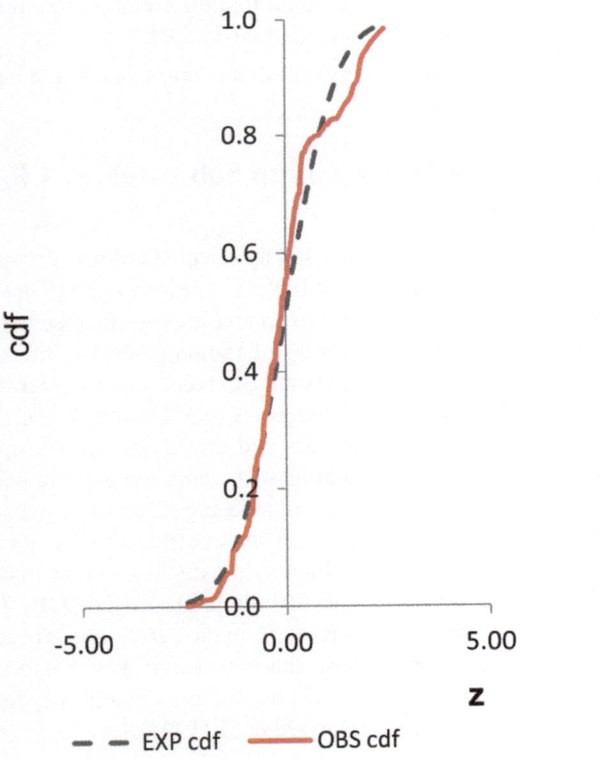

Figure 1. Cumulative distribution function (cdf) for the natural logarithms of the mammal Am $CR_{wo\text{-}media}$ dataset (N = 139). OBS cdf = observed cdf; EXP cdf = expected cdf for a lognormal distribution.

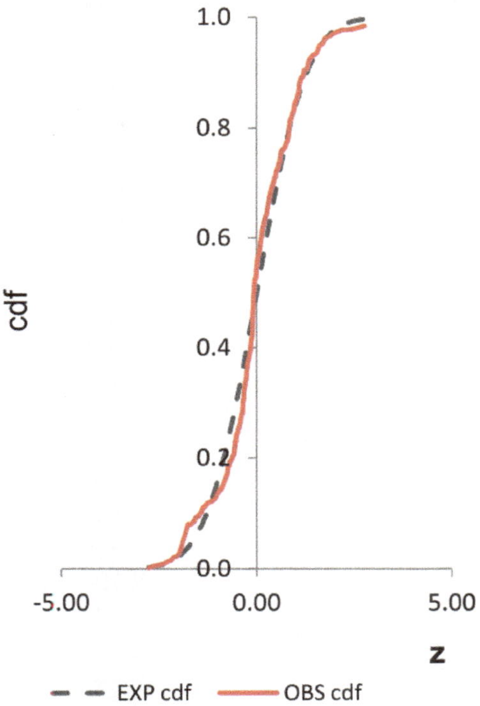

Figure 2. Cumulative distribution function for the natural logarithms of the shrub Cs $CR_{wo\text{-}media}$ dataset (N = 354). OBS cdf = observed cdf; EXP cdf = expected cdf for a lognormal distribution.

As expected, the calculated ranges for the RDB are consistently broader than those reported in the WTD. For the examples considered, the extent of the difference in range values is relative to the proportion of the WTD data which are summarised values, with greater variation between ranges being observed when the underlying dataset contains predominantly summarised data. For example, the data underlying the Am mammal data shown in Table 3 are all summarised data. The maximum value within the WTD of 0.17 is an arithmetic mean with an associated standard deviation of 0.36. It is therefore not surprising that the maximum value calculated within the RDB is considerably higher.

Some of the currently available assessment models utilise 95th percentile values in the screening level assessment tiers. In the ERICA Tool the 95th percentile is estimated from the arithmetic mean and standard deviation assuming a lognormal distribution. Given that the WTD geometric statistics are directly estimated from the arithmetic summary statistics, it is unsurprising that the two approaches to estimating the 95th percentile ($Lognorm_{95}$ and GM_{95}) give similar values. However, for the reconstructed database, the GM_{95} values are higher (by up to a factor of circa 2) than the $Lognorm_{95}$ values, with the exception of Pu mammal.

Testing the Robustness of the RDB Approach

The predictive capability of the RDB approach was assessed using three datasets for which all individual values were available: (i) ^{90}Sr activity concentrations in small mammals from the Chernobyl exclusion zone (additional data from the study described by Beresford et al., 2008d); (ii) ^{137}Cs activity concentrations in invertebrates from coastal sand dunes close to the Sellafield reprocessing plant (UK) (Wood et al., 2008, Wood et al., 2009a and Wood et al., 2009b); and (iii)

^{210}Pb activity concentrations in rabbits (RIFE, 1996, RIFE, 1998, RIFE, 1999, RIFE, 2000, RIFE, 2002, RIFE, 2003 and RIFE, 2004). Table 4 compares summary statistics estimated directly from the individual data with those generated using the RDB approach having input arithmetic means and associated standard deviations estimated for sub-groups of the data (e.g. by species etc.). These sub-group arithmetic means and standard deviations were also used to generate overall summary statistics using the approach adopted within the WTD (Table 4). There was good agreement between the arithmetic mean and standard deviation values derived using all three approaches, with the WTD approach giving the closest agreement to the actual data. For geometric mean and standard deviation, the RDB approach provided a better estimate than the WTD approach. Whilst not predicting the absolute range observed in the source data the RDB approach gave better estimates than those derived from the summarised data (i.e. as per the WTD) alone.

Table 4. Comparison of summary statistics derived from source data or using the WTD and RDB approaches.

Element	Wildlife group	Approach	*N*	Arithmetic mean ± SD	Geometric mean (SD)	Range
Cs	Invertebrate	Source data	72	(2.4 ± 3.0)E-2	1.1E-2 (3.8)	2.6E-4–1.3E-1
		WTD	72	(2.4 ± 3.0)E-2	1.5E-2 (2.7)	1.4E-2–6.5E-2
		RDB	72	(2.5 ± 2.9)E-2	1.4E-2 (3.0)	1.2E-3–1.2E-1
Pb	Mammal (rabbit)	Source data	21	(2.3 ± 2.2)E-2	1.6E-2(2.5)	2.8E-3–9.0E-2
		WTD	21	(2.3 ± 2.2)E-2	1.7E-2(2.2)	5.9E-3–4.4E-2
		RDB	21	(2.3 ± 2.0)E-2	1.5E-2 (2.5)	3.4E-3–6.8E-2
Sr	Mammal	Source data	49	3.8 ± 3.4	2.6 (2.6)	1.9E-1–17
		WTD	49	3.8 ± 3.4	2.8 (2.2)	6.9E-1–5.4
		RDB	49	3.7 ± 3.0	2.7 (2.3)	3.5E-1–13

Given that the RDB approach uses a probabilistic approach to generate a reconstructed dataset, there is a need to evaluate the potential variability in the result obtained. The Cs mammal data (not including Rangifer species, which is the approach used to summarise mammal data within the WTD) were used to generate a reconstructed dataset five times. The range in resultant arithmetic mean values was less than 15% with the arithmetic standard deviation value varying by 60%; geometric mean and standard deviation values were similar across all five simulations. The Cs mammal dataset was comparatively large (N = 2463) so repeat simulations were also undertaken for two relatively small subsets (Arctic fox (N = 10) and moose (N = 3)). Less than 20% variation was observed for any of the arithmetic and geometric summary parameters for the Arctic fox data. Whilst the mean values and the geometric standard deviation were generally similar (within 3%) across the simulations for the smaller moose datasets, the arithmetic standard deviation varied by an order of magnitude. We are aware that McCullough (2008) questioned the implementations of the Wichmann-Hill random number generator algorithm (Wichman and Hill, 1982) within Excel™ 2007. It is unclear whether Microsoft has addressed the issues raised by McCullough, but the results of our repeat testing suggest that any issues concerning Excel's random number generation do not significantly affect our implementation of the methodology described above. If considerably larger datasets were being considered then we recommend that different random number generator options are tested (L'Ecuyer, 2012).

These evaluations give us some confidence in the outputs of the RDB approach.

Terrestrial Wildlife Group Sub-category $CR_{wo\text{-}media}$ Values

The $CR_{wo\text{-}media}$ data summarised by selected wildlife group sub-categories are presented in Table 5. The approach to database reconstruction has enabled us to test for significance between sub-categories for a selection of radionuclide-wildlife group combinations. In some instances, there are no significant differences between sub-categories (e.g. Cs and Sr transfer to broadleaf and coniferous trees and Cs transfer to arthropods), perhaps demonstrating that in such cases the generic wildlife group $CR_{wo\text{-}media}$ value is a suitable predictor of transfer. For all mammal comparisons, with the exception of Pu, Rangifer species had significantly higher transfer than other mammal groups. This appears to justify the approach taken by IAEA (2013) to exclude Rangiferdata from the derivation of mammal $CR_{wo\text{-}media}$ values on the basis that this would skew the resultant summary statistics due to the unusual transfer pathway for this mammal sub-category (Howard et al., 1991).

Table 5. $CR_{wo\text{-}media}$ summary statistics for wildlife group sub-categories, calculated using the RDB approach.

Element	Wildlife group	Wildlife sub-category	*N*	Arithmetic mean ± SD	Geometric mean (SD)[a]	Reference ID[b] (*ni*)
Am	Arthropod	Carnivorous	6	(7.2 ± 4.4)E-2	6.2E-2 (1.6)*	170(3), 488(3)
		Detritivorous	29	(1.2 ± 1.5)E-1	6.8E-2 (3.2)*	170(7), 172(4), 223(2), 488(16)
		Herbivorous	9	(1.9 ± 5.6)E-1	6.1E-3 (11.1)#	170(3), 407(6)
Am	Mammal	Carnivorous	13	(1.1 ± 2.9)E-1	5.8E-3 (11.6)#,+	197(9), 488(4)
		Herbivorous	27	(8.0 ± 32)E-2	1.2E-3 (29.4)+	184(13), 407(8), 488(6)
		Omnivorous	84	(3.1 ± 5.4)E-2	1.2E-2 (5.2)#	221(28), 245(47), 488(9)
		Rangifer spp.[c]	9	(1.2 ± 0.6)E-1	1.0E-1 (1.76)*	197(9)
Cs	Arthropod	Carnivorous	15	(2.4 ± 4.7)E-1	4.1E-2 (6.7)*	170(6), 195(6), 488(3)
		Detritivorous[d]	56	(1.1 ± 2.7)E-1	3.1E-2 (4.1)*	169(8), 170(7), 172(4), 223(3), 257(18), 488(16)
		Herbivorous[d]	5	(3.7 ± 2.8)E-2	2.9E-2 (2.0)*	170(5)
Cs	Bird	Carnivorous	11	(1.5 ± 1.8)E-1	6.0E-2 (5.5)#	190(7), 405(4)
		Herbivorous	57	1.0 ± 1.5	3.2E-1 (4.8)*	163(5), 190(2), 228(40), 258(4), 263(1), 405(4), 486(1)
		Omnivorous	79	(6.1 ± 19)E-1	1.8E-1 (4.3)*,#	189(55), 190(9), 405(13), 486(2)
Cs	Mammal	Carnivorous	231	(5.4 ± 19)E-1	1.4E-1 (4.1)*	190(12), 275(5), 405(12), 06(119), 486(1), 488(8)
		Herbivorous	1879	3.8 ± 8.4	1.8 (3.5)#	163(202), 184(14), 190(73), 208(1), 209(1221), 228(26), 230(9), 242(25), 268(11), 288(12), 294(266), 405(15), 486(4)
		Omnivorous	333	3.3 ± 6.0	1.0 (6.2)+	168(104), 190(75), 268(74), 289(25), 405(22), 486(15), 488(18)
		Rangifer spp.[c]	916	17 ± 16	11 (3.1)*	160(1), 163(414), 164(7), 218(2), 228(459), 241(33)
Cs	Tree	Broadleaf	252	(1.4 ± 2.0)E-1	6.3E-2 (4.1)*	190(21), 210(970), 265(9), 470(1), 471(3), 472(27), 473(11), 474(5), 475(7), 477(4), 478(3), 484(65), 485(1), 519(1)
		Coniferous	235	(1.4 ± 2.5)E-1	6.2E-2 (3.8)*	189(90), 472(33), 474(2), 475(5), 476(3), 484(102)
Pu	Arthropod	Carnivorous	9	(1.5 ± 0.9)E-2	1.2E-2 (2.3)*	170(3), 488(6)
		Detritivorous	68	(3.2 ± 4.7)E-2	8.2E-3 (7.1)*	170(7), 216(23), 223(6), 488(32)
		Herbivorous	8	(1.3 ± 0.9)E-3	9.9E-4 (2.1)#	261(2), 407(6)
Pu	Mammal	Carnivorous	29	(5.3 ± 6.1)E-3	2.1E-3 (5.0)*	197(9), 405(12), 488(8)
		Herbivorous	56	(6.0 ± 21)E-2	2.3E-3 (11.5)*	184(14), 222(1), 268(2), 405(15), 407(12), 488(12)
		Omnivorous	113	(5.8 ± 29)E-2	4.0E-3 (6.7)*	221(22), 245(47), 268(4), 405(22), 488(18)
		Rangifer spp.[c]	9	(4.2 ± 4.0)E-3	2.9E-3 (2.4)*	197(9)
Sr	Bird	Carnivorous	10	(1.9 ± 2.4)E-1	9.0E-2 (4.4)#	190(6), 405(4)
		Herbivorous	7	(3.1 ± 2.7)E-1	2.1E-1 (5.6)*,#	190(1), 263(1), 405(4), 486(1)
		Omnivorous	74	(5.1 ± 10)E-1	2.5E-1 (2.8)*	189(55), 190(6), 405(13)

Sr	Mammal	Carnivorous	164	(8.6 ± 15)E-1	3.5E-1 (3.8)$^{+}$	190(8), 405(12), 406(144)
		Herbivorous	108	2.6 ± 3.0	7.7E-1 (7.0)$^{\#}$	163(3), 190(53), 228(26), 268(11), 405(15)
		Omnivorous	202	1.8 ± 2.3	8.7E-1 (3.7)$^{\#}$	190(59), 245(47), 268(74), 405(22)
		Rangifer spp.[c]	435	6.5 ± 4.1	4.6 (2.8)*	160(1), 163(136), 218(2), 228(296)
Sr	Tree	Broadleaf	114	(4.4 ± 7.1)E-1	1.3E-1 (5.3)*	190(7), 473(11), 478(3), 480(3), 482(20), 484(45), 485(1)
		Coniferous	74	(5.6 ± 15)E-1	8.2E-2 (6.0)*	479(1), 480(1), 482(6), 484(66)

[a]Means with the same symbol are not significantly different ($p > 0.05$), significance was tested using general linear model with natural log data.

[b]For consistency with ICRP, 2009 and IAEA, 2013 the reference ID numbers for the underlying database as described by Copplestone et al. (2013) are used (see Annex 1 for source reference information).

[c]Rangifer spp. data are not included in the herbivorous mammal data.

[d]IAEA (2013) has data from Crossley et al. (1973) [Reference ID 175] wrongly categorised by feeding type. These data have been removed and are not considered here.

Previous studies have suggested that the transfer of Cs to carnivorous vertebrates (such as canine and feline species) is higher than to vertebrates at lower trophic levels (Lowe and Horrill, 1991, Gaare and Staarland, 1994 and Pendleton et al., 1964). However, the data for mammals in Table 5 show a significantly higher transfer to herbivorous and omnivorous species than to carnivorous species. Investigation of the WTD source literature revealed that over 50% of the mammals classified as carnivorous are actually insectivorous bat species and small mammals, such as species of mole and shrew, rather that 'classical' carnivorous mammals such as canine species. For birds, the $CR_{wo\text{-}media}$ value for herbivorous species is significantly higher than that for carnivorous, again carnivorous bird data are dominated by insectivorous species (Lanius collurio andFicedula sp.) and all carnivorous bird data originated from the Chernobyl exclusion zone. Most of the herbivorous bird data are for Lagopus lagopus, which inhabits areas with relatively high radiocaesium transfer.

Terrestrial Habitat Sub-category $CR_{wo\text{-}media}$ Values

Table 6 summarises and compares CR data by habitat sub-category. In general, organisms in coastal sand dunes have lower $CR_{wo\text{-}media}$ values than other terrestrial sites as reported in previous studies (Wood et al., 2008, Wood et al., 2009a and Wood et al., 2009b). However, all the coastal sand dune data originate from two sites close to the Sellafield reprocessing plant where sea-to-land transfer of actinides and aerial deposition of other radionuclides are thought to be the main transport routes rather than root uptake (Wood et al., 2009a). Conversely, $CR_{wo\text{-}media}$ values for forest tend to be higher than those for the other habitats with which they can be compared (forest data originates from throughout Europe and one study in North America). It is necessary to evaluate sub-category values with caution; the habitat sub-category $CR_{wo\text{-}media}$ values have been calculated using the data for the broad wildlife group and may be influenced by the proportion of data coming from different wildlife sub-categories (and vice-versa).

Table 6. $CR_{wo\text{-}media}$ summary statistics for habitat sub-categories, calculated using the RDB approach.

Element	Wildlife group	Habitat sub-category	*N*	Arithmetic mean ± SD	Geometric mean (SD)[a]	Reference ID[b] (*ni*)
Am	Arthropod	Forest	34	(2.0 ± 4.3)E-1	7.9E-2 (3.6)*	170(28), 172(4), 223(2)
		Coastal sand dunes	40	(6.5 ± 14)E-2	2.7E-2 (3.5)$^{\#}$	488(40)
		Semi-natural grassland	8	(4.0 ± 7.1)E-2	4.8E-3 (8.6)$^{+}$	382(2), 407(6)
Am	Mammal	Forest	62	(2.7 ± 2.2)E-2	1.4E-2 (4.0)*	172(15), 245(47)
		Coastal sand dunes	19	(3.9 ± 2.3)E-4	3.2E-4 (1.9)$^{\#}$	488(19)
		Semi-natural grassland	45	(1.0 ± 2.9)E-1	1.9E-2 (5.7)*	197(9), 221(28), 407(8)

Cs	Amphibian	Forest	7	(4.7 ± 1.9)E-1	4.4E-1 (1.5)*	188(7)
		Coastal sand dunes	39	(9.8 ± 8.1)E-2	7.5E-2 (2.1)#	486(39)
		Wetland	91	(4.9 ± 4.6)E-1	2.7E-1 (6.2)*	188(4), 205(82), 256(6)
Cs	Arthropod	Forest	64	(1.2 ± 2.6)E-1	4.0E-2 (4.0)*	170(39), 172(4), 223(3), 257(18)
		Coastal sand dunes	40	(2.5 ± 5.3)E-2	7.8E-3 (4.4)#	488(40)
		Semi-natural grassland	10	(2.4 ± 2.0)E-2	1.9E-2 (2.0)*,#	382(3), 388(7)
Pu	Arthropod	Forest	29	(4.0 ± 4.1)E-2	2.4E-2 (2.9)*	170(23), 223(6)
		Coastal sand dunes	80	(2.8 ± 3.7)E-2	1.6E-2 (3.1)*,#	488(80)
		Semi-natural grassland	10	(5.5 ± 7.5)E-2	6.2E-3 (13)#	382(4), 407(6)
Pu	Mammal	Forest	111	(5.7 ± 12)E-3	2.3E-3 (4.1)#	172(15), 245(47), 405(49)
		Coastal sand dunes	38	(7.9 ± 4.3)E-4	7.1E-4 (1.6)+	488(38)
		Semi-natural grassland	21	(1.4 ± 3.2)E-1	1.4E-2 (17)*	197(9), 407(12)
Sr	Shrub	Forest	12	(4.2 ± 3.2)E-1	3.1E-1 (2.6)*	467(11), 468(1)
		Semi-natural grassland	60	(9.2 ± 5.8)E-2	7.7E-2 (1.8)#	164(60)
		Wetland	45	(5.5 ± 2.6)E-2	4.9E-2 (1.7)+	164(45)

[a]Means with the same symbol are not significantly different ($p > 0.05$), significance was tested using general linear model with natural log data.

[b]For consistency with ICRP (2009) and IAEA (2013) the reference ID numbers for the underlying database as described by Copplestone et al. (2013) are used (see Annex 1 for source reference information).

Stable Element Versus Radioisotope

Databases, such as the WTD, often amalgamate data by element, regardless of isotope (Copplestone et al., 2013). Increasing use of analytical techniques, such as ICP-MS, is producing total element data for application in radiological assessments (e.g. Barnett et al., 2013a, Beresford, 2010, Sheppard, 2013 and Yankovich et al., 2013). Table 7demonstrates significant differences between stable elements and radioisotopes forRangifer species Pb $CR_{wo\text{-}media}$ values and shrub Sr $CR_{wo\text{-}media}$ values. Whilst we cannot explain the difference for Sr shrub data, we note that there is a bias in data sources. All of the stable Sr shrub $CR_{wo\text{-}media}$ data come from North America, predominantly Canada, whereas the majority of the ^{90}Sr data originate from Russia; Vaccinium spp. dominate both the stable Sr and ^{90}Sr entries. The difference in Rangifer species $CR_{wo\text{-}media}$ values for Pb is perhaps unexpected given that there is known to be a comparatively high transfer of ^{210}Pb via the aerial deposition – lichen – reindeer pathway (e.g. Thomas et al., 1994). Inspection of the lichen data within the WTD suggests that the $CR_{wo\text{-}media}$ for lichen is higher for ^{210}Pb than stable Pb.

Table 7. Stable element and radioisotope $CR_{wo\text{-}media}$ value summary statistics, calculated using the RDB approach.

Element	Wildlife group	Isotope	N	Arithmetic mean ± SD	Geometric mean (SD)[a]	Reference ID[b] (n_i)
Pb	Rangifer spp.	Stable Pb	66	8.0 ± 3.9	6.5 (2.3)*	163(65), 218(1)
		^{210}Pb	204	2.2 ± 1.0	1.9 (1.7)#	214(24), 258(180)
Sr	Shrub	Stable Sr	131	1.1 ± 0.9	8.3E-1 (2.0)*	347(60), 348(60), 467(11)
		^{90}Sr	176	(5.1 ± 5.3)E-2	2.2E-2 (3.8)#	164(111), 252(64), 468(1)

[a]Means with the same letter are not significantly different ($p > 0.05$); significance tested using general linear model with natural log data.

[b]For consistency with ICRP (2009) and IAEA (2013) the reference ID numbers for the underlying database as described by Copplestone et al. (2013) are used (see Annex 1 for source reference information).

CONCLUSIONS

Large variation between predicted and measured whole-body activity concentrations has been observed in various studies (e.g. Johansen et al., 2012 and Wood et al., 2009b). This is highly likely to be due to the differences in site characteristics and the gross simplification in many models of representing transfer using one global $CR_{wo-media}$ value for a given radionuclide-organism combination. A potential solution is to disaggregate summarised datasets, such as that presented in IAEA (2013), to estimate more refined $CR_{wo-media}$ values (e.g. for specific ecosystem types, wildlife groups etc.). The approach presented in this paper for analysing summarised datasets using a database reconstruction method has been demonstrated to be robust. It has enabled the statistical analysis of differences between ecosystem and wildlife group sub-categories and between stable elements and their radioisotopes.

$CR_{wo-media}$ value summary statistic derivation is confounded by the underlying dataset available to the IAEA. IAEA (2013) acknowledges that the methods used to estimate geometric statistics from the available data will result in approximations. Although we have shown that the WTD approach for calculating arithmetic summary statistics is fit-for-purpose, that for estimating geometric summary statistics is inadequate. We note that the ICRP have recommended geometric mean values for Reference Animals and Plants using the WTD approach (ICRP, 2009). We recommend that the approach derived in this paper be adopted to derive more robust geometric summary statistics.

Based on our evaluation of the current database, a number of the comparisons of $CR_{wo-media}$ values presented in Section 3 show statistically significant differences between habitat, wildlife group and isotope sub-categories (Table 5, Table 6 and Table 7). In some instances, the differences may be due to biases and limitations in the underlying database, casting doubt on the application of more refined $CR_{wo-media}$ values. Bayesian approaches, as discussed by Hosseini et al. (2013), may present an option for defining more refined $CR_{wo-media}$ values when few data are available.

The limited comparison between stable element and radioisotope data in Section 3.5indicates significant differences for the two element-organism combinations considered, although these differences may be due to factors other than the isotope under consideration. An evaluation of stable Cs and ^{137}Cs $CR_{wo-media}$ values for freshwater fish from the WTD (Beresford et al., 2013) also showed significant differences, but again this may have been due to bias in the dataset. Rowan (2013) identified higher transfer of^{137}Cs compared to stable Cs transfer to freshwater fish in a Canadian river, although the findings of Rowan are most probably explained by the pulsed releases of ^{137}Cs into the river. However, Barnett et al. (2013b) identified higher transfer of ^{137}Cs for forest plants and animals compared to stable Cs measured in the same samples. The differences observed by Barnett et al. (2013b) cannot be readily explained by data bias or site characteristics. There is clearly a need to undertake further research on the limitations of using stable element data for deriving radionuclide $CR_{wo-media}$ values, especially given the increase in the use of stable element data for this purpose, due to the cost-effectiveness of ICP-MS analysis (e.g. Barnett et al., 2013b, Beresford, 2010, Sheppard, 2013 and Sheppard et al., 2010), and the dominance of stable element data within the WTD as demonstrated by Copplestone et al. (2013) for a selection of elements.

Environmental radiation protection models such as the ERICA Tool (Brown et al., 2008) adopt a tiered approach for assessing the impact of ionising radiation on wildlife. Tier 1 is a simple and highly conservative 'screening' assessment in which, if certain criteria are met, the assessor can exit the assessment process with a high level of confidence that there are no significant radiation impacts on biota and that no further action is required. Tier 2 provides a less conservative screening assessment in which the assessor can modify modelling parameters to produce a more realistic assessment. At Tier 3, the assessor can additionally undertake probabilistic assessment in an attempt to produce a realistic assessment of risk, with quantified uncertainty.

Uncertainty in modelling parameters leads to risk in decision making (Chen et al., 2011). Given the uncertainty in $CR_{wo-media}$ data, we suggest that summarised $CR_{wo-media}$ values are used with caution above the initial, highly conservative, screening-level assessments. This is consistent with the recommendation that site-specific data should be used for higher tier assessments (Brown et al., 2008 and USDoE, 2002). However, generic $CR_{wo-media}$ values may have applicability in higher tier assessments for radionuclides contributing little to internal dose (Howard et al., 2013b). Alternative methods should be used to quantify transfer at higher assessment tiers if data are not available for the site (e.g. the phylogenetic approach proposed by Beresford et al. (2013), which accounts for the effect of site).

ACKNOWLEDGEMENTS

The authors would like to thank all of those who contributed data to the database initiated by the IAEA under the EMRAS II programme in collaboration with the IUR and ICRP (seeYankovich et al., 2013, Copplestone et al., 2013, Howard et al., 2013a and ICRP, 2009). Thanks are also expressed to Dr Peter Henrys from NERC Centre for Ecology & Hydrology (CEH), for his advice on statistical analysis. CEH involvement in this work was funded under a Natural Environment Research Council Knowledge Exchange grant (www.ceh.ac.uk/PROTECT/) and the EURATOM STAR network of excellence in radioecology (www.star-radioecology.org).

Annex 1. Full source information for reference IDs used within the wildlife transfer database and quoted within Table 5, Table 6 and Table 7

Reference ID	Source
160	Bakunov, N.A., Panasenkova, O.I., Drichko, V.F., ^{90}Sr, ^{137}Cs and Natural Radionuclides in the Ecosystem of a Deep Lake., Russian J. Ecol. 30 (1998) 361–363. (in Russian).
163	Beresford, N.A. et al., Approaches to estimating the transfer of radionuclides to Arctic biota, Radioprotection 40 (2005) S285–S290.
164	Beresford, N.A., Wright, S.M., Brown, J.E., Sazykina, T., “Review of approaches for the estimation of radionuclide transfer to reference Arctic biota”. (EPIC Deliverable 2) Centre for Ecology and Hydrology, Merlewood (2002).
168	Christaldi, M., Ieradi, L.A., Mascanzoni, D., Mattei, T., Environmental impact of the Chernobyl accident: mutagenesis in bank voles from Sweden, Int. J. Radiat. Biol. 59 (1991) 31-40.
169	Cooper, K., The effect of chronic radiation on invertebrate diversity and abundance within the chernobyl exclusion zone. Msc thesis (Restoration Ecology), University of Liverpool (2002)
170	Copplestone, D., Coniferous Woodland Ecosystem – Lady Wood. The food chain transfer of radionuclides through semi natural habitats. Section 3. PhD Thesis. University of Liverpool (1996) 77–164.
172	Copplestone, D., Johnson, M.S., Jones, S.R., Toal, M.E., Jackson, D., Radionuclide behaviour and transport in a coniferous woodland ecosystem: vegetation, invertebrates and wood mice, Apodemus sylvaticus, Sci. Total Environ. 239 (1999) 96–109.
175	Crossley, D.A.J., “Comparative movement of ^{106}Ru, ^{60}Co and ^{137}Cs in arthropod food chains” (Proc. Symp. On Radioecology. Proc. of the 2nd National Symposium, USAEC, Washington.) (NELSON, D.J., EVANS, F.C., Eds.). United States Atomic Energy Commission Report, CONF-670503, Washington (1973) 687–695.
184	Ferenbaugh, J.K., Fresquez, P.R., Ebinger, M.H., Gonzales, G.J., Jordan, P.A., Radionuclides in soil and water near a low level disposal site and potential ecological and human health impacts, Environ. Monit. Assess. 74 (2002) 243-254.
188	Gaschak, S., International Radioecology Laboratory, Slavutych, Ukraine. (pers.comm.).
189	Gaschak, S. et al., “Radioecology of small birds in the Chornobyl zone”. (Proc Int. Conf. on Radioactivity in the Environment, Nice) (STRAND, P., BORRETZEN, P., JOLLE, T. Eds.) Norwegian Radiation Protection Authority, Østerås (2005) 494–497
190	Gaschak, S., Chizhevsky, I., Arkhipov, A., Beresford, N.A., Barnett, C.L., “The transfer of Cs-137 and Sr-90 to wild animals within the Chernobyl exclusion zone”, (Proc. Int. Conf. on the Protection of the Environment from the Effects of Ionizing Radiation. 6–10 October 2003, Stockholm) International Atomic Energy Agency, Vienna (2003) 200–202
195	Gilhen, M., Current radionuclide activity concentrations in the Chernobyl Exclusion Zone and an assessment of the ecological impact. MSc Thesis. School of Biological Sciences, University of Liverpool (2001).
197	Hanson, W.C., “Transuranic elements in arctic tundra ecosystems”, Transuranic elements in the environment. DOE/TIC-22800. (Hanson, W.C., Ed.) U.S Department of Energy, Washington D.C., (1980) 441–458.
205	Jagoe, C.H., Majeske, A.J., Oleksyk, T.K., Glenn, T.C., Smith, M.H., Radiocesium concentrations and DNA strand breakage in two species of amphibians from the Chernobyl exclusion zone, Radioprotection – Colloques 37 (2002) C1 873–878.
208	Johanson, K. J, “Radiocaesium in game animals in Nordic countries”. Nordic Radioecology – the transfer of radionuclides through Nordic ecosystems to man. (DAHLGARRD, H., Ed.) Elsevier, Amsterdam (1994) 287–301.
209	Johanson, K.J., Bergstrom R., Radiocesium transfer to man from moose and roe deer in Sweden, Sci. Total Environ. 157 (1994) 309–316.
210	Johanson, K.J., Bergstrom, R., Eriksson, O., Erixon, A., Activity concentrations of Cs-137 in moose and their forage plants in mid-Sweden, J. Environ. Radioact. 22 (1994) 251–267.
214	Kauranen, P., Miettinen, J.K., Po-210 and Pb-210 in the Arctic food chain and the natural radiation exposure of Lapps, Health Phys. 16 (1969) 287–295.
216	Little, C.A., “Plutonium in a grassland ecosystem“, Transuranic elements the environment. DOE/TIC-22800. (HANSON, W.C., Ed.) U.S Department of Energy, Washington D.C., (1980) 420–440.
218	Lubashevsky, N. et al., Radioactive contamination of the Yamal Peninsula and assessment of radiation protection of its population. Ecology 4 (1993) 39–45 (in Russian).
221	Markham, O.D., Puphal, K.W., Filer, T.D., Radionuclides in soil and water near a low level disposal site and potential ecological and human health impacts, Environ. Monitor. Assess. 7 (1978) 422–428.
222	Mietelski, J.W., Plutonium in the environment of Poland (a review). Plutonium in the environment. (KUDO, A., Ed.). Elsevier, Amsterdam (2001) 401–412.

223	Mietelski, J.W. et al., Cs-137, K-40, Sr-90, Pu-238, Pu-239 + 240, Am-241 and Cm243 + 244 in forest litter and their transfer to some species of insects and plants in boreal forests: Three case studies, J. Radioanal. Nucl. Chem. 262 (2004) 645–660.
228	Miretsky, G., Alekseev, P.V., Ramzaev, O.A., Teodorovich, I.E., Shuvalov, I.E., "New radioecological data for the Russian Federation (from Alaska to Norway)", Environmental Radioactivity in the Arctic and Antarctic, (STRAND, P., HOLM, E. Eds.) Norwegian Radiation Protection Authority, Østerås. (1993) 69–272.
230	Nelin, P., Radiocesium uptake in moose in relation to home-range and habitat composition, J. Environ. Radioact. 26 (1995) 189–203.
241	Ramzaev, P.V., Hygienic investigation of radiation situation in the Far Northof the USSR attributed to global fallout. Dissertation of Doctor of Medical Science. Institute for Radiation Hygiene, Leningrad (1967) (in Russian).
242	Rantavaara, A.H., "Transfer of radiocesium through natural ecosystems to foodstuffs of terrestrial origin in Finland." Transfer of radionuclides in natural and semi-natural environments. (DESMET, G., NASSIMBENI, P., BELLI, M. Eds.) Elsevier Applied Science, New York (1990) 202–209.
245	Ryabokon, N.I., Smolich, I.I., Kudryashov, V.P., Goncharova, R.I., Long-term development of the radionuclide exposure of murine rodent populations in Belarus after the Chernobyl accident, Radiat. Environ. Biophys. 44 (2005) 169–181.
252	Sheppard, S.C., Evenden, W.G., Characteristics of plant concentration ratios assessed in a 64-site field survey of 23 elements, J. Environ. Radioact. 11 (1990) 15–36.
256	Stark, K., Avila, R., Wallberg, P., Estimation of radiation doses from ^{137}Cs to frogs in a wetland ecosystem, J. Environ. Radioact. 75 (2004) 1–14.
257	Toal, M.E., Copplestone, D., Johnson, M.S., Jackson, D., Jones, S.R., Quantifying ^{137}Cs aggregated transfer coefficients in a semi natural woodland ecosystem adjacent to a nuclear reprocessing facility, J. Environ. Radioact. 63 (2002) 85–103.
258	Troitskaya, M.N., Hygienic assessment of increased levels of exposure of population of the Far North. Dissertation of Doctor of medical sciences. Institute for Radiation Hygiene, Leningrad (1981) (in Russian).
261	Whicker, F.W., Little, C.A., WInsor, T.F., "Plutonium behaviour in the terrestrial environs of the Rocky Flats installation", Environmental surveillance around nuclear installations. 5-9th November, 1973. Warsaw. IAEA-SM-180/45 IAEA, Vienna (1974) 89–103.
263	Wood, M.D. et al., Application of the ERICA Integrated Approach at the Drigg coastal sand dunes, J. Environ. Radioact. 99 (2008) 1484–1495.
265	Anjos, R.M., Mosquera, B., Sanches, N., Cambui, C.A., Mercier, H., Caesium, potassium and ammonium distribution in different organs of tropical plants, Environ. Exper. Bot. 65 (2009) 111–118.
268	Beresford, N.A. et al., Estimating the exposure of small mammals at three sites within the Chernobyl exclusion zone – a test application of the ERICA Tool, J. Environ. Radioact. 99 (2008) 1496–1502.
275	Gwynn, J.P., Fuglei, E., Dowdal, M., Cs-137 in arctic foxes (Alopex lagopus) on Svalbard, J. Environ. Radioact. 92 (2007) 30–40.
288	Mortvedt, J.J., Plant and soil relationships of Uranium and Thorium decay series radionuclides – a Review, J. Environ. Qual. 23 (1994) 643–650.
289	Paller, M.H., Jannick, T.G., Wike, L.D., Concentration ratios for small mammals collected from the exposed sediments of a ^{137}Cs contaminated reservoir, J. Environ. Radioact. 90 (2006) 224–235.
294	Steinnes, E., Gaare, E., Engen, S., Influence of soil acidification in southern Norway on the ^{137}Cs exposure to moose?, Sci. Total Environ. 407 (2009) 3905–3908.
347	COGEMA Resources Canada Inc. (AREVA), McClean Lake Operation Status of the Environment Report, Assessment period 2003–2005. Saskatoon, Saskatchewan (2006).
348	AREVA Resources Canada Inc. (AREVA), McClean Lake Operation Status of the Environment Report, Assessment period 2006–2008. Saskatoon, Saskatchewan (2009).
382	Dragovic, S., Howard, B.J., Caborn, J.A., Barnett, C.L., Mihailovic, N., Transfer of natural and anthropogenic radionuclides to ants, bryophytes and lichen in a semi-natural ecosystem, Environ. Monitor. Assess. 166 (2010) 667–686.
388	Dragovic, S., Jankovic Mandic, L.J., Transfer of radionuclides to ants, mosses and lichens in semi-natural ecosystems, Radiat. Environ. Biophys. 49 (2010) 625–634.
405	Gashchak, S., Beresford, N.A., Personal communication (2009).
406	Gashchak, S., Beresford, N.A., Maksimenko, A., Vlaschenko A.S., Strontium-90 and caesium-137 activity concentrations in bats in the Chernobyl exclusion zone, Radiat. Environ. Biophys 49 (2010) 635–644.
407	Giles M.S., Twining J.R., Williams A.R., Jeffree R.A., Domel R.U., "Rehabilitation of Former nuclear test sites in Australia", Final Report of the Technical Assessment Group for the Maralinga Rehabilitation Project – Study No. 2 Radioecology, Technical Assessment Group, AGPS, Canberra (1990).

467	Higley, K.A., Estimating transfer parameters in the absence of data, Radiat. Environ. Biophys. 49 (2010) 645–656.
468	Panchenko, S.V., Panfilova, A.A., "Regarding the role of the forest ecosystems in exposure of the population". Problems of forest radioecology, (PANCHENKO S.V, Ed.) MOGUL, Moscow (2000) 228–293 (in Russian).
470	Alexakhin, R.M., Naryshkin, M.A., Radionuclide migration in forest biogeocenoses, (PREVOLOTSKY A.N., Ed.), Nauka, Moscow (1977) 148 (in Russian).
471	Bogachev, A.V., Ca and ^{90}Sr migration in the soil-plant system, Problems of Forest Radioecology, (Panchenko S.V, Ed.) Gidrometeoizdat, Moscow 302 (2000) 89–101 (in Russian).
472	Dvornik, A.V., Ipatyev, V.A., "Modelling and predictive estimates of the radionuclide accumulation by woody plants and forest-derived foodstuffs", Forest. Human. Chernobyl. Forest ecosystems after the accident at the Chernobyl NPP: condition, prediction, response of the population, ways of rehabilitation, (Ipatyev, V.A. Ed.), Institute of Forest of National Academy of Science, Gomel Retchinsk 454 (2005) 178–213 (in Russian).
473	Bulko, N.I., "The dynamics of radioactive contamination levels of the soil and tree layer", Forest. Human. Chernobyl. Forest ecosystems after the accident at the Chernobyl NPP: condition, prediction, response of the population, ways of rehabilitation, (IPATYEV, V.A. Ed.), Gomel Retchinsk 454 (1999) 94–137 (in Russian).
474	Ipatyev, M.A., Bulko, N.I., Mitin, N.V., Shabaleva, M.A., Didenko, L.G., "The hydromeliorative method for decreasing radionuclide concentrations in forest ecosystems", Radioecological Phenomena of Forest Ecosystems, The Institute of Forest of the NAS of Belarus, Gomel, Belarus (2004) 137–166 (in Russian).
475	Ipatyev, M.A., Bulko, N.I., Mitin, N.V., Shabaleva, M.A., Didenko, L.G., "The silvicultural (phytologic) method for decreasing radioactivity levels in forest ecosystems", Radioecological Phenomena of Forest Ecosystems, The Institute of Forest of the NAS of Belarus, Gomel, Belarus (2004) 67–104 (in Russian).
476	Bulko, N.I., Ipatyev, V.A., Forest ecosystems after the accident at the Chernobyl NPP: condition, prediction, response of the population, ways of rehabilitation, Forest. Human. Chernobyl. (IPATYEV, V.A. Ed.), The Institute of Forest of the NAS of Belarus, Gomel, Belarus 454 (2005) 7–303 (in Russian).
477	Martinovich, B.S., Golushko, R.M., Vlasov, V.K., Afinogenov, A.M., Interspecific differences in radionuclide accumulation by woody plants in the Chernobyl zone emissions and their causality, Radioactivity after nuclear detonations and accidents 8 (2000) 187–194 (in Russian).
478	Molchanov, A.A. et al., Some regularities of distribution of fission products deposited in composition of global fallout in forest vegetation, Lesovedenie (1968) 18–23 (in Russian).
479	Mukhamedshin, K.D., Chilimov, A.I., Bezuglov, V.K., Snytkin, G.V., "Certification of forest resources by the radiation characteristic as the basis to obtain safe forest products in areas affected by radionuclides" Problems of Forest Radioecology (PANCHENKO, S.V., Ed), MOGUL, Moscow. 302, (2000) 7–46. (in Russian).
480	Perevolotsky, A.N., ^{137}Cs and ^{90}Sr distribution in forest biogeocenoses, (Prevolotsky, A.N. Ed.), Institute for Radiology, Gomel (2006) 124–127 (in Russian).
482	Perevolotsky, A.N., Effects of cultivation conditions on ^{137}Cs and ^{90}Sr accumulation levels in wood and bark of the major stand-forming species, (Prevolotsky, A.N. Ed.), Gomel (2006) 267–273 (in Russian).
484	SHCHEGLOV, A.I., Biogeochemistry of technogenic radionuclides in forest ecosystems of the central regions of the East European Plain, Doctor of Sciences Thesis, Moscow State University Moscow (1997) (in Russian).
485	Yushkov, P.I., ^{90}Sr and ^{137}Cs accumulation and distribution in birch near the liquid wastes disposal site of the Beloyarskaya NPP Ekologiya 7 (2000) 106–112 (in Russian).
486	Wood, M.D., Assessing the impact of ionizing radiation in temperate coastal sand dunes: measurement and modelling. Ph.D. Thesis, University of Liverpool (2010).
488	Wood, M.D., Leah, R.T., Jones, S.R., Copplestone, D., Radionuclide transfer to invertebrates and small mammals in a coastal sand dune ecosystem, Sci. Total Environ. 407 (2009) 4062–4074.
519	Livens, F.R., Horrill, A.D., Singleton, D.L., Distribution of radiocesium in the soil-plant systems of upland areas of Europe, Health Phys. 60 (1991) 539–544.

REFERENCES

1. Albrecht, J., Abalos, M., Rice, T.M., 2007. Heavy metal levels in ribbon snakes (Thamnophis sauritus) and anuran larvae from the Mobile-Tensaw River Delta, Alabama, USA. Arch. Environ. Contam. Toxicol. 53 (4), 647–654.
2. Barnett, C.L., Beresford, N.A., Walker, L.A., Baxter, M., Wells, C., Copplestone, D., 2013a. Element and radionuclide concentrations in representative species of the ICRP's reference animals and plants and associated soils from a forest in north-west England. NERC-Environmental Inf. Data Centre. http://dx.doi.org/10.5285/e40b53d4-6699-4557-bd55-10d196ece9ea.
3. Barnett, C.L., Beresford, N.A., Walker, L.A., Baxter, M., Wells, C., Copplestone, D., 2013b. Transfer parameters for ICRP reference animals and plants collected from a forest ecosystem. Radiat. Environ. Biophys. (in press).

4. Beresford, N.A., Wright, S.M., Barnett, C.L., Wood, M.D., Gaschak, S., Arkhipov, A., Sazykina, T.G., Howard, B.J., 2005. Predicting radionuclide transfer to wild animals: an application of a proposed environmental impact assessment framework to the Chernobyl exclusion zone. Radiat. Environ. Biophys. 44 (3), 161–168.
5. Beresford, N.A., Barnett, C.L., Brown, J., Cheng, J.-J., Copplestone, D., Filistovic, V., Hosseini, A., Howard, B.J., Jones, S.R., Kamboj, S., Kryshev, A., Nedveckaite, T., Olyslaegers, G., Saxén, R., Sazykina, T., Vives i Batlle, J., Vives-Lynch, S., Yankovich, T., Yu, C., 2008a. Inter-comparison of models to estimate radionuclide activity concentrations in non-human biota. Radiat. Environ. Biophys. 47, 491–514.
6. Beresford, N.A., Barnett, C.L., Howard, B.J., Scott, W.A., Brown, J.E., Copplestone, D., 2008b. Derivation of transfer parameters for use within the ERICA tool and the default concentration ratios for terrestrial biota. J. Environ. Radioact. 99 (9), 1393–1407.
7. Beresford, N.A., Balonov, M., Beaugelin-Seiller, K., Brown, J., Copplestone, D., Hingston, J.L., Horyna, J., Hosseini, A., Howard, B.J., Kamboj, S., Nedveckaite, T., Olyslaegers, G., Sazykina, T., Vives i Batlle, J., Yankovich, T., Yu, C., 2008c. An international comparison of models and approaches for the estimation of radiological exposure to non-human biota. Appl. Radiat. Isot 66, 1745–1749.
8. Beresford, N.A., Gaschak, S., Barnett, C.L., Howard, B.J., Chizhevsky, I., Strømman, G., Oughton, D.H., Wright, S.M., Maksimenko, A., Copplestone, D., 2008d. Estimating the exposure of small mammals at three sites within the Chernobyl exclusion zone e a test application of the ERICA tool. J. Environ. Radioact. 99, 1496–1502.
9. Beresford, N.A., 2010. The transfer of radionuclides to wildlife. Radiat. Environ. Biophys. 49 (4), 505–508.
10. Beresford, N.A., Yankovich, T.L., Wood, M.D., Fesenko, S., Andersson, P., Muikku, M., Willey, N.J., 2013. A new approach to predicting environmental transfer of radionuclides to wildlife: a demonstration for freshwater fish and caesium. Sci. Total Environ. 463e464, 284–292.
11. Brown, J.E., Alfonso, B., Avila, R., Beresford, N.A., Copplestone, D., Prohl, G., Ulanovsky, A., 2008. The ERICA tool. J. Environ. Radioact. 99 (9), 1371–1383.
12. Chen, H., Wood, M.D., Maltby, E., 2011. Uncertainty analysis in a GIS-based multicriteria analysis tool for river catchment management. Environ. Modell. Softw. 26 (4), 395–405.
13. Copplestone, D., Beresford, N.A., Brown, J., Yankovich, T., 2013. An international database of radionuclide concentration ratios for wildlife: development and uses. J. Environ. Radioact. 126, 288–298. http://dx.doi.org/10.1016/ j.jenvrad.2013.05.007.
14. Crossley, D.A.J., 1973. Comparative movement of 106Ru, 60Co and 137Cs in arthropod food chains. In: Nelson, D.J., Evans, F.C. (Eds.), Proc. Symp. On Radioecology. Proc. of the 2nd National Symposium, USAEC, Washington. United States Atomic Energy Commission Report CONF- 670503, Washington, pp. 687–695.
15. Gaare, E., Staarland, H., 1994. Pathways of fallout radiocesium via reindeer to man. In: Dahlgaard, H. (Ed.), Nordic Radioecology: the Transfer of Radionuclides through Nordic Ecosystems to Man. Elesvier, Amsterdam, pp. 303–334.
16. Gochfeld, M., Burger, J., 1987. Factors affecting the distribution of heavy metals e age effects and the metal concentration patterns in common terns, Sterna hirundo. Biol. Trace Elem. Res. 12, 389–399.
17. Hinton, T.G., Garnier-Laplace, J., Vandenhove, H., Dowdall, M., Adam-Guillermin, C., Alonzo, F., Barnett, C.L., Beaugelin-Seiller, K., Beresford, N.A., Bradshaw, C., Brown, J., Eyrolle, F., Fevrier, L., Gariel, J.-C., Gilbin, R., Hertel-Aas, T., Horemans, N., Howard, B.J., Ikäheimonen, T., Mora, J.C., Oughton, D., Real, A., Salbu, B., Simon-Cornu, M., Steiner, M., Sweeck, L., Vives i Batlle, J., 2013. An invitation to contribute to a strategic research agenda in radioecology. J. Environ. Radioact 115, 73–82.
18. Hosseini, A., Stenberg, K., Avila, R., Beresford, N.A., Brown, J.E., 2013. Application of the Bayesian approach for derivation of PDFs for concentration ratio values. J. Environ. Radioact. 126, 376–387. http://dx.doi.org/10.1016/ j.jenvrad.2013.04.007.
19. Hosseini, A., Thorring, H., Brown, J.E., Saxen, R., Ilus, E., 2008. Transfer of radionuclides in aquatic ecosystems e default concentration ratios for aquatic biota in the ERICA tool. J. Environ. Radioact. 99 (9), 1408–1429.
20. Howard, B.J., Beresford, N.A., Hove, K., 1991. Transfer of radiocesium to ruminants in natural and semi-natural ecosystems and appropriate countermeasures. Health Phys. 61, 715–725.
21. Howard, B.J., Beresford, N.A., Copplestone, D., Telleria, D., Proehl, G., Fesenko, S., Jeffree, R.A., Yankovich, T.L., Brown, J.E., Higley, K., Johansen, M.P., Mulye, H., Vandenhove, H., Gashchak, S., Wood, M.D., Takata, H., Andersson, P., Dale, P., Ryan, J., Bollhöfer, A., Doering, C., Barnett, C.L., Wells, C., 2013a. The IAEA handbook on radionuclide transfer to wildlife. J. Environ. Radioact. 121, 55–74.
22. Howard, B.J., Wells, C., Beresford, N.A., Copplestone, D.C., 2013b. Exploring methods to prioritise concentration ratios when estimating weighted absorbed dose rates to terrestrial reference animals and plants. J. Environ. Radioact. 126, 326–337. http://dx.doi.org/10.1016/j.jenvrad.2013.04.007.
23. IAEA, 2009. Quantification of Radionuclide Transfer in Terrestrial and Freshwater Environments for Radiological Assessments. IAEA-TECDOC-1616. International Atomic Energy Agency, Vienna, p. 622.
24. IAEA, 2010. Handbook of Parameter Values for the Prediction of Radionuclide Transfer in Terrestrial and Freshwater Environments. IAEA-TRS-472. International Atomic Energy Agency, Vienna.
25. IAEA, 2013. Handbook of Parameter Values for the Prediction of Radionuclide Transfer to Wildlife. Technical Reports Series. International Atomic Energy Agency, Vienna (in press).

26. ICRP, 2009. Environmental protection: transfer parameters for reference animals and plants. ICRP Publication 114. Ann. ICRP 39 (6).

27. Jeffree, R.A., 1991. An experimental-study of 226Ra and 45Ca accumulation from the aquatic medium by fresh-water turtles (Family e Chelidae) under varying Ca and Mg water concentrations. Hydrobiologia 218 (3), 205–231.

28. Johansen, M.P., Barnett, C.L., Beresford, N.A., Brown, J.E., Cerne, M., Howard, B.J., Kamboj, S., Keum, D.K., Smodis, B., Twining, J.R., Vandenhove, H., Vives i Batlle, J., Wood, M.D., Yu, C., 2012. Assessing doses to terrestrial wildlife at a radioactive waste disposal site: inter-comparison of modelling approaches. Sci. Total Environ. 427e428, 238–246.

29. L'Ecuyer, P., 2012. Random Number Generation. In: Springer Handbooks of Computational Statistics. Springer, Berlin Heidelberg, pp. 25–71.

30. Lowe, V.P.W., Horrill, A.D., 1991. Caesium concentration factors in wild herbivores and the fox (Vulpes vulpes L). Environ. Pollut. 70, 93–107.

31. Mann, R.M., Sanchez-Hernandez, J.C., Serra, E.A., Soares, A., 2007. Bioaccumulation of Cd by a European lacertid lizard after chronic exposure to Cd-contaminated food. Chemosphere 68 (8), 1525–1534.

32. McCullough, B.D., 2008. Microsoft Excel's 'Not the Wichmann-Hill' random number generators. Comput. Stat. Data 52, 4587–4593.

33. Pendleton, R.C., Lloyd, R.D., Mays, C.W., Church, B.W., 1964. Trophic level effect on the accumulation of caesium-137 in cougars feeding onmule deer. Nature 204, 707–709.

34. RIFE, 1996. Radioactivity in Food in the Environment (RIFE-1). Available from: http://www.cefas.defra.gov.uk/publications-and-data/scientific-series/ radioactivity-in-food-and-the-environment-(rife).aspx.

35. RIFE, 1998. Radioactivity in Food in the Environment (RIFE-3). Available from: http://www.cefas.defra.gov.uk/publications-and-data/scientific-series/ radioactivity-in-food-and-the-environment-(rife).aspx.

36. RIFE, 1999. Radioactivity in Food in the Environment (RIFE-4). Available from: http://www.cefas.defra.gov.uk/publications-and-data/scientific-series/ radioactivity-in-food-and-the-environment-(rife).aspx.

37. RIFE, 2000. Radioactivity in Food in the Environment (RIFE-5). Available from: http://www.cefas.defra.gov.uk/publications-and-data/scientific-series/ radioactivity-in-food-and-the-environment-(rife).aspx.

38. RIFE, 2002. Radioactivity in Food in the Environment (RIFE-7). Available from: http://www.cefas.defra.gov.uk/publications-and-data/scientific-series/ radioactivity-in-food-and-the-environment-(rife).aspx.

39. RIFE, 2003. Radioactivity in Food in the Environment (RIFE-8). Available from: http://www.cefas.defra.gov.uk/publications-and-data/scientific-series/ radioactivity-in-food-and-the-environment-(rife).aspx.

40. RIFE, 2004. Radioactivity in Food in the Environment (RIFE-9). Available from: http://www.cefas.defra.gov.uk/publications-and-data/scientific-series/ radioactivity-in-food-and-the-environment-(rife).aspx.

41. Rowan, D.J., 2013. Bioaccumulation factors and the steady state assumption for cesium isotopes in aquatic foodwebs near nuclear facilities. J. Environ. Radioact. 121, 2–11.

42. Rudge, S.A., Johnson, M.S., Leah, R.T., Jones, S.R., 1993. Biological transport of radiocesium in a seminatural grassland ecosystem 1. Soils, vegetation and invertebrates. J. Environ. Radioact. 19 (3), 173–198.

43. Sakai, H., Saeki, K., Ichihashi, H., Kamezaki, N., Tanabe, S., Tatsukawa, R., 2000. Growth-related changes in heavy metal accumulation in green turtle (Chelonia mydas) from Yaeyama Islands, Okinawa, Japan. Arch. Environ. Contam. Toxicol. 39 (3), 378–385.

44. Scott, D.E., Whicker, F.W., Gibbons, J.W., 1986. Effect of season on the retention of 137Cs and 90Sr by the yellow-bellied slider turtle (Pseudemys scripta). Can. J. Zool. 64 (12), 2850–2853.

45. Sheppard, S.C., Long, J.M., Sanipelli, B., 2010. Measured elemental transfer factors for boreal hunter/ gatherer scenarios: fish, game and berries. J. Environ. Radioact. 101 (11), 902–909.

46. Sheppard, S.C., 2013. Transfer factors toWhitetail deer: comparison of stomach-content, plant-sample and soil-sample concentrations as the denominator. J. Environ. Radioact. 126, 434–437. http://dx.doi.org/10.1016/j.jenvrad.2012.12.003.

47. Thomas, P.A., Sheard, J.W., Swanson, S., 1994. Transfer of 210Po and 210Pb through the lichen-caribou-wolf food chain of northern Canada. Health Phys. 66, 666–677.

48. Tuovinen, T.S., Roivainen, P., Makkonen, S., Kolehmainen, M., Holopainden, T., Juutilainen, J., 2011. Soil-to-plant transfer of elements is not linear: results for five elements relevant to radioactive waste in five boreal forest species. Sci. Total Environ. 410, 191–197.

49. USDoE, 2002. A Graded Approach for Evaluating Radiation Doses to Aquatic and Terrestrial Biota Technical Standard DOE-STD-1153-2002. United States Department of the Environment, Washington D.C.

50. Vives i Batlle, J., 2012. Radioactivity in the marine environment. In: Meyers, R.A. (Ed.), Encyclopedia of Sustainability Science and Technology. Springer Science & Business Media, LLC, pp. 8387–8425.

51. Wichman, B.A., Hill, I.D., 1982. Algorithm as 183: an efficient and portable pseudorandom number generator. Appl. Stat. 31, 188–190.

52. Whicker, F.W., Pinder, J.E., Bowling, J.W., Alberts, J.J., Brisbin, I.L., 1990. Distribution of long-lived radionuclides in an abandoned reactor cooling reservoir. Ecol. Monogr. 60 (4), 471–496.

53. Wood, M.D., Marshall, W.A., Beresford, N.A., Jones, S.R., Howard, B.J., Copplestone, D., Leah, R.T., 2008. Application of the ERICA integrated approach at the Drigg coastal sand dunes. J. Environ. Radioact 99 (9), 1484–1495.

54. Wood, M.D., Leah, R.T., Jones, S.R., Copplestone, D., 2009a. Radionuclide transfer to invertebrates and small mammals in a coastal sand dune ecosystem. Sci. Total Environ. 407 (13), 4062–4074.

55. Wood, M.D., Beresford, N.A., Barnett, C.L., Copplestone, D., Leah, R.T., 2009b. Assessing radiation impact at a protected coastal sand dune site: an intercomparison of models for estimating the radiological exposure of non-human biota. J. Environ. Radioact. 100, 1034–1052.

56. Wood, M.D., Beresford, N.A., Semenov, D.V., Yankovich, T.L., Copplestone, D., 2010. Radionuclide transfer to reptiles. Radiat. Environ. Biophys. 49 (4), 509–530.

57. Yankovich, T.L., Beresford, N.A., Fesenko, S., Fesenko, J., Phaneuf, M., Dagher, E., Outola, I., Andersson, P., Thiessen, K., Ryan, J., Wood, M.D., Bollhöfer, A., Barnett, C.L., Copplestone, D., 2013. Establishing a database of radionuclide transfer parameters for freshwater wildlife. J. Environ. Radioact. 126, 299–313. http://dx.doi.org/10.1016/j.jenvrad.2012.07.014.

58. Yankovich, T.L., Beresford, N.A., Wood, M.D., Aono, T., Andersson, P., Barnett, C.L., Bennett, P., Brown, J.E., Fesenko, S., Johansen, M., Hosseini, A., Howard, B.J., Phaneuf, M., Tagami, K., Takata, H., Twining, J.R., Uchida, S., 2010. Whole-body to tissue concentration ratios for use in biota dose assessments for animals. Radiat. Environ. Biophys. 49 (4), 549–565.

CHAPTER 4 SOIL GAS RADON ASSESSMENT AND DEVELOPMENT OF A RADON RISK MAP

G. Cinelli, L. Tositti, B. Capaccioni, E. Brattich, and D. Mostacci

Keywords: Vulsini Volcanic district, Soil gas radon, Geology, Radon risk map

INTRODUCTION

Natural radioactivity is widely distributed in the lithosphere as well as in all the various environmental compartments as a result of nucleosynthesis and biogeochemical cycling, providing a large fraction of the background radiation dose to human population. It is mainly characterized by a small number of primordial radionuclides among which the most relevant ones are ^{40}K and the members of the three natural radioactive families of ^{238}U, ^{232}Th and ^{235}U. All the three families present an intermediate radon isotope which, due to the noble gas properties, can be easily remobilized from the mineral matrices where it is produced by radioactive decay. Radon isotopes of natural origin are, respectively, ^{222}Rn (half-life $t_{1/2}$ = 3.8 day), ^{220}Rn ($t_{1/2}$ = 55.6 s) and ^{219}Rn ($t_{1/2}$ = 3.96 s), in order of decreasing half-life and hence, on a first approximation, radiologic importance. The parent radionuclides of radon isotopes are present in all the crustal materials and their derivatives such as soil, industrial wastes coming from ore smelting, mineral extraction and industrial use, fossil fuel employment and cycles, waste recycling and building materials, from which they are released into the atmosphere (UNSCEAR 2008; Eisenbud and Gesell 1997).

Public exposure to natural ionizing radiation is largely due to radon. The estimated value of worldwide average annual exposure to the various components of natural radiation show that^{222}Rn contribution constitutes as much as 50 % of the overall radiation dose reaching values of about 1.15 mSv/year per capita (UNSCEAR 2008). As a general rule, radon exposure is largely due to its accumulation within confined environments with reduced or no air exchange, leading to the inhalation of potentially hazardous amounts of airborne alpha emitters both in the gaseous and in the particulate form with very well recognized epidemiological noxious effects (Porstendörfer 1994; UNSCEAR 2006; WHO 2008).

The cumulative effect of several factors, such as lithology, geomorphology, local/regional geotectonics and finally building materials and techniques as well as living habits (ventilation), lead to indoor radon accumulation and its inherent health risk.

Its transfer from the parent material into the atmosphere is controlled by a number of physical factors, such as porosity and degree of fracturing, temperature and pressure gradients, and moisture. Radon emitted from the ground surface or from materials of crustal origin in outdoor air is rapidly dispersed leading to low atmospheric concentration levels, while in confined environments, such as buildings, dwellings, tunnels, caves and mines, radon accumulates leading to potentially hazardous indoor concentration levels in the absence of mitigation actions.

The new Euratom Directive on Basic Safety Standards by the European Union published in January 2014 (EC 2013) presents several new aspects concerning natural radioactivity with respect to the 1996 edition, e.g., the radon action plan in which "...Member States shall establish a national action plan addressing long-term risks from radon exposures in dwellings, buildings with public access and workplaces for any source

Citation: Cinelli, G., Tositti, L., Capaccioni, B., Brattich, E., and Mostacci, D. Soil gas radon assessment and development of a radon risk map, Environmental Geochemistry and Health, April 2015, Volume 37, Issue 2, pp 305–319. DOI:10.1007/s10653-014-9649-9.ss of radon ingress, whether from soil, building materials or water… Member States shall identify areas where the radon concentration (as an annual average) in a significant number of buildings is expected to exceed the relevant national reference level…."

In the past (EC 1996), those areas have been usually called "radon-prone areas",[1] even if there was no authoritative definition of a radon-prone area. According to Bossew et al. (2013), "Qualitatively, this concept denotes areas where observed or expected values of a ^{222}Rn-related variable are high with respect to reference values or with respect to the mean over the domain". In general, radon-prone areas are identified according to two main strategies: (a) direct measurements of indoor radon concentration and (b) indirect methods including soil gas radon survey and gamma-dose assessment based on γ-spectrometry from laboratory, field and aerial surveys all implying the existence of a more or less known transfer factor from the crustal environment into the buildings (Dubois and Bossew 2006; García-Tavalera et al. 2013). Since each single methodology is usually not sufficient to the scope, hybrid approaches are often used suggesting the need for integrated information as an optimal tool for radon area classification. The process is finalized once geostatistical elaborations of the measured parameters have been suitably performed. For instance, maps based on indoor radon measurements and integrating geological information have been used in Great Britain (Miles and Appleton 2005) and Belgium (Cinelli et al. 2010), whereas maps based on soil gas measurements have been developed in Germany (Kemski et al. 2009) and Czech Republic (Barnet et al. 2008). At European level, the Radioactivity Environmental Monitoring (REM) group of the Joint Research Centre (JRC) of the European Commission started the European Atlas of Natural Radiation (EANR) (De Cort et al. 2011) some years ago. The European indoor radon map (EIRM) displays annual mean indoor radon concentrations in ground floor rooms of dwellings on a defined reference grid with a resolution of 10 km × 10 km (Gruber et al. 2013b). In parallel to this effort, a European Geogenic RadonMap (EGRM) is under development by the JRC: This map aims to display a quantity closer to geogenic hazard, i.e., which measures "what earth delivers" in terms of radon irrespective of anthropogenic factors and temporally constant over a geological timescale (Gruber et al. 2013a).

In order to assess the radon risk in buildings in a given area on the basis of soil radon or of radon-related variables, it is necessary to set up indexes accounting for the effective radioactivity levels as well as for the physical properties of solids through which radon transfer occurs. This approach based on radon potential assessment and on the use of Radon indexes such as those authoritatively introduced by Barnet and coworkers in the Czech Republic (Barnet et al. 2008) first and presently extending to the other European countries, allows to predict the indoor radon in new buildings and to estimate the radiological risk from this relevant but ubiquitous radiation source.

This work presents the results of an investigation concerning NORM[2] distribution in one of the areas with the highest natural background radiation in Italy. In particular, the study concerns the Vulsini Volcanic district in northern Lazio, a well-known quaternary volcanic area subject of a previous paper recently published by the authors aimed at the assessment of both the regional NORM level and distribution as related to the specific magmatic processes and of the associated radon risk (Capaccioni et al. 2012). In this area, volcanic products have relevant U, Th and K contents ranging, respectively, from 6 to 32 ppm, from 31 to 120 ppm and from 0.7 to 8 % by weight. Beside the lithological and radiological assessment in connection with the different Vulsinian volcanic rocks, this paper includes a limited, but significant number of indoor radon measurements covering both historical and modern buildings in order to collect preliminary information on radon exposure in this region. Markedly, high values were recorded in buildings (46–3,269 Bq/m^3) and in cellars (30,000 Bq/m^3) pointing at the need of a more systematic investigation related to the territory rather than to specific situations and therefore reflecting radon risk areal distribution for the local population with a more rigorous approach. Moreover, Capaccioni et al. (2012) pointed out the strong relationships between the high indoor radon level and the local rock formations able to affect both indoor radon buildup, as a part of the local landscape, and building material, especially tuffs, whose use in this area is historically recognized since ancient times. In spite of the evidence concerning the high radiation background in the investigated region, the relationships between rocks radioactivity and soil gas radon in a given area is not obvious, since many factors and processes may contribute to influence the latter. In particular, soil gas radon depends on uranium–radium concentration in the residual mineral fraction, the degree of remobilization of members of the radioactive families by weathering and/or post depositional chemical processes, porosity, faulting and advection in case of secondary magma degassing from a deep source. However, since the major source of indoor radon is in the soil and in the bedrock surrounding and under the buildings, our investigation on the Vulsini district was extended to the collection of data on soil gas radon in this region.

The present paper is therefore focused on the results obtained from a campaign of soil gas radon measurements mainly carried out in the urban area of Bolsena, the most important town of the Vulsinian volcanic district. Its main aims are integrating previous information on this high background radiation area, evaluating local levels of soil gas radon, creating both a soil gas radon map and a conjunct radon risk map integrating soil gas radon data, geological information and radiation protection issues, and, finally, the identification of radon-prone areas, as suggested by the International Commission for Radiological Protection (ICRP) and the EU Council Directive 96/29/EURATOM (1996) and the new Euratom Directive on Basic Safety Standards published in January 2014 (EC 2013).

GEOLOGICAL SETTING

The Vulsini Volcanic district (Nappi et al. 1995; Capaccioni et al. 2012), which was active in the period 570–127 ka (Gillot et al. 1991), is located in the northern part of the Quaternary potassic volcanic belt of the Roman Magmatic province (central-southern Italy). Four volcanic complexes have been recognized in the evolution of the district: Paleo-Bolsena, Bolsena, Latera and Montefiascone (Nappi et al. 1991). They developed with alternating effusive and explosive eruptions, with Strombolian, Plinian and Ignimbrite-forming phases. Volcanic products are widely differentiated including leucite, basanite and shoshonite magmatic suites (Nappi and Valentini 2005).

The Bolsena volcanic complex mainly took place in the eastern part of the Vulsini district after an extensive phase of subsidence which affected the final activity of the Paleo-Bolsena volcanic complex, responsible for a thick sequence of volcano-lacustrine deposits within the Bolsena caldera (Nappi and Valentini 2005). The Bolsena volcanic complex developed during two eruptive cycles (Nappi and Marini 1986). The first one starts with an initial effusive and/or Strombolian phase and ends with a minor explosive and effusive phase. The second cycle also consists of a moderate initial effusive and/or Strombolian phase but ends with a large, paroxysmal explosive activity, producing a widespread tuff deposit. In details, the oldest products of Bolsena complex are represented by leucite-bearing lava flows outcropping in the N and E sectors. The final phase of the first cycle is characterized by pyroclastic falls, small scale pyroclastic flows, welded tuffs and several outward and inward trachytic lava flows. Phases of volcanic-tectonic collapses took place after this moderate explosive to effusive activity and part of the NE Bolsena caldera was outlined by complex faulting. N–S and NNW–SSE lines of weakness formed throughout the E side of the present Bolsena Caldera and high potassic series magmas were tapped. The leucite-bearing lava flows and scoria cones associated with this activity can be considered as the initial phase of the second Bolsena cycle. On the contrary, the final stage of the Bolsena complex gives rise to the pyroclastic sequence of the Orvieto-Bagnoregio Ignimbrite (333 ka, Nappi et al. 1991).

The detailed geological formations present around Bolsena village are shown in Fig. 1.

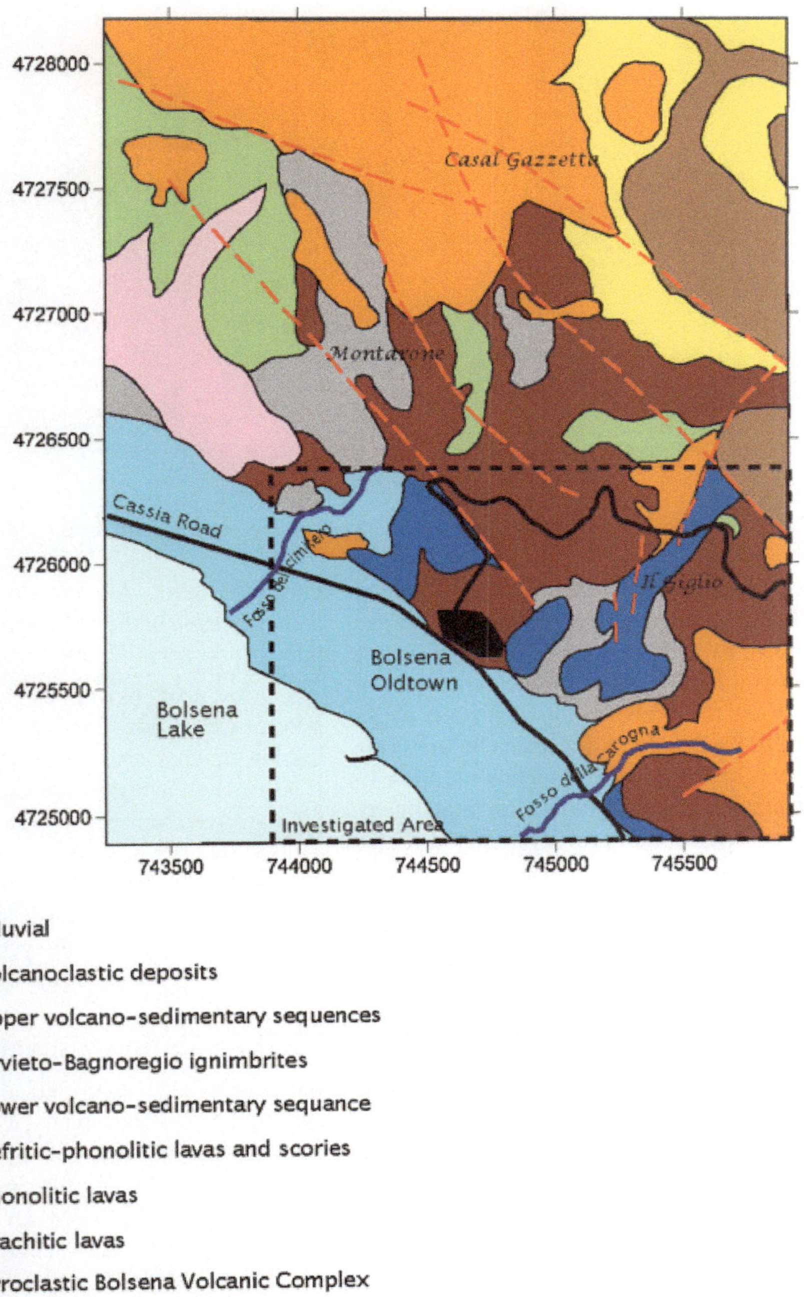

Figure 1. Geological sketch map of the area around Bolsena village (after Renzulli 1988, modified).

As outlined in a previous paper (Capaccioni et al. 2012), concentrations of natural radionuclides in local volcanic outcrops are rather high compared to average Earth's crust substantially enhancing the regional radiation background. In particular, uranium and thorium concentrations, typically high in this kind of magmatic lithologies, have been found to range from 80 to 394 Bq/kg and from 126 to 487 Bq/kg, respectively (Capaccioni et al. 2012; Cinelli2012). This agrees with the high indoor radon detected (ibidem) and conducive of high soil gas radon supported by both the local mineral matrices as well as from faulting and degassing as the declining phase of the secondary volcanic activity.

INSTRUMENTS AND METHODS

Data

A soil gas radon campaign was carried out in March 2011 covering an area of about 2 km^2 with 63 sampling stations distributed within the urban area of Bolsena and including part of its outskirt, following a square grid-based sampling design (see Fig. 2), with cell sizes about 100 m. All the stations occupied were georeferenced following the WGS 84 (UTM 32T) geographic coordinate system (Fig. 2) using a GPS (Garmin).

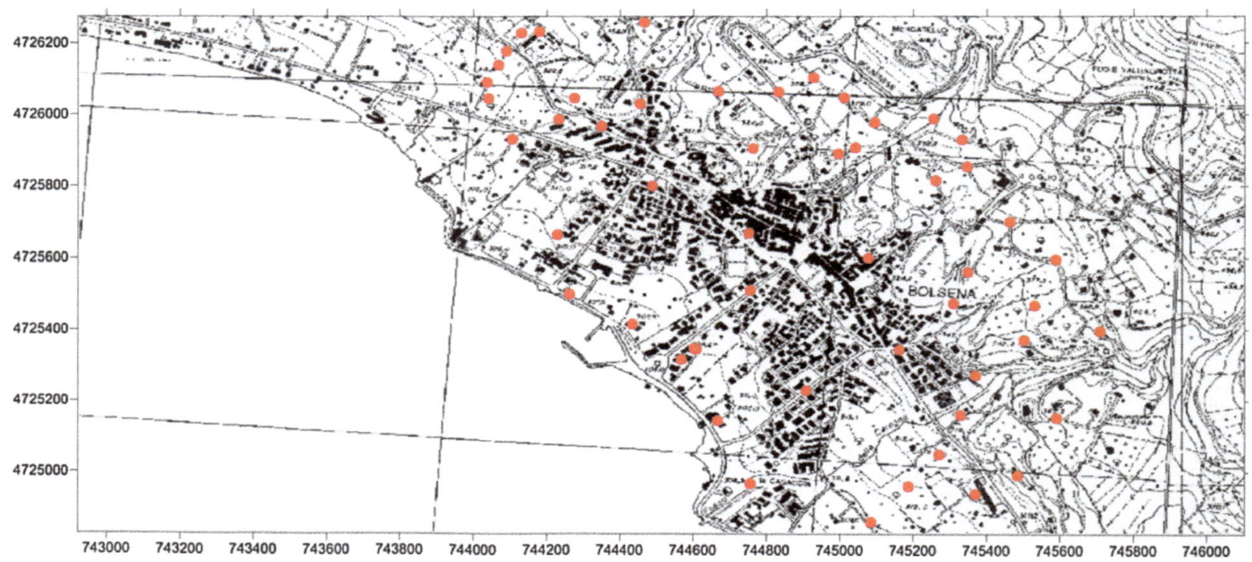

Figure 2. Locations in and around Bolsena where soil gas radon concentrations are measured; the*red points* indicate the measurement points.

Soil gas radon was measured by coupling a RAD-7 radon monitor (Durridge Co.) to a standard soil probe. The soil gas probe was inserted down to an approximate depth of 60–70 cm where in this area you find the hard rock basement, so it was not possible to insert the probe to the suggested depth of 1 m (Barnet et al. 2008). Briefly, the instrument works by circulating air from the ground through a membrane filter to retain airborne particulate matter containing radon progeny and through desiccant (drierite) to prevent radon artifacts during measurements. Purified air from soil interstices is hence pumped inside the RAD-7 measuring chamber where radon gas is detected through α-decay of its daughter ^{218}Po therein produced. In order to measure soil gas radon, the instrument was operated in sniff mode (RAD-7 2009). Since secular equilibrium between ^{222}Rn and ^{218}Po is reached in about 15 min, a single measurement must have an average duration of 25–30 min with readings taken every 5 min. The measurement is terminated when the relative difference between two consecutive readings is lower than 15 %. The final result is estimated as the average of the last two readings.

Eight soil samples, 1 kg each, were collected to estimate permeability, a parameter required by the radon risk modeling suggested by Barnet et al. (2008). It was possible to derive a rough estimate of the permeability very easily from the weight percentage of fine fraction (<63 μm). Soils with the weight percentage of the fine fraction <15 % were designed as high permeable soils, in the range 15–65 % as medium permeable and in the case of the fine fraction above 65 % as low permeable ones (Barnet et al. 2008).

Sieve analysis was carried out to determine the weight percentage of fine fraction. A wet-sieving process has been used in which the material is mixed with water until it becomes a suspension which is placed on the sieve (mesh size: 63 μm). Above the sieve, a water spray nozzle is placed which supports the sieving process additionally to the sieving motion. The rinsing is carried out until the liquid which is discharged through the receiver is clear. Sample residues on the sieves are dried at 105 °C (until the weight remained constant), and the fraction <63 μm can be calculated.

High-resolution γ-spectrometry

Soil samples, crushed and sieved at 2,000-μm mesh, were analyzed by γ-spectrometry with a p-type coaxial Hyper Pure Germanium crystal detectors (HPGe), with an energy range 0–2,000 keV. The detector has a relative efficiency of 38 % and a resolution (FWHM) of 1.8 at 1,330 keV, respectively. The system was calibrated for energy and efficiency using a multiple nuclide source (QCY48, Amersham) in a jar geometry (diameter: 56 mm; thickness: 10 mm). Spectra were analyzed with the GammaVision-32 software (version 6.07, Ortec). Quantitative analysis on samples was carried out by subtracting the spectrum of water in the same geometry, while uncertainty on peaks (k = 1, 68 % level of confidence) was calculated propagating the combined error over the efficiency fit previously determined with the counting error. Minimum detectable activity was calculated making use of the Traditional ORTEC method (ORTEC 2003) with a peak cut-off limit of 40 %.

^{238}U and ^{232}Th were determined using the emissions of their radioactive descendants ^{226}Ra and^{228}Ac. The correction of the ^{226}Ra peak at 186 keV was carried out assuming a secular equilibrium between ^{226}Ra–^{238}U and natural ^{235}U/^{238}U isotopic ratio (Gilmore 2008). Under these two hypotheses, the ^{226}Ra peak was corrected by dividing by 1.7337. The results were also checked according to the method, described by De Corte et al. (2005), based on the correction of the peak at 186 keV for the contribution of ^{235}U using ^{234}Th peak at 63.3 keV, assuming natural^{235}U/^{238}U isotopic ratio and ^{238}U–^{234}Th in equilibrium. The correction of ^{234}Th peak at 63.3 keV for the ^{232}Th peak at 63.8 keV has been made using the ^{228}Ac peak at 338.3 keV. The two methods led to very close corrected activity concentrations of ^{226}Ra, with differences <5 %.

Conversion from specific activity (Bq/kg) to bulk elemental weight fraction was obtained with the following conversion factors (Stromswold 1995):

- 1 % K = 309.7 Bq/kg
- 1 ppm U = 12.35 Bq/kg
- 1 ppm Th = 4.072 Bq/kg.

To reach appropriate counting statistics, samples were counted for 80,000 s. Certified reference materials (DH-1a and UTS-3, CANMET) were used to verify the quality of the measurements.

Geostatistics

Geostatistics offers a way to describe the spatial continuity of natural phenomena and provides adaptations of classical regression techniques to take advantage of this continuity (Isaaks and Srivastava 1989). It is thus natural that this collection of methods and tools was applied to analyze the spatial structure of soil gas radon concentration (Dubois and Bossew 2006). Kriging is the most common estimation procedure used in geostatistics (Langley 1971). It predicts unknown values using known values and a variogram model. By means of the variogram, an important component of the Kriging method, the spatial correlation between data is measured. The software Surfer11 (SURFER 2012) was used to study the spatial structure.

Radon Index

The geogenic radon potential is the essential parameter describing the subsurface as the main source for indoor radon independently on the building characteristics (Kemski et al. 2001); radon production and radon supply are the essential criteria for evaluating the geogenic radon potential. A way to define the radon potential is the Radon Index (RI) based on multivariate cross-tabulation (Gruber et al. 2013a). In this approach, scores are assigned to combinations of input quantities; the resulting RI is a categorical-ordinal quantity, i.e., in ordered classes as (I, II, III, IV) or (low, medium, high). The RI has been defined in this way in several countries such as the USA (EPA 1993), the Czech Republic (Barnet et al. 2008) and Germany (Kemski et al.2001).

The radon risk classification in Czech Republic is based on the assessment of two main parameters: the soil gas radon (^{222}Rn) concentration and the permeability of soil and rock for gasses. If the numerical value of permeability is not available (as in our case), it is sufficient to estimate it as low, medium or high and the radon index of the building is assessed using the classification reported in Table 1 (Barnet et al. 2008) .[3]

Table 1. Radon index (risk) assessment (Barnet et al. 2008)

Radon index (RI) category	**Soil gas radon concentration C (kBq/m^3)**		
Low	c < 30	c < 20	c < 10
Medium	30 ≤ c < 100	20 ≤ c < 70	10 ≤ c < 30
High	c ≥ 100	c ≥ 70	c ≥ 30
	Low	Medium	High
	Permeability		

Radon Mapping Methodology

Geostatistical elaboration for a soil gas radon and a radon risk mapping was carried out based on the following criteria:

a. The area was subdivided into square cells with a surface of 100 m × 100 m, each cell being characterized by a coordinate pair associated to its center;

b. Geological information available in Renzulli map (Renzulli 1988) was attributed to the center of each square cell through available georeferencing in GIS system;

c. Choosing the variogram estimator in the software Surfer 11 (SURFER 2012), an experimental variogram is computed for the total database and for each geological group;

d. Calculation of mean radon concentration was referred to the cell center. Mean radon concentration was predicted applying Kriging to the experimental values (or ln-transformed data) considering only the nugget effect in the variogram model which makes Kriging practically equivalent to the simple moving average. In the algorithm, the following values of constraining conditions were chosen:

- 15: the maximum number of data to be used to calculate the mean at the cell center;
- 10: the minimum number of data to be used to calculate the mean at the cell center; fewer data can lead to doubtful results;
- 500 m: the distance (radius) from cell center that the code looks up to find data points when calculating the mean at the cell center;

e. Radon risk mapping required the calculation of a Radon Index (RI), which in the present work, was estimated following Barnet methodology (2008) based on the soil gas radon concentration and permeability given as low, medium or high. In the hypothesis of locally normal or log-normal distribution for soil gas radon data, the probability to be in an area with high Radon Index (P (hRI)) has been calculated using the following expression:

$$P(hRI) = \int_{C_p}^{\infty} \exp\left(-\frac{(x-\bar{x})}{2\times\sigma_g}\right) \times \frac{1}{\sigma_g \times \sqrt{2\pi}} \delta x \quad (1)$$

where $\bar{x}$ is the mean of soil gas radon concentration calculated at the cell center in the case of normal distribution or the logarithmic mean in case of lognormal distribution; σ_g is the standard deviation of the group of data considered in the case of normal distribution or the logarithmic standard deviation in case of lognormal distribution; C_p is the soil gas radon concentration threshold, given the permeability class, to be in the high radon index category (Table 1) if the distribution is normal or the ln (Cp) if the distribution is lognormal.

RESULTS AND DISCUSSION

Soil gas radon data from the Bolsena area presented in this work range between 7 and 176 kBq/m³ (Table 2). Table 3 reports a comparison of the data collected in the Bolsena area with data from other locations including regional, national and international places among those available from the literature. It can be observed that Bolsena mean data are intermediate with respect to other situations reported in Table 3. It can be seen that the arithmetic mean is twice the mean for Italy, while it appears very close to data from Ciampino–Marino (the Alban Hills), i.e., at the southernmost tips of the Latium Quaternary Volcanic complex, which is characterized by the same potassic and ultrapotassic volcanism as the Volsini Volcanic district (see Capaccioni et al. (2012) for details on the high radiation background in this area).

Table 2. Main statistics parameters of soil gas radon concentrations (kBq/m³) and the ln-transformed data (Bq/m³) considering the full database and the geological groups separately

	Total	Volcanic products	Alluvial	Ln-transformed data		
				Total	Volcanic products	Alluvial
Valid N	63	36	27	63	36	27
Mean	56.2	66.9	42.0	10.7	10.9	10.4
Median	52.4	66.2	36.9	10.9	11.1	10.5
Minimum	7.0	9.3	7.0	8.9	9.1	8.9
Maximum	176.0	176.0	90.9	12.1	12.1	11.4
1. Quartile	29.6	42.9	24.2	10.29	10.67	10.09
3. Quartile	75.6	86.3	63.2	11.23	11.36	11.05
SD	33.5	35.6	24.6	0.72	0.66	0.71
Skewness	0.93	0.81	0.49	−0.82	−1.13	−0.7
Excess Kurtosis	1.47	1.27	−0.73	0.33	1.53	0.048
p value S–W test[a]	0.0084	**0.1886**	**0.1257**	0.0055	0.0086	**0.0942**
p value *t* test		0.0028			0.0054	

[a]Shapiro–Wilk test

Table 3. Comparison of soil gas radon concentration (kBq/m³) obtained in the present work with those obtained in Italy and in the Czech Republic published in the literature

^{222}Rn (kBq/m³)	Mean	Median	Min	Max	SD	LQ	UQ
Italy[a]	26.6	13.7	0.4	1,200	39.5	5.5	32.6
Volcanic areas[a]	43.4	28.5	0.4	393.3	45.0	12.2	59.9
Bolsena (this work total database)	56.2	52.4	7.0	176.0	33.5	29.6	75.6
Ciampino–Marino[b]	52.0	30.5	1.5	367.3	47.2	23.3	64.8
Austria[c]	75		40	600			

Czech Republic[c]	28.1	–	1	1,664	40.4	–	–
Protezozoic-Paleozoic volcanites[d]	28.5	21.7	–	233.8	28.7	10.9	37.1
Tertiary volcanites[c]	21.14	16.20	–	197.2	25.8	6.90	26.0
France[c]	58.0			598	42.0		
Germany[c]	55.0		<5	>1,000			
Igneus rocks[c]	110.0		<5	>1,000			

[a]Beaubien et al. (2003)

[b]Etiope and Lombardi (1994)

[c]Dubois (2005)

[d]Barnet et al. (2008)

Figure 3a, b depicts the soil gas radon data, and the ln-transformed data obtained from Bolsena survey, respectively. The data reported in Fig. 3a shows two peaks, respectively, at about 30 and 60 kBq/m^3 which may suggest a bimodal distribution. This is expected to be observed in connection with two distinct geochemical matrices with different uranium–radium concentration levels: Soil gas radon detected in the two subsets will reflect both parent lithologies described by Nappi et al. (1982) and/or possibly different remobilization processes due to chemical weathering. This finding seems to be in agreement with the observations given by Cinelli (2012) who showed that Volsinian volcanic lithology in this area are typically characterized by high NORM content. In particular, according to the similarity observed between the soil gas radon from Bolsena and Ciampino–Marino previously mentioned, it seems reasonable to associate the lower level soil gas radon peak to the alluvial component and the higher one to the volcanic products, respectively, depicted in green and red in Fig. 3a and b.

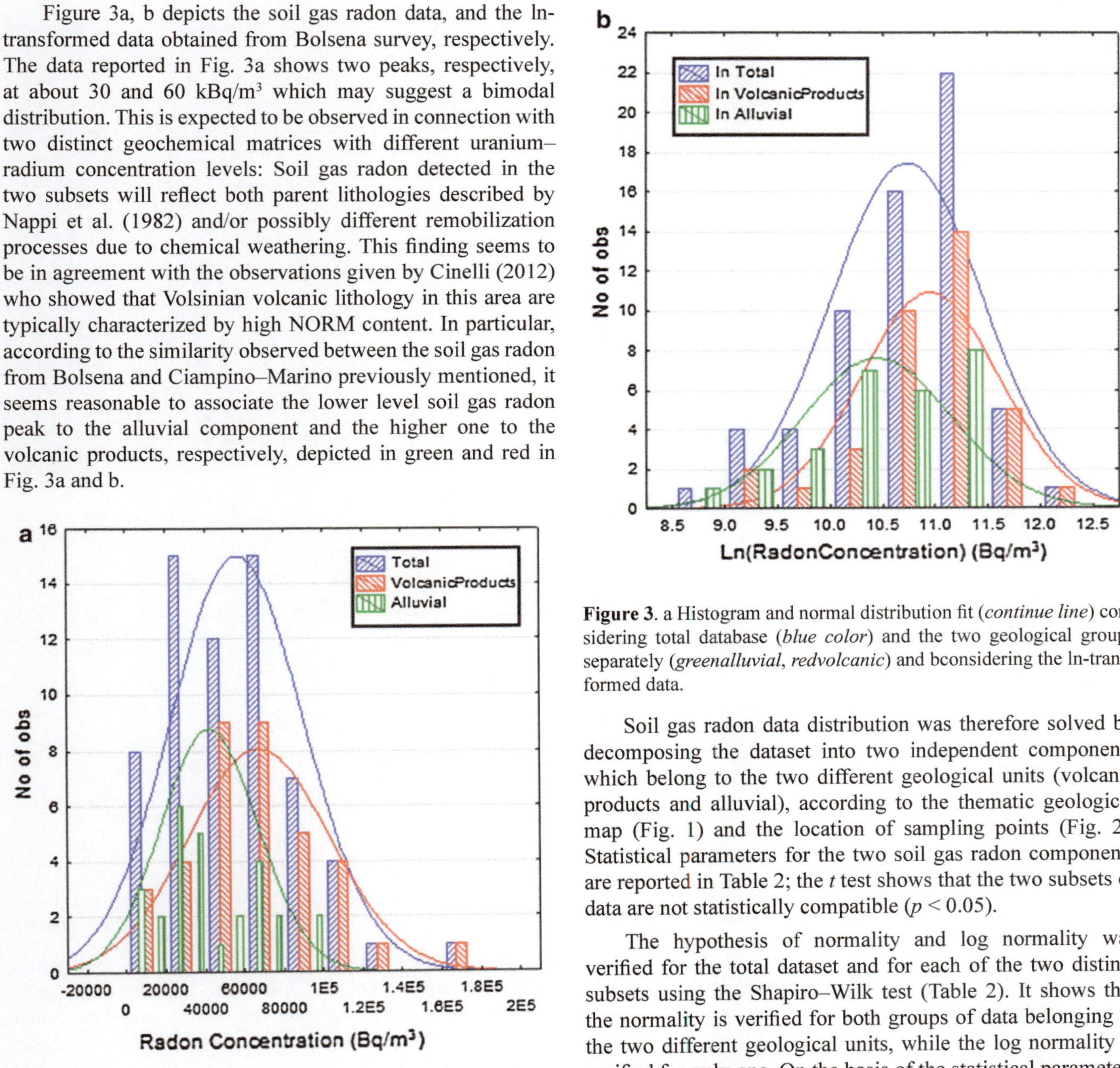

Figure 3. a Histogram and normal distribution fit (*continue line*) considering total database (*blue color*) and the two geological groups separately (*greenalluvial*, *redvolcanic*) and bconsidering the ln-transformed data.

Soil gas radon data distribution was therefore solved by decomposing the dataset into two independent components which belong to the two different geological units (volcanic products and alluvial), according to the thematic geological map (Fig. 1) and the location of sampling points (Fig. 2). Statistical parameters for the two soil gas radon components are reported in Table 2; the t test shows that the two subsets of data are not statistically compatible ($p < 0.05$).

The hypothesis of normality and log normality was verified for the total dataset and for each of the two distinct subsets using the Shapiro–Wilk test (Table 2). It shows that the normality is verified for both groups of data belonging to the two different geological units, while the log normality is verified for only one. On the basis of the statistical parameters (Table 2), the histograms (Fig. 3a, b) and the q–q plots (Fig. 4), the two subsets belonging to the two different geological units could be approximated with a normal distribution. The model distribution is used to evaluate the percentage of cases higher than Cp (Eq. 1). In this context, the bad fits to low-concentration data, or to data above *Cp*, have no consequence. The important point is that the model should correctly predict the quantile corresponding to *Cp*, which is reasonably achieved by the normal distribution.

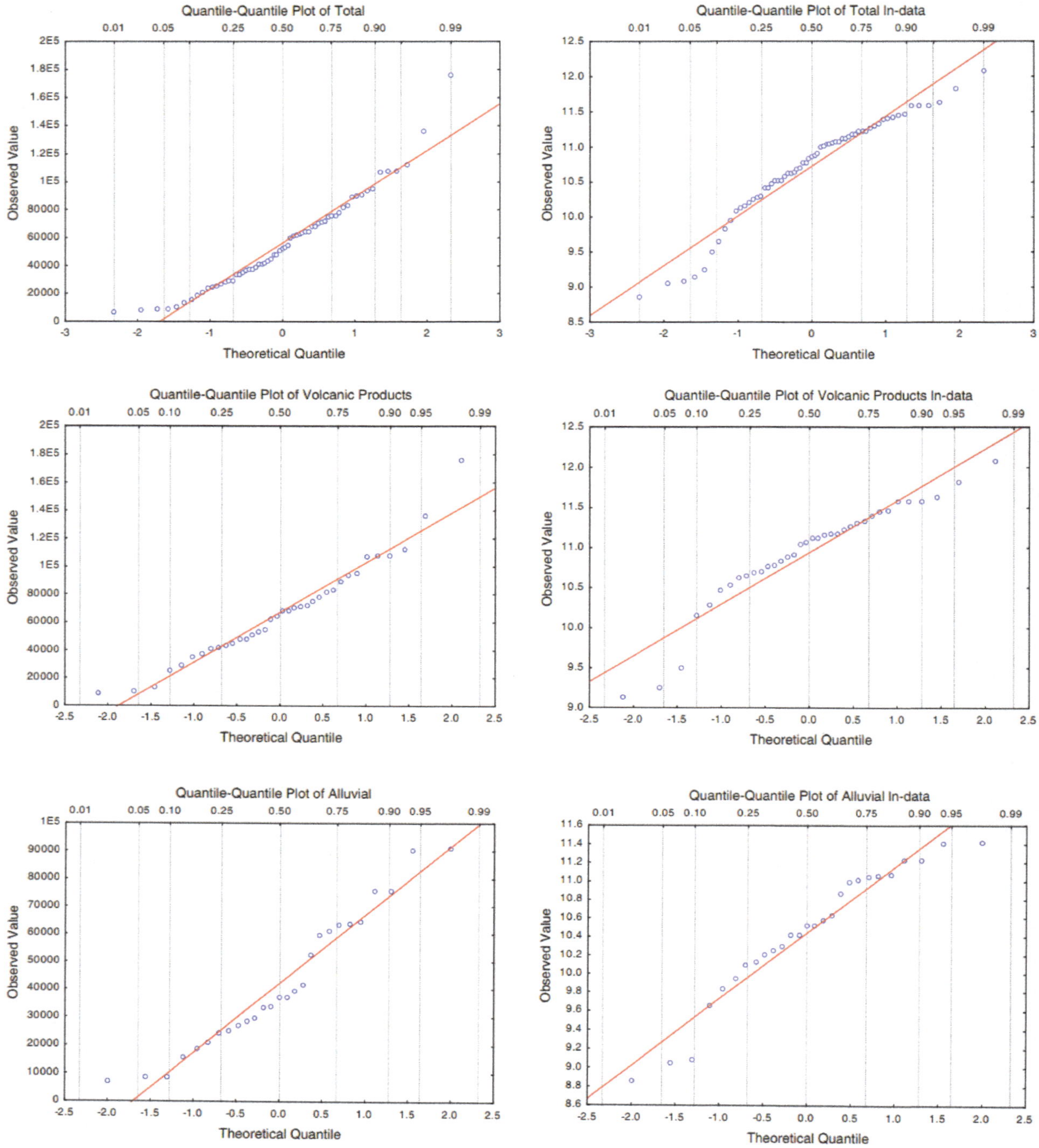

Figure 4. On the *left* normal quantile–quantile plots for soil gas radon concentrations (C) measured in the total, volcanic products and alluvial areas. On the *right* normal quantile–quantile plots for ln-transformed soil gas radon concentrations (C) measured in the total, volcanic products and alluvial areas.

Comparison between Experimental Results and Modeled Soil Gas Radon Data

For the sake of completeness, soil gas radon data measured in Bolsena were compared with the value estimated applying a soil-pore diffusion model proposed by Nero (1988) on the basis of the parent ^{226}Ra measured in a small set of soil samples by high-resolution γ-spectrometry. The model includes both diffusive and advective transport of radon and admits a simple analytical solution under the hypotheses of semi-infinite homogeneous isotropic soil, with a one-dimensional vertical steady-state transport. For a purely diffusive transport, assuming radon concentration to be negligible in free air, the models predicts a simple concentration profile versus depth in the soil:

$$C(z) \approx \left(1 - e^{z\sqrt{\lambda_{Rn}/D_e}}\right) \cdot C(-\infty) \qquad (2)$$

where C is the radon concentration in pores (Bq/m^3), D_e the effective diffusion coefficient (m^2/s), λ_{Rn} the decay constant of radon (s^{-1}), and $C(-\infty) = G/\lambda_{Rn}$, G being the volumetric radon generation rate in the soil pores (Bq m^{-3} s^{-1}) defined as follows

$$G = A_{Ra} \cdot \rho \cdot f \cdot \lambda_{Rn} \cdot \left(\frac{1-\varepsilon}{\varepsilon}\right) \tag{3}$$

where A_{Ra} is the activity concentration (Bq kg^{-1}) of ^{226}Ra, f the emanation factor (dimensionless), defined as the ratio between the radon activity emanating in the air-filled pores to the total radon production in the material, and ρ is the bulk density of the material (kg m^{-3}). The important parameters were set equal to: ρ 2,650 kg/m^3, ε 0.434, D_e 2 × 10^{-6} m^2/s for "normal" soil, 5 × 10^{-6} m^2/s for "dry" soil and 2 × 10^{-7} m^2/s for "wet" soil as proposed in Nero (1988), respectively. The ^{226}Ra activity was fixed equal to 142 Bq/kg, the average value of the activity concentrations measured in soil samples (132, 127, 169 Bq/kg) by γ-spectrometry analysis. The emanation coefficient was fixed equal to 0.33, measured by gamma spectrometry ad 1 minus the ratio between the mean specific activity of radon decay products ^{214}Pb and ^{214}Bi w.r.t. the parent ^{226}Ra (mean value of analyzed soil samples 0.25, 0.27 and 0.47). The concentration profile reported in Fig. 5 shows that the theoretical soil radon values, calculated in an ideal soil where only the diffusive transport is considered, at depth of 60–70 cm, are in good agreement with the average value of the measured data, i.e., about 56 kBq/m^3 (Table 2). However, the model is too much schematic to be used to replace soil radon measurements.

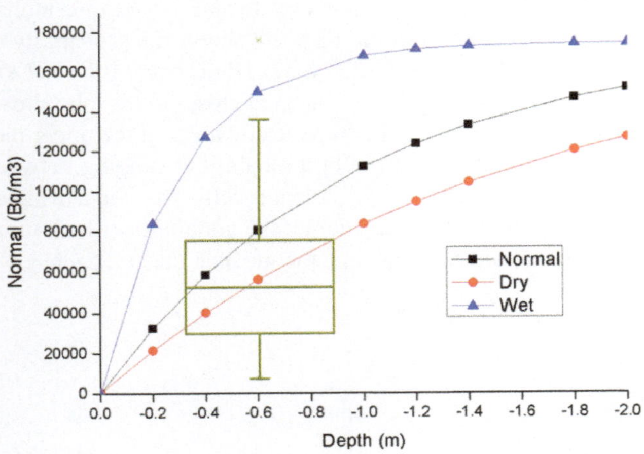

Figure 5. Calculated diffusive profile in an ideal soil, using ^{226}Ra activity and emanation coefficient from average soil samples. *Box–whisker* plots superimposed to modeled profiles represent the experimental soil gas radon data described in this work: The *box* ranges between 25/75th percentiles and the *whisker* coefficient is 1.5, while crosses indicate outliers.

Geostatistical Elaboration and Soil Gas Radon Concentration Mapping

Soil gas radon variograms have been elaborated both for the full database and for the two distinct geological groups previously extracted. They show significant statistical fluctuations; therefore, the choice of the variogram model is not obvious (see isotropic variograms in Fig. 6). Also anisotropic experimental variograms calculated using an angular tolerance of 30° show no variation with direction. As no spatial correlation is seen, the choice is oriented to the constant variogram model (pure nugget).

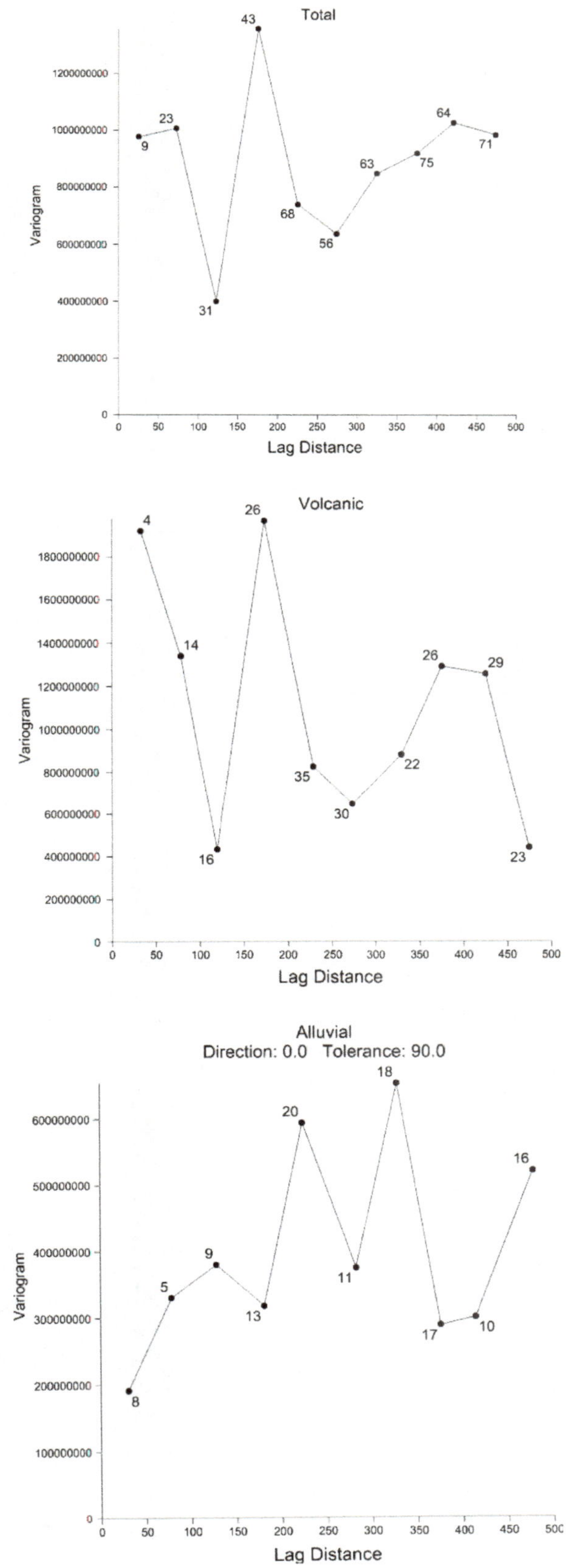

Figure 6. Empirical variograms of Rn concentration considering the total database and the two geological subgroups: volcanic and alluvial.

With this variogram model, soil gas radon maps were produced according to the methodology previously described in the "Radon mapping methodology". Figure 7 shows the mean soil gas radon concentration over 0.1 × 0.1 km cells across the sampled area.

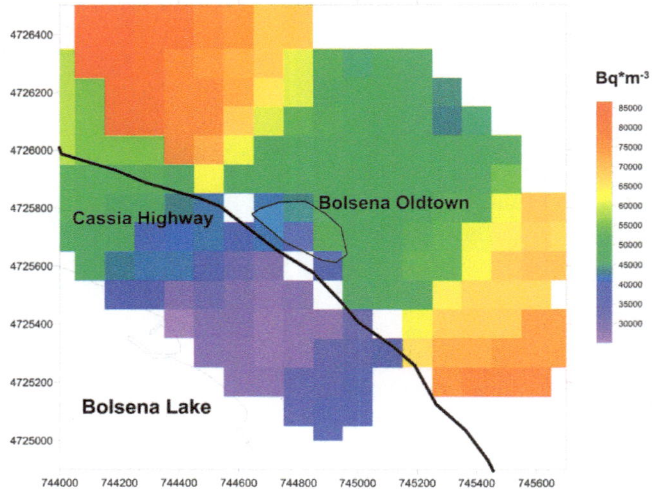

Figure 7. Map of soil gas radon concentrations in Bq/m³ based on geology and soil gas radon measurements.

The graphical output of the geostatistical elaboration clearly shows that the spatial distribution of the soil gas radon data locates the lower concentration levels near the lake in correspondence of likely alluvial areas, while higher concentrations are located close to the old Bolsena village in correspondence with the volcanic outcrops, in agreement with previous comments.

Radon Risk Assessment

The radon-related information collected cumulatively in Bolsena and in the Volsini Volcanic district suggests the need to assess the level of radon risk in this region. The soil gas radon and permeability data collected were therefore employed to calculate the probability of being in an area with high Radon Index (defined in 3.5 and Table 1) considering separately the two geological groups, alluvial and volcanic products. The soils of the examined area were designed as medium permeable soils on the basis of the measurements of the weight percentage of the fine fraction carried out on the representative soil samples (thus C_p = 70 kBq/m³ in Eq. (1)). As a consequence of the constant variogram model, the standard deviation σ_g of the whole geological group can be applied to the local subgroups (10–15 data) used to establish the cell mean concentration. Figure 8 shows the probability of being in an area of high Radon Index (PhRI) over 0.1 × 0.1 km cells across the studied area. The area closer to the lake shows a PhRI below 30 %, while the volcanic area, in the upper part of the map, is characterized by probabilities ranging between 30 % and 70 %. White color indicates cells where in a distance (radius) of 500 m from cell center the code did not look up to find 10 data points to calculate the mean at the cell center.

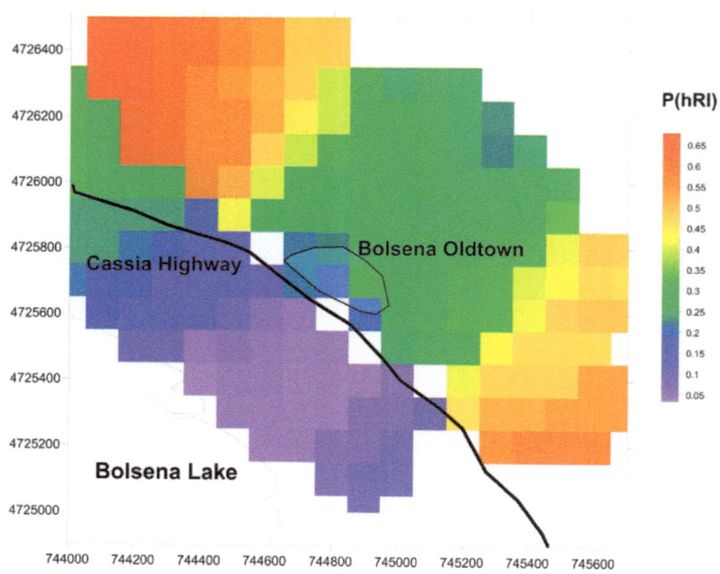

Figure 8. Map of probability to be in an area of high Radon Index—P(hRI) in %.

The central part of the volcanic area presents lower values than the external part. Observing Fig. 1, it can be noted that while the central part of the sampling area is characterized by products coming from the Bolsena volcanic complex, the external part is described by volcanic products from the Orvieto volcanic complex. Considering data from Bolsena and, respectively, Orvieto volcanic complexes soil gas radon concentration mean values of 64 and 80 kBq/m^3 can be found. Grouping together data measured in rocks coming from Bolsena and from Orvieto, the mean ^{226}Ra activity concentrations are 187 and 231 Bq/kg, respectively (Capaccioni et al.2012). Being the ^{226}Ra the precursor of radon, the highest ^{226}Ra activity concentration found in rocks from the Orvieto volcanic complex explains the higher value of soil gas radon concentrations in the lateral part (Orvieto complexes) and hence the higher percentage of high radon risk. We did not consider Bolsena and Orvieto as separate groups for mapping, because of the low number of data.

CONCLUSIONS

A series of sixty-three soil gas radon measurements were carried out in Bolsena, the principal urban settlement in the Volsini Volcanic district, characterized by a higher than average natural radioactivity background in connection with Quaternary potassic volcanic lithologies.

Soil gas radon concentration ranges between 7 and 176 kBq/m^3, indicating a large degree of variability in the NORM content and behavior of the parent soil material, related in particular to the occurrence of two different lithologies. The soil gas radon concentration measured in this study is consistent with the results of a calculation based on laboratory measurements of ^{226}Ra and emanation factor, using the schematic diffusion of Nero (1988).

Soil gas radon mapping confirmed the existence of two different areas: lower soil gas radon area, close to the lake of Bolsena is consistent with an alluvial lithology, while close to the old Bolsena village, there is a dominance of the acidic high radioactive contribution of volcanic rocks from the Vulsini district with higher soil radon.

The result of the radon risk assessment, based on soil gas radon and permeability data, is a map where the alluvial area is characterized by a probability of being in an area with high Radon Index lower than 20 %, while the probability is higher than 30 % in the northernmost part of the map characterized by volcanic products, until reaching a probability above 50 % in the external areas described by products from the Orvieto volcanic complex.

Considering these results, as well as the high indoor radon building found in the same area (Capaccioni et al. 2012), an appropriate action should be undertaken to prevent radon pollution in new buildings. Our maps are a first sketch of the definition of the areas which should be protected.

FOOTNOTES

[1]ICRP suggested (Publication 65, paragraph 76, 102) that Radon Prone Areas might be those parts of the country where at least 1 % of dwellings have radon levels more than ten times the national average as determined by appropriate statistical sampling (EC 1997).

[2]NORM: acronym for Naturally Occurring Radioactive Materials.

[3]More precisely, the Czech procedure applies to a given building site, and the radon concentration representative of the site is the third quartile of at least 15 measurements on the same site. Having done one single measurement per site, we take it as representative of the site.

ACKNOWLEDGMENTS

The authors wish to thank the two reviewers for their constructive comments which improved the manuscript. Riccardo Panzeri is thanked for his helpful work in situ. We would like to thank the inhabitants of Bolsena village, the public administration and in particular to Dr. Pietro Tamburini for their collaboration.

REFERENCES

1. Barnet, I., Pacherová, P., & Neznal, M. (2008). Radon in geological environment—Czech experience Czech Geological Survey Special Papers, No. 19, Prague, (pp. 19–28).
2. Beaubien, S. E., Ciotoli, G., & Lombardi, S. (2003). Carbon dioxide and radon gas hazard at the Alban hill area (Central Italy). *Journal of Volcanology and Geothermal Research, 123*, 63–80.
3. Bossew, P., Stojanovska, Z., Zunic, Z. S., & Ristova, M. (2013). Prediction of Indoor Radon Risk from Radium concentration in soil: Republic of Macedonia Case Study. *Romanian Journal of Physics* 58 (Suppl): S29–S43, Bucharest.
4. Capaccioni, B., Cinelli, G., Mostacci, D., & Tositti, L. (2012). Long-term risk in a recently active volcanic system: Evaluation of doses and indoor radiological risk in the quaternary Vulsini Volcanic District (Central Italy). *Journal of Volcanology and Geothermal Research, 247–248*, 26–36. doi:10.1016/j.jvolgeores.2012.07.014.
5. Cinelli, G. (2012). *Indoor and outdoor Natural Radioactivity in the Vulsini Volcanic District (central Italy): Estimation of radiological risk.* PhD thesis in Earth Science, University of Bologna. http://amsdottorato.unibo.it/4458/1/cinelli_giorgia_tesi.pdf.
6. Cinelli, G., Tondeur, F., & Dehandschutter, B. (2010). Development of an indoor risk map of the Wallon region of Belgium, integrating geological information. *Environmental Earth Sciences,62*, 809–819.
7. De Cort, M., Gruber, V., Tollefsen, T., Bossew, P., & Janssens, A. (2011). Towards a European Atlas of Natural Radiation: Goal, status and future perspectives. *Radioprotection, 46*, 737–743.
8. De Corte, F., Umans, H., Vandenberghe, D., De Wispelaere, A., & Van den Haute, P. (2005). Direct gamma-spectrometric measurement of the 226Ra 186.2 keV line for detecting 238U/226Ra disequilibrium in determining the environmental dose rate for the luminescence dating of sediments. *Applied Radiation and Isotopes, 63*, 589–598.
9. Dubois, G. (2005). An overview of radon surveys in Europe. Radioactivity environmental monitoring

emissions and health unit institute for environment and sustainability JRC—European commission 2005. EUR 21892 EN, EC.

10. Dubois, G., & Bossew, P. (2006). From babel to the round table of Camelot: On setting up a common language and objective for European radon risk mapping. Part I. Radon risk maps, different maps for different purposes. In: I. Barnet, M. Neznal, P. Pacherova (Eds.) *Proceedings of the 8th international workshop on the geological aspect of radon risk mapping*, pp. 39–48. 26–30 September 2006, Prague, Czech Republic.EC (European Commission) (1990). Commission recommendation 90/143/Euratom of 21 February 1990 on the protection of the public against indoor exposure to radon. Official Journal L-80 of 27/03/90. European Commission, Bruxelles.
11. EC (European Commission). (1996). Council Directive 96/29/Euratom of 13 May 1996 laying down basic safety standards for the protection of the health of workers and the general public against the dangers arising from ionizing radiation. Official Journal L-159 of 27/06/96. European Commission, Bruxelles.
12. EC (European Commission). (1997). Radiation Protection 88 Recommendations for the implementation of title VII of the European Basic Safety standards Directive (BSS) concerning significant increase in exposure due to natural radiation sources.
13. EC (European Commission). (2013). Council Directive 2013/59/Euratom of 5 December 2013 laying down Basic Safety Standards for Protection against the Dangers Arising from Exposure to Ionising Radiation. Official Journal L13 of 17/01/2014 European Commission, Bruxelles.
14. Eisenbud, M., & Gesell, T. (1997). Chapter 6: Natural radioactivity. In M. Eisenbud & T. Gesell (Eds.), *Environmental radioactivity* (pp. 134–200). London: Academic Press.
15. EPA (US Environmental Protection Agency). (1993). EPA Map of Radon Zones (Report 402-R-93-071) http://www.epa.gov/radon/zonemap.html. Accessed 13 June 2014.
16. Etiope, G., & Lombardi, S. (1994). Soil Gas ^{222}Rn in Sedimentary Basins in Central Italy: Its Implications in Radiation Protection Zoning. *Radiation Protection Dosimetry, 56*(1–4), 231–233.
17. García-Tavalera, M., García-Pérez, A., Rey, C., & Ramos, L. (2013). Mapping radon-prone areas using: Radiation dose rate and geological information. *Journal of Radiological Protection, 33*, 605–620.
18. Gillot, P. Y., Nappi, G., Santi, P., & Renzulli, A. (1991). Space-time evolution of the Vulsini Volcanic Complexes, central Italy. EUG VI, Strasburg, 24–28 March 1991. Terra abstract, 3–1, 446.
19. Gilmore, G. (2008). Practical gamma-ray spectrometry. Wiley.
20. Gruber, V., Bossew, P., De Cort, M., & Tollefsen, T. (2013a). The European map of the geogenic radon potential. *Journal of Radiological Protection, 33*, 51–60.
21. Gruber, V., Tollefsen, T., Bossew, P., & De Cort, M. (2013b). The European indoor radon map and beyond. *Carpathian Journal of Earth and Environmental Sciences, 8*(2), 169–176.
22. Isaaks, E. H., & Srivastava, R. M. (1989). *An introduction to applied geostatistics* (p. 561). New York: Oxford University Press.
23. Kemski, J., Klinger, R., Siehl, A., & Valdivia-Manchelo, M. (2009). From radon hazard to risk prediction-based on geological maps, soil gas and indoor measurements in Germany.*Environmental Geology, 56*, 1269–1279.
24. Kemski, J., Siehl, A., Stegemann, R., & Valdia-Manchego, M. (2001). Mapping the geogenic radon potential in Germany. *Science of the Total Environment, 272*(1–3), 217–230.
25. Langley, R. (1971). Practical statistics. Dover.
26. Miles, J. C. H., & Appleton, J. D. (2005). Mapping variation in radon potential both between and within geological units. *Journal of Radiological Protection, 25*, 256–276.
27. Nappi, G., Chiodi, M., Rossi, S., & Volponi, E. (1982). L'Ignimbrite di Orvieto nel quadro dell'evoluzione vulcanico-tettonica dei vulsini orientali caratteristiche geologiche e tecniche.*Bollettino della Società Geologica Italiana, 101*, 327–342.
28. Nappi, G., & Marini, A. (1986). I cicli eruttivi dei Vulsini Orientali nell'ambito della vulcano tettonica del complesso. *Member Social Geology Italy, 35*, 679–687.
29. Nappi, G., Renzulli, A., & Santi, P. (1991). Evidence of incremental growth in the vulsinian calderas (Central Italy). *Journal of Volcanology and Geothermal Research, 47*, 13–31.
30. Nappi, G., Renzulli, A., Santi, P., & Gillot, Y. P. (1995). Geological evolution and geochronology of the Vulsini volcanic district (central Italy). *Bollettino della Società Geologica Italiana, 114*, 599–613.
31. Nappi, G., & Valentini, L. (2005). Structural evolution of the Vulsini Volcanic District, (Central Italy). *Acta Vulcanologica, 17*(1–2), 81–94.
32. Nero, A. V., Jr. (1988) *Radon and its decay products in indoor air*. In: Nazaroff, W.W., Nero, A. V. Jr. (Eds.) NewYork: Wiley, pp. 1–53.
33. ORTEC. (2003). *Gamma-vision 32 A66-B32 user's manual*. ORTEC USA, Part No. 783620 Manual Revision D.
34. Porstendörfer, J. (1994). Properties and behavior of radon and thoron and their decay products in the air. *Journal of Aerosol Science, 25*(2), 219–263.
35. RAD7 Radon Detector. (2009). User manual, Durrige Company Inc.
36. Renzulli, A. (1988) Rilevamento geo-petrografico e studio geochimico del Complesso Vulcanico di Bolsena (Vulsini orientali): relazioni tra vulcanismo e magmatismo. Tesi di Laurea in Scienze Geologiche, Università degli Studi di Urbino, pp 201 (con carta geologica dell'area alla scala 1:12.500).
37. Stromswold, D. C. (1995). Calibration facilities for borehole and surface environmental radiation measurements. *Journal of Radioanalytical and Nuclear Chemistry, 194*(2), 393–401.

38. SURFER. (2012). User's guide, golden software.

39. UNSCEAR (United Nations Scientific Committee on the effects of Atomic Radiation). (2006). Sources and Effects of Ionizing Radiation. Report to General Assembly, Annex E, United Nations, New York, NY.

40. UNSCEAR (United Nations Scientific Committee on the effects of Atomic Radiation). (2008). Sources and effects of ionizing radiation. Report to General Assembly, Annex B, United Nations, New York.

41. WHO (World Health Organization). (2008).http://www.who.int/ionizing_radiation/env/radon/en/index.html.

CHAPTER 5

DEVELOPMENT OF A NEURAL NETWORK APPROACH TO CHARACTERISE 226RA CONTAMINATION AT LEGACY SITES USING GAMMA-RAY SPECTRA TAKEN FROM BOREHOLES

Adam Varley, Andrew Tyler, Leslie Smith and Paul Dale

Keywords: Borehole gamma spectroscopy, Radium contamination, Monte Carlo and Neural networks

INTRODUCTION

Origin and Regulation of Radium Contaminated Land

At the start of 20th century, radium was being used for a multitude of purposes, including medicines, confectionaries and what would prove to its most beneficial use: a seemingly unbroken light source known as "Undark" (Kathren, 1998). Since these early explorations, not only has our understanding improved into the radioactive emissions released by radium and its decay series but also the detrimental mechanisms with which they interact with living tissue (Rundo, 1993 and Paschoa, 1998). In the United Kingdom (UK), many redundant radium artefacts are now classified and controlled as low or intermediate level (HMSO, 1996).

Although the majority of radium production ended in the UK by the 1930's, radium salts were still imported for medical, industrial and military purposes into the 1960's (Tyler et al., 2013). In the absence of contemporary legislation, considerable quantities of highly radioactive radium waste were discarded by means of burial (Harvie, 1999). Only in 1960 was the use, keeping and disposal of radioactive sources controlled by statute through the Radioactive Substances Act 1960 and later the Radioactive Substances Act 1993 (HMSO, 1996). Examples of these legacy burial sites have also been identified in other parts of Europe and North America (Adams, 1993, Landa, 1993 and Adsley et al., 2004).

It has been conservatively estimated that in the UK alone there are between 150 and 250 Radium Contaminated Legacy Sites (RCLS), but the number could be closer to 1000 (DECC, 2012). Considering the possible extent of contamination and the risk to society they pose, legislation has now been passed in UK allowing environmental regulatory agencies to identify, assess and, if needs be, designate radioactively contaminated land (Tyler et al., 2013).

Characterisation of Radium Contamination

Following the potential identification of any land as being contaminated with radium, the land has to be accurately characterised providing a foundation for subsequent dose calculations and risk assessments. This will determine whether actions are required in terms of remediation. Estimates of the source's activity, burial depth and lateral extent must be provided. Furthermore, knowledge of the localised extent of the source can be instrumental in proposed remediation strategies.

Citation: Adam Varley, Andrew Tyler, Leslie Smith, Paul Dale, Development of a neural network approach to characterise 226Ra contamination at legacy sites using gamma-ray spectra taken from boreholes, Journal of Environmental Radioactivity, Volume 140, February 2015, Pages 130-140, ISSN 0265-931X, http://dx.doi.org/10.1016/j.jenvrad.2014.11.011.

Localised extent can be defined by source geometries where: the contamination can be considered more of a point source (in extreme cases referred to as a "hot" particle) or dissociated (or more appropriately an extended homogenous source). This will have implications on exposure pathways, transport processes, received dose and ultimately risk. In general, a point source (PS) is considered to be more hazardous, since human contact may result in a much higher dose than extended homogenous source (EHS) of similar activity. In the scenario where the risk a PS poses is considered too high, it should either be removed and disposed of or isolated to prevent human exposure (Dale et al., 2008). However, areas of contamination cannot always be categorised as singular PS or EHS. Often, many PS of similar activity (usually low activity) can be identified, either attributed to a number of small radioactive items or larger items mechanically broken up (Patton et al., 2013). This eventuality can be thought of as a Heterogeneous Source (HS), but separating HS from EHS via non-invasive methods can be very challenging. The aim of this work is to characterise highly radioactive PS.

Detection of Radium Contamination

For the most part, *in situ*, mobile and airborne gamma-spectrometry are the workhorses for large scale radioactive contamination land characterisation as alternative analytical methods tend to be expensive and time consuming, and can often be unrepresentative (Aage et al., 1999, Guillot, 2001, IAEA, 2003, Tyler, 2008 and Kock et al., 2012). The majority of this research has been focussed on ^{137}Cs detection for extended sources (Tyler et al., 1996, Boson et al., 2009 and Carrazana González et al., 2012) and "hot" particle detection (Maučec et al., 2004a, Davies et al., 2007 and Tyler et al., 2010). Up to now, however, very few researchers have focussed their efforts on characterising RCLS (Thummerer and Jacob, 1998, Adsley et al., 2004 and Haddad et al., 2014). Yet, with an increasing awareness of the potential number of contaminated sites in existence, it is essential that efficient methods be developed for their rapid and accurate characterising.

At any RCLS, the principal contaminant tends to be ^{226}Ra and its progeny which is a reflection of the long half-life of ^{226}Ra and its persistence in the environmental. Direct gamma-spectrometry of ^{226}Ra in the environment is challenging as it only has one relatively weak low energy gamma ray from which to infer its activity (186 keV). Subsequently its daughter products (^{214}Bi and ^{214}Pb) are conventionally used as a proxy measure. However, this can be inherently problematic as secular equilibrium is not always encountered as a result of ^{222}Rn emanation. To address this issue, many studies assume the fulfilment of equilibrium introducing systematic uncertainty to any ^{226}Ra activity estimations (Thummerer and Jacob, 1998 and Hendriks et al., 2001). Before reliable approximations of depth, activity and localised distribution of ^{226}Ra can be made, four inherent confounding factors must first be respected:

- If the photon flux received by a detector is low, gaining acceptable counting uncertainty on the measurement can be impractical.
- ^{226}Ra and daughter products form part of the ^{238}U decay series where concentration variations can vary considerably over the scale of meters.
- As a source is buried an exponential decrease in unscattered photons is observed with the vast majority of photons that reach the detector being scattered.
- At energies below 150 keV, photons, although numerous, tend to undergo photoelectric absorption making the composition of the geological matrix an important control on photon flux (Tyler, 1999 and Tyler, 2008). Backscattered photons (<250 keV) can also be challenging to interpret.

These factors, acting in combination, influence the confidence with which a source in the presence of a typically heterogeneous background radiation field can be resolved. Moreover, once a source has been identified, considerable uncertainties relating to its localised extent and activity can remain. It is for these reasons *in situ* and mobile gamma-spectroscopy of ^{226}Ra PS, below observed activity thresholds (<70 MBq), is considered impractical below depths of about 70 cm. This is because the majority of the source signal, particularly the intense low energy peaks below 609 keV, is enveloped by background noise with increasing source depth. Measurements beyond this depth must therefore be addressed with borehole measurements (Wilson and Conaway, 1991,Meisner et al., 1995, Adsley et al., 2004 and Bugai et al., 2005).

The Borehole Measurement

Borehole measurements are customarily taken as a depth series, when the detector is lowered into the borehole. Ensuing spectra can then provide knowledge into layers of contamination if sufficient spatial coverage is performed to validate extrapolation (Adsley et al., 2004 and Bugai et al., 2005). Otherwise, the shape and magnitude of standalone spectra offer insight into localised source arrangements (Giles and Dooley, 1998). Subtle changes occurring within the spectrum's overall shape, suggestive of alterations in source geometry and activity, could potentially correspond to the presence of contamination. Identifying such changes is invaluable in the search for hazardous "hot" particles in close proximity of the borehole (Wilson et al., 1997). For a detailed review of borehole measurements refer to Kobr et al. (2005).

The source geometries, Extended Homogeneous source (EHS), Point Source (PS) and for completeness Heterogeneous Source (HS) are illustrated alongside the detector in a borehole geometry (Fig. 1). First consider a PS, where *D* is the mass thickness of shielding (g cm^{-2}) and is its angle perpendicular to the axis of detector. The measure mass thickness was preferred over Euclidean distance, since it takes into account the amount of shielding, related to the density of soil, which can significantly vary with depth and lateral position (Tyler, 2008). Secondly, an EHS can be described by *Ed* indicating its vertical depth with its midpoint at the centre of the detector's active volume. For completeness the final geometry HS, is a differing number of PS at variable *D* from the detector; this eventuality will be considered by this study as EHS.

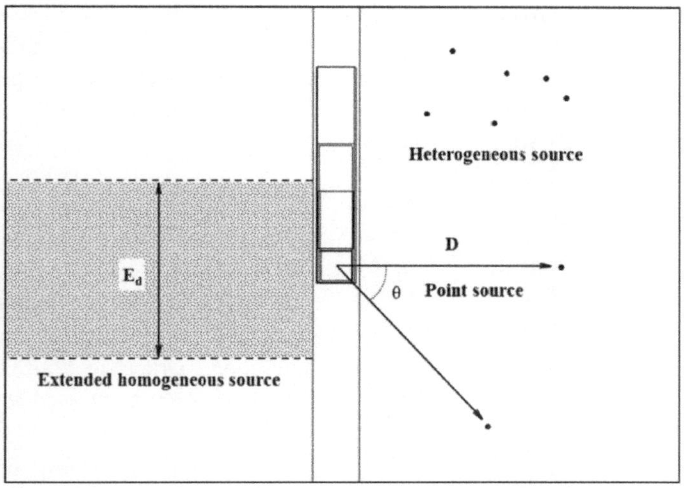

Figure 1. Cross-section of the detector in the borehole including the source geometries of interest: Extended homogeneous source, Point source and Heterogeneous source.

Exploring the parameters, *Ed* and *D*, as spectral shape drivers is the fundamental aim of this study. Nevertheless, other parameters known to influence spectral shape, although not the primary focus in this study, such as soil density and the constituent that make up background must be added by way of assessing the uncertainties that will be introduced to any conclusions of activity and geometry.

Spectral Processing

Without contamination present, changes in the shape and magnitude of borehole spectra will almost exclusively be due to deviations in background activity (^{40}K, ^{238}U series and^{232}Th series) and shielding influences brought about by changes in soil density and composition (Fig. 2). If a site is contaminated, it is the fundamental goal of a surveyor to differentiate between these benign background fluctuations in spectral shape and those initiated by the presence of ^{226}Ra contamination, particularly presented from a PS at great distance from the detector. However, establishing information from spectra that have relatively sparse counts contributed from contamination can be very difficult. Additionally, in most cases there is likely to be a continuum of activities, shielding arrangements and source geometries within contaminated sites resulting in a similar continuum of detector response (Wei et al., 2010). Therefore, characterisation methods applied for ^{226}Ra contamination must be robust enough to cope with fluctuations in background but at the same time be sensitive enough to provide reliable estimates of activity and depth (Fig. 2).

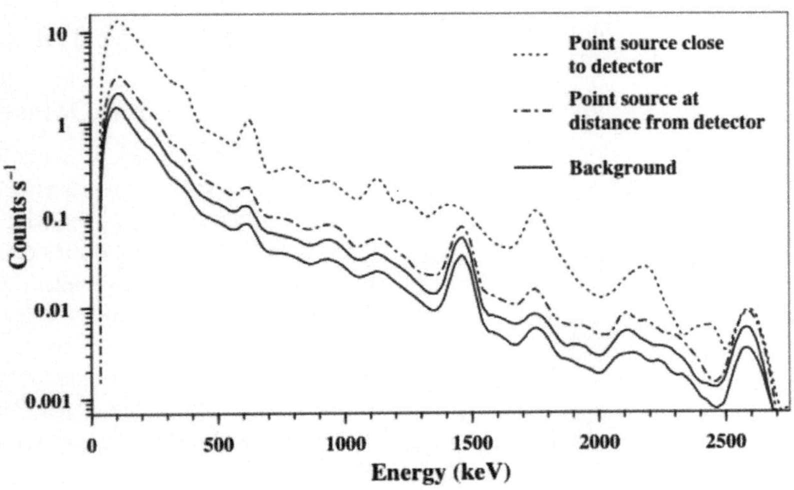

Figure 2. Changes in spectral shape brought about by the introduction of a point source at different distances from the detector. Note the similarity in signal presented by a point source at distance and typical background spectra.

The important spectral unfolding process, providing insight into relative spectral contributions, is not an instructive one and firstly requires extensive knowledge of the individual detectors response to known source geometries which must be provided by a robust calibration procedure. Complications often arise when trying to account for, by analytical calibration methods, the extensive environmental scenarios that can lead to spectral changes particularly for extended sources. Monte Carlo simulations (MCS) present a more suitable way to account for environmental variables such as density, soil composition and source geometry (Forster et al., 1990 and Hendriks et al., 2002).

Once a dynamic calibration dataset has been collected, relating it to field observations can be problematic. A commonly applied method of interpreting the signal from a detector is gross counting. This approach provides only a relative measure of the total flux of photons (or dose rate) and little information of source distribution since energy discrimination is not performed (Adsley et al., 2004). A more adequate method that relies on the differential attenuation of two or more of the numerous intense full energy peaks, ^{214}Bi (609, 1120, 1764 and 2240 keV) and to a lesser extent ^{214}Pb (295, 351 keV), can be used to establish the amount of shielding between the source and detector (Miller et al., 1994, Trnková et al., 2010 and Haddad et al., 2014). However, the method can be severely hindered by the need to strip out background counts and poor counting statistics, often peaks in low-resolution detectors cannot be formed. Alternatively, a more sophisticated approach, coined "Full Spectral Analysis", can be applied. This method attempts to add linear combinations of calibration data to the vast majority of the channels of a field spectrum by a Poisson weighted least squares fitting procedure (Hendriks et al., 2001 and Maučec et al., 2004b) or Non-negative least squares algorithm (Caciolli et al., 2012 and Guastaldi et al., 2013) followed by a χ^2 goodness of fit test. Unfortunately, this method requires sufficiently low counting uncertainty across the spectrum to reliably fit individual spectral contributions; a scenario that is not always obtainable in the field. Moreover, fitting calibration spectra for this application may become complicated by the fact there is a continuum of contamination and multiple source distribution under investigation.

It is well understood that gamma-spectrometry data taken from the environment will contain similarities in spectral shape, or, more precisely, channels will regularly exhibit correlation from one measurement to next. This will be predominantly due to background contributions to each individual spectrum (Fig. 2). Difficulties can arise when trying to apply conventional statistical approaches to a dataset when this redundant cross-channel correlation has not been taken into consideration (Fagan et al., 2012). Principal Component Analysis (PCA) is a method commonly used to explore the underlying structure of a multivariate dataset and was employed in this study to contend with variation in background.

The mathematical derivation (Hotelling, 1933 and Chatfield and Collins, 1980) and in depth discussions regarding the different implementation of PCA (Hovgaard, 1997 and Runkle, 2006) can be found in the literature. Essentially, PCA multiplies the spectral matrix by its, mean-centred, singular value decomposed matrix producing a set of uncorrelated variables. Generally the first few sets of loadings associated with their corresponding Principal components (PCs) of the decomposed matrix can then be considered as representative of the source signal and can be set aside for further statistical analysis (Im et al., 2007). Another convenient outcome of the PCA process is that the number of dimensions is significantly reduced as lower order elements are generally discounted as noise contributions.

The second step utilised the pattern recognition capabilities of a Neural Network (NN) to classify source geometry and approximate activity, mass depth (*D*) and vertical depth (*Ed*) from higher order PCs. The basic design framework of neural networks (NNs) is analogous to the human brain and they have been used to solve many complex non-linear problems across a variety of fields including gamma-ray spectroscopy (Yoshida et al., 2002, Dragovic et al., 2005 and Dragović et al., 2006). They have even been used to map counts directly to activity and source burial depth (Wei et al., 2010).

An NN is composed of a number of processing units known as nodes that are, by convention, separated into three distinct layers: the input, hidden and output. The input layer is a collection of the nodes defining the explanatory variables of the problem. The hidden layer can in fact be made up of one or more layers and the output layer, contains the desired response variables. The hidden layer provides the NN the ability to learn non-linear transformations. Each node has its own weight set, with the weights defining the strength of the connections between neurons in adjacent layers (Yoshida et al., 2002). The weights are established during a training phase where the error between predicted outputs and desired output of the specified training set is minimised in an iterative fashion (Medhat, 2012). For a detailed review of the workings of NNs refer to Gurney (2003).

The aims of this study were:

- Investigate whether PS and EHS can be distinguished from each other in the borehole geometry.
- Apply optimised method to an RCLS providing estimates of activity and source distribution.

MATERIALS AND METHODS

Field Site: Headland Dataset

Dalgety bay, Fife, Scotland, is a former military site where wartime and post-wartime activities have led to specific areas of the site becoming associated with ^{226}Ra contamination (Tyler et al., 2013). Following the sites decommissioning a new town was built on the area (also called Dalgety Bay) with a Sailing club located on the on the west coast where much of the radium contamination was believed to be deposited (Fig. 3). Public access along the coast provide the opportunity for the general public to come into contact with potentially harmful sources via either direct contact, ingestion or inhalation (Dale et al., 2008 and Tyler et al., 2013).

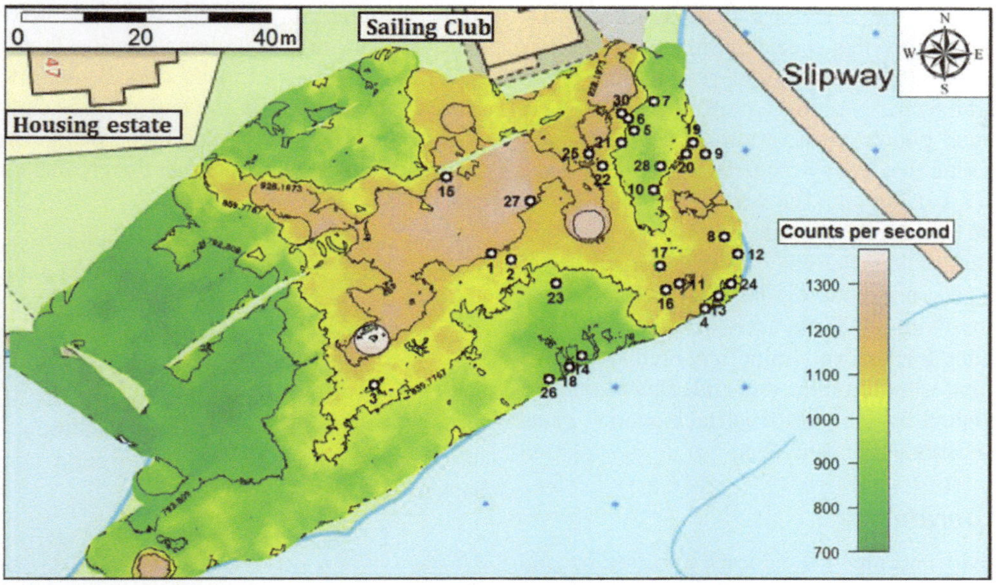

Figure 3. Maps of the headland with gross counts using a 76 × 76 mm handheld Lanthanum bromide detector overlaid. The surface was interpolated using ordinary Kriging. Locations and numbers of boreholes have been included.

An intrusive survey was undertaken and borehole measurements were obtained from an area on the headland around the sailing club previously suspected of having contamination at depths beyond the capabilities of conventional surface measurements (Tyler et al., 2011). Cores were not necessarily concentrated around the highest surface signal as indicated by the *in situ* survey (Fig. 3), as surface sources and contaminated material were recovered from many of these locations. Another feature is a large proportion of the cores were situated either on the edge of the headland and around the main sailing clubhouse (middle top) as re-deposition of contamination by sea erosion and contact with the general public were the primary concerns of the original survey.

Due to the heterogeneous composition of the soil matrix, a relatively small diameter auger (60 mm diameter) was used since penetration into the contaminated site with an auger with a larger diameter was likely to have been unviable. A total 30 augered holes with varying depths (0.2–1.6 m) were taken over identified hotspots and a 51 × 51 mm Sodium iodide (NaI:Tl) detector, encased in plastic tubing, was lowered into each hole. Spectra with 1024 channels representing an energy range of 20–3000 keV were recorded using Ortec›s Maestro software, at 0.1 m depth intervals for at least 600 s to attain reasonable counting statistics. This dataset is referred to as the "Headland dataset" (HD) for the remaining discussions.

Monte Carlo

Monte Carlo codes offer a robust alternative to either labour intensive and expensive experimental calibration or mathematically cumbersome deterministic approaches (Stromswold, 1995 and Maučec et al., 2009). For example, acquiring representative laboratory spectra can be hindered by the need to strip out the laboratory background which can vary slightly over long acquisition times due to problems of radon exhalation. This can, for example, introduce significant error when using relatively weak calibration sources at large distances. Field calibration although more characteristic of the background at the HD site presents practical problems of burying the source and being confident of its distance from the detector and the exact amount of shielding (i.e. density of soil) between the source and the detector. Numerous studies, facing similar challenging calibration situations, have opted for and successfully applied Monte Carlo Simulations (MCS) to a variety of environmental measurements (Maučec et al., 2004a and Allyson and Sanderson, 1998). The code used in this study was Monte Carlo N-Particle eXtented (MCNPX) (Briesmeister, 1993).

MCNPX Optimisation

The simulations used in this study only retained key features of the NaI:Tl detector, such as the active volume, aluminium outer canning and protective plastic piping, since this was found to accurately account for scattering within the real detector. Beck's "standard" soil composition was used for all simulations since the actual soil composition was not known (Beck et al., 1972). Decay data was obtained from the National Nuclear Data Centre (2013) and only emissions with relative abundance of 1% were used in the simulations for all radionuclides.

Although MCS possess clear advantages over conventional calibration procedures, there is a major drawback, in that the time it can take to obtain acceptable uncertainty on average particle fluxes can be unfeasible (Likar et al., 2004). This is because each particle must be tracked from birth until death where during its lifetime a large number of irrelevant interactions take place consuming computer time. Although there are a number of accessible variance reduction techniques available to use in MCNPX, for example population control methods, if the modeller does not exercise considerable precaution, bias can be introduced to the final tally results (Allyson, 1994 and Serov et al., 1998).

This study used a more straightforward procedure. Firstly Multigroup/adjoint calculations were utilised, to estimate the vertical and lateral extent needed to accurately reconstruct an entire environmental spectrum from extended sources;

commonly described as the detector's Field Of View (De Groot et al., 2009). In short, this special treatment of photons sees the problem effectively reversed, with photons starting in the detector and gaining energy until a cut off of 2614 keV (the highest environmental photon energy) was reached (Maučec et al., 2004b). Covering the density range that was likely to be present at the site (1.1–1.8 g cm^{-2}), it was found that the soil thickness needed to accurately recreate a borehole spectrum was 0.5 m above and below the detector 0.55 m parallel to the borehole. After this, a method outlined by Hendriks et al. (2002) was used involving only electrons in close proximity to the detector being tracked and sampling bremsstrahlung energies for those that were terminated outside this proximity. This was accomplished by the use of surface source write/ surface source read cards within MCNPX.

Benchmark Experiments

To validate the code defining the geometry, materials and response of the detector a benchmark investigation to a known source geometry and activity was undertaken. At the time of measurement, no borehole calibration facility was available. A set of flat concrete pads doped with ^{40}K, ^{238}U and ^{232}Th geared more towards *in situ* and airborne calibration were used instead. The MCNPX Gaussian Energy Broadening (GEB) feature was used to reconstruct the broadened peaks generated by the detector.

Spectra from the concrete calibration pads and MCS are in good agreement (Fig. 4). The^{232}Th and ^{238}U pads were reproduced well. Minor discrepancies were found in the simulated Compton continuum of the ^{40}K pad where it was overestimated compared to the pad, this was noted by another study (Hendriks et al., 2002). This is likely to be caused by the different positions of pads at the calibration facility resulting in incomplete removal of background contribution by the background pad.

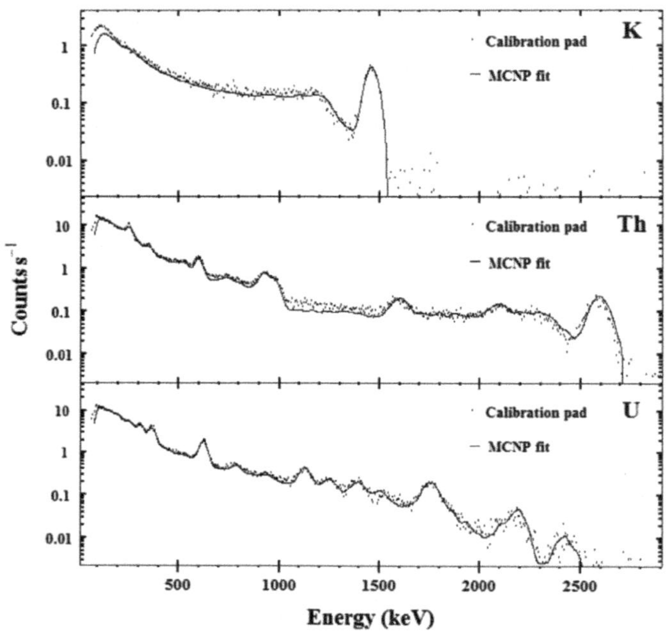

Figure 4. Benchmark experiment results showing MCNPX fitted data (lines) to calibration pad (Potassium, Thorium and Uranium) data (dots).

Spectral Compilation

Before any spectral interpretation of the HD could be performed, enough data spanning the range of environmental variables thought to be present at the site had to be generated so as to embody the relevant spectral shapes. Additionally, establishing the overall spread of the spectral population obtained by sensibly varying model parameters provides uncertainty estimates for any conclusions made about the parent source distribution. This step is also essential prior to training an NN as extrapolations outside of datasets are known to be very unreliable (Moreira et al., 2010).

This procedure could not be performed purely in MCNPX because of time constraints, because on average it took approximately 4 h for each simulation to attain acceptable statistical uncertainty even with optimisation. Instead a resampling procedure of a discrete range of MCNPX generated spectra, encompassing only changes in source geometry and density variation, was undertaken. This permitted more straightforward parameters, such as spectral drift and relative spectral contribution (or activity) to be sampled and adjusted afterwards allowing a larger and more robust spectral dataset to be produced. The rest of this section details this methodology.

All source and background spectra were simulated within MCNPX covering representative densities from 1.1 to 1.8 g cm^{-3} with intervals of 0.1 g cm^{-3}, typical of the densities range found within the cores taken at the site. Energies below 300 keV were disregarded to avoid systematic uncertainties associated with variations in geological matrix (Hendriks et al., 2002 and Caciolli et al., 2012). Fig. 5A demonstrates good agreement in count rate below 300 keV between MCS and field spectra "28 90 cm" although this was not the case for spectra obtained. Good agreement in spectral shape was nonetheless maintained above 300 keV for the remaining measurements.

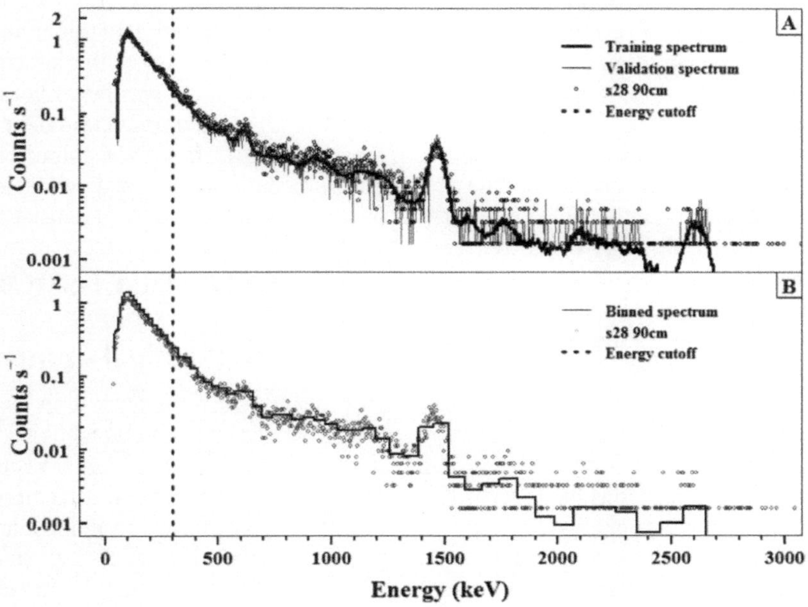

Figure 5. A) Example simulated background alongside a field measurement taken from core 28 at 90 cm. Note that the "Training spectrum" is far more statistically defined than either the Poisson noise induced "Validation spectrum" and "s28 90 cm". B) Full Width at Half Maximum binning intervals used on all spectra.

A base count rate of ~24 counts per second (for the energy range above 300 keV) was used as the mode count rate of a lognormal distribution established from a background core with minimum and maximum count rates of 13 and 65 counts s^{-1} respectively. Whilst the probability of reaching background count rates of 65 counts s^{-1} was considered extremely unlikely at Dalgety bay headland, it was thought best to take a conservative approach with the little spatial coverage of background data that was available. Although, this would raise the limit of detection and uncertainty on final activity and depth predictions the spectral shape recognition capabilities of the proposed method was anticipated to negate such fluctuations. Relative contributions from each of the natural decay series were found to be reasonable well correlated within background cores demonstrated by Pearson's linear correlation coefficient above 0.8. This deviation was accounted for within the model.

The background dataset was then spiked using selected simulated source spectra of corresponding density and a randomly sampled activity. Spectral drift was introduced into each spectrum by sampling a Gaussian distribution with a standard deviation of 3 keV (at 1461 keV) typically found within the temperature and magnetic field variations within the environment for the detector in question. The MCS were recorded to a much higher statistical accuracy, typically >95%, to form the "Training dataset (Fig. 5). Field results were known to have a greater noise element due to the limited counting time and detector volume (Minty and Hovgaard, 2002). Accordingly, Poisson noise was introduced into individual bins depending on a sampled count rate (>600 s). The addition of noise established the "Validation dataset" and was considered to be more representative of the error structure of the HD (Fig. 5A).

Clearly using over 1000 energy bins presents a large relative variation within individual bins from one spectrum to the next, particularly as counts become sparse at higher energies. To reduce this surplus noise without too much loss of energy distinction, the energy range 300–2918 keV was irregularly binned according to the estimated Full Width at Half Maximum established using the same Gaussian Energy Broadening model fit implemented in MCNPX (Briesmeister, 1993). Higher energy spectral features can be observed more easily as the sparse nature of counts is diminished, for instance the ^{208}Th (2614 keV) and ^{214}Bi (1764 keV) peaks (Fig. 5B). Conversely, at low energy where the FWHM is lower spectral structure is not lost, observe the low energy ^{214}Bi (609 keV) can still be observed.

All relevant sample data: source Activity (*A*), PS depth (*D*) and vertical depth (*Ed*) was recorded for individual spectra. PCA was then carried out on the combined simulated dataset and HD to allow comparison. All steps mentioned were carried out using the base features in the software package R (R Development Core Team, 2012).

Neural Network: Training Procedure

To optimise the performance of the NN and ensure that the trained network was learning general patterns within the problem rather than adapting to the training data itself, three separate data sets were produced: the training set, a test set and cross validation set (Dragovic et al., 2005). All datasets were mean centred and scaled relative to the variance. Initially, each NN was trained and tested with statistically defined MCNP spectra (spectral drift was added to ensure SCs remained similar). The essential stage of cross validation was performed using data with Poisson noise introduced "Validation dataset" which was known to be more characteristic of the noisy HD (Fig. 5). The transformation used in the hidden layer was a sigmoidal function and the algorithm used to train the network was resilient backpropogation (Riedmiller and Braun, 1993). The R package RSNNS was used to construct and train all NNs (Bergmeir and Benítez, 2012).

The architecture of an NN may be different from one problem to the next depending on the problem's level of complexity. It was discovered early on to reach the optimised level of performance for this problem it was better to divide the procedure into three separate networks since this eliminated crosstalk effects between the output neurons specifying the activity and depth parameters of an EHS and a PS. The first NN's purpose was to classify spectra into one of the three classes: background, EHS or PS. The final networks were then used to make estimates regarding activity (kBq or Bq kg^{-1}), burial depth (g cm^{-2}) and lateral extent (cm). Crucially, they were only trained and tested with spectra that were identified by the classification network. To ensure that the correct architecture for each network was selected an exhaustive search was conducted to: establish the number of PCs to use in the input layer, the number of hidden nodes and hidden layers, and the number of learning epochs. Decisions made regarding the design of the network were based around minimising the error within the validation dataset. This was checked again using confusion matrices for classification results (Zell et al., 1993) and R^2 values for any regression results produced by the EHS and PS networks (Moreira et al., 2010). Between 1000 and 2000 training data were found to adequately train all the networks. Test and validation sets were 30% of the training set.

Uncertainty on regression results was estimated by resampling the predicted output values 50 times using the original background parameters. These values were then fed back into the original network alongside the training data and the standard deviation of the injected values was used as the uncertainty. Caution was taken not to bias the latent variables used by PCA with introduction of new values, since this would have influenced final NN outputs. To avoid this eventuality the procedure was looped where error spectra values were introduced into the original dataset one at a time.

RESULTS AND DISCUSSION

Analysis of Principal Components

90% of the total variance within the dataset was explained by the first 5 principal components, which suggests the latter PCs possess largely noise elements. Visual analysis of the PC 1 and PC 2 loadings demonstrates the merit of the PCA transform: at this early stage of analysis point source effective depth is being separated within PC space with shielding thickness variation (Fig. 6). This is confirmed by the shallow point source depth (larger lighter points towards the bottom of the plot), in contrast to deeper sources (smaller darker points) towards the top left of the plot. Interestingly, distance from the background pack (Crosses) would appear to infer activity.

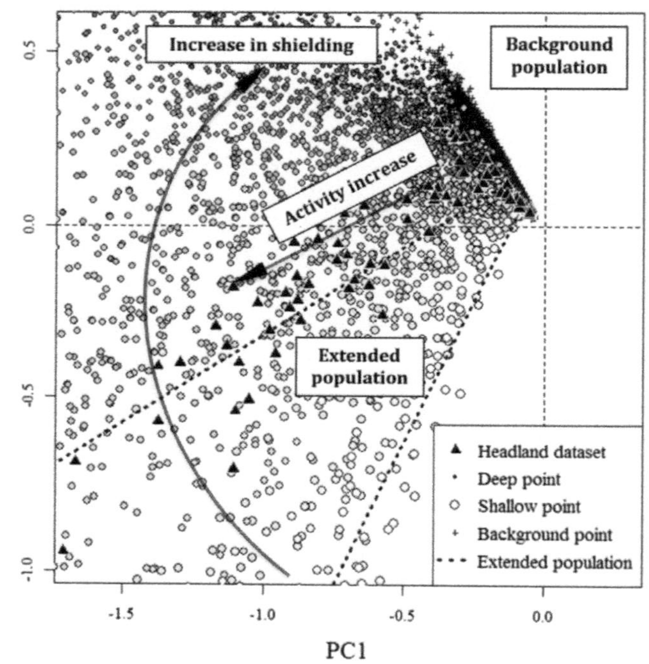

Figure 6. Plot of Principal components 1 and 2 loadings. Background spectra (Black crosses) are tightly clustered in the top right of the plot. Differing sizes and shades of circular points indicate varying thicknesses of shielding and greater distance from the background pack infers greater activity. The extended population are bound by the black dotted lines. The headland dataset are represented by black triangles.

Arguably conventional separation techniques, such as a Mahalanobis distance metric could be used to delineate a boundary between source and background (Runkle, 2006). Moreover, a linear regression between PC1 and PC2 could be performed to establish a relationship with depth and activity (Adams et al., 2012). However, a number of problems may be encountered using these approaches. Firstly, separation via parametric methods (i.e. Mahalanobis distance) invariably contains a distribution-based assumption, normally a multivariate Gaussian distribution, to define separation limits from the background dataset. This assumption is often not correct leading to misclassification. Secondly and most crucially, separation of the extended source population, encompassed by the black lines in Fig. 6, from point sources in the intermediate range (2–20 g cm^{-2}) is not possible through a linear regression technique, and this is of particular importance since a large proportion of the HD lie within this region. Furthermore analyses of lower order PCs, using a similar approach, becomes increasingly challenging. This suggests that to reliably separate extended sources from point sources more information from lower order PCs is needed but the relationship is likely to be non-linear. To confront these issues three separate NN were used to establish structure within the PC loadings.

Classification Network

The first NN was used to classify spectra into one of the three classes. It was established by using the first 5 PCs, a hidden layer with 16 neurons and 1500 learning epochs gave the smallest Relative Mean Squared Error (RMSE) on the cross validation dataset (~15%) in the case of the classification network. It must be noted at this early stage, throughout this work comparatively large errors were encountered on output neurons for the cross validation sets due to the noise introduced during spectral compilation (Section2.3). Another outcome was that networks were trained using relatively few iterations compared to other studies (Moreira et al., 2010 and Dragović et al., 2006).

The final output of the classification NN (CNN) was decided by the "Winner takes all" approach and the overall performance assessed by calculating the misclassification rate (Zell et al., 1993). The highest misclassification was witnessed on the background results (10.2%) due to the low activities used at large depths for both PS and EHS within the cross validation set. It was decided to include these levels in order to attain detection limits. Generally PS's were classified well above a certain threshold, dependent on the activity and depth, representing the minimum detectable activity (MDA) where source becomes misclassified as background as source count contributions became negligible (Fig. 7A). EHS were also characterised well, however misclassified shallow depth PS (5–20 g cm^{-2}) can be seen distributed along on the MDA boundary (<10 Bq kg^{-1}) (Fig. 7B). As expected as the extent depth (*Ed*) becomes less and the overall volume of the contaminated layer is reduced, leading to less source contributions, the MDA increases to about 30 Bq kg^{-1}. The most significant case of misclassification can be seen subtended within PS results between 5 and 20 g cm^{-2} and below 10 kBq in which a 37% classification rate was found (Fig. 7A). This implies the two populations must still significantly overlap within PC space and the NN struggles to separate as too few source counts were contributed to the already noisy background spectra. The second reason is that the spectral shape, regardless of noise, in these specific geometries is too similar, using only energies above 300 keV, for the NN to separate. It is likely a combination of the two has led to this misclassification uncertainty. If energies below 300 keV could be sufficiently characterised these populations could be more effectively resolved. This however presents a real challenge.

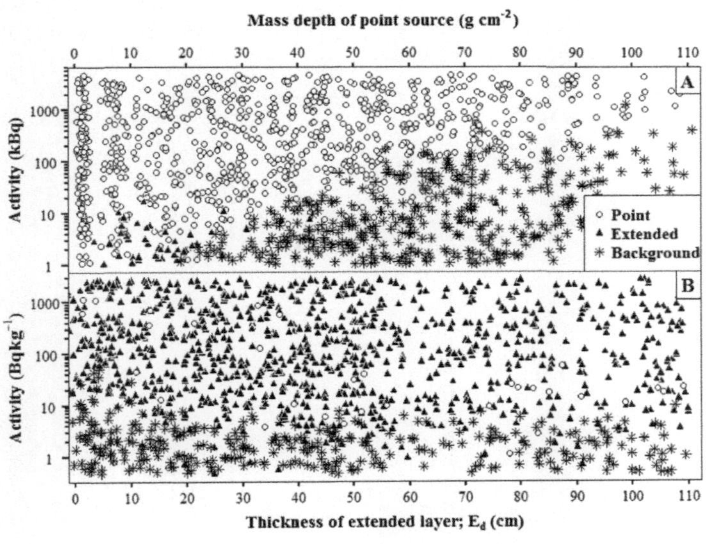

Figure 7. Classification Neural Network output for A) Point source and B) Extended source. Discrete depths have been jittered slightly to give a better sense of population density. The legend in plot A conceals largely background-misclassified points.

This method presents a real improvement in comparison to a traditional parametric approach where this degree of separation would not be possible (Fig. 6). Consideration must also be drawn to the areas of significant misclassification, for example, PS's under 10 kBq at depths below 20 g cm^{-2}. This circumstance does not pose a great risk compared to more active PS which are more than likely be classified correctly (Fig. 7A).

Point and Extended Neural Networks

Quantification of activity and depth (both *D* and *Ed*) was performed using two final NNs: Point (PNN) and Extended (ENN). Interestingly both required only 3 PCs as inputs to accurately estimate depth, but it was soon recognised that to stabilise activity estimates a fourth input neuron specifying total counts should be included. The number of hidden neurons and the size of training set needed to accurately map the problem in both NN cases were roughly similar to the CNN (Table 1). Again, a relatively small number of iterations were required to attain RMSE minima on the cross validation datasets (<25 000) and it was documented during training that both networks were found to diverge rapidly after convergence: indicative of sudden overtraining (Medhat, 2012).

Table 1. Input parameters and R^2 values (and accompanying p-values in brackets) produced for the cross validation dataset for Point Neural Network and Extended Neural Network.

Neural network	Iteration number	Number of neurons in hidden layer	Size of training set	R^2 value	
				Depth	Activity
Point	25,000	16	1000	0.942 (<0.001)	0.910 (<0.001)
Extended	8000	10	2000	0.670 (<0.001)	0.965 (<0.001)

During the training of preliminary networks it was established by limiting the maximum activity of training and test sets to realistic environmental constraints, for example PS (<5 MBq) and EHS (<3 kBq kg^{-1}), uncertainties on more probable lower activity sources could be reduced. Such activity constraints are well within activities found during intrusive surveys of Dalgety bay headland (Patton et al., 2013).

Drawing attention to accuracy of the models, the overall ability of both NN's to generalise a relationship was good for activity estimates. This is supported by high R^2 values (PNN = 0.955 (<0.001) and ENN = 0.937 (<0.001)) for both NN's. PS depth prediction was additionally very good (R^2 value of 0.942 (<0.001)). Predictions made by the ENN for vertical depth (*Ed*) were not as reliable (R^2 value of 0.670(<0.001)). This suggests that very subtle changes in spectral shape occur as the thickness of the layer contamination is varied, and these cannot be identified as easily as the change in spectral shape of PS with variable depth. This is understandable since the majority of photons that reach the detector will have originated from areas close to the detector. Thus with increasing thickness of contamination relatively less signal is received due to the inverse square law. Consequentially, accurate measurements of *Ed* are unlikely and predictions made by the ENN for this parameter should be treated with caution.

Analysis of the Headland Dataset

To demonstrate the capacity of the method, analysis of two cores from the HD is included (Fig. 8). Firstly, confidence within the ENN predictions is provided by comparing the similarity in shape of the total count rate (Fig. 8A.1 and Fig. 8B.1) and activity estimates (Bq kg^{-1}) (Fig. 8A.2 and Fig. 8B.2) with core depth for both the cores. Interestingly, the majority of the HD measurements (~70%) that were identified as having contamination were predicted to be EHS. This outcome supports general intrusive findings at the headland where the majority of contaminated material is well distributed ash and clinker from the burning of radioactive artefacts (Patton et al., 2013).

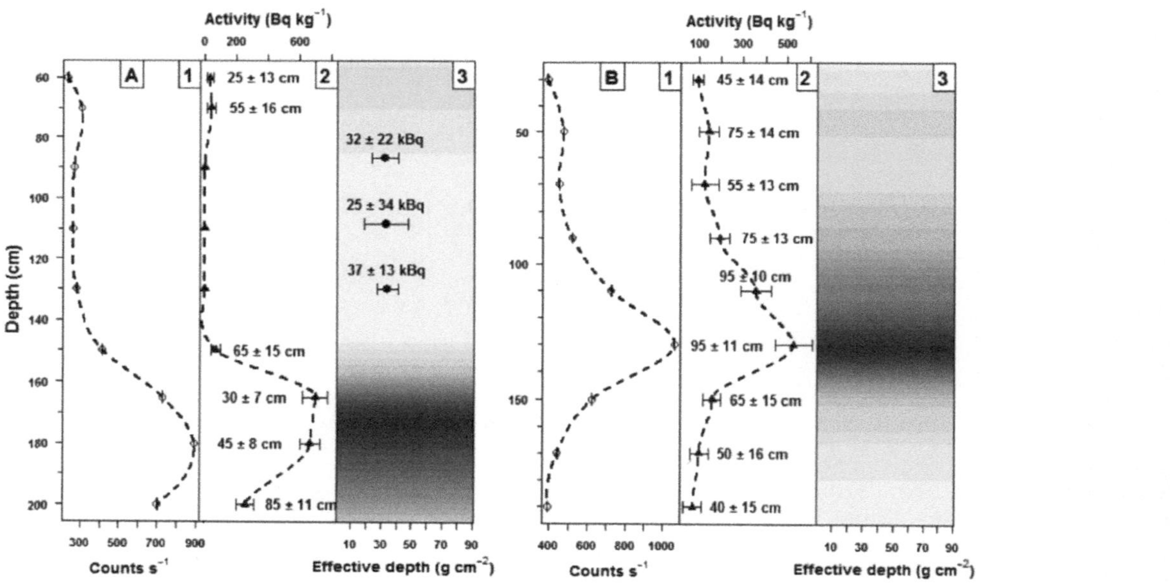

Figure 8. Neural network results for cores "s7" (A) and "s21" (B) taken from the Headland dataset. Individual core results have been separated into three individual plots 1, 2 and 3. Plot 1 provides total count rate (20–3000 keV) as a function of depth (error bars are hidden behind points). Plot 2 gives Extended Neural Network predictions for activity (Bq kg^{-1}) on the x axis and vertical depth (cm) estimates are accompanying text values. Plot 3 offers a visual representation of the core with darker shading indicating higher activity homogeneous contamination (similar to plot B) and whether a point source is present and at what depth ($x$axis) and activity (accompanying text values) it occurs.

An important finding was the identification of a relatively thick (~90 cm) elevated activity extended layer (357 ± 69 Bq kg^{-1}) at 130 cm within "s21" (Fig. 8B.2). This coincides with a large spike in total count rate (Fig. 8B.1). In the original survey this was disputed to be a point source due to the Gaussian nature of the total count rate increase within the depth series. Even with further analysis using the differential peak method the source signal could not be classified. This scenario clearly demonstrates the value of the current approach.

The highest predicted extended activities (600–700 Bq kg^{-1}) were found in a relatively thin contaminated section of core "s7" at 160–180 cm (Fig. 8A.2). This area did not contribute the highest total count rate (>1000 counts per second) though; as seen in core "s21" (Fig. 8B.1). This highest count rate was caused by a thicker (95 ± 11 cm) less active (520 ± 85 Bq kg^{-1}) layer. This shows that using this technique can provide insight into the thickness of a layer meaning that more accurate estimations of activity can be made instead of assuming a completely distributed source. Another key feature that the CNN identified at core depths between 90 and 130 cm was the presence of PS's in between two extended layers (Fig. 8A.3). The PNN provided clarification that these sources were at relatively short distances away from the detector (~35 g cm^{-2}) and at low activities (~30 kBq). Although PS were identified by the network, the consistency of the activities and depth would suggest the detector is in a pocket of low contaminated soil with larger activities at greater distances from the detector. Algorithmic identification of this situation would be very challenging. This emphasises the importance of human interpretation. To verify this notion further cores would have to be taken. This scenario highlights a real limitation of the borehole measurement without substantial spatial coverage. Similar geometries that are beyond the scope of the technique to differentiate, and that would require further spatial coverage would be for example, localised areas of homogeneous contamination that are not distributed symmetrically around the borehole and measurements above or below an extended layer.

Attention must be drawn to the errors associated with predictions of activity and depth from the NN's (Fig. 9). Standard deviations from both networks showed similar patterns, generally with increasing burial depth and decreasing activity the relative standard deviation increased. This is particularly prevalent with the point source estimations at effective depths of 30–40 g cm^{-2} and less than 20 kBq (Fig. 9A), and low activity (<100 Bq kg^{-1}) sections (<40 cm) of contamination (Fig. 9B), and this practically renders these readings unusable. This is understandable as source spectral shape would have become increasingly difficult to differentiate from background as source counts became too few.

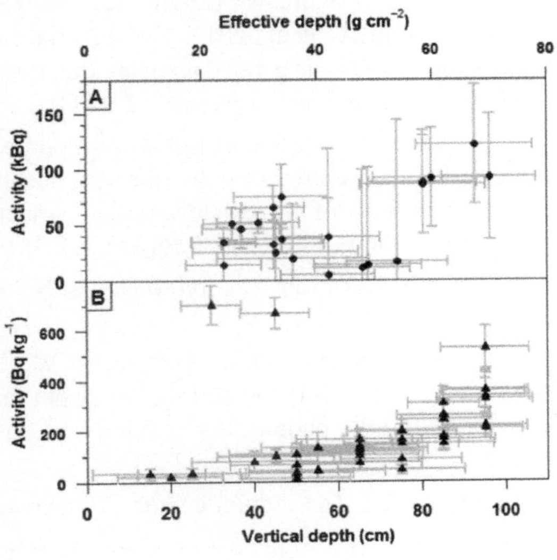

Figure 9. Estimated uncertainties associated with Headland dataset source measurements A) Point Source and B) Extended Homogeneous Source.

Interestingly, the deepest and highest activity predictions for PS occurred at the base of two cores that were positioned close together, suggestive of high activity at depth. Without further boreholes to confirm this, the actual activities are challenging to deduce as they are so far away from the detector.

There are practical ways to alleviate some of the uncertainty associated with field results, indicated by the large error bars (Fig. 9). Firstly reduction in counting uncertainty across the energy range could be attained by using another detector. NaI(Tl) detectors have relatively low energy resolution and the size used in this survey was particularly small (51 × 51 mm). If a larger, higher resolution detector was used, such as a larger volume Lanthanum bromide, uncertainties could be reduced (Yongpeng and Bin, 2012).

Another way to reduce uncertainty would be to collect more background results to provide a better understanding of the background population. This study was limited by this fact resulting in a conservative estimate of background population being made. This would have would have invariably raised the limit of detection and introduced more uncertainty on final activity and depth predictions. Other than collecting further background cores at the site, cores could have also been drilled deeper beyond contamination (providing little stratification of background constituents was present), giving more reliable background estimates for individual cores. However, this was not possible at much of the site as hard rock restricted further augering.

CONCLUSIONS

^{226}Ra contamination at depths typically below 50 cm cannot be reliably measured using conventional surface gamma-ray measurements. Borehole gammaspectroscopy is used for the purpose of characterisation, where details of the geometric nature of contamination and activity estimates are vital if formal risk assessments are to be developed in order to protect the general public. Current methods of spectral processing, however, either do not have the ability to perform the task or prove unreliable.

An approach has been described based upon feature extraction using PCA, followed by NN's to relate key features of representative MCS to obtained field results. This method provided a reliable means to characterise the geometric nature of contamination, offer activity and depth estimates of point sources, and give insight into potential layers of homogeneous contamination. The potential of the technique was demonstrated by analysis of core data taken from Dalgety Bay Headland where prediction from the majority of cores suggested that contamination was mostly dissociated: supporting intrusive survey findings.

Nevertheless, limitations associated with the nature of the borehole measurement still remain and cannot realistically be solved unless adequate spatial coverage is performed, making some predictions very uncertain, particularly of PS at distance. The use of improved detector technology and better understanding of the background could, however, alleviate some of the estimated uncertainty associated with predictions from the method.

ACKNOWLEDGEMENTS

The authors would like to thank the Scottish Environmental Protection Agency and the Natural Environmental Research Council (NE/I018956/1) for funding the work, and the Dalgety Bay Sailing Club for allowing access onto the site. Additional thanks must be given to Mike Davies and Pete Burgess for useful suggestions.

REFERENCES

1. Aage, H.K., Korsbech, U., Bargholz, K., Hovgaard, J., 1999. A new technique for processing airborne gamma ray spectrometry data for mapping low level contaminations. Appl. Radiat. Isotopes 51, 651–662.
2. Adams, A., 1993. The origin and early development of the Belgian radium industry. Environ. Int. 19, 491–501.
3. Adams, J.C., Joyce, M.J., Mellor, M., 2012. The advancement of a technique using principal component analysis for the non-intrusive depth profiling of radioactive contamination. Nucl. Sci. IEEE Trans. 59, 1448–1452.
4. Adsley, I., Davies, M., Murley, R., Pearman, I., Scirea, M., 2004. 3D GPS mapping of land contaminated with gamma-ray emitting radionuclides. Appl. Radiat. Isotopes 60, 579–582.
5. Allyson, J.D., 1994. Environmental Gamma-ray Spectrometry: Simulation of Abso-lute Calibration of In-situ and Airborne Spectrometers for Natural and Anthropogenic Sources. PhD thesis. Glasgow University, p. 274.
6. Allyson, J.D., Sanderson, D.C.W., 1998. Monte Carlo simulation of environmental airborne gamma-spectrometry. J. Environ. Radioact. 38, 259–282.
7. Beck, H., De Campo, J., Gogolak, C., 1972. In Situ Ge (Li) and Na (Tl) Gamma-ray Spectrometry. US Department of Energy, Environmental Measurements Labo-ratory, HASL-258, New York.
8. Bergmeir, C., Benítez, J.M., 2012. Neural networks in R using the Stuttgart neural network simulator: RSNNS. J. Stat. Softw. 46, 1–26.
9. Boson, J., Plamboeck, A.H., Ramebäck, H., Ågren, G., Johansson, L., 2009. Evaluation of Monte Carlo-based calibrations of HPGe detectors for in situ gamma-ray spectrometry. J. Environ. Radioact. 100, 935–940.
10. Briesmeister, J.F., 1993. MCNP-a General Monte Carlo N-particle Transport Code. LA-12625.
11. Bugai, D., Kashparov, V., Dewiere, L., Khomutinin, Y., Levchuk, S., Yoschenko, V., 2005. Characterization of subsurface geometry and radioactivity distribution in the trench containing Chernobyl clean-up wastes. Environ. Geol. 47, 869–881.
12. Caciolli, A., Baldoncini, M., Bezzon, G.P., Broggini, C., Buso, G.P., Callegari, I., et al., 2012. A new FSA approach for in situ g ray spectroscopy. Sci. Total Environ. 414, 639–645.
13. Carrazana González, J., Cornejo Díaz, N., Jurado Vargas, M., 2012. Application of the Monte Carlo code DETEFF to efficiency calibrations for in situ gamma-ray spectrometry. Appl. Radiat. Isotopes 70, 868–871
14. Chatfield, C., Collins, A.J., 1980. Principal Component Analysis. In Anonymous Introduction to Multivariate Analysis. Springer, pp. 57–81.
15. Dale, P., Robertson, I., Toner, M., 2008. Radioactive particles in dose assessments. J. Environ. Radioact. 99, 1589–1595.
16. Davies, M., McCulloch, G., Adsley, I., 2007. Experience of monitoring beaches for radioactive particles. J. Radiol. Prot. 27, A51.
17. De Groot, A., Van der Graaf, E., De Meijer, R., Maučec, M., 2009. Sensitivity of in-situ g-ray spectra to soil density and water content. Nucl. Instrum. Methods Phys. Res. A Accel. Spectrom. Detect. Assoc. Equip. 600, 519–523.
18. DECC, 2012. Radioactive Contaminated Land Statutory Guidance Environmental Protection Act 1990: Part 11A. Contaminated Land. Department of Energy and Climate Change 2012.
19. Dragovic, S., Onjia, A., Stankovic, S., Anicin, I., Bacic, G., 2005. Artificial neural network modelling of uncertainty in gamma-ray spectrometry. Nucl. Instrum. Methods Phys. Res. A Accelerators Spectrom. Detect. Assoc. Equip. 540, 455–463.
20. Dragović, S., Onjia, A., Bačić, G., 2006. Simplex optimization of artificial neural networks for the prediction of minimum detectable activity in gamma-ray spectrometry. Nuclear Instrum. Methods Phys. Res. A Accelerators Spectrom. Detect. Assoc. Equip. 564, 308–314.
21. Fagan, D.K., Robinson, S.M., Runkle, R.C., 2012. Statistical methods applied to gamma-ray spectroscopy algorithms in nuclear security missions. Appl. Radiat. Isotopes 70, 2428–2439.
22. Forster, R., Little, R., Briesmeister, J., Hendricks, J., 1990. MCNP capabilities for nu-clear well logging calculations. Nucl. Sci. IEEE Trans. 37, 1378–1385.
23. Giles, J., Dooley, K., 1998. High resolution gamma-spectroscopy well logging system. J. Radioanalytical Nucl. Chem. 233, 125b–130.
24. Guastaldi, E., Baldoncini, M., Bezzon, G., Broggini, C., Buso, G., Caciolli, A., et al., 2013. A multivariate spatial interpolation of airborne g-ray data using the geological constraints. Remote Sens. Environ. 137, 1–11.
25. Guillot, L., 2001. Extraction of full absorption peaks in airborne gamma-spectrometry by filtering techniques coupled with a study of the derivatives. Comparison with the window method. J. Environ. Radioact. 53, 381–398.
26. Gurney, K., 2003. An Introduction to Neural Networks. CRC Press, p. 139.
27. Haddad, K., Al-Masri, M.S., Doubal, A.W., 2014. Determination of ^{226}Ra contami-nation depth in soil using the multiple photopeaks method. J. Environ. Radioact. 128, 33–37.
28. Harvie, D.I., 1999. The radium century. Endeavour 23, 100–105.
29. Hendriks, P., Limburg, J., De Meijer, R., 2001. Full-spectrum analysis of natural g-ray spectra. J. Environ. Radioact. 53, 365–380.

30. Hendriks, P.H.G.M., Maučec, M., de Meijer, R.J., 2002. MCNP modelling of scintillation-detector g-ray spectra from natural radionuclides. Appl. Radiat. Isotopes 57, 449–457.

31. HMSO, 1996. CM 2919 (1995) Review of Radioactive Waste Management Policy-final Conclusions.

32. Hotelling, H., 1933. Analysis of a complex of statistical variables into principal components. J. Educ. Psychol. 24, 417.

33. Hovgaard, J., 1997. Airborne Gamma-ray Spectroscopy. Airborne Gamma-ray Spectrometry.

34. IAEA, 2003. Guidelines for Radioelement Mapping Using Gamma Ray Spectrometry Data. Nuclear Fuel Cycle and Materials Section, International Atomic Energy Agency, p. 173.

35. Im, H., Lee, Y., Park, Y.J., Song, B.C., Cho, J., Kim, W., 2007. Noise reduction in prompt gamma spectra acquired in short times. Nucl. Instrum. Methods Phys. Res. A Accelerators Spectrom. Detect. Assoc. Equip. 574, 272–279.

36. Kathren, R.L., 1998. NORM sources and their origins. Appl. Radiat. Isotopes 49, 149–168.

37. Kobr, M., Mareš, S., Paillet, F., 2005. Geophysical well logging. In: Anonymous Hydrogeophysics. Springer, pp. 291–331.

38. Kock, P., Lanke, J., Samuelsson, C., 2012. A real-time statistical alarm method for mobile gamma spectrometry–Combining counts of pulses with spectral dis-tribution of pulses. Nucl. Instrum. Methods Phys. Res. A Accel. Spectrom. Detect. Assoc. Equip. 681, 55–60.

39. Landa, E.R., 1993. A brief history of the American Radium Industry and its ties to the Scientific Community of its early twentieth century. Environ. Int. 19, 503–508.

40. Likar, A., Vidmar, T., Lipoglavsek, M., Omahen, G., 2004. Monte Carlo calculation of entire in situ gamma-ray spectra. J. Environ. Radioact. 72, 163–168.

41. Maučec, M., de Meijer, R.J., Rigollet, C., Hendriks, P.H.G.M., Jones, D.G., 2004a. Detection of radioactive particles offshore by g-ray spectrometry Part I: Monte Carlo assessment of detection depth limits. Nucl. Instrum. Methods Phys. Res. A Accel. Spectrom. Detect. Assoc. Equip. 525, 593–609.

42. Maučec, M., de Meijer, R.J., van der Klis, M.M.I.P., Hendriks, P.H.G.M., Jones, D.G., 2004b. Detection of radioactive particles offshore by g-ray spectrometry Part II: Monte Carlo assessment of acquisition times. Nucl. Instrum. Methods Phys. Res. A Accel. Spectrom. Detect. Assoc. Equip. 525, 610–622.

43. Maučec, M., Hendriks, P.H.G.M., Limburg, J., de Meijer, R.J., 2009. Determination of correction factors for borehole natural gamma-ray measurements by Monte Carlo simulations. Nucl. Instrum. Methods Phys. Res. A Accel. Spectrom. Detect. Assoc. Equip. 609, 194–204.

44. Medhat, M.E., 2012. Artificial intelligence methods applied for quantitative analysis of natural radioactive sources. Ann. Nucl. Energy 45, 73–79.

45. Meisner, J., Nicaise, W., Stromswold, D., 1995. CsI (Tl) with photodiodes for identi-fying subsurface radionuclide contamination. Nucl. Sci. IEEE Trans. 42, 288–291.

46. Miller, K.M., Shebell, P., Klemic, G.A., 1994. In-situ Gamma-Ray spectrometry for the measurement of uranium in surface soils. Health Phys. 67, 140–150.

47. Minty, B., Hovgaard, J., 2002. Reducing noise in gamma-ray spectrometry using spectral component analysis. Explor. Geophys. 33, 172–176.

48. Moreira, M.C.F., Conti, C.C., Schirru, R., 2010. A new NaI(Tl) four-detector layout for field contamination assessment using artificial neural networks and the Monte Carlo method for system calibration. Nucl. Instrum. Methods Phys. Res. A Accel. Spectrom. Detect. Assoc. Equip. 621, 302–309.

49. National Nuclear Data Center, 2013. Nuclear Datasheets.

50. Paschoa, A.S., 1998. Potential environmental and regulatory implications of naturally occurring radioactive materials (NORM). Appl. Radiat. Isotopes 49, 189–196.

51. Patton, N., Gemmill, J., Milne, J., 2013. Appropriate Person Report. Scottish Envi-ronmental Protection Agency.

52. R Development Core Team, 2012. R: a Language and Environment for Statistical Computing.

53. Riedmiller, M., Braun, H., 1993. A Direct Adaptive Method for Faster Back-propagation Learning: the RPROP Algorithm, pp. 586–591.

54. Rundo, J., 1993. History of the determination of radium in man since 1915. Environ. Int. 19, 425–438.

55. Runkle, R., 2006. Analysis of spectroscopic radiation portal monitor data using principal components analysis. IEEE Trans. Nucl. Sci. 53, 1418–1423.

56. Serov, I.V., John, T.M., Hoogenboom, J.E., 1998. A new effective Monte Carlo Midway coupling method in MCNP applied to a well logging problem. Appl. Radiat. Isotopes 49, 1737–1744.

57. Stromswold, D., 1995. Calibration facilites for borehole and surface environmental radiation measurements. J. Radioanal. Nucl. Chem. 194, 393–401.

58. Thummerer, S., Jacob, P., 1998. Determination of depth distributions of natural ra-dionuclides with in situ gamma-ray spectrometry. Nucl. Instrum. Methods Phys. Res. A Accelerators Spectrom. Detect. Assoc. Equip. 416, 161–178.

59. Trnkova, L., Trojek, T., Thinova, L., 2010. Gamma spectrometric measurements of depth-related radionuclide distribution in walls. Appl. Radiat. Isotopes 68, 832–835.

60. Tyler, A.N., 1999. Monitoring anthropogenic radioactivity in salt marsh environ-ments through in situ gamma-ray spectrometry. J. Environ. Radioact. 45, 235–252.

61. Tyler, A.N., 2008. In Situ and Airborne Gamma-ray Spectrometry. Radioactivity in the Environment. Elsevier, pp. 407–448.

62. Tyler, A.N., Sanderson, D.C.W., Scott, E.M., Allyson, J.D., 1996. Accounting for spatial variability and fields

of view in environmental gamma ray spectrometry. J. Environ. Radioact. 33, 213–235.

63. Tyler, A.N., Scott, E.M., Dale, P., Elliott, A.T., Wilkins, B.T., Boddy, K., et al., 2010. Reconstructing the abundance of Dounreay hot particles on an adjacent public beach in Northern Scotland. Sci. Total Environ. 408, 4495–4503.

64. Tyler, A.N., Ruffell, A., Dale, P., 2011. Dalgety Bay Headland Investigation (Prepared for Scottish Environmental Protection Agency).

65. Tyler, A., Dale, P., Copplestone, D., Bradley, S., Ewen, H., McGuire, C., et al., 2013. The radium legacy: contaminated land and the committed effective dose from the ingestion of radium contaminated materials. Environ. Int. 59, 449–455.

66. Wei, W., Du, Q., Younan, N.H., 2010. Particle swarm optimization based spectral transformation for radioactive material detection and classification. Comput. Intell. Meas. Syst. Appl. 1–6.

67. Wilson, R., Conaway, J., 1991. Simulations of a Spectral Gamma-ray Logging Tool Response to a Surface Source Distribution on the Borehole Wall. Los Alamos National Laboratory Publication, pp. 1118–1122.

68. Wilson, R.D., Koizumi, C.J., Meisner, J.E., Stromswold, D.C., 1997. Spectral Shape Analysis for Contaminant Logging at the Hanford Site. Los Alamos National Laboratory Publication, pp. 457–461.

69. Yongpeng, W., Bin, T., 2012. Monte-carlo simulation of response functions for nat-ural gamma-rays in LaBr3 detector system with complex borehole configura-tions. Plasma Sci. Technol. 14, 481.

70. Yoshida, E., Shizuma, K., Endo, S., Oka, T., 2002. Application of neural networks for the analysis of gamma-ray spectra measured with a Ge spectrometer. Nucl. Instrum. Methods Phys. Res. A Accelerators Spectrom. Detect. Assoc. Equip. 484, 557–563.

71. Zell, A., Mache, N., Huebner, R., Mamier, G., Vogt, M., Herrmann, K., et al., 1993. SNNS-Stuttgart Neural Network Simulator, pp. 1–155.

SECTION II - DOSIMETRY AND RADIATION-INDUCED THERAPY

CHAPTER 6 RADIOLOGICAL DOSE RECONSTRUCTION

Jacqueline Garnier-Laplace, Karine Beaugelin-Seiller, Claire Della-Vedova, Jean-Michel Métivier, Christian Ritz, Timothy A. Mousseau and Anders Pape Møller

INTRODUCTION

The nuclear disaster at the Fukushima Daiichi nuclear power plant (NPP) following the massive earthquake and devastating tsunami on 11 March 2011 was rated at 7 which is the highest level on the international nuclear disaster scale, putting it on par with the accident at Chernobyl. Vast amounts of radioactive materials were released, estimated as ca. 10–15% (i.e. 400–630 PBq) and 35% (i.e. 58 PBq) of the total iodine and cesium radioisotopes emitted by the Chernobyl accident, respectively[1,2]. The effect of these radioactive releases on abundance, condition and rate of reproduction in birds and other animals has been the subject of investigation during 2011–2014 within the 50-km area northwest of Fukushima Daiichi NPP[3,4,5,6,7]. In total, 400 sampling points (in 2011, 300 points) in areas within and outside the 20-km exclusion zone were visited annually to observe abundance and diversity of birds and other organisms, as well as their reproductive state; a number of environmental variables including ambient radiation level at the exact census points were also recorded. In total this database contains information for 1500 point censuses (300 identical points from 2011 to 2014 with an additional 100 more points from 2012 to 2014).

Different analyses from this dataset have been published, showing reduced species richness and abundance in areas of relatively high ambient radiation level[7,8], as also shown for the Chernobyl Exclusion Zone – CEZ[4,9,10,11,12]. These analyses were performed taking into account a number of potentially confounding environmental variables such as descriptors of the census conditions (e.g., time, cloud cover, wind, temperature) and of landscape (i.e. cover type such as e.g., farmland, grass, coniferous trees)[4,6,7,9,10,11,12]. Analyses based on Generalized Linear Mixed Models (GLMM) with Poisson distributed data, least squares analyses and non-parametric Spearman rank order correlations showed similar conclusions[6]. Thus the conclusions appeared to be independent of statistical analyses. The most recent analyses of the entire dataset collected in the Fukushima area by Møller *et al.*[6] showed the abundance of birds decreased with increasing level of ambient radiation, with significant variation among species, and the relationship between abundance and radiation became increasingly negative over time.

Among the 154 bird species present in the inventory at Chernobyl and Fukushima, species with small body size and hence relatively high food consumption rates were more negatively impacted by radiation at Fukushima and Chernobyl[7]. Secondary consumers showed stronger negative effects of radiation on abundance than herbivores, and more so at Fukushima than at Chernobyl[7]. There was no overall effect of migration behavior, but migratory species were more negatively impacted in Chernobyl, while residents were more negatively impacted in Fukushima[7] perhaps reflecting the effects of high acute exposures to resident species during the initial phase of the disaster. Species with carotenoid and pheomelanin plumage pigments associated with antioxidant status showed stronger negative effects, especially in Chernobyl compared to Fukushima, while species with eumelanic coloration, which is not related to antioxidant status, did not show such an effect. These differences between Chernobyl and Fukushima may reflect differences in duration of exposure, differences in radioactive isotopes still being present in the radioactive deposits at the census periods, and differences in

Citation: Jacqueline Garnier-Laplace, Karine Beaugelin-Seiller, Claire Della-Vedova, Jean-Michel Métivier, Christian Ritz, Timothy A. Mousseau, and Anders Pape Møller. Radiological dose reconstruction, Scientific Reports, 5, Article number: 16594 (2015). DOI:10.1038/srep16594.ss potential accumulation of mutations since sampled individuals are offspring from a much smaller number of generations in Fukushima than in Chernobyl[7,13].

Recently, Garnier-Laplace *et al.*[14] proposed a re-assessment of inter-species radio sensitivity emphasizing that organisms in their natural environment from the CEZ appeared to be ca. eight times more sensitive to radiation than they were under laboratory conditions. This is not surprising given that organisms under field conditions may suffer from poor nutrition and/or unfavorable abiotic factors, and parasitism and predation with strong effects on abundance and species diversity, while lab populations are usually kept under optimal conditions, partly as a consequence of legislation related to research ethics. Additionally the duration of exposure is clearly a major feature that distinguishes laboratory and field experiments, since for the same exposure dose rate, the resulting absorbed doses are drastically different with ultimately much higher doses in the field than in the laboratory. Finally, any shift in sensitivity between field and laboratory may be due to the presence of other stressors such as stable contaminants and/or to selection of strains through phenotypic acclimation, DNA methylation, genetic adaptation across generations, or multigenerational phenotypic effects (e.g., maternal effects)[15,16,17].

On the basis of ecological data describing bird diversity and abundance in the 50-km contaminated area around Fukushima published by Møller*et al.*[6,7], the objectives of the present study were to reconstruct the total dose (and dose rates) of individual birds and to analyse whether this new approach might better explain the intensity and type of observed effects on bird abundance and species diversity. More precisely, we reassessed the entire dataset by substituting the ambient radiation level previously used by Møller *et al.*[6,7] by the total doses reconstructed for birds. As noticed by Beresford *et al.*[18,19], the ambient radiation level is assumed to be a biased radiation dose indicator, especially when several species of free-ranging animals may be impacted. For a given contaminated environment, where ambient radiation level is constant, radiological dose rate absorbed by living organisms may vary by several orders of magnitude since animal biodiversity is characterized by a variety of species-specific morphological and ecological features (e.g., types of habitats, diet) that may greatly influence the range of absorbed dose. Any dose (rate) reconstruction needs to assess its two elementary components: the external dose (rate) from the radio-contaminated habitat and the internal dose (rate) from internalization of radionuclides. In this study, both components were assessed on the basis of (i) the stylized morphological and ecological features of the species and (ii) the radioactive concentration of the soil using GPS coordinates from each census point combined with the radioactive contamination maps of the Fukushima area, the latter being based on field monitoring in soils performed by Japanese university scientists, from June-July 2011[20]. We re-analysed the ecological dataset with reconstructed total dose for bird individuals (sum of internal dose and external dose) at census points to investigate its relationship with temporal and spatial records of bird abundance and species richness. We also examined the relationship between absorbed dose and the abundance and diversity of birds and we compared estimated critical radiotoxicity endpoints (e.g., dose giving 50% effects on the abundance) with various radiation effect benchmarks published by international organisations.

RESULTS

Comparison between Ambient Radiation Levels and Estimated Bird Dose Rates and Total Doses

The ratio between the reconstructed absorbed dose rates for adults of all bird species and the measured ambient radiation levels according to site, year and species, varied from 0.1 to 20. For example, the minimum value for this ratio was obtained in 2011 for *Anas poecilorhyncha* at site ID99 (Fig. 1a), where the ambient level was measured at 19 μGy h^{-1} and the maximum ratio (x20) was obtained in 2014 for site ID1 (Fig. 1a) and *Phasianus colchicus.* Table 1 reports the ranges of variation in ambient radiation levels among sites per year and the way that this heterogeneity is reflected in the calculated dose rates among species. Globally, whatever year, where ambient dose rate varied by two orders of magnitude among sites, variation in absorbed dose rates among species and among sites also varied by two orders of magnitude, the minimum value being estimated for *Anas poecilorhyncha* and the maximum for *Phasianus colchicus* and *Eophona personata.* Additionally, for a given site, the absorbed dose rate varied eight-fold among the 57 species mainly due to variation in Concentration Ratio values selected for Cs isotopes. For a given species, the absorbed dose rate varied by a factor of 44 among the 300 sites. The empirical distribution of the maximum values per species obtained for the full dataset of the reconstructed dose rates for adult birds is given in Fig. 2.

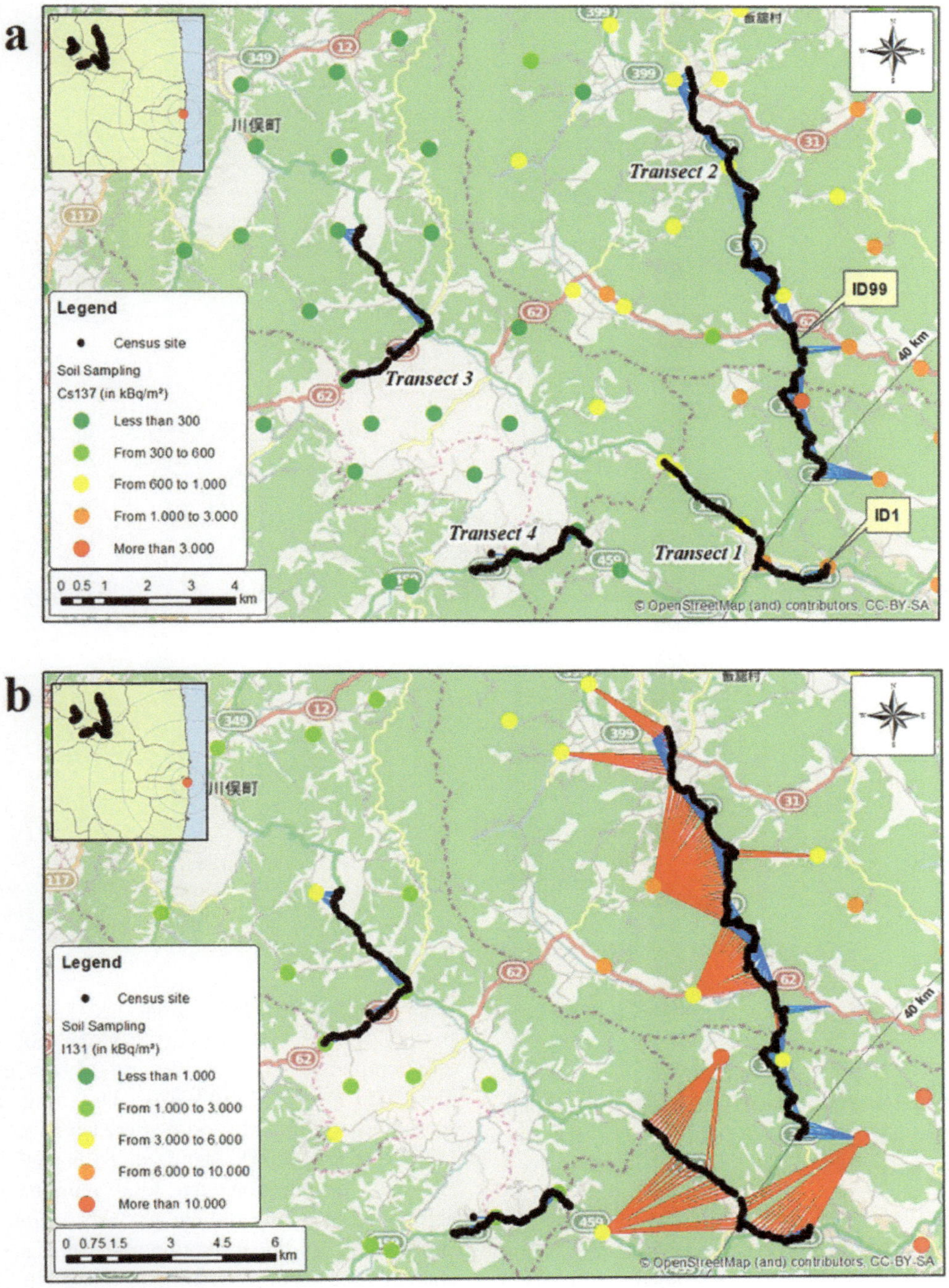

Figure 1: Location of the 300 census sites for birds distributed along four transects. Each census site was associated with soil activity ((a) ^{137}Cs equal to ^{134}Cs and (b) ^{131}I) equal to that measured at the nearest soil sampling point. Note that several neighbor census sites were associated with the same measurement point. Maps were created with GIS software (ArcGIS 10.1) http://support.esri.com/en/downloads/patches-servicepacks/view/productid/66/metaid/2064 with geographical background using data available under the Open Database Licence ("© OpenStreetMap and contributors"; cartography licensed as CC BY-SA) http://www.openstreetmap.org/copyright.

Table 1: Range of variation in measured ambient radiation among the 300 census sites per year and corresponding range of variation among the 57 species of calculated dose rates for adult birds.

Year	Ambient radiation range among sites (μGy/h^{-1})	Absorbed dose rates among sites and among species (μGy/h^{-1})
2011	0.55–31	0.28–97
2012	0.21–28	0.24–84
2013	0.18–21	0.21–74
2014	0.16–13	0.19–66

All values are rounded to 2 significant digits.

Figure 2: Empirical cumulative probability distribution of maximum estimated dose rates for the 57 species, 300 sites and four census years.

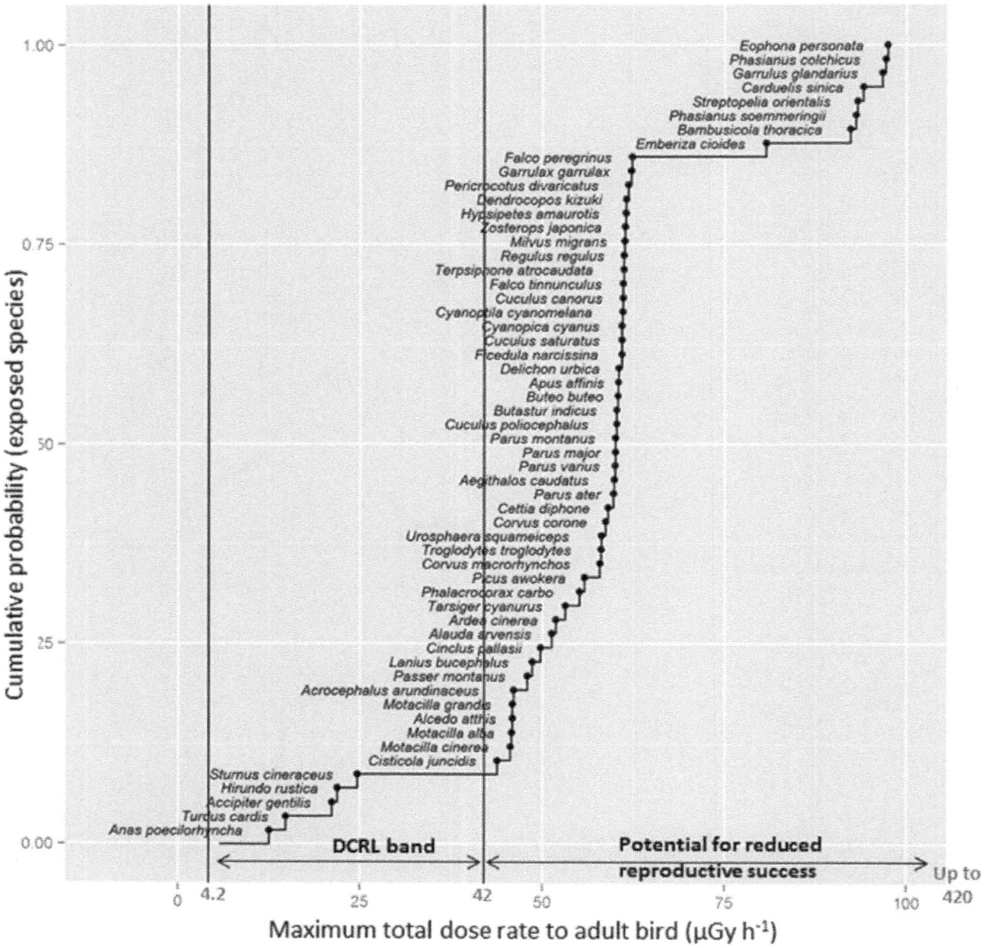

The adult bird exposure levels were compared to ranges of biological effects reported by ICRP21.

Testing the Relationships between Bird Abundance and Simpson's Index of Diversity, Respectively, and Total Doses

When averaged for the full dataset (i.e. 57 species x 300 sites x 4-yr), the estimated total dose was 0.13 Gy (range: 0.0031–1.23 Gy; N=1190). The average observed total number of birds per site was 6.17 (range: 0–49; N=1200). The average observed Simpson's Index of diversity was 0.66 (range: 0–1; N=1200).

The total number of birds decreased significantly with increasing total dose (log_{10}-transformed) (Table 2; z=−4.060, p<0.0001; standardised partial slope (SE)=−0.299 (0.074)), altitude (z=−5.980, p<0.0001; standardised partial slope (SE)=−0.275 (0.046)), grass as land cover (z=−4.980, p<0.0001; standardised partial slope (SE)=−0.173 (0.035)) and temperature (z=−2.400, p=0.016; standardised partial slope (SE)=−0.182 (0.076)). The total number of birds increased significantly with increasing "cover by farmland" (z=5.790, p<0.0001; standardised partial slope (SE)=0.266 (0.046)). In addition, the total number of birds differed significantly among the categories of wind speed, and had a significant curvilinear relation with time (z=5.050, p<0.0001; standardised coefficient (SE)=0.352 (0.070)). Total dose (log_{10}-transformed) was among predictors having the greatest effects on the total number of birds. Using the unstandardised partial slope of total dose (log_{10}-transformed) (Table 2), we estimated a loss of 22.6% with CI 95% [12.4; 31.6] (i.e. the loss being calculated as [exp (−0.256)− 1]) of the total number of birds per unit of log_{10}-transformed total dose (in Gy), i.e. each time the total dose increases by a factor 10 (Fig. 3a).

Table 2: Total number of birds: effects of log_{10}total dose and confounding variables.

Random effects:				
Groups	Variance	SD		
Site	0.052	0.228		
CensDayTra[a]	0.023	0.150		
Fixed effects:				
	Estimate	SE	z	p

(Intercept)	1.666	0.048	34.650	<0.0001
log_{10} Total dose	**−0.299**	**0.074**	**−4.060**	**<0.0001**
	(−0.256)[b]	**(0.063)[b]**		
Time	−0.054	0.047	−1.160	0.246
Time^2	**0.352**	**0.070**	**5.050**	**<0.0001**
Cloud cover	0.016	0.053	0.290	0.769
Temperature	**−0.182**	**0.076**	**−2.400**	**0.016**
Wind 1[c]	0.079	0.096	0.820	0.410
Wind 2	−0.041	0.068	−0.600	0.549
Wind 3	**−0.290**	**0.101**	**−2.880**	**0.004**
Wind 4	**−0.471**	**0.170**	**−2.770**	**0.006**
Wind 5	−0.020	0.139	−0.140	0.886
Altitude	**−0.275**	**0.046**	**−5.980**	**<0.0001**
Grass	**−0.173**	**0.035**	**−4.980**	**<0.0001**
Farmland	**0.266**	**0.046**	**5.790**	**<0.0001**
Coniferous	0.011	0.015	0.720	0.470

Effect size was standardised by two SD. Parameters with a significant effect ($p<0.05$) are highlighted in bold.

[a]CensDayTra is the combination of Census day and Transect categories.

[b]Unstandardised partial slope values obtained after model fit with the same fixed and random effects, but without standardization of the input variables.

[c]Wind 0 was the reference category.

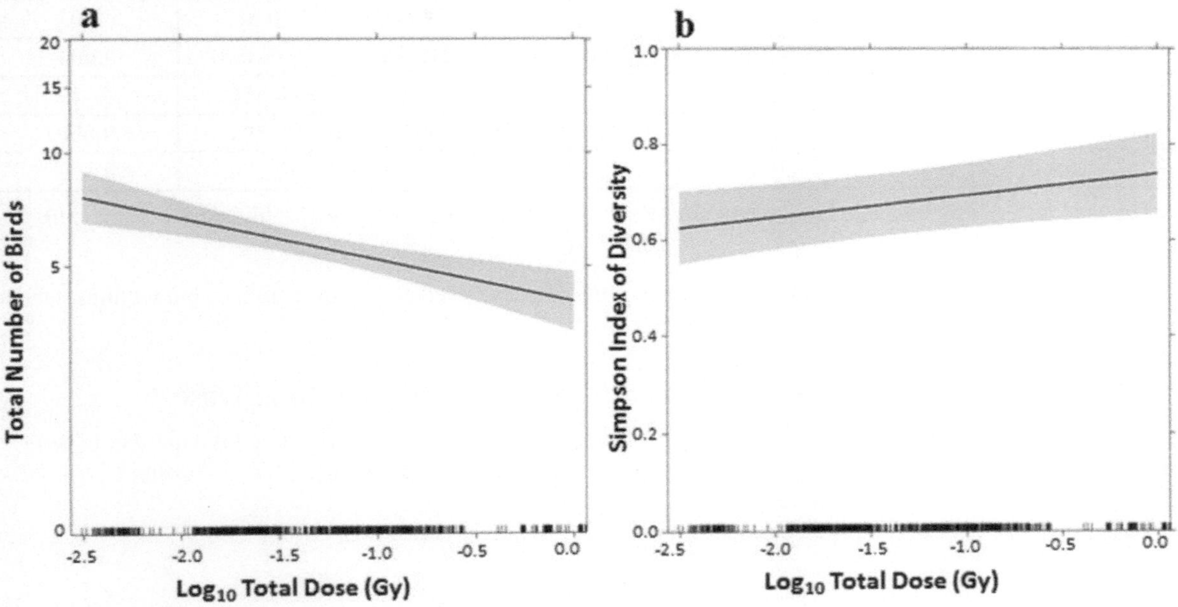

Figure 3: (a) Effect display44 for the calculated total dose (log_{10}-transformed) predictor of total number of birds (TNB), in the fitted GLMM. After controlling for the possible confounding variables, the total number of birds decreased by 22.6% per unit of log_{10} total dose. Note that the vertical axis is on a scale of the linear predictor with axis tick marks labelled on the scale of the response (TNB). The decrease is highly significant ($z=-4.06$, $p<0.0001$; unstandardised partial slope (SE)=−0.256 (0.063)). (b) Effect display for the calculated total dose (log_{10}-transformed) predictor of Simpson's index of diversity, in the fitted LMM. After controlling for the possible confounding variables, the probability that two individuals belonged to different species increases linearly by 4.5% per unit of log_{10} total dose. The increase is significant ($t=2.3$, $p<0.025$; unstandardised partial slope (SE)=−0.045 (0.020)); Grey bands in the panels represent the 95% confidence intervals around the fits.

Species diversity expressed as the Simpson's index of diversity increased significantly with increasing total dose (log_{10}-transformed) (Table 3; $t=2.302$, $p=0.025$; partial standardized slope (SE)=0.053 (0.02)) and with "cover by farmland" ($t=6.594$, $p<0.0001$; partial standardised slope (SE)=0.089 (0.014)) and decreased with increasing time ($t=-5.643$, $p<0.0001$; partial standardised slope (SE)=−0.084 (0.015)) and increasing altitude ($t=-2.888$, $p=0.004$; partial standardised slope (SE)=−0.040 (0.014)). In addition, bird species diversity differed significantly among wind speed categories. After controlling for all the other predictors, the probability of observing two individuals of different species increased linearly by ca. 4.5% with CI 95% [0.6; 8.4] (unstandardised coefficient) per unit of log_{10}-transformed total dose (in Gy) (Fig. 3b).

Table 3: Simpson's index of diversity: effects of $\log_{10}$ total dose and confounding variables.

Random effects:					
Groups	Variance	SD			
Site	0.002	0.042			
Census Day	0.001	0.028			
Transect	0.004	0.063			
Residual	0.026	0.160			
Fixed effects:					
	Estimate	SE	df	t	p
(Intercept)	0.687	0.035	3.40	19.846	<0.001
Total Dose Log	**0.053**	**0.023**	**55.30**	**2.302**	**0.025**
	(0.045)[b]	**(0.020)[b]**			
Time	**−0.084**	**0.015**	**145.90**	**−5.643**	**<0.0001**
Time^2	0.008	0.023	974.40	0.323	0.747
Cloud cover	0.006	0.015	123.20	0.389	0.698
Temp	−0.001	0.019	18.20	−0.033	0.974
Wind1[a]	0.009	0.026	48.10	0.335	0.739
Wind2	0.007	0.023	26.80	0.306	0.762
Wind3	**−0.150**	**0.031**	**309.90**	**−4.806**	**<0.0001**
Wind4	**−0.125**	**0.043**	**20.90**	**−2.901**	**0.009**
Wind5	−0.026	0.037	19.20	−0.682	0.503
Altitude	**−0.040**	**0.014**	**318.90**	**−2.888**	**0.004**
Grass	0.005	0.011	292.60	0.456	0.649
Farmland	**0.089**	**0.014**	**299.20**	**6.594**	**<0.0001**
Coniferous	0.010	0.011	282.60	0.928	0.354

Effect size was standardised by two SD. Parameters with a significant effect ($p<0.05$) are highlighted in bold.

[a]Wind 0 was the reference category.

[b]Unstandardised partial slope values obtained after model fit with the same fixed and random effects, but without standardization of the input variables.

Further Investigating the Relationship between Bird Abundance and Total Dose

Dose –response modelling based on a subset of randomly selected total doses and corresponding total number of birds estimated from the previously fitted GLMM (Table 2) allowed us to predict that a total absorbed dose of 0.55 Gy with CI 95% [0.45; 0.70] caused a 50% loss in the total number of birds (Fig. 4).

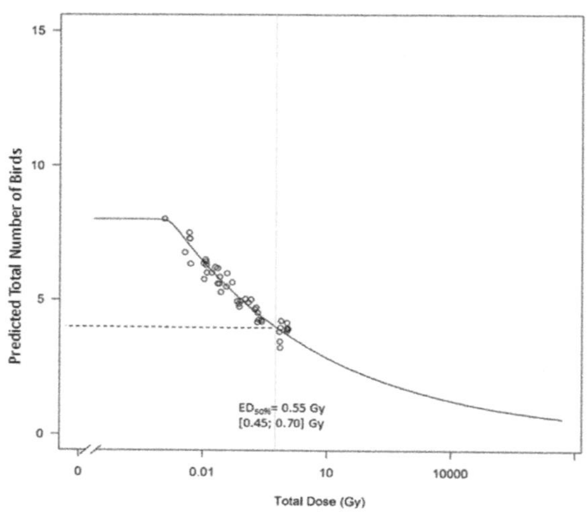

Figure 4: Log logistic model fitted to randomly predicted total number of birds derived from the global GLMM, and its ED_{50} prediction and associated 95% Confidence Interval (ED_{50} is the total absorbed dose causing a 50% reduction in the total number of birds).

DISCUSSION

In this study, substituting the ambient dose rate measured at the census point (from 0.16 to 31 μGy h^{-1}) by the transformed dose variable using radiological dose rate reconstructed for adult birds of each species (from 0.3 to 97 μGy h^{-1}), we confirmed that the overall abundance of birds at Fukushima during 2011–2014 decreased with increasing absorbed doses (Fig. 3a). As such, this relationship is directly consistent with exposure levels cited in the literature that are known to induce physiological disturbances in terrestrial vertebrates or more specifically in birds. The International Committee for Radiological Protection recommended in its Publication 108[21] (which is dedicated to concepts and approach for radiological protection of the environment) to use Derived Consideration Reference Levels (DCRL) values corresponding to the "*band of dose rates within which there is likely to be some chance of deleterious effects occurring to individuals of such type of organism*". For birds, the DCRL range is 0.1–1 mGy d^{-1} (or 4–42 μGy h^{-1}). On the basis of an expert judgement from a critical literature review, ICRP[21] also reported the dose rate ranges where various significant effects were described in birds: mortality in adults (>1000 mGy d^{-1} or 42,000 μGy h^{-1}), long-term effects on developing embryos (e.g. reduction in life-span) (100–1000 mGy d^{-1} or 4,200 to 42,000 μGy h^{-1}), increased morbidity (10–100 or 420 to 4,200 μGy h^{-1}), and reduced reproductive success (1–10 mGy d^{-1} or 42 to 420 μGy h^{-1}). We considered the empirical cumulative distribution of the maximum exposure levels per species across the 300 sites and the four years, along with the assumption that radio sensitivity is similar among bird species. Comparing with ICRP bands previously described, we found that 90% of the 57 species constituting the observed bird community were likely chronically exposed at a dose rate that could potentially affect their reproductive success (Fig. 2). This finding is valid when reasoning at the bird community level in the studied area, but needs to be refined if we want to rank species at risk since the most exposed species is not necessarily the most radiosensitive.

More precisely, we were able to quantify a loss of 22.6% of the total number of individuals per increment of one unit $\log_{10}$ in the total dose over the four-year post-accident period in the study area. On the basis of the present dataset and the global GLMM we implemented, we were able to predict a value of 0.55 Gy for the total dose inducing 50% loss in the total number of birds at a census site (ED_{50}) (Fig. 4). This value can be compared to the transitional vertebrate Predicted No Effect Dose Rate (PNEDR) proposed by Garnier-Laplace *et al.*[22] for chronic exposure to ionising radiation which equals 2 μGy h^{-1}. This benchmark, being derived from a minimalist dataset, was considered as indicative of the order of magnitude only, rather than being a definitive number. When multiplied by the exposure duration of birds in this study, this benchmark can be converted into a range which extends from 5.4 mGy in 2011 to 58 mGy in 2014. This range is consistently 10 to 100 times lower than the estimated ED_{50} of 0.55 Gy. Since the Simpson's biodiversity index analysis was more quantitative than qualitative, it remains difficult to identify whether this loss in number of individuals was peculiar for a specific species.

We demonstrated that the relationship between total doses and species diversity, estimated as Simpson's index, increased significantly with total doses (Fig. 3b). One could speculate that an increase in diversity may result indirectly from a decrease in abundance, as a result of homogenization of abundances for various species. Møller *et al.*6concluded that in the Fukushima area, although bird species on average declined in abundance with increasing ambient levels, several species increased in abundance due to changes in land-use and/or to competitive release. From ecological surveys implemented in the Chernobyl Exclusion Zone[4,9,10] in sites covering ambient radiation levels ranging from 0.01 to 4500 μGy h^{-1}, statistical analyses provided evidence of dramatic effects on species richness and abundance of "forest" birds and skewed age and sex ratios in many birds populations. It would be informative to reassess the data collected in previous years concerning effects on the biota of Chernobyl Exclusion Zone using the same approach we have implemented in the present study to reconstruct in an ecologically relevant way the radiological dose to biota. As demonstrated for this study in the Fukushima area, our method potentially enhances the relevance and consistency of the analysis of causal relationship between levels of exposure (dose or dose rate) and type and intensity of observed effects. Other studies published after the Fukushima accident, such as those dedicated to the pale blue grass butterfly[23,24], earthworms[25] and wild macaques[26], might also benefit from a re-analysis that includes a rigorous dose assessment.

Importantly, the method presented here to obtain relatively refined estimates of bird individual dose, have permitted a much finer-scale analysis of the factors shaping the biological endpoints of interest, in this case, species level performance within the context of the broader bird community exposed to radioactive substances accidentally released into the environment. However, like any modeling approach, our dose estimates were based on assumptions and models, and present therefore limitations and uncertainties.

One among them is the use of real measured soil activity concentrations at the closest soil sampling stations to any bird census point. Such input data used to reconstruct the bird dose takes into account roughly the spatial heterogeneity of radioactive deposits and avoids more complex and uncertain spatial interpolation. Moreover, bird dose reconstruction ideally needs to be combined with the spatial home range for individuals of the 57 species. This home range is generally known to vary depending on habitat type/quality, population density, behavior, physiology, etc.[27]. To our knowledge meaningful data for species home ranges for individuals only exist for a few of the 57 species of interest in this study. So our approach seems a reasonable compromise to address such lack of knowledge. Additionally, we calculated a maximum cumulated dose per species since we adopted the hypothesis that all species were present at the time of the accident and that dose accumulation was not limited by life span. Life span per species is difficult to estimate robustly since it can be influenced by environmental conditions. We considered that cumulative dose over a 4-yr period for the maximum was still quite realistic for the 57 species. Analysis of longer term data will require an additional assumption to limit the accumulated dose in a realistic manner with regard to species' life spans.

Another important source of uncertainty for dose estimates is that we ignored the early life stages for dose reconstruction in adult birds. It would have been highly speculative to calculate the dose absorbed by eggs and nestlings although eggs and nestlings are known to be particularly radiosensitive compared to adults. This may have particular relevance here given that the period of highest exposures overlapped with the breeding season for many species. For any given species, the dose assessment for eggs and nestlings requires data on nest material, duration of incubation and rearing duration of chicks in the nest. Such information varies greatly across species and may have been modified over the four-year census period since they are sensitive to changes in environmental factors. To give the order of magnitude of the uncertainty introduced by voluntary omission of early life stages in bird dose assessment, we can refer to a recent field study performed in May-June 2012 by Bonisoli-Alquati *et al.*3 dedicated to nestling barn swallows *Hirundo rustica* in Fukushima 80 km NW of the contaminated area. The authors measured external dose (rate) of nestlings by using thermoluminescent dosimeters left in the nest and found that it varied from 0.15 to 4.9 mGy (0.23 to 7.52 μGy h^{-1}). Nest materials contributed dominantly to the dose of nestlings. This value represents ca. 50% of the dose rate we calculated for adult barn swallows in 2012, the latter varying from 0.4 to 18 μGy h^{-1} across the 300 census sites. However, when converted into total dose by multiplying by the duration over which these dose rates apply, the contribution represents less than 5% of the total dose, which is the basic variable used in our statistical analysis. Adult barn swallows considered in our study in 2012 had absorbed from 4.8 to 210 mGy since the accident, depending on the site at which they were observed. Although this contribution of early stage dose to total dose may vary across the 57 species of this study, we can reasonably assume that it is of minor importance. Moreover this effect is balanced by our conservative choice to calculate the total dose only for birds present at the moment of the accident. Finally, it seems reasonable to assume that any such effects will add noise to the data and not result in systematic bias in the conclusions.

Another limitation to our present dose calculation is the use of the simple Concentration Ratio (CR) concept to model the internal dose of adult birds. This commonly used approach generally leads to a range of CR values spanning several orders of magnitude across species of birds. For example for cesium, IAEA[28] reported a range of variation from 0.0014 to 16 (Bq kg^{-1} fresh wet: Bq kg^{-1}, dry weight soil) on the basis of a dataset of 180 observations. In the present study where we followed recommendations from IAEA[28] and Brown *et al.*[29] for filling data gaps, we were able to reduce the uncertainty by selecting fit-for-purpose data per species, i.e. using species-specific CR values when possible or adopting taxonomically based extrapolation rules for combinations (species, radionuclide) where data were lacking. These rules consist of selecting a CR value acquired first for a similar genus, then for another species with similar diet and lastly among vertebrate classes such as mammals considered of "similar taxonomy". We selected the CR method for our analysis since our dose estimates mainly dealt with the late phase of the Fukushima accident, over 4 years since July 2011, when soil radionuclide concentrations were not subject to rapid changes over time. We recognize however that it is much less appropriate for the 2011 dose estimation due to the rapid changes of soil concentrations of short-lived radioisotopes in the early phase after the accident. According to the United Nations Science Committee on the Effects of Atomic Radiation (UNSCEAR)[2], these short-lived radioisotopes contributed to high dose rates, but of very short duration (typically a few days) due to rapid radioactive decay. For 2011, uncertainties that would have been introduced by the use of dynamic models would have been much larger since this type of models requires more parameters.

Although assumptions are needed to properly perform dose calculations as discussed above, reconstructed doses as proposed in this paper are likely the most appropriate variable reflecting the intensity of the radiological exposure. Dose reconstruction allows for accounting of differences in morphology and ecology among species in a comparable manner, as well as spatial heterogeneity in soil radioactive contamination. Our estimates of absorbed doses for adult birds are in agreement with these previous publications. Garnier-Laplace *et al.*30calculated dose rates of birds for the first 3-week period after the Fukushima accident and reported a value of 1.5 mGy d^{-1} (63 μGy h^{-1}) accounting for ^{134}Cs, ^{137}Cs and ^{131}I and a series of short-lived radioisotopes. This value fits very well within the bounds of the inter-species range calculated for the present study in 2011 (0.3 to 97 μGy h^{-1}). UNSCEAR2 also assessed the dose rate absorbed by terrestrial birds during the first two months after the accident. Based largely on measured data, the Committee estimated the 95th percentile of the dose rate distribution in the area of Koriyama City (50 to 100 km west of the Fukushima Daiichi site) in June 2011 at 1.5 μGy h^{-1}. Using a similar methodology as the one used here, the Committee also estimated a dose rate of 21 μGy h^{-1} for duck in June 2011 in Okuma town, an area with relatively high deposition density inside the Fukushima exclusion zone.

This paper encourages performing ad hoc statistical data treatment of field datasets where ambient dose levels are substituted by radiological dose (rates) to biota of interest. This would help advance the understanding of radiation effect mechanisms and their relation with exposure modalities such as acute vs. chronic exposure to various radiation types, along with realistic ecological conditions in the field where a number of environmental factors are to be taken into account. Additionally, it is of major importance to collect information on dose-effect relationships acquired in radioactively contaminated area for ecologically relevant endpoints, i.e. those with potential consequences in terms of ecosystem structure and function and population demography. Such knowledge will help to elucidate findings from the first comparison of species' radiosensitivity between controlled laboratory conditions and natural environments performed by Garnier-Laplace *et al.*[14], where the meta-analysis failed to discriminate among the various reasons that could drive the apparent higher radio sensitivity of species in the field. For instance, field exposure-effect relationships can be modified due to the combination of radiotoxicity effects on growth rate/reproduction and of genetic diversity, competition, predation and abiotic factors including other pollutants in addition to radionuclides. This point was also recently highlighted in Bonisoli-Alquati *et al.*[3], along with the issue of challenging effect benchmarks published by a number of international organisations to be used as references for ionising radiation in ecological risk assessments.

Inclusion of information concerning the duration of exposure to ionising radiation by migrants and residents would extend the present study. The absence of such information is likely to result in conservative conclusions in the present study. Likewise CR data were derived from studies varying extensively in sampling effort from a single to numerous individuals. Such differences in sampling effort must be addressed because they are known to strongly bias statistical analyses of comparative data[31]. Finally, the findings of our present study are clearly consistent with the present knowledge of dose-effect relationship for ionising radiation. It reinforces the need for continuing ecological surveys in the Fukushima affected area, but also at Chernobyl and other sites exposed to ionising radiation. The merger of advanced ecological methods with sophisticated dose reconstruction models presented in this paper has never been attempted before and is promising for improving the understanding of ecological consequences of chronic exposure to ionising radiation.

METHODS

Study Sites and Bird Census Methods

We re-analysed a data subset described in Møller *et al.*[6]. Briefly, it reports breeding bird censuses at 300 sampling sites visited once a year at the beginning of July 2011–2014. To avoid giving less weight to the year 2011 in the present reassessment based on a global data analysis (300 census points x 4 years), we did not use the 100 sites that were added to the original study from 2012 to 2014. Each sampling site was localized using GPS coordinates and altitude. The 300 census sites were spaced by ca. 100 m and are for logistic and legal reasons distributed along four transects (Fig. 1). The dataset reports specific abundances for 57 species of birds using the point count census method. The repeatability and reliability of this approach has been tested in previous studies in Chernobyl and elsewhere[32,33], but also in numerous other studies since the initial study by Blondel *et al.*[34]. Various environmental descriptors collected per site by Møller *et al.*[6] were also used as potential covariates in the present analysis with the same justification as in the original study. This list is as follows: the time of day at the start of counts at each point, the time squared to reflect the curvilinear relation between bird behavioral activity and time of day[33], cloud cover, temperature, wind force, and ground coverage 50 m around the census point to represent the type of habitats (as % of grass, bush, tree, deciduous forest, farmland (i.e. arable land), coniferous forest cover, recorded to the nearest 10%). In addition, radiation was measured at ground level at each survey point after having conducted the survey (thus making the survey blindly with respect to radiation level) using a hand-held dosimeter (Model: Inspector, International Medcom, Inc, Sebastopol, CA, USA). We measured levels several (2–3) times at each site one measurement right after another and averaged the measurements (see Møller *et al.*6 for detailed methods).

Basic Lines for Reconstruction of Total Radiological Doses Absorbed by Different Bird Species

The biological effects of ionising radiation are generally dependent on the dose absorbed, which is linked to the energy deposited in the body of living organisms from two pathways. One pathway is external irradiation from the surrounding contamination such as e.g. from contaminated soils, mainly due to gamma rays, but also possibly to beta radiation for small organisms (of sizes <1 cm). A second pathway is internal irradiation due to internalization of radionuclides, whatever the physiological process involved. The radiation dose for an organism is the total quantity of energy absorbed from ionising radiation per unit mass of tissue (1 Gy = 1 J kg^{-1} of tissue), and the dose rate refers to the energy absorbed over time (e.g., μGy h^{-1}). Radioactive decay results in different types of emissions that vary in energy among different radionuclides, and the effectiveness of radiation in causing biological damage is related to the type of radiation emitted. Exposure from alpha radiation [with high linear energy transfer (LET)] is more damaging than low LET gamma rays and beta radiation per unit of absorbed dose. Radiation weighting factors are used to tackle this issue. As effects of exposure to ionising radiation are additive, a thorough dose assessment should consider all exposure pathways for all radionuclides present, including any radioactive daughter products.

Here, the basic equations utilize radionuclide activity concentration data in soil and birds in order to estimate the external and internal absorbed dose rates (in μGy h^{-1}) by birds of a given species, along with radionuclide-, species- and irradiation pathway-specific dose conversion coefficients (DCCs). The latter were determined per radionuclide and daughter(s) for adult stage of each species with the EDEN v3.1 software[35].

The dose rate due to internal irradiation absorbed by the bird species *j*due to internalization of the radionuclide *r* (*IDR(j,r)* expressed in μGy h^{-1}) is calculated according to equation (1):

$$IDR(j, r) = DCC_{int}(j, r).\ CR(j, r).\ A_{soil}(r) \quad (1)$$

where

- $DCC_{int}(j,r)$ is the radionuclide-specific dose conversion coefficient for internal exposure of the species *j*, defined as the ratio between the dose rate to the bird species *j* and the activity concentration of radionuclide*r* in this bird (μGy h^{-1} per Bq kg^{-1} fresh weight);
- *CR(j,r)* is the concentration ratio of the radionuclide *r* by the bird species *j* and corresponds to the ratio between the activity concentration of the radionuclide in the bird species at the whole body level and the activity concentration of the same radionuclide in soil (kg dry weight soil/ kg fresh weight bird); this CR is known to be sensitive to the diet of the bird[22];
- $A_{soil}(r)$ is the activity of the radionuclide *r* in soil (Bq kg^{-1} of soil dry weight).

The dose rate due to external irradiation absorbed by the bird species *j*due to the presence of the radionuclide *r* in its neighborhood (*EDR(j,r)*expressed in μGy h^{-1}) is calculated according to equation (2):

$$EDR(j, r) = [DCC_{on-soil}(j, r).\ T_{on-soil}(j) + DCC_{off-soil}(j, r).\ (1 - T_{on-soil})].\ A_{soil}(\quad (2)$$

where

- $DCC_{on\text{-}soil}(j,r)$ is the dose conversion coefficient for the species *j*externally exposed when located on soil, to the radionuclide *r* present in soil (µGy h^{-1} per Bq kg^{-1} of soil);
- $T_{on\text{-}soil}(j)$ is the fraction of the time that the species *j* spends on soil (dimensionless);
- $DCC_{off\text{-}soil}(j,r)$ is the dose conversion coefficient for the species *j*externally exposed when located at a given distance from the soil surface to the radionuclide *r* present in soil (µGy h^{-1} per Bq kg^{-1} of soil).

Finally, the total dose rate absorbed by the bird species *j* exposed to all the radionuclides of interest is the sum of equations (1) and (2) applied for all radionuclides:

$$TDR(j) = \sum_{r}[IDR(j, r) + EDR(j, r)] \tag{3}$$

To estimate the total dose to birds, we assumed all species to be exposed to ionising radiation from the day of the accident (11 March 2011). Therefore, the total dose absorbed by each species *j* at a given site *i* calculated at the census date *k* noted TD_{ijk} was obtained according to:

$$TD_{ijk} = \sum_{k} TDR_{ijk} \times D_k \tag{4}$$

where TDR_{ijk} is the dose rate for species *j* at site *i* and census date *k*, and D_k is the duration of the period between the census date and the accident for year 2011 and the period between two successive census (ca. 365 days) for year 2012, 2013 and 2014.

Therefore we used the maximum estimates of the total dose for individuals yet hatched in 2011 when the accident occurred, resulting from an exposure duration of 112, 478, 843 and 1208 days for 2011, 2012, 2013 and 2014 census respectively.

Bird Species Characteristics and Assumptions Needed for Dose Calculation

For each of the 57 species, we hypothesize that the individuals were present at the census point for breeding at the moment of the accident. We acknowledge that whatever the species, this assumption leads to a fairly realistic dose estimate for resident species, and to an overestimation that we consider to be the highest for migratory species exhibiting the shortest period of residence in the area. We assume the dose absorbed by individuals at the adult stage to be a reasonable proxy to represent the intensity of the stress potentially associated with the exposure to ionising radiation for the species, even though stages other than adults are ignored. For dose calculation for adults, a simplified representation of the body as ellipsoids of known mass and size (geometric characteristics) was adopted, along with the media elementary composition. DCCs were calculated on this basis for ^{134}Cs, ^{137}Cs and ^{131}I. In addition, each species was qualified by a simplified diet, either herbivorous or omnivorous to adopt the fit-for-purpose values of concentration ratios to quantify radionuclide aggregated transfer from soil to bird. Finally, a bird's life style was simplified by allocating to each species the associated fraction of time spent at a defined distance from soil, according to their mode of life.

Soil Radioactive Contamination Data

The GPS coordinates defining each census point were used as input data to select the corresponding concentrations of radionuclides in soils on the basis of the monitoring performed by Japanese universities June-July 2011[20]. During these surveys, activities of ^{134}Cs, ^{137}Cs and ^{131}I in samples of 5-cm layer bare soils were measured systematically at more than 2,000 sampling stations mainly located in the 80-km region from the Fukushima Daiichi NPP. The soil activity at the census point was assumed to be equal to the one measured at the nearest soil sampling point. Activity expressed in Bq m^{-2} was transformed into Bq kg^{-1} considering a conversion factor of 65 kg m^{-2} (sampling of a 5-cm soil layer with a density of 1300 kg m^{-3} in MEXT[36]). Several neighbor census points were associated with the same measurement point as shown in Fig. 1. The distances between bird census points and soil sampling points varied from 12 m to 1.6 km for cesium isotopes (and from 32 m to 3.3 km for iodine) and were ca. of the same order of magnitude as the spatial resolution of soil sampling (systematic grid of 2×2 km^2). Radioactive decay was considered calculating the time elapsed between the accident date and the census date, with a physical decay of 2.2 y, 30.2 y and 8 d for ^{134}Cs, ^{137}Cs and ^{131}I respectively. Considering only those three radioisotopes was of very small influence in our dose estimates. On the basis of maximum soil deposition concentrations for ^{134}Cs, ^{137}Cs, ^{131}I, ^{129m}Te, ^{110m}Ag, ^{89}Sr, ^{90}Sr, ^{238}Pu, ^{240}Pu reported by Saito*et al.*20, we estimated the two cesium isotopes contributed to 78 to 97% of the total dose rate estimates for the two species characterized by the minimum (*Anas poecilorhyncha*) and maximum (*Phasianus colchicus*) absorbed dose rate in 2011, and that their contribution tended to 100% from 2012 onwards. At the first census, four months after the accident, ^{131}I only accounted for a maximum of 0.15% of the total dose rates of birds due to the short half-life of this isotope (8.02 days).

Statistics

The total doses (TD_{ijk}), reconstructed per species *j* per site *i* and census year *k*, were weighted by the observed relative species abundances (A_{ijk}/TNB_{ik}) and then summed for all the species in order to obtain a unique value (TD_{ik}) per site and per year as follows:

$$TD_{ik} = \sum_{(j=1)}^{nj}\left[TD_{ijk} \times \frac{A_{ijk}}{TNB_{ik}}\right] \tag{5}$$

where A_{ijk} is the abundance of species *j* observed at a site *i* during year*k*; TNB_{ik} is the total number of birds observed at a census site *i* for year*k*, corresponding to the sum of all individuals of all species at site *i*during census year *k* and *nj* is the number of species in the whole study.

This weighted average total dose is a representative indicator of the radiological stress intensity at a site *i* during year *k*.

Simpson's index of diversity[37] for a site *i* at a year *k* is defined as:

$$SID_{ik} = 1 - \sum_{j=1}^{nj} \left(\frac{A_{ijk}}{TNB_{ik}} \right)^2 \quad (6)$$

This index represents the probability that two individuals randomly observed in a census site *i* of year *k* will belong to different species.

Generalized Linear Mixed Models (GLMM), assuming Poisson error distribution, and Linear Mixed Models (LMM) were used to assess the effect of total dose on total number of birds and Simpson's index of diversity, respectively. After checking for multicollinearity (i.e. omitting variables with Pearson correlation coefficient ≥ 0.87), the possible confounding variables included in models were time, squared time (because bird activity can be curvilinear with time), cloud cover, temperature, wind (as a categorial variable), altitude, %Grass, %Farmland, and %Coniferous. The main predictor, i.e. total dose was logarithm (base 10) transformed in order to improve linearity with total number of birds and Simpson's index of diversity. To facilitate interpretation of regression coefficients, inputs variables were standardized by dividing by two standard deviations[38,39].

Site and the combination of census day and transect were included as random effects in the GLMM, while site, census day and transect were considered in the LMM. These specific random structures were selected after comparing several models, using the Akaike Information Criterion (AIC). LMMs were fitted using restricted maximum likelihood estimation; GLMMs were fitted using maximum likelihood estimation. Effects of predictors on total number of birds and Simpson's index of diversity were assessed using model-based approximate Wald z-statistic test and t test with Satterthwaite's approximation to degrees of freedom[40]. The significance level was fixed at 5%. All analyses were performed with the R software, version 3.1.2[41] and RStudio environment version 0.98.1091[42]. GLMM and LMM were fitted using the package *lme4*[43].

Since the effect of total dose was assessed as significant on total number of birds, we estimated the level giving 50% loss in total abundance (i.e. the ED_{50} critical radiotoxicity endpoint). From the fitted GLMM the dose-response relationship between total dose and total number of birds was predicted for a subset of doses, which were chosen in such a way that they were uniformly distributed over the range of calculated doses. Predicted values for total number of birds were augmented with random errors to recover the variation in the original data. Such predicted dose-response curves were generated many times. For each curve, ED_{50} was subsequently estimated using a constrained log-logistic model and these estimates were summarized to give the final estimate.

ACKNOWLEDGEMENTS

We are grateful to Professor N. Beresford from CEH, UK for kindly having provided guidance to select fit-for-purpose values for concentration ratios of cesium in birds. For the original field study, funding was provided in part by the US National Science Foundation, the National Geographic Society, the Samuel Freeman Charitable Trust, and the University of South Carolina College of Arts and Sciences and Office of Research.

REFERENCES

1. IRSN. *Fukushima, one year later. Initial analyses of the accident and its consequences*. Report IRSN/DG/2012-003 (IRSN, Fontenay-aux-Roses, France, 2012).
2. UNSCEAR. *Sources, Effects and Risk of Ionizing Radiation*. Vol. I: 2013 Report to the General Assembly, Scientific Annex A: Levels and effects of radiation exposure to the nuclear accident after the 2011 great east-Japan earthquake and tsunami. Report UNSCEAR/A/68/46 (UNSCEAR, Vienna, Austria, 2014).
3. Bonisoli-Alquati, A. *et al.* Abundance and genetic damage of barn swallows from Fukushima. *Sci. Rep.* 5, Article number 9432 (2015), doi: 10-1038/srep09432.
4. Møller, A. P. *et al.* Abundance of birds in Fukushima as judged from Chernobyl. *Environ. Pollut.* 164, 36–39 (2012).
5. Møller, A. P., Nishiumi, I., Suzuki, H., Ueda, K. & Mousseau, T. A. Differences in effects of radiation on abundance of animals in Fukushima and Chernobyl. *Ecol. Indicators* 24, 75–81 (2013).
6. Møller, A. P., Nishiumi, I. & Mousseau, T. A. Cumulative effects on interspecific differences in response of birds to radioactivity from Fukushima. *J. Ornithol.* in press (2015a).
7. Møller, A. P., Mousseau, T. A., Nishiumi, I. & Ueda, K. Ecological differences in response of bird species to radioactivity from Chernobyl and Fukushima. *J. Ornithol.* in press (2015b).
8. Mousseau, T. A. & Møller, A. P. Chernobyl and Fukushima: Differences and similarities, a biological perspective. *Trans. Am. Nucl. Soc.* 107, 200–203 (2012).
9. Møller, A. P. & Mousseau, T. A. Species richness and abundance of birds in relation to radiation at Chernobyl. *Biol. Lett.* 3, 483–486 (2007a).
10. Møller, A. P. & Mousseau, T. A. Determinants of interspecific variation in population declines of birds from exposure to radiation at Chernobyl. *J. Appl. Ecol.* 44, 909–919 (2007b).
11. Møller, A. P. & Mousseau, T. A. Efficiency of bio-indicators for low-level radiation under field conditions. *Ecol. Indicators* 11, 424–430 (2011a).
12. Møller, A. P. & Mousseau, T. A. Conservation consequences of Chernobyl and other nuclear accidents. *Biol. Cons.* 114, 2787–2798 (2011b).
13. Mousseau, T. A. & Møller, A. P. Genetic and ecological studies of animals in Chernobyl and Fukushima. *J. Hered.* 105, 704–709 (2014).
14. Garnier-Laplace, J. *et al.* Are radiosensitivity data derived from natural field conditions consistent with data from controlled exposures? A case study of Chernobyl wildlife chronically exposed to low dose rates. *J. Environ. Radioact.* 121, 12–21 (2013).
15. Mousseau, T. A. & Fox, C. W. The adaptive significance of maternal effects. *Trends Ecol. Evol.* 13, 403–407 (1998).

16. Mousseau, T. A. Intra- and interpopulation genetic variation: explaining the past and predicting the future In *Adaptive Genetic Variation in the Wild* (eds Mousseau, T. A., Sinervo, B. & Endler, J. A.) 219–250 (Oxford University Press, 2000).

17. Parisot, F. *et al.* DNA alterations and effects on growth and reproduction in *Daphnia magna* during chronic exposure to gamma radiation over three successive generations. *Aquatic Toxicol.* 163, 27–36 (2015).

18. Beresford, N. A. *et al.* Comment on "Abundance of birds in Fukushima as judged from Chernobyl" by Møller et al. (2012). *Environ. Pollut.* 169, 136 (2012a).

19. Beresford, N. A. *et al.* Response to authors' reply regarding "Abundance of birds in Fukushima as judged from Chernobyl" by Møller et al. (2012). *Environ. Pollut.* 169, 139–140 (2012b).

20. Saito, K. *et al.* Detailed deposition density maps constructed by large-scale soil sampling for gamma-ray emitting radioactive nuclides from the Fukushima Daiichi Nuclear Power Plant accident. *J. Environ. Radioact.* 139, 308–319 (2015).

21. ICRP. Environmental Protection – the Concept and Use of Reference Animals and Plants, ICRP Publication 108, *Ann. ICRP* 38 (4-6) (2008).

22. Garnier-Laplace, J. *et al.* A multi-criteria weight of evidence approach for deriving ecological benchmarks for radioactive substances. *J. Radiol. Prot.* 3, 215–233 (2010).

23. Hiyama, A. *et al.* The biological impacts of the Fukushima nuclear accident on the pale grass blue butterfly. *Sci. Rep.* 2, 570 (2012).

24. Hiyama, A. *et al.* The Fukushima nuclear accident and the pale grass blue butterfly: evaluating biological effects of long-term low-dose exposures. *BMC Evol. Biol.* 13, 168 (2013).

25. Fujita, Y., Yoshihara, Y., Sato, I. & Sato, S. Environmental radioactivity damages the DNA of earthworms of Fukushima Prefecture, Japan. *Eur. J. Wildlife Res.* 60, 145–148 (2014).

26. Ochiai, K. *et al.* Low blood cell counts in wild Japanese monkeys after the Fukushima Daiichi nuclear disaster. *Sci. Rep.* 4, 5793 (2014).

27. Haskell, J. P., Ritchie, M. E. & Olff, H. Fractal geometry predicts varying body size scaling relationships for mammal and bird home ranges. *Nature*, 418(6897), 527–530 (2002).

28. IAEA. *Handbook of parameters values for the prediction of radionuclide transfer to wildlife.* IAEA-TRS-479, (IAEA, Vienna, Austria, 2014).

29. Brown, J. E., Beresford, N. A. & Hosseini, A. Approaches to providing missing transfer parameter values in the ERICA Tool - How well do they work? *J. Environ. Radioact.* 126, 399–411 (2013).

30. Garnier-Laplace, J., Beaugelin-Seiller, K. & Hinton, T. G. Fukushima wildlife dose reconstruction signals ecological consequences. *Environ. Sci. Technol.* 45, 5077–5078 (2011).

31. Garamszegi, L. Z. & Møller, A. P. Effects of sample size and intraspecific variation in phylogenetic comparative studies: A meta-analytic review. *Biol. Rev.* 85, 797–805 (2010).

32. Møller, A. P. & Mousseau, T. A. Rigorous methodology for studies of effects of radiation from Chernobyl on animals and humans. *Biol. Lett.* 5, 356–359 (2011c).

33. Voříšek, P., Klvanova, A., Wotton, S. & Gregory, R. D. *A best practice guide for wild bird monitoring schemes. European Bird Census Council, publication supported by a grant of the European Commission*, (Czech Society for Ornithology/The Royal Society for the Protection of Birds, 2008).

34. Blondel, J., Ferry, C. & Frochot, B. La méthode des indices ponctuels d'abondance (I. P. A.) ou des relevés d'avifaune par "stations d'écoute". *Alauda* 38, 55–71 (1970).

35. Beaugelin-Seiller, K., Jasserand, F., Garnier-Laplace, J. & Gariel, J. C. Modeling radiological dose in non-human species: Principles, computerization, and application. *Health Phys.* 90, 485–493 (2006).

36. MEXT – Japanese Ministry of Education, Culture, Sports, Sciences and Technology, Calculation Results and Basis regarding Internal Exposure Studied in Summarizing the "Tentative Approach". (2011), Available at http://radioactivity.nsr.go.jp/en/contents/4000/3346/24/1306601_0512_1.pdf (Accessed 2d June 2015).

37. Magurran, A. E. *Measuring biological diversity* (Blackwell, Oxford, United Kingdom, 2004).

38. Gelman, A. Scaling regression inputs by dividing two standard deviations. *Stat. Med.* 27, 2865–2873 (2008).

39. Gelman, A. *et al.* arm: data analysis using regression and multilevel/hierarchical models. R package, version 1.8-4 (2015), Available at http://cran.r-project.org/web/packages/arm/ (Accessed 2d June 2015).

40. Kuznetsova, A., Bruun Brockhoff, P. & Bojesen Christensen, R. H. lmerTest: Tests in Linear Mixed Effects Models. R package, version 2.0-29.8 (July 2015), Available at http://CRAN.R-project.org/package=lmerTest (Accessed 2d June 2015).

41. R Development Core Team. R: A language and environment for statistical. (2014) R Foundation for Statistical Computing, Vienna, Austria, Available at http://www.r-project.org/ (Accessed 8th September 2015).

42. RStudio. RStudio: Integrated development environment for R (version 0.98.1091) [Computer Software]. Boston, MA. Retrieved November 6, 2014. R Foundation for Statistical Computing, Vienna, Austria. Available at http://www.rstudio.com/ (Accessed 8th September 2015).

43. Bates, D. & Maechler, M. Lme4 : linear mixed-effects models using Eigen and S4 classes. R package, version 1.1-7 (2014), Available at http://cran.r-project.org/web/packages/lme4/ (Accessed 2d June 2015).

44. Fox, J. Effect displays in R for generalised linear models. *J Stat Softw* 8, 1–27 (2003).

CHAPTER 7

BAYESIAN MODEL SELECTION VALIDATES A BIOKINETIC MODEL FOR ZIRCONIUM PROCESSING

Daniel Schmidl, Sabine Hug, Wei Bo Li, Matthias B Greiter, and Fabian J Theis

Keywords: Bayesian inference, Model selection, MCMC sampling, Compartmental model, Internal dosimetry, Systems biology

BACKGROUND

Radioactive zirconium (Zr) isotopes are produced in large quantities in nuclear fission reactors; one of the most common fragments in uranium fission is the radioactive ^{95}Zr. For example, the estimated released ^{95}Zr activity of the Fukushima and Chernobyl accidents is considered to have detrimental health effects not only via irradiation, but also via the intake of edibles[1, 2]. The estimation of radiation doses is indispensable for risk analysis. This is true for occupational exposure[3] and patients undergoing diagnostic and therapeutic nuclear medicine[4] as well as for the public in general[5]. To calculate the radiation dose a mathematical model is required for quantifying the deposition of radioactivity from the incorporated radionuclide inside the human body. In internal dosimetry, this model is called biokinetic model as defined by the International Commission on Radiological Protection (ICRP) in[5]. Also, the ICRP put forward the current standard model, which we will simply denote the ICRP model. The parameters of this model were mostly derived from animal data. In order to obtain more reliable dose estimates for humans, the Helmholtz Zentrum München (HMGU) developed a new, physiologically more plausible biokinetic model[6]. It is based on the processing of non-radioactive Zr isotopes in 16 investigations with 12 healthy human subjects. The measurements were taken in vivo in plasma and urine up to 100 days after administration by application of the double tracer technique. Moreover, a global statistical analysis method has been developed and the uncertainty and sensitivity of the HMGU model parameters were analyzed[7, 8].

The biokinetic models mentioned above incorporate basic processes in the human physiological system[3, 5, 9, 10]. Mathematically, this is characterized as follows: All major human organs and tissues are simplified in the model structure as separate compartments that represent kinetically homogeneous amounts of radionuclides; the connections between organs and tissues are described via transfer rates, i.e. model parameters that represent the exchange rates between the individual mutually exclusive compartments. These multi-compartmental systems along with their transfer parameters describing the kinetic behavior of radionuclides in the human body are called compartmental models[5, 11]. Throughout this paper we use the terms biokinetic model and compartmental model interchangeably. The transfer of substances into and out of compartments is governed by the law of mass balance. Transfer parameters are frequently evaluated on the basis of experimental data obtained from laboratory animals and, to a lesser extent, human beings[10]. Although animal data is not directly comparable to human data, the former can nevertheless be very helpful as prior information.

In this publication, we address the problem of model inference and model selection. A Bayesian approach enables us to cover model and measurement uncertainties for a compartmental model based on human data, while

Citation: Schmidl, D., Hug, S., Li, W. B., Greiter, M. B., and Theis, F. J. Bayesian model selection validates a biokinetic model for zirconium processing, BMC Systems Biology, (2012); 6: 95. DOI:10.1186/1752-0509-6-95.

simultaneously taking into account the prior information. The Bayesian framework provides a fully probabilistic approach[12]. It is grounded on the probability distribution of a problem specific parameter space conditioned on the given data. This specifies a measure of belief for all possible parameter values. Similarly – albeit not identical – to confidence intervals, Bayesian analyses provide credible sets for the parameters at stake, holding regions and limits of high parameter probability[13]. However, as they are intrinsically driven by prior informations, some care has to be taken in their interpretation[14].

For an overall assessment of the two competing biokinetic models for Zr, the previous model parameter uncertainty analysis[7, 8] is not sufficient, because uncertainties arising from the model structure were not taken into account. This shortcoming was addressed by our Bayesian approach. Considering the models themselves as a random variable allows to compute the probability for each of the models conditioned on given data. The ratio of the marginal likelihoods of two models, i.e. the ratio of the probability for the data to be produced by the specific model, is known as the Bayes factor, a quantity introduced by Jeffreys[15]. Performing model selection using Bayes factors is particularly useful when dealing with a few models only. While classical model selection approaches using statistics such as the AIC or likelihood ratio tests are based on single best parameter estimates[16], the Bayes factor takes into account all possible parameters values and thus deals with model uncertainty and avoids overfitting issues[17, 18]. Moreover, in contrast to classical tests, the Bayes factor provides evidence for either one of the (possibly non-nested) models by definition. With the introduction of Markov chain Monte Carlo (MCMC) methods[19–21] as tools for sampling from probability distributions, a remarkable increase in Bayesian analyses was noticed. However, due to very complex probability surfaces these approaches often struggle with sampling efficiency[22]. In order to avoid resulting convergence issues of the MCMC approach, we combined a technique called thermodynamic integration with a novel copula-based Metropolis-Hastings sampler[23]. This provides numerically stable results for the inference process.

The HMGU and ICRP models were compared based on in vivo plasma and urine data of 16 investigations of 12 human subjects[6] using Bayes factors. More precisely, the models were evaluated for each investigation individually and for the concatenated data of all investigations. The latter allows to infer transfer rates (including credible intervals) for an average individual. We furthermore provide an analysis based on the (i) plasma data and (ii) urine data individually. Throughout the analysis, the HMGU model turned out to be superior compared to the ICRP model with respect to covering the specific data. This means the HMGU model more precisely explains the given observations and therefore the processing of zirconium in the human body. We then used the HMGU model to analyze the accretion of zirconium in bones: not only did we observe a delayed aggregation but also to lesser extents than predicted by the ICRP model. Lastly, the Bayesian framework yielded credible bounds for retrospective dose assessment of an average individual, this is, based on the concatenated data of all 16 investigations. We provide a user-friendly estimation table for the prediction of initially ingested zirconium concentrations for ex post measurements. This impacts the estimation of intake and radiation dose, especially the bone dose, when aiming for personalized occupational monitoring data.

METHODS

Biokinetic Models for Zirconium Processing

We infer the biokinetics of zirconium as it is processed in the human body. The currently used compartmental model was recommended by the ICRP in[5, 10, 24] (Figure1A). It consists of eleven compartments and 15 transfer rates. Zirconium enters the body via the stomach compartment $y_9$and is processed until it reaches any of the two final compartments urine, y_7, or feces, y_8. Some of the transfer rates and compartments of the ICRP model are however physiologically questionable: The direct mass transport from the two bone compartments to the urinary bladder contents and upper large intestine compartments or the distinction between trabecular bone surface and cortical bone surface as such. In order to address these shortcomings, we have recently proposed the alternative HMGU model[6] combining the two bone compartments into one single compartment and replacing these mass flows by physiologically more plausible transfer rates (Figure1B). Altogether both models share eight transfer rates, which we denoted by $x_1,\dots,x_8$. Transfers present in just one of the models have a unique index to facilitate distinction.

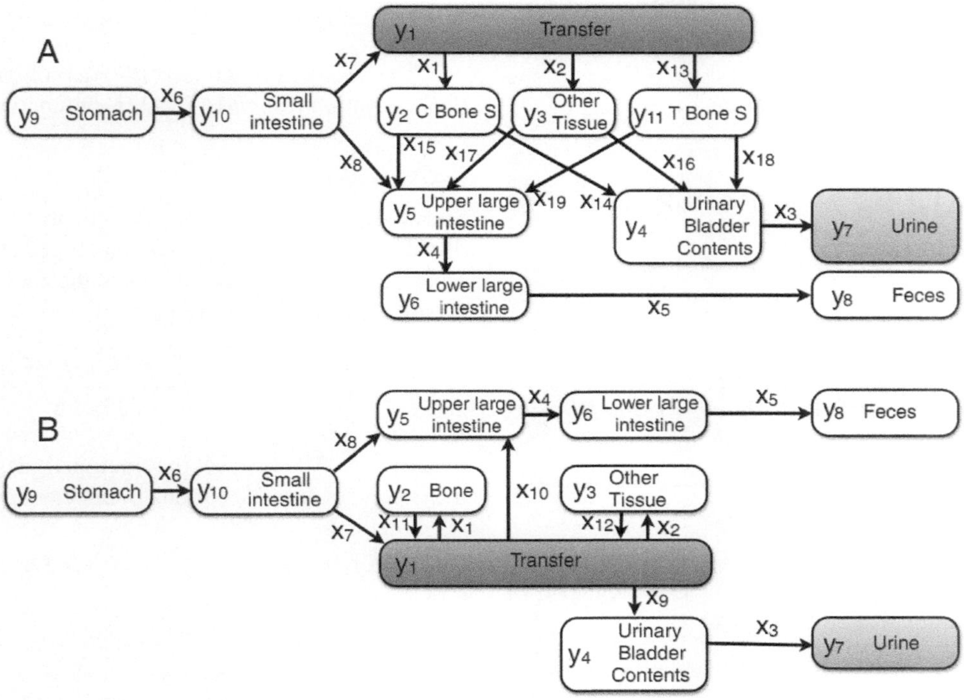

Figure 1. Models for the biokinetics of zirconium. A: ICRP model. The model consists of eleven compartments $y_1,\ldots,y_{11}$ and 15 time independent transfer rates $x_1,\ldots,x_8,x_{13},\ldots,x_{19}$. B: HMGU model. The model consists of ten compartments $y_1,\ldots,y_{10}$ and twelve transfer rates $x_1,\ldots,x_{12}$. In both models zirconium enters the body in the stomach compartment y_9 and diffuses through the system until it reaches either one of the two final compartments urine, y_7, or feces, y_8. The gray compartments y_1 and y_7 are directly related to the datasets measured.

The dynamics of both models are described by a system of coupled linear first-order ordinary differential equations (ODEs): For each compartment y_j with time-dependent concentration $y_j(t)$, the rate of change of y_j is given by

$$\frac{d}{dt}y_j(t) = \sum_{\alpha\in\mathcal{A}^+_{y_j}} x_\alpha y_{[x_\alpha]}(t) - \sum_{\beta\in\mathcal{A}^-_{y_j}} x_\beta y_j(t) \qquad (1)$$

where $\mathcal{A}^+_{y_j}$ is the set of indices of all transfer rates x_α flowing into compartment y_j, $\mathcal{A}^-_{y_j}$ the set of indices of all transfer rates flowing out of compartment y_j and $y_{[x_\alpha]}$ is the compartment which is connected to y_j by the transfer rate x_α. For instance $\mathcal{A}^+_{y_5} = \{8, 10\}$, $y_{[x_8]} = y_{10}$ and $y_{[x_{10}]} = y_1$ in the HMGU model. We have $y_9(0)=100\%$ and therefore $y_{j\neq 9}(0)=0\%$, this is, the complete amount of zirconium is initially contained in the stomach compartment.

Experimental Data

The human biokinetic data was measured in a stable tracer study executed at the Helmholtz Zentrum München (HMGU) [6, 25]. It includes 16 investigations of 12 healthy humans with ingestion of a investigation-specific amount of isotopically enriched stable zirconium. The administered amount was based on the individuals weight, aiming at a dose of 0.09mg stable tracer per kg body weight. Tracer concentrations were determined in blood plasma and urine. For the plasma data, samples were taken several times during the first day in increasing intervals, and more scarcely later on. Urine was collected completely in 12-24h periods on several days. The last samples were taken at 100d after tracer administration. Tracer concentrations were normalized to the respective tracer amount ingested in each investigation, such that the total ingested amount corresponds to 100% at t=0 in the stomach compartment y_9. For model development, the transfer compartment was taken to be identical with blood plasma, and concentrations therein were expressed as % per kg plasma. The plasma concentration was scaled by the total amount of plasma in the body to get absolute concentrations[26]. Urine data was expressed as excretion rate in % per day.

Model likelihood

Technical limitations, such as missing in vivo measurement techniques for all involved compartments as well as noisy data introduce model uncertainties to biological systems[27]. Comparing different kinds of models based on single parameter estimates as done in maximum-likelihood approaches is thus very critical. For statistical model evaluation we here applied a Bayesian approach, taking into account the full parameter distribution: For each investigation i we assume that the data

$$\mathcal{D}_i = (y_1^{i,1}, y_1^{i,2}, \ldots, y_1^{i,n_i^b}, \dot{y}_7^{i,1}, \dot{y}_7^{i,2}, \ldots, \dot{y}_7^{i,n_i^u})$$

follows the solution $\mathbf{c}_{x^k}(t)$ of the differential equation given in (1) for any of the two models $\mathcal{M}^k$ and some corresponding parameter vector x^k, where the model index k∈{HI}. Here, $\mathcal{M}^I$ is the ICRP model and $\mathcal{M}^H$ the HMGU model. Corresponding to the notation in Figure1A and 1B, $x^I = (x_1,\ldots,x_8,x_{13},\ldots,x_{19})$ and $x^H = (x_1,\ldots,x_{12})$. While $y_1^{i,\cdot}$ indicates measurements in plasma, i.e. in the transfer compartment y_1, $\dot{y}_7^{i,\cdot}$ designates measurements of the excretion rate in the urine compartment y_7. There are n_i^b measurements in plasma and n_i^u measurements in urine for investigation i. Assuming furthermore that all data points contain normally distributed measurement errors, the investigation i and model k specific likelihood function has the form

$$\mathcal{L}_i(\boldsymbol{x}^k, k|\mathcal{D}_i) = \underbrace{\prod_{\alpha=1}^{n_i^b} \Phi\left(y_1^{i,\alpha} | c_{\boldsymbol{x}^k}^b(t_\alpha), \sigma_i^b\right)}_{\mathcal{L}_i^b(\boldsymbol{x}^k, k|\mathcal{D}_i)}$$

$$\times \underbrace{\prod_{\beta=1}^{n_i^u} \Phi\left(\dot{y}_7^{i,\beta} | \frac{d}{dt} c_{\boldsymbol{x}^k}^u(t_\beta), \sigma_i^u\right)}_{\mathcal{L}_i^u(\boldsymbol{x}^k, k|\mathcal{D}_i)},$$

where $c_{\boldsymbol{x}^k}^b(t_\alpha)$ denotes the solution to Equation (1) for the transfer compartment y_1 at time point t_α, corresponding to the measurement at $y_1^{i,\alpha}$, for the parameter vector $\boldsymbol{x}^k$. Furthermore, $\frac{d}{dt} c_{\boldsymbol{x}^k}^u(t_\beta)$ is the derivative of the solution for the urine compartment y_7 at time point t_β, corresponding to the measurement $\dot{y}_7^{i,\beta}$, while $\Phi(\cdot|\mu\sigma)$ is the univariate probability density function of the normal distribution with mean μ and standard deviation σ.

The standard deviations for plasma, σ_i^b, and for urine σ_i^u, are fitted investigation-specifically by simulated annealing[28] before starting the MCMC sampling process. They correspond to the combined strength of all deviations from the ODE, e.g. to the size of the measurement error as well as to the magnitude of the difference between the ODE solution and the data points that is due to natural internal fluctuations not considered by an ODE approach. The biological variability between the individual investigations is accounted for by the fact that we fit different σ_i^b and σ_i^u for each investigation i and thus get investigation-specific likelihoods. This leads to individual credible intervals for each parameter in each investigation in the MCMC sampling procedure later on.

The complete data (i.e. concatenated data) likelihood is given by $\mathcal{L}_{ALL}(\boldsymbol{x}^k, k|\mathcal{D}) = \prod_{i=1}^{16} \mathcal{L}_i(\boldsymbol{x}^k, k|\mathcal{D}_i)$ for the complete data $\mathcal{D} = \{\mathcal{D}_1, \ldots, \mathcal{D}_{16}\}$ where in all $\mathcal{L}_i(\boldsymbol{x}^k, k|\mathcal{D}_i)$ the same fitted investigation independent $\sigma_i^b = \sigma^b$ and $\sigma_i^u = \sigma^u$ are used.

For the calculation of $\mathcal{L}_i(\boldsymbol{x}^k, k|\mathcal{D}_i)$ Equation (1) has to be solved based on $\boldsymbol{x}^k$. Since (1) is of first order, it can be written as

$$\frac{d\mathbf{y}_{\boldsymbol{x}^k}(t)}{dt} = A(\boldsymbol{x}^k) \cdot \mathbf{y}_{\boldsymbol{x}^k}(t), \tag{2}$$

where $\mathbf{y}_{\boldsymbol{x}^k}(t)$ is the vector of all the compartments of model k and the time independent matrixA($\boldsymbol{x}^k$) represents all the interactions between these compartments, depending on the transfer rate values $\boldsymbol{x}^k$. The analytical solution is then given by

$$\mathbf{y}_{\boldsymbol{x}^k}(t) = e^{A(\boldsymbol{x}^k)t} \cdot \mathbf{y}_{\boldsymbol{x}^k}(t=0). \tag{3}$$

The matrix exponential $e^{A(xk)t}$ was computed by eigenvalue decomposition using MATLAB's eigfunction.

Bayes Factors

Specifying model specific, investigation independent prior distributions p($\boldsymbol{x}^k$|k) based on combined human/animal data yields the posterior distributions of the parameters for model k according to Bayes' theorem:

$$p(\boldsymbol{x}^k|\mathcal{D}_i, k) = \frac{\mathcal{L}_i(\boldsymbol{x}^k, k|\mathcal{D}_i) p(\boldsymbol{x}^k|k)}{p(\mathcal{D}_i|k)}, \tag{4}$$

where $p(\mathcal{D}_i|k)$ denotes the marginal density obtained by integrating over the according parameter space $\boldsymbol{X}^k$, i.e.

$$p(\mathcal{D}_i|k) = \int_{\boldsymbol{X}^k} \mathcal{L}_i(\boldsymbol{x}^k, k|\mathcal{D}_i) p(\boldsymbol{x}^k|k) \, d\boldsymbol{x}^k. \tag{5}$$

The quantity $p(\mathcal{D}_i|k)$ is called data evidence and is the basis for the model selection process. For comparing two models k and k', we can view the model index as a random variable, apply Bayes' theorem again and take ratios to cancel the denominator, yielding

$$\frac{p(k|\mathcal{D}_i)}{p(k'|\mathcal{D}_i)} = \frac{p(\mathcal{D}_i|k)}{p(\mathcal{D}_i|k')} \cdot \frac{p(k)}{p(k')}. \tag{6}$$

The ratio of the two likelihoods in Equation (6) is known as the Bayes factor

$$B_{k,k'}^i = \frac{p(\mathcal{D}_i|k)}{p(\mathcal{D}_i|k')}. \tag{7}$$

We had no initial preference for any of the models and thus chose a uniform model prior. The Bayes factor in Equation (7) then coincides with the posterior odds ratio between the models k and k' conditioned on the data $\mathcal{D}_i$ [18, 29].

The Bayes factor compares the posterior probability $p(k|\mathcal{D}_i)$ that the data $\mathcal{D}_i$ have arisen according to model k versus the probability $p(k'|\mathcal{D}_i) = 1 - p(k|\mathcal{D}_i)$ that $\mathcal{D}_i$ have arisen according to model k', in contrast to single parameter measures such as the AIC or the likelihood ratio test[16]. The models may be non-nested. Due to the evaluation of each model on its whole parameter space $\boldsymbol{X}^k$(cf. Equation (5)), the Bayes factor naturally penalizes model complexity and thus prevents overfitting issues[30–32]. An interpretation of the likelihood ratio in the Bayes factor was given by Jeffreys[15]. Most importantly, a Bayes factor $B_{k,k'}^i > 3$ substantially favors model k, while $B_{k,k'}^i > 100$ decisively favors model k. Clearly, for $B_{k,k'}^i < 1$, model k' is favored with evidence $B_{k',k}^i = 1/B_{k,k'}^i$.

Prior Information

Since the problem of radiation protection has been extensively researched, quite a large number of animal studies have been conducted. These yielded excessive prior knowledge for the Bayesian modeling approach. As the ICRP model is the recommended model used for dose estimation, there naturally exists information on the distribution types of the parameters involved in the model together with confidence intervals[7]. Four parameters have a lognormal distribution, five a triangular distribution and six have a normal distribution. From the confidence intervals, the parameters of the normal and lognormal distributions were calculated. For the HMGU model detailed prior information is also available from previous studies[7, 8]. Here, eight parameters have a lognormal distribution and four a triangular one. It is noteworthy that of the eight parameters shared in both models, x_8 is the only one having different distributions in the ICRP and HMGU model. Due to a lack of prior knowledge of the dependency structure between the parameters, the multivariate prior distribution $p(\boldsymbol{x}^k|k)$ of model k was taken to be the product of the univariate prior distributions $p(x_r^k|k)$ for each parameter x_r^k, i.e. $p(\boldsymbol{x}^k|k) = \prod_r p(x_r^k|k)$. Each univariate prior distribution was truncated at zero. While Bayes factors were computed inter alia for each investigation separately (see Results and discussion), the same prior information was applied throughout all investigations. This is reasonable since the priors contain information from a huge variety of preceding experiments.

Thermodynamic Integration

Computing the marginal of Equation (5) by numerical integration generally turns out to be a daunting task. There exist a variety of approaches to tackle this problem. Popular choices include Chib's method, which is based on a Gibbs sampling scheme and therefore not always easily applicable[33] or the Reversible Jump MCMC algorithm proposed by Green[34], based on an across model search. Since the latter involves sampling of an additional model parameter, the sampling generally takes longer than sampling within the different models only. We therefore applied a within model sampling technique called thermodynamic integration (TI). It was proposed by Lartillot and Philippe[35] and Friel and Pettitt[36] and successfully applied e.g. in Xu et al.[37]. The method splits apart the computation into several intermediate steps by introducing an auxiliary "temperature" parameter $\tau \in [0,1]$ that governs the influence of the parameter likelihood. The basis of this approach is the power posterior, which is the usual posterior modified such that the likelihood is exponentiated by the temperature parameter and then normalized accordingly to obtain a probability density:

$$p_\tau(\mathcal{D}_i|k) = \frac{\mathcal{L}_i(\boldsymbol{x}^k, k|\mathcal{D}_i)^\tau p(\boldsymbol{x}^k|k)}{z(\mathcal{D}_i|k,\tau)}. \tag{8}$$

More precisely, the quantity of interest is the normalization constant

$$z(\mathcal{D}_i|k,\tau) = \int_{X^k} \mathcal{L}_i(\boldsymbol{x}^k, k|\mathcal{D}_i)^\tau p(\boldsymbol{x}^k|k)\, \mathrm{d}\boldsymbol{x}^k \tag{9}$$

since it yields a way to compute the terms of the Bayes factor (cf. Equation (7)) by differentiating its logarithm

$$\frac{d}{d\tau}\log z(\mathcal{D}_i|k,\tau) = \int_{X^k} \log \mathcal{L}_i(\boldsymbol{x}^k, k|\mathcal{D}_i) \times \frac{\mathcal{L}_i(\boldsymbol{x}^k, k|\mathcal{D}_i)^\tau p(\boldsymbol{x}^k|k)}{z(\mathcal{D}_i|k,\tau)}\, \mathrm{d}\boldsymbol{x}^k = \mathbb{E}_{p_\tau}\left[\log \mathcal{L}_i(\boldsymbol{x}^k, k|\mathcal{D}_i)\right] \tag{10}$$

and then integrating both sides with respect to τ

$$\log(p(\mathcal{D}_i|k)) = \int_0^1 \mathbb{E}_{p_\tau}\left[\log \mathcal{L}_i(\boldsymbol{x}^k, k|\mathcal{D}_i)\right] \mathrm{d}\tau, \tag{11}$$

according to Calderhead and Girolami[38]. This means that the natural logarithm of the marginal likelihood can be computed as the integral over the expectation of the logarithmized data likelihood within the model with respect to the power posterior. The parameter τ governs the flatness of the power posterior surface and, much as in the concept of path sampling[39], stabilizes the computation of Equation (5)[36]: choosing a discretization $0=\tau_1<\tau_2<\ldots<\tau_{N-1}<\tau_N=1$, we can compute the natural logarithm of the marginal likelihood $p(\mathcal{D}_i|k)$ by numerically approximating the integral in Equation (11) by

$$\log(p(\mathcal{D}_i|k)) \approx \sum_{n=1}^{N-1} \tfrac{1}{2}(\tau_{n+1}-\tau_n)\left\{\mathbb{E}_{p_{\tau_{n+1}}}\left[\log \mathcal{L}_i(\boldsymbol{x}^k, k|\mathcal{D}_i)\right] + \mathbb{E}_{p_{\tau_n}}\left[\log \mathcal{L}_i(\boldsymbol{x}^k, k|\mathcal{D}_i)\right]\right\}. \tag{12}$$

Also, the expectation with respect to the power posterior in Equation (12) is approximated in the usual way by substituting it with the Monte Carlo estimate

$$\mathbb{E}_{p_{\tau_n}}\left[\log \mathcal{L}_i(\boldsymbol{x}^k, k|\mathcal{D}_i)\right] \approx \frac{1}{M}\sum_{m=1}^{M} \log \mathcal{L}_i\left(\boldsymbol{x}^k_{(m)}, k|\mathcal{D}_i\right), \tag{13}$$

where $\boldsymbol{x}^k_{(m)}$ denotes a sample drawn from $p_{\tau_n}(\mathcal{D}_i|k)$. For all our applications we chose a temperature schedule with N=30 steps according to $\tau_n = \left(\frac{n-1}{N-1}\right)^5, n = 1,\ldots,N$ to estimate $\log(p(\mathcal{D}_i|k))$ for each k and i as suggested by Calderhead and Girolami[38].

Copula-based Monte Carlo Sampling

The model, investigation, and temperature specific underlying Markov chain Monte Carlo (MCMC) samples were drawn using the recently introduced copula-based Metropolis-Hastings (MH) algorithm[23]. Copulas are constructs from probability theory for assessing and sampling from multivariate distributions. They are widely used in finance and ecology[40, 41]. For any absolutely continuous multivariate cumulative distribution function (cdf) $F(x_1,\ldots,x_d)$ with marginal cdf's $F_i(x_i), i=1,\ldots,d$, joint density function $f(x_1,\ldots,x_d)$ and marginal density functions$f_i(x_i), i=1,\ldots,d$, we decompose

$$f(x_1,\ldots,x_d) = c\,(F_1(x_1),\ldots,F_d(x_d))\cdot f_1(x_1)\cdot\ldots\cdot f_d(x_d), \tag{14}$$

where $c(u_1,\ldots,u_d)$ is a unique copula density function defined on $[0,1]^d$ with uniformly distributed marginals on [0,1]. This copula function covers the full dependency structure of the variables. In other words, every joint distribution function can be decomposed into the marginal behavior of its individual variables and a function covering its dependency structure[42]. The MH proposal function then generates problem specific proposals with an according dependence structure drawn from a pair copula distribution. Fitting the copula distribution was done in preruns containing 1,000,000 unthinned samples each. They were generated for each investigation and model separately. For back-and-forth conversion of the prerun samples and proposals[23], we naturally applied the according prior distributions of the models at hand. Choosing different conversion functions is possible, but affects the sampling performance. Before starting the final MCMC sampling procedure, the maximum a posteriori parameter estimates were computed by simulated annealing and used as initial MCMC sampling values. This makes a burn-in period dispensable. For thinning the Markov chains, i.e. for drawing approximately independent samples in the MCMC procedure, we applied the autocorrelation-based Effective Sample Size (ESS) proposed by Kass[43]. The ESS holds the number of samples left when the Markov chain is thinned such that two consecutive samples can be considered approximately independent. The copula-based MH approach is able to deal with the dependence structure in the high dimensional sampling space and allows for high proposal acceptance rates at simultaneously high ESS's. Finally, all Bayes factors were computed based on 30,000 proposals of the copula-based MH algorithm at each τ_n throughout all applications.

RESULTS AND DISCUSSION

In this section, we present the results of our analysis. We address the question which model is superiorly fitting the data. First, several general results, such as investigation dependency of the Bayes factor and effects of parameter correlations are shown, before turning to the results of the model selection, and their consequences for the HMGU and ICRP models.

Investigation Specificity of Transfer Rates

In radiation protection the transfer rates for the biokinetics of radionuclides in the human body are derived from data collected in various independent experiments[5]. We measured plasma and urine levels in 16 different investigations. This poses the question whether the models should be compared based on the complete dataset, or whether statistical evaluation should be done for each investigation individually. While the former approach results in one overall Bayes factor, the latter yields 16 investigation specific, not directly comparable Bayes factors. All investigations follow the same pulse-like time courses in the transfer compartment y_1 while the excretion rates in the urine compartment y_7 exhibit an exponential decay behavior (Figure2). However, zirconium tracer concentrations showed up to a 50-fold difference between maximal plasma concentrations, i.e. for investigation 10 (1.616%) and 6 (0.033%).

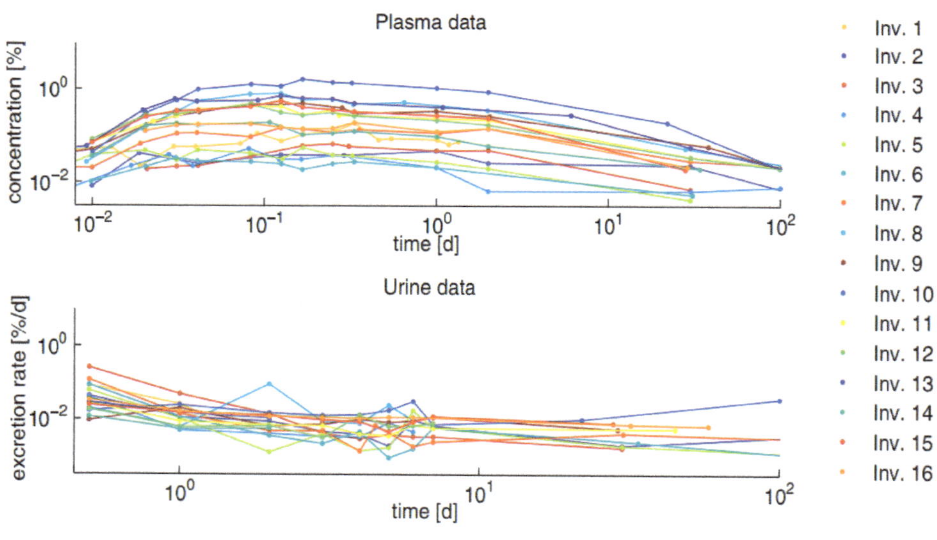

Figure 2. The experimental data. Plasma and urine data for investigations 1-16 on log-log-timescale.

To test the hypothesis whether the diversity in concentration also effects transfer rates and therefore the estimated Bayes factors, we pairwise compared the posterior sample marginals of the MCMC run (corresponding to the samples of $\tau=1$) for parameter x_7 of the ICRP model between all investigations by means of a Kolmogorov-Smirnov test. Here x_7 was chosen as it directly affects the observed plasma levels[8]. Except for one pair, all p-values were $<6\cdot10^{-8}$, meaning that the chance of falsely rejecting the hypothesis of comparable marginals is negligible. Therefore, as the posterior marginal distributions are quite different, it can be deduced that the basis for the Bayes factor, the joint posterior distribution, can differ quite strongly w.r.t. the individuals. This indicated that each investigation should be treated separately. Nevertheless, in order to infer the transfer rates of an average subject, as currently used by the ICRP, the concatenated data had to be used. We therefore compared the HMGU and ICRP model based on both the concatenated data $\mathcal{D} = \{\mathcal{D}_1, \ldots, \mathcal{D}_{16}\}$ and, in order to account for the biological diversity, the individual investigation specific datasets $\mathcal{D}_i$ $(i = 1, \ldots, 16)$. This could also be the basis for further analysis of influence factors such as weight or gender.

MCMC-based Parameter Estimation

Throughout, the analysis was based on 30,000 proposals for each of the 30 temperature levels in all 17 cases (one for each investigation and one for n). For the HMGU model the average ESS including one standard error, i.e. taken over all temperature levels and investigations, is 5832±405. In case of the ICRP model we obtained in average 5808±252 (approximately independent) samples from the Markov chains. This naturally implied high acceptance rates for both models. The sampling procedure thus captured the power posteriors very well.

From the posterior samples, we could derive new credible intervals for the parameters at hand as well as a new MAP estimate for an average subject which can be used if single parameter values are required. As can be seen in Figure3, the fit of the time courses covered the data, indicating that both models are in principle able to fit the data. This justifies our ODE approach with additive noise. However, from the fits alone it is not obvious which model is superior. Note that the credible intervals in Figure3 represent only the uncertainty based on the parameters, in contrast to measurement uncertainties accounted for by the σ_i^b s and σ_i^u s, which are not shown. Clearly, this uncertainty in the parameters is specific to the individual investigations or the complete data, respectively.

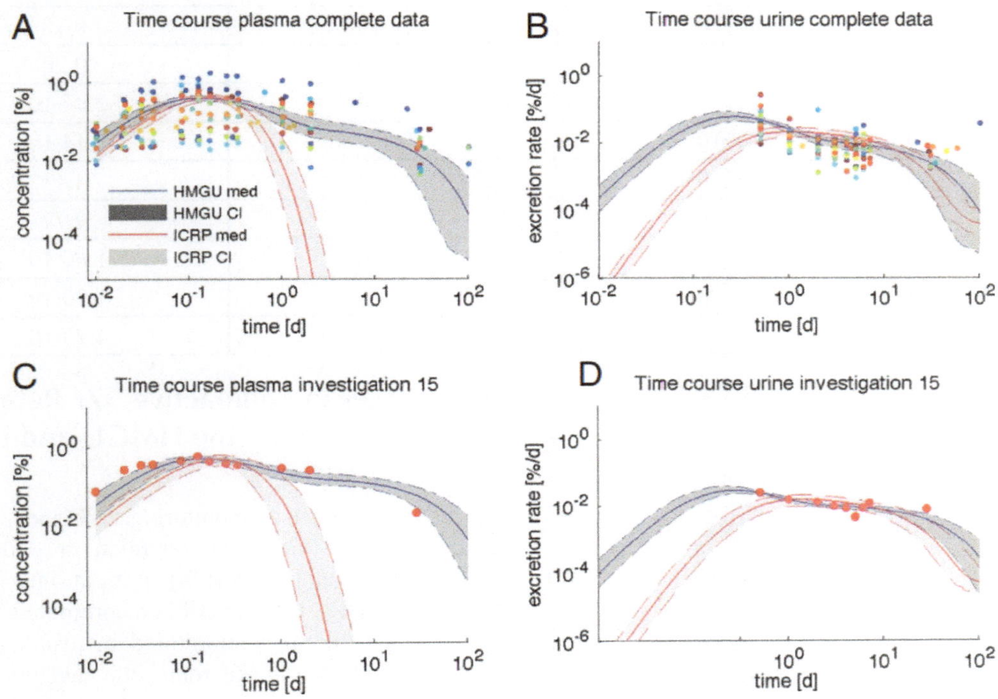

Figure 3. Posterior time courses. Sample median (solid line) and 90% credible interval (CI, shaded area) for the numerical solution of the time courses based on the τ=1 HMGU (blue) and ICRP (red) MCMC samples for the complete plasma data (A), urinary excretion rate over time of the complete data (B), plasma data of exemplary investigation 15 (C), and urinary excretion rate over time of exemplary investigation 15 (D) on a log-log scale. The median and CI represent the uncertainty in the parameters, in contrast to measurement uncertainty (not shown). Colored markers are the data points. The median and the 90% credible interval were computed pointwisely at each time point over all MCMC-based solutions. For readability we truncated plasma plots at $1 \cdot 10^{-5}$[%] and urine plots at $1 \cdot 10^{-6}$[%/d].

Parameter Correlations and Model Identifiability

The posterior probabilities of both the HMGU and ICRP model showed strong correlation between the parameters x_7 and x_8 throughout all investigations. The estimated Kendall's τ's based on the preruns were $\hat{\tau}_{HMGU}$ =0.8027±0.01 and $\hat{\tau}_{ICRP} = 0.3452 \pm 0.02$. This can be explained as follows: At time point t = 0 the stomach compartment $y_9$is the only compartment with non-zero Zr concentration. It is exclusively connected to the small intestines y_{10} in all models. Therefore, all Zr compounds have to pass through y_{10}, which further on distributes them to the observed transfer compartment y_1 via x_7 or to the upper large intestines y_5 via x_8. Aberrations in one of the parameters x_7 or x_8 thus have a direct effect on the amount of zirconium predicted for y_1. This affects the according posterior distributions. The same effect is found for the complete data $\mathcal{D}$. Despite the parameter dependencies, the posterior distributions of the ICRP and HMGU model are identifiable for all 16 investigations, this is, the investigation specific maximum a posteriori estimates are well defined and inferable.

Bayesian Model Comparison

Using the concept of thermodynamic integration we compared the HMGU and the ICRP model based on (i) the concatenated data $\mathcal{D} = \{\mathcal{D}_1, \ldots, \mathcal{D}_{16}\}$ and (ii) the individual investigation specific datasets $\mathcal{D}_i$ $(i = 1, \ldots, 16)$. This results in a total of 17 Bayes factors. We found that all Bayes factors favored the HMGU model; in 14 out of the 17 cases even decisively.

Table 1. Bayes factors

Inv.	$B^A_{H,I}$	$B^p_{H,I}$	$B^u_{H,I}$
1	$7.17 \cdot 10^1$	$7.12 \cdot 10^1$	1.05
2	$1.15 \cdot 10^2$	$2.93 \cdot 10^2$	$3.94 \cdot 10^3$
3	$5.95 \cdot 10^4$	$5.23 \cdot 10^4$	1.34
4	$1.07 \cdot 10^3$	$2.64 \cdot 10^3$	$3.47 \cdot 10^1$
5	$2.19 \cdot 10^2$	$4.73 \cdot 10^2$	$1.34 \cdot 10^2$
6	$4.64 \cdot 10^3$	$3.93 \cdot 10^3$	$2.38 \cdot 10^3$
7	$2.18 \cdot 10^2$	$2.30 \cdot 10^2$	$1.34 \cdot 10^3$
8	$3.75 \cdot 10^1$	$1.28 \cdot 10^2$	0.22
9	$4.62 \cdot 10^2$	$2.32 \cdot 10^2$	0.18
10	$8.62 \cdot 10^2$	$1.16 \cdot 10^2$	0.20
11	$1.17 \cdot 10^5$	$1.81 \cdot 10^1$	$2.94 \cdot 10^3$
12	$1.78 \cdot 10^2$	5.48	$1.14 \cdot 10^1$
13	$7.19 \cdot 10^2$	$1.41 \cdot 10^1$	4.41
14	$3.58 \cdot 10^1$	7.43	9.77
15	$6.29 \cdot 10^3$	$2.17 \cdot 10^1$	$1.60 \cdot 10^2$
16	$6.22 \cdot 10^2$	$1.34 \cdot 10^1$	$1.20 \cdot 10^4$
ALL	$1.20 \cdot 10^{11}$	$3.43 \cdot 10^4$	$4.73 \cdot 10^7$

Bayes factors for the HMGU versus the ICRP model ($B^A_{H,I}$) for investigation 1,…,16 and the complete data model (ALL) as well as the according Bayes factors for the plasma ($B^p_{H,I}$) and urine ($B^u_{H,I}$) data. The HMGU model is favored substantially, when $B^{\cdot}_{H,I} > 3$ and decisively, when $B^{\cdot}_{H,I} > 100$. Also, $1/B^{\cdot}_{H,I} = B^{\cdot}_{I,H}$.

In order to take a closer look at the contribution of the plasma and urine data to the above results, we computed additional Bayes factors based on the likelihoods $\mathcal{L}^b_i(\boldsymbol{x}^k, k|\mathcal{D}_i)$ and $\mathcal{L}^u_i(\boldsymbol{x}^k, k|\mathcal{D}_i)$ individually. Here, i = 1,…,16, ALL and k ∈ {I,H}, where I represents the ICRP and H the HMGU model. The time courses already suggested better coverage of plasma data by the HMGU model (Figure3); for urine the situation is not that clear. This was confirmed by the Bayes factors: all 17 Bayes factors based on plasma data favored the HMGU model; in ten cases even decisively (Table1, third column). For the urine data, three investigations slightly favored the ICRP model (Table1, fourth column). In summary, all decisive Bayes factors are in favor of the HMGU model. While the HMGU model was never decisively rejected, the ICRP model was decisively rejected in the majority of cases. Hence, in depth analysis showed that the HMGU model is superior to the ICRP model with respect to zirconium processing in the human body. This not only holds investigation-specifically, but also based on the complete data. We additionally considered an extension of the HMGU model which, however, did not show any significant improvements.

Differences in Radioactive ^{95}Zr Retention in Bone Predicted by the HMGU and ICRP Models

In internal exposure monitoring, biokinetic models were used to predict the organ retention or daily excretion of incorporated radionuclides[44]. With an interval of 120 days the radioactivity of ^{95}Zr possibly incorporated by occupational workers was routinely monitored by whole body counters. Depending on the intake route, the radiation dose of bone surfaces or colon was taken as regulatory limit for a decision if an individual is requested for person-specific monitoring[45]. In this monitoring procedure, the biokinetic model structure and parameters are used implicitly in the background. The organ retention function is the solution of the model in each compartment; the organ doses are directly related to the integral of radioactivity of ^{95}Zr in source organs over 50 years.

In order to compare the retention of ^{95}Zr as predicted by the ICRP and HMGU models, the 90% credible intervals for the time courses in the bone compartments were calculated based on the posterior samples. It is found that there is a significant difference between the two models (Figure4), where for the ICRP model we added the concentrations in the two bone compartments. The time courses were derived for stable isotopes of Zr and thus had to take the radioactive decay of ^{95}Zr with half-life of 64.032 d[46] into account. The decrease of retention in bone using the HMGU model consequently reduces the radiation dose estimate in bone in comparison to the ICRP bone dose which is currently used in monitoring.

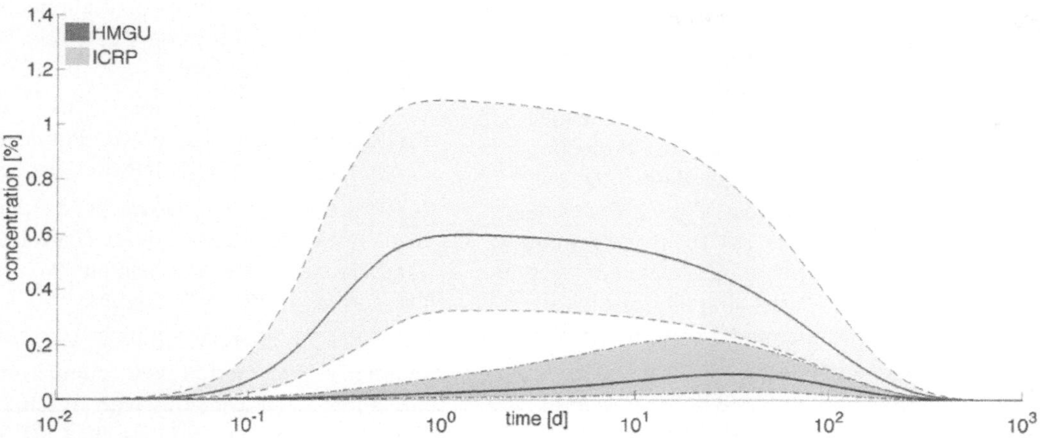

Figure 4. Zirconium retention in bones. Median (solid lines) as well as 90% credible intervals (shaded areas) for the retention of ^{95}Zr in the bone compartment(s) as predicted by the HMGU and ICRP models, taking into account radioactive decay.

Retrospective Dose Assessment

Internal doses due to incorporated radionuclides have to be estimated with the help of biokinetic models based on indirect measurements, using for example bioassays for blood or urinary excretion. Normally, bioassay or in vivo data (e.g. radioactivity accumulated in skull or knee detected by a partial body counter) are measured after an accidental intake of radionuclides. Uncertainties of estimated doses are significant and have a large impact on the remediation and thus action costs. In contrast to conventional uncertainty analysis as performed in[7], our Bayesian approach naturally integrates the uncertainties of measured data and parameters simultaneously. This trait of the Bayesian approach is useful as it provides an estimate for the intake and its credible intervals.

For example, if the urinary excretion after accidental exposure is measured, we can compute credible intervals for the initial intake of radionuclide ^{95}Zr by exploiting the posterior distribution together with the linearity of the HMGU model. In order to be as general as possible we used the posterior samples based on the complete data. Given a posterior sample$\boldsymbol{x}^H$, a measurement $\dot{y}_7^t$ in [μg/d] for the urinary excretion rate of zirconium at time point tcorresponds to a unique solution $\mathbf{c}_{\boldsymbol{x}^H}(t)$ of the HMGU ODE system. Due to the linearity of the ODE's, the initial concentration $\mathbf{c}_{\boldsymbol{x}^H}(0)$ is by definition zero for all except the stomach compartment y_9. The latter reads $y_9(0) = \dot{y}_7^t \cdot 100\%/c^9_{\boldsymbol{x}^H}(t)$ where $c^9_{\boldsymbol{x}^H}(t)$ denotes the value of $\mathbf{c}_{\boldsymbol{x}^H}(t)$ in the stomach compartment at time point t. Now, assuming that for arbitrary posterior samples $\boldsymbol{x}^H$ the measurement $\dot{y}_7^t$ is contained in the 90% credible interval of the solution $\mathbf{c}_{\boldsymbol{x}^H}(t)$ with initial condition $y_9(0)$ as given above, lower and upper bounds for credible regions of the initial amount of zirconium taken in at t_0=0 emerge. These are based on the posterior samples. The estimated extrapolation factors for multiplication with a urine measurement (in [μ g/d]) after time t (in [h]) are contained in Table2 and yield the initial amount of zirconium contained in the stomach at t_0=0. For example, if an amount of $\dot{y}_7^{2d} = 50\mu g/d$ was measured after two days, we find from Table2 that the 90% credible interval for the ingested amount lies between 0.029g and 0.059g. Since the above calculations are based on non-radioactive Zr isotopes, the results have to be corrected for dose assessment with respect to radioactive decay of the radionuclide in question, i.e. in many cases ^{95}Zr.

Table 2. Urine predictions for the HMGU model

Time *t*	**6h**	**12h**	**18h**	**24h**	**30h**
lbf for IC	1233.91	1820.44	2614.48	3369.70	4100.16
mf for IC	1763.73	2225.90	3153.70	4228.19	5340.23
ubf for IC	2512.54	2832.49	3978.27	5650.86	7516.00
Time t	36h	42h	48h	54h	60h
lbf for IC	4778.27	5352.64	5800.77	6153.80	6450.74
mf for IC	6364.76	7250.67	7977.31	8557.87	9006.97
ubf for IC	9122.11	10655.01	11878.81	12960.61	13903.07

Shown are the lower bound factor (lbf), median factor (mf), and upper bound factor (ubf) for multiplication with a urine measurement (in [μ g/d]) after time t (in [h]) on a 60h grid yielding the initial intake concentration (IC) at $t_0 = 0$.

CONCLUSIONS

We were the first to evaluate two competing biokinetic ODE models for zirconium processing in the human body after ingestion. These models were the current model recommended by the International Commission on Radiological Protection (ICRP) and a model developed by the Helmholtz Zentrum München (HMGU). The analysis was based on a Bayesian approach, i.e. individual Bayes factors for 16 investigations as well as a Bayes factor based on the concatenated dataset. In order to obtain reliable Monte Carlo sampling results, we combined the numerically stable thermodynamic integration with an efficient copula-based Metropolis-Hastings algorithm. In summary, the HMGU model was unequivocally superior with 14 of 17 Bayes factors being even decisive when compared to the well-established ICRP model. Also, when restricting the data on plasma and urine measurements only, we found that the HMGU model was clearly favored. The HMGU model thus best covers human data.

In contrast to the ICRP model, the HMGU model predicted a delayed accumulation of zirconium in bones which might be experimentally tested in animals in the future. Furthermore, we showed that the HMGU model can be applied for retrospective dose assessment, where the initially ingested amount of zirconium can be reconstructed including credible intervals from ex post urine measurements. This provides a simple hands-on tool that facilitates the decision if measures have to be taken in case of accidental exposure. In future applications the superior HMGU model together with its posterior samples can readily be used as the basis for dose estimation in internal dosimetry. The Bayesian framework for the compartmental model analysis developed in the present work is directly applicable to a personalized dose assessment and the uncertainty quantification if a person-specific monitoring is requested. More generally, the presented methodology is suitable for any ODE-based model selection task, such as the modeling of protein signaling, gene regulation, or drug processing[47], nowadays frequently put forward in systems biology[48, 49] or pharmacogenetics[50].

ACKNOWLEDGEMENTS

The authors wish to thank Nikola Müller and Andreas Raue for careful reading of the manuscript and helpful discussions. This work was supported by the Federal Ministry of Education and Research (BMBF) in its MedSys initiative (project "SysMBO"), and the European Union within the ERC grant "LatentCauses".

REFERENCES

1. Eidgenössisches Nuklearsicherheitsinspektorat Informationsdienst: Radiologische Auswirkungen aus den kerntechnischen Unfällen in Fukushima vom 11.3.2011. 2011, Brugg, ENSI, Industriestrasse 19 5200 Brugg, Switzerland, http://www.ensi.ch/de/dossiers/fukushima-2/ensi-bericht-zu-fukushima-iv-radiologische-auswirkungen/
2. United Nations Scientific Committee on the Effects of Atomic Radiation: Sources and Effects of Ionizing Radiation. 2008, United Nations Publications, New York
3. ICRP: Limits for Intakes of Radionuclides by Workers Part 1. ICRP Publication 30. 1979, Pergamon Press, Ann.ICRP 8(4), Oxford
4. ICRP: Radiation Dose to Patients from Radiopharmaceuticals. ICRP Publication 53. 1987, Pergamon Press, Ann. ICRP 18(1–4), Oxford
5. ICRP: Age-dependent Doses to Members of the Public from Intake of Radionuclides (Part 1 : Ingestion dose coefficients) ICRP Publication 56. 1989, Pergamon Press, Ann. ICRP 20(2), Oxford
6. Greiter M, Giussani A, Höllriegl V, Li W, Oeh U: Human biokinetic data and a new compartmental model of zirconium – A tracer study with enriched stable isotopes. Sci Total Environ. 2011, 409: 3701-3710. 10.1016/j.scitotenv.2011.06.031.
7. Li W, Greiter M, Oeh U, Hoeschen C: Reliability of a new biokinetic model of zirconium in internal dosimetry Part I , Parameter uncertainty analysis. Health Phys. 2011, 101 (6): 660-676. 10.1097/HP.0b013e3181fbfba9.
8. Li W, Greiter M, Oeh U, Hoeschen C: Reliability of a new biokinetic model of zirconium in internal dosimetry Part II , Parameter sensitivity analysis. Health Phys. 2011, 101 (6): 676-692.
9. Guyton A, Hall J: Textbook of Medical Physiology (11th ed.). 2006, Elsevier Saunders, Philadelphia
10. ICRP: Report on the Task Group on Reference Man. ICRP Publication 23. 1975, Pergamon Press, Oxford
11. Jacquez J: Compartmental analysis in biology and medicine (3rd ed.). 1996, MI: BioMedware, Ann Arbor
12. Clyde C, George E: Model Uncertainty. Stat Sci. 2004, 19: 81-94. 10.1214/088342304000000035.
13. Marin J, Robert C: Bayesian core: a practical approach to computational Bayesian statistics. 2007, Springer Verlag, New York
14. Bland J, Altman D: Bayesians and frequentists. BMJ. 1998, 317: 1151-1160.
15. Jeffreys H: Some tests of significance, treated by the theory of probability. Proc Camb Philol Soc. 1935, 31: 203-222. 10.1017/S030500410001330X.
16. Davison A: Statistical Models. 2003, Cambridge University Press, Cambridge
17. Aris-Brosou S: How Bayes tests of molecular phylogenies compare with frequentist approaches. Bioinformatics. 2003, 19: 618-624. 10.1093/bioinformatics/btg065.
18. Kass R, Raftery A: Bayes factors. J Am Stat Assoc. 1995, 90: 773-795. 10.1080/01621459.1995.10476572.
19. Gelfand AE, Smith AFM: Sampling-based approaches to calculating marginal densities. J Am Stat Assoc. 1990, 85: 398-409. 10.1080/01621459.1990.10476213.
20. Liu J: Monte Carlo strategies in scientific computing. 2008, Springer Verlag, New York
21. Robert C, Casella G: Monte Carlo statistical methods. 2004, Springer Verlag, New York
22. Ramsay J, Hooker G, Campbell D, Cao J: Parameter estimation for differential equations: a generalized smoothing approach. J R Stat Soc Series B Stat Methodol. 2007, 69: 741-796. 10.1111/j.1467-9868.2007.00610.x.

23. Schmidl D, Czado C, Theis F: A vine copula based adaptive MCMC sampler for efficient inference of dynamical systems. Bayesian Anal. accepted

24. ICRP: Age-dependent Doses to Members of the Public from Intake of Radionuclides (Part 2: Ingestion dose coefficients). ICRP Publication 67. 1993, Pergamon Press, Ann. ICRP 23(3–4), Oxford

25. Greiter M, Höllriegl V, Oeh U: Method development for thermal ionization mass spectrometry in the frame of a biokinetic tracer study with enriched stable isotopes of zirconium. Int J Mass Spectrom. 2011, 304: 1-8. 10.1016/j.ijms.2011.02.013.

26. Alberts B, Johnson A, Lewis J, Raff M, Roberts K, Walter P: Molecular biology of the cell (4th ed.). 2002, Garland Science, New York

27. Raue A, Kreutz C, Maiwald T, Bachmann J, Schilling M, Klingmüller U, Timmer J: Structural and practical identifiability analysis of partially observed dynamical models by exploiting the profile likelihood. Bioinformatics. 2009, 25: 1923-1929. 10.1093/bioinformatics/btp358.

28. Kirkpatrick S, Gelatt C, Vecchi M: Optimization by simulated annealing. Science. 1983, 220: 671-680. 10.1126/science.220.4598.671.

29. Chib S, Jeliazkov I: Marginal likelihood from the Metropolis-Hastings output. J Am Stat Assoc. 2001, 96: 270-281. 10.1198/016214501750332848.

30. Lodewyckx T, Kim W, Lee M, Tuerlinckx F, Kuppens P, Wagenmakers E: A tutorial on Bayes factor estimation with the product space method. J Math Psychol. 2011, 55: 331-347. 10.1016/j.jmp.2011.06.001.

31. Myung I, Pitt M: Applying Occam's razor in modeling cognition: A Bayesian approach. Psych Bull Rev. 1997, 4: 79-95. 10.3758/BF03210778.

32. Pitt M, Myung I, Zhang S: Toward a method of selecting among computational models of cognition. Psychol Rev. 2002, 109: 472-491.

33. Chib S: Marginal likelihood from the Gibbs output. J Am Stat Assoc. 1995, 90: 1313-1321. 10.1080/01621459.1995.10476635.

34. Green P: Reversible jump Markov chain Monte Carlo computation and Bayesian model determination. Biometrika. 1995, 82: 711-732. 10.1093/biomet/82.4.711.

35. Lartillot N, Philippe H: Computing Bayes factors using thermodynamic integration. Syst Biol. 2006, 55: 195-207. 10.1080/10635150500433722.

36. Friel N, Pettitt N: Marginal likelihood estimation via power posteriors. J R Stat Soc Series B Stat Methodol. 2008, 70: 589-607. 10.1111/j.1467-9868.2007.00650.x.

37. Xu T, Vyshemirsky V, Gormand A, von Kriegsheim A, Girolami M, Baillie G, Ketley D, Dunlop A, Milligan G, Houslay M, Kolch W: Inferring signaling pathway topologies from multiple perturbation measurements of specific biochemical species. Sci Signal. 2010, 3: ra20-10.1126/scisignal.2000517.

38. Calderhead B, Girolami M: Estimating Bayes factors via thermodynamic integration and population MCMC. Comput Stat Data Anal. 2009, 53: 4028-4045. 10.1016/j.csda.2009.07.025.

39. Gelman A, Meng X: Simulating normalizing constants: from importance sampling to bridge sampling to path sampling. Stat Sci. 1998, 13: 163-185

40. Min A, Czado C: Bayesian inference for multivariate copulas using pair-copula constructions. Journal of Financial Econometrics. 2010, 8: 511-546.

41. Salvadori G: Extremes in nature: an approach using copulas. 2007, Springer Verlag, New York

42. Kurowicka D, Joe H: Dependence Modeling: Vine Copula Handbook. 2010, World Scientific Publishing Co. Pte. Ltd, Singapore

43. Neal R: Probabilistic Inference Using Markov Chain Monte Carlo Methods. 1993, Tech. rep., University of Toronto, http://www.cs.toronto.edu/~radford/review.abstract.html

44. ICRP: Individual Monitoring for Internal Exposure of Workers. ICRP Publication 78. 1997, Pergamon Press, Ann. ICRP 27(3–4), Oxford

45. Bundesministerium für Umwelt Naturschutz und Reaktorsicherheit: Richtlinie für die physikalische Strahlenschutzkontrolle zur Ermittlung der Körperdosis. Teil 2: Ermittlung der Körperdosis bei innerer Strahlenexposition (Inkorporationsüberwachung) (§§40, 41 und 42 StrlSchV). 2007, Bonn

46. ICRP: Nuclear Decay Data for Dosimetric Calculations. ICRP Publication 107. 2008, Pergamon Press, Ann. ICRP 38(3), Oxford

47. Krumsiek J, Pölsterl S, Wittmann D, Theis F: Odefy-From discrete to continuous models. BMC Bioinformatics. 2010, 11: 233-10.1186/1471-2105-11-233.

48. Becker V, Schilling M, Bachmann J, Baumann U, Raue A, Maiwald T, Timmer J, Klingmüller U: Covering a broad dynamic range: information processing at the erythropoietin receptor. Science. 2010, 328 (5984): 1404-1408. 10.1126/science.1184913.

49. Raia V, Schilling M, Böhm M, Hahn B, Kowarsch A, Raue A, Sticht C, Bohl S, Saile M, Möller P, Gretz N, Timmer J, Theis F, Lehmann WD, Lichter P U K: Dynamic mathematical modeling of IL13-induced signaling in Hodgkin and primary mediastinal B-cell lymphoma allows prediction of therapeutic targets. Cancer Res. 2011, 71 (3): 693-704. 10.1158/0008-5472.CAN-10-2987.

50. Zhao W, Elie V, Roussey G, Brochard K, Niaudet P, Leroy V, Loirat C, Cochat P, Cloarec S, Garaix F, Bensman A, Fakhoury M, Jacqz-Aigrain E, André J: Population pharmacokinetics and pharmacogenetics of tacrolimus in de novo pediatric kidney transplant recipients. Clin Pharmacol Ther. 2009, 86 (6): 609-618. 10.1038/clpt.2009.210.

CHAPTER 8 SPACE RADIATION RISKS FOR ASTRONAUTS

Francis A. Cucinotta

INTRODUCTION

In this paper we discuss predictions of risks and the probability of causation (PC) also known as attributable risk for space radiation exposure for astronauts participating in one or more missions on the International Space Station (ISS). In low Earth orbit (LEO), astronauts are exposed to galactic cosmic rays (GCR) – made up of high-energy protons and high-energy and charge (HZE) nuclei, protons and electrons in Earth's radiation belts, and solar particle events (SPEs) – comprised largely of low- to medium-energy protons. The lack of human epidemiology data for these radiation types makes risk predictions highly uncertain. Also, the risks of low dose radiation for circulatory disease and early and late effects in the central nervous system are an emerging concern for space travel. NASA limits astronaut exposures to a 3% risk of exposure induced death (REID) for cancer, and protects against uncertainties in risks projections using an assessment of 95% confidence intervals (CI) of risk estimates[1]–[3]. NASA has followed recommendations from the National Council of Radiation Protection and Measurements (NCRP) for setting astronaut radiation limits [4], [5]. In addition, improvements in other areas of spaceflight safety and ground-based occupational safety[6]–[8] should be considered in the context of radiation risk limits. The principle of As Low As Reasonably Achievable (ALARA) is a requirement to limit exposures even below radiation limits [4], [5].

The uncertainties in estimating risks and dose limits for astronauts have been recognized by several reports from the National Research Council (NRC) [9]–[11] and NCRP [5], [12]. The uncertainty is largely due to the lack of information on the radiobiology of GCR HZE particles that produce distinct biological effects from ground-based radiation such as X-rays or gamma rays, and for which no human data is available. This uncertainty led the NCRP to recommend that methods used for LEO radiation risk assessments [5] are not of sufficient accuracy for long-term exposure to GCR, and to a full NCRP report [12] advising NASA on the information needed to accurately estimate risks and set exposure limits. In the face of the obstacles of large radiobiological uncertainties while needing to support current missions and future mission planning, NASA developed an approach to estimate the 95% CL in cancer risk estimates using an approach developed by the NCRP [12], [13] that was extended to the space radiation exposures [2], [14], [15]. This approach formed the basis for the current NASA radiation exposure limits [1] and supported by a NRC review [10].

Experimental studies have shown that HZE nuclei produce both qualitative and quantitative differences in biological effects compared to terrestrial radiation [5], [12], [16]–[23], leading to large uncertainties in predicting exposure health outcomes to humans. Animal studies of tumor induction by HZE particles have shown high values for relative biological effectiveness (RBE) and qualitatively distinct dose responses [16]–[19] compared to gamma rays, higher rates of metastatic tumors [19], [20] and increases in tumor grade [21], [22]. The shape of the dose response for tumor induction by HZE particles is similar to older studies with fission neutrons which suggested more lethal tumors were induced compared to gamma rays [23], [24]. Concepts from the multi-stage model of cancer development suggest that HZE particles likely affect both tumor initiation and promotion with higher frequency compared to gamma rays, and that non-targeted effects [25]–[27] play an important role at the doses to be incurred on space missions. Qualitative differences in cancer risks are not accounted for in current uncertainty assessment by NASA [2], [11]. In this report I describe sensitivity analysis on how increased tumor lethality for highly ionizing particles could modify risk estimates for ISS missions. The potential impacts of qualitative differences between HZE particles and low LET radiation were not considered in our earlier reports [2], [3].

Citation: Cucinotta FA (2014) Space Radiation Risks for Astronauts. PLoS ONE, 9(4): e96099. DOI:10.1371/journal.pone.0096099.

Beyond efforts related to risk limitation prior to a mission, there is a concern for cancers observed in crew member's post-mission and their possible association with prior space radiation exposures. The PC is a conditional probability of risk used as an indicator of a potential causal relationship between radiation exposure and occurrence of cancer in a population. PC estimates above 50% suggest an observed cancer was more likely to be attributed to radiation exposure than not [28]–[30]. The calculation of PC with concomitant uncertainty analysis provide an estimate that an observed cancer was caused by occupational exposure, however, should be augmented with considerations of an individual's family history of disease, possible individual exposure to other carcinogens, and of individual based biomarkers.

In the remainder of this report, I first summarize the NASA cancer risk assessment model (denoted as NSCR-2012) [2] and its application to PC estimates and years of expected life-loss for ISS missions. Predictions focus on an individual that would participate in multiple ISS missions where radiation limits may be approached or projected to be exceeded, including current interest in 1-year missions on the ISS. For a reasonable worse-case, a 1-year mission is considered near the average solar minimum combined with other 6-month missions to the ISS in other times of a solar cycle. The next solar minimum should occur around 2019 to 2021, however the depth of the solar modulation is difficult to predict at this time with the most recent solar minimum in 2009–2010 one of the deepest on record [2]. Previously [3] results of a meta-analysis of circulatory diseases in populations exposed to low LET radiation [31] and methods to extrapolate these results for space radiation exposures [3], were used in REID estimates of ischemic heart disease (IHD) and cardiovascular disease (CVD), and to make predictions of the combined REID for cancer and circulatory diseases for space missions. In this report, I introduce a method to revise the uncertainty analysis in the NSCR-2012 model[2], [3] to study the effects of increased tumor lethality for highly ionizing radiation. For the first time, risk predictions for astronauts participating in 1-year or multiple ISS missions are made, including sex and age specific comparisons for an average U.S. population and a population of never-smokers (NS) [2], [32].

METHODS

Cancer Risk Projection Model

The instantaneous cancer incidence or mortality rates, λ_I and λ_M, respectively are modeled as functions of the tissue averaged absorbed dose D_T, or dose-rate D_{Tr}, sex, age at exposure a_E, and attained age a or latency L, which is the time after exposure $L=a-a_E$. The λ_I (or λ_M) is a sum over rates for each tissue that contributes to risk, λ_{IT} (λ_{MT}). These dependencies vary for each cancer type that could be increased by radiation exposure. The total risk of exposure induced cancer (REIC) is calculated by folding the instantaneous radiation cancer incidence-rate with the probability of surviving to time t, which is given by the survival function $S_0(t)$ for the background population times the probability for radiation cancer death at previous time, summing over each mission exposure, and then integrating over the remainder of a lifetime:

$$REIC(a_E,D_T)= \sum_{j=1}^{N_m} \int_{a_{Ej}} dt \lambda_{Ij}(a_{E_j},t,D_{Tj}) S_0(t) e^{-\sum_{k=1}^{N_m} \int_{a_E}^{t} dz \lambda_{M_k}(a_{E_k},z,D_Tk)} \quad (1)$$

where z is the dummy integration variable. In Eq. (1), N_m is the number of missions (exposures), and for each exposure, j, there is a minimum latency of 5-years for solid cancers and circulatory diseases, and 2-years for leukemia assumed. After adjustment for low dose and dose-rates through introduction of the dose and dose-rate effectiveness factor (DDREF) and radiation quality through the NASA defined quality factor (QF) function, the tissue-specific cancer incidence rate for an organ dose equivalent, H_T, can be written as a weighted average of the multiplicative and additive transfer models, often called a mixture model:

$$\lambda_{IT}(a_E,a,H_T) = [v_T ERR_T(a_E,a)\lambda_{0IT}(a)+(1-v_T)EAR_T(a_E,a)] \frac{H_T}{DDREF} \quad (2)$$

where v_T is the tissue-specific transfer model weight, λ_{0IT} is the tissue-specific cancer incidence rate in the reference population, and where ERR_T and EAR_T are the tissue specific excess relative risk and excess additive risk per Sievert (Sv), respectively, that are described in other reports [33]–[35].

Space Radiation Organ Dose Equivalent

For calculations of space radiation tissue specific cancer risks, Eq. (2) is used for the cancer incidence risk rate with the organ dose equivalent estimated using the NSCR-2012 model [2],[3]. The NASA QF depends on two physical parameters: particle charge number, Z and kinetic energy per nucleon, E. However, a key parameter that describes the density of a particle track is Z^{*2}/β^2 where Z^* is the effective particle charge number and β is the particle velocity scaled to the speed of light, is used to simplify the description [2]. In the NASA approach [2] distinct QFs for estimating solid cancer and leukemia risk are used, Q_{solid} and $Q_{leukemia}$, respectively. Here a cancer risk cross section representing the biological effect probability per particle is written as [2]:

$$\Sigma(Z,E) = \Sigma_0[P(Z,E)+\frac{\alpha_\gamma}{\Sigma_0}(1-P(Z,E))L] \quad (3)$$

With L the particle LET, and

$$P(Z,E)=\left(1-e^{-Z^{*2}/\kappa\beta^2}\right)^m(1-e^{-E/0.2}) \quad (4)$$

where the central estimates of the three parameters of the model (Σ_0/α_γ, m, and κ) that are listed in Table 1 are estimated based on subjective estimates of results from radiobiology experiments [2]. A QF function is then defined by

Table 1. Parameters for central estimates of NASA quality factor (QF) parameters from Eq.'s (3) to (5) for solid cancer and leukemia risks.*

Parameter	Solid Cancer	Leukemia
m	3	3
κ	550 (1000)	550 (1000)
$\Sigma_0/\alpha_\gamma \mu m^2$ Gy	7000/6.24	1750/6.24
E_{TD}, MeV/u	0.2	0.2

*Values in parenthesis for when distinct values for light ions (Z ≤ 4) are to be used.
doi:10.1371/journal.pone.0096099.t001

$$Q_{NASA} = (1 - P(Z,E)) + \frac{6.24(\Sigma_0/\alpha_\gamma)P(Z,E)}{L} \quad (5)$$

For calculations for a specific GCR particle type described by Z and E, Eq. (2) is replaced by

$$\lambda_{ZIT}(F_T, a_E, a) = \lambda_{I\gamma T}(a_E, a)$$
$$\{D_T(E,Z)(1 - P(Z,E)) + (\Sigma_0/\alpha_\gamma)P(Z,E)F_T(Z,E)\} \quad (6)$$

where $\lambda_{\gamma I}$ is the inner bracketed terms in Eq. (2) that contains the ERR and EAR functions for individual tissues. Calculations are made using the NASA models of the GCR environments and radiation transport in spacecraft materials and tissue, which estimate the energy spectra,$\varphi_k(E)$ of each particle k for 190 isotopes of the elements from Z=1 to 28, neutrons, and contributions from pions, electrons, muons, and gamma rays [2]. The model agrees with flight measurements for dose and dose equivalent to within ±15% as shown in prior reports [2],[36]–[38], which is accounted for in the model uncertainty analysis. The fluence spectra, $F(X_{tr})$where $X_{tr}=Z^{*2}/\beta^2$ can be found by transforming the energy spectra, $\varphi_k(E)$ for each particle, k of mass number and charge number, A_k and Z_k respectively as:

$$F(X_{tr}) = \sum_k \left(\frac{\partial X_{tr}}{\partial E}\right)^{-1} \phi_k(E) \quad (7)$$

The Jacobian in Eq. (8) is evaluated using the Barkas [39] form for the effective charge number given by

$$Z^* = Z(1 - e^{-125\beta/Z^{2/3}}) \quad (8)$$

The tissue specific cancer incidence rate for GCR or SPEs can then be approximated by:

$$\lambda_{IT} \approx \lambda_{I\gamma T}$$
$$\left\{\sum_k \int dE \phi_{kT}(E) L_k(E)(1 - P(Z_k,E)) + (\Sigma_0/\alpha_\gamma)\int dX_{tr} F(X_{tr}) P(X_{tr})\right\} \quad (9)$$

where $L_k(E)$ is the LET of particle k, and the summation is over all particles types contributing to exposure. A 50% percentile M or F anatomical model is used in organ dose evaluations [36]. A summation over all cancer types is made in evaluating the radiation contribution to the survivor function in evaluating tissue specific risks, and a further summation over all cancer types to evaluate the over-all cancer risk.

Hazard Rate for Cancer Mortality

The Hazard rates for cancer mortality λ_M are modeled following the method introduced by the U.S. National Academy of Sciences, Committee on the Biological Effects of Ionizing Radiation (BEIR VII) report [34], whereby the incidence rate of Eq.(2) is scaled by the age, sex, and tissue specific ratio of rates for mortality to incidence in the population under study:

$$\lambda_{MT}(a_E, a, H_T) = \frac{\lambda_{0MT}(a)}{\lambda_{0IT}(a)} \lambda_{IT}(a_E, a, H_T) \quad (10)$$

Qualitative Differences Due to Increased HZE Particle Tumor Lethality

Studies of tumors in mouse and rats [16]–[24] by highly ionizing radiation, suggest that solid tumors induced by HZE particles are qualitatively distinct from background tumors or tumors induced by low LET with observations of higher tumor grade, and increased propensity for metastatic tumors. An upper limit on the possibility of higher tumor lethality would be to use REIC estimates for REID estimates on space missions. However this estimate would be too large due to the presence of low LET particles such as protons that make up a significant fraction of space radiation organ doses. To make a more realistic estimate we assume the increased lethality follows a radiation quality dependence similar to the RBE for cancer induction. The cancer mortality rate is modified as.

$$\lambda_{MT} \approx \frac{\lambda_{0MT}(a)}{\lambda_{0IT}(a)} \lambda_{I\gamma T}$$
$$\left\{\sum_k \int dE \phi_{kT}(E) L_k(E)(1 - P(X_{tr})) + (\Sigma_0/\alpha_\gamma) F_{lethal} \int dX_{tr} F(X_{tr}) P(X_{tr})\right\} \quad (11)$$

where the second term in Eq. (11) is increased by a tumor lethality fraction, F_{lethal} for highly ionizing particles. The first term in Eq. (11) dominates for low LET radiation and is not altered under our considerations of increased tumor lethality for highly ionizing radiation. For our sensitivity study of F_{lethal} we considered a probability distribution function (PDF) to represent the uncertainty in the increased lethality for HZE particles and secondary particles from neutrons. The PDF is modeled as a normal distribution considering median values of 1.25 or 1.5 and using a 25% variance, and compared to results without any increase in tumor quality for densely ionizing radiation.

Expected Years of Life-Loss and Probability of Causation

The tissue specific life-loss expectancy, LLE_T for cancer death from radiation exposure can be estimated in terms of conditional survival probabilities for the unexposed and exposed populations:

$$LLE_T = \frac{\int_{a_E} dt S_0(a_E,t) - \int_{a_E} dt S_T(a_E,t,H_T)}{REID_T(H_T)} \tag{12}$$

The PC is the fraction of the incidence of a disease in a population (exposed and non-exposed) that is due to radiation exposure. Thus the PC represents the incidence of a disease in the population that would be eliminated if there were no radiation exposure. The PC is estimated from Eq. (1) by limiting the upper limit of integration to the year of disease diagnosis, a_{Diag} for both the exposed population and the reference population, with the PC defined in terms of the conditional tissue specific excess relative risk, ERR_T:

$$PC = \frac{ERR_T(a_{Diag},H_T)}{1+ERR_T(a_{Diag},H_T)} \tag{13}$$

where the conditional ERR_T is defined by

$$ERR_T(a_{Diag},H_T) = \frac{\sum_{j=1}^{Nm} \int_{a_{Ej}}^{a_{Diag}} dt \lambda_{IT}(a_{E_j},t,H_{T_j}) S_0(t) e^{-\sum_{k=1}^{Nm} \int_{a_{Ek}}^{a_{Diag}} dz \lambda_{Mk}(a_{E_k},z,H_{Tk})}}{\int_{a_E}^{a_{Diag}} dt \lambda_{IT0}(a_E,t) S_0(t)} - 1 \tag{14}$$

Uncertainties for Multiple ISS Missions

The NSCR model considers PDFs to represent the uncertainties in values for the QF, DDREF, epidemiology data (statistical, bias, and dosimetry errors) and transfer weights for assigning proportions assigned to additive and multiplicative models, and the physics uncertainties in organ dose evaluation. PDFs describing these uncertainties were described in our earlier reports [2], [3]. Monte-Carlo sampling over the combined model is implemented using standard methods [2], [13].

For evaluation of multiple ISS missions, for each Monte-Carlo trial the random deviates representing the QF, DDREF and epidemiology and transfer uncertainties are held fixed over all missions considered for a given astronaut career. However, in considering physics uncertainties related to particle spectra and doses at specific organs, assuming these uncertainties are correlated across all missions or vary from mission to mission could be considered. Factors that arise include systematic errors in organ dose evaluation or use of retrospective dosimetry, or possible errors in future mission projections with an uncertainty that varies for each prediction. Because the physical uncertainties are much smaller than the QF and DDREF uncertainties, these choices lead to nearly identical results. We assumed the physical uncertainties were independent for each mission in the predictions described next.

RESULTS

We considered an array of risk calculations for female and male astronauts with ages between 40 and 50 years at the time of an ISS mission. Calculations are made for average of either solar minimum, solar maximum or median solar cycle conditions for a 51.6×380 km circular orbit. Solar modulation parameters for these environments were described in our earlier report[2]. Calculations assume an average shielding of the ISS is equivalent to 20 g/cm^2 of aluminum based on previous analysis [34]. Trapped radiation exposures decrease rapidly with increasing depth and GCR dominated organ exposure at the average or larger shielding depths, and change modestly with increasing shielding beyond 20 g/cm^2 [2], [3]. The distribution spectra of %REID per year for solid cancer and leukemia versus the radiation quality descriptive parameter, Z^{*2}/β^2, is shown in **Figure 1** for average spacecraft shielding conditions for a 40-y female NS with average solar minimum conditions. The parameter Z^{*2}/β^2 describes the relationship between biological effectiveness and particle track more effectively than LET and is used differentially in the NASA quality factor for light ($Z \leq 2$) and heavy particles ($Z>2$)[2]. A prominent peak occurs near 26^2 corresponding to relativistic iron particles with similar peaks near values of integer Z^2 observed for other HZE particles. However, the REID distribution at large values of Z^{*2}/β^2 (>100) also includes contributions from stopping hydrogen and helium particles produced as secondary radiation inside spacecraft or tissue through nuclear reactions and atomic slowing down. **Figure 1** illustrates that HZE particles and high LET secondaries produced by neutrons and the slowing down of charged particles dominate cancer risks for ISS missions.

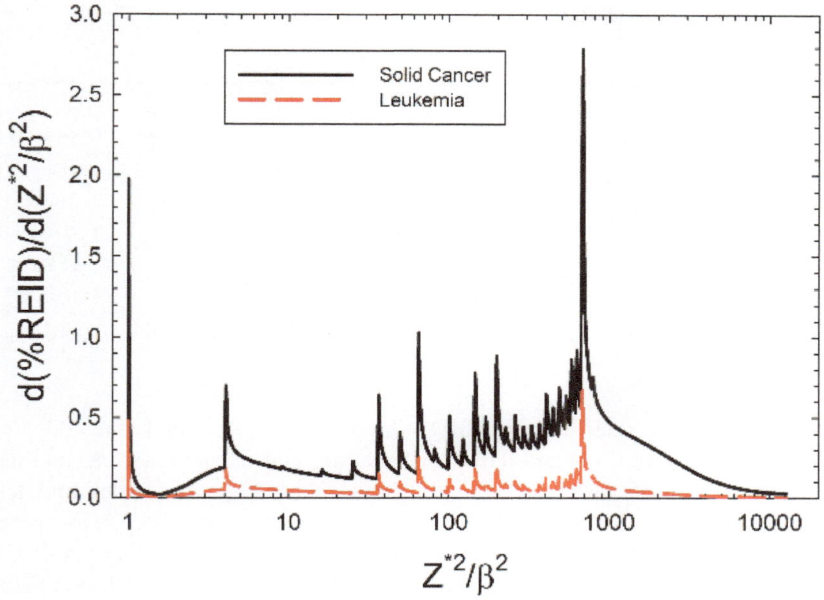

Figure 1. Distribution of the percent risk of exposure induced death (%REID) for solid cancer and leukemia versus particles type as represented by Z^{*2}/β^2 for 45-y female never smokers. Results are for exposure to space radiation on an 1-year ISS mission near solar minimum with 20 g/cm^2 aluminum shielding.

In order to illustrate the age dependence of REIC and REID predicted by the NSCR-2012 model for F and M populations, **Figure 2** shows central estimates of REID from cancer versus ages of exposure from 20 to 60 y for 1-year ISS missions for average solar minimum conditions. **Figure 2** includes results for average U.S. and NS population. Our previous report described our NS model to represent most astronauts that are life-time abstinent from the use of tobacco products [2]. The higher risks for the U.S. population compared to the NS populations is an important considerations for crew selection when considering possible maximum mission duration within NASA safety standards.

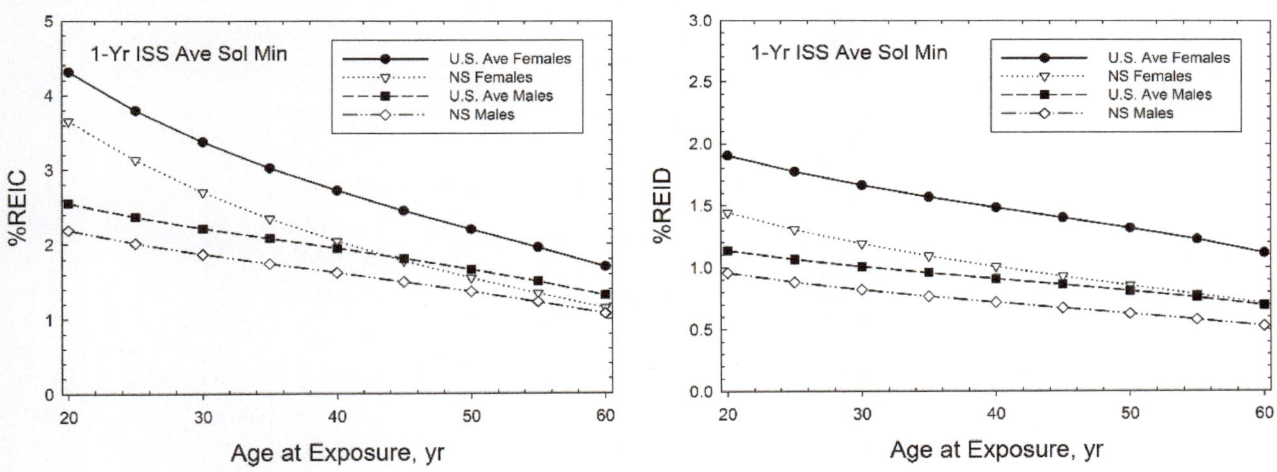

Figure 2. Central estimates of the percent risk of exposure induced cancer (% REIC) (left panel) and percent risk of exposure induced death (%REID) (right panel) versus age at exposure for 1-year ISS missions near solar minimum. Predictions for F and M of the U.S average population or a never-smoker (NS) population are shown.

Table 2 shows organ average dose equivalents for solid cancer, leukemia and circulatory disease risk estimates. Results are shown for 1-year exposure for three solar conditions corresponding to the average solar maximum, solar minimum, and solar median for a fixed altitude of 380 km. In practice the ISS would possibly orbit the Earth at a slightly higher altitude near solar maximum and lower altitude near solar minimum. GCR dominate organ dose equivalent over trapped radiation exposure for altitudes of at least 400 km and vary by only a few percent for nearly circular orbits within a few 10's of km altitude of 380 km. At higher altitudes (>400 km) the trapped proton contributions to organ dose equivalents become appreciably larger and would increase total exposures by a significant amount.

Table 2. Summary of International Space Station (ISS) organ dose equivalents for solid cancer, leukemia and circulatory disease risk estimates for different solar cycle conditions for females (males).

Missions	Solid Cancer, Sv	Leukemia, Sv	Circulatory Disease, Gy-Eq
1-Y Solar Min	0.187 (0.175)	0.109 (0.104)	0.132 (0.126)
1-Y Solar Med	0.146 (0.138)	0.084 (0.08)	0.10 (0.096)
1-Y Solar Max	0.10 (0.094)	0.054 (0.052)	0.072 (0.064)
1-Y Solar Min and 0.5-Y Solar Med	0.26 (0.244)	0.151 (0.144)	0.182 (0.174)
1-Y Solar Min, 0.5-Y Solar Med, and 0.5-Y Solar Max	0.31 (0.291)	0.178 (0.171)	0.215 (0.205)

Predictions are for single or multiple ISS missions. Solar cycle conditions considered are average solar minimum (Solar Min), average solar maximum (Solar Max), or median solar cycle (Solar Med), with solar modulation parameters for these conditions described in [2].

doi:10.1371/journal.pone.0096099.t002

Predictions of tissue specific REID, total cancer REID and the additional REID contributions from CVD and IHD are shown in Figure 3 for the case of two ISS missions of total duration of 18 months (6 months for solar median conditions, and 12 months near solar minimum). Central estimates and upper 95% CI of REIC and REID for cancer are slightly reduced (~2%) when CVD and IHD are included in calculations due to the role of competing risks. Risks for females are about 20% higher than males due to the added contributions from breast, ovarian, and uterine cancers, and an important difference in lung cancer risks for males and females. Also, organ dose equivalents for females are a few percent larger than males due to less body mass. Predictions of CVD and IHD are similar for M and F and NS and U.S. average populations [25], and increase overall REID by about 40% on average.

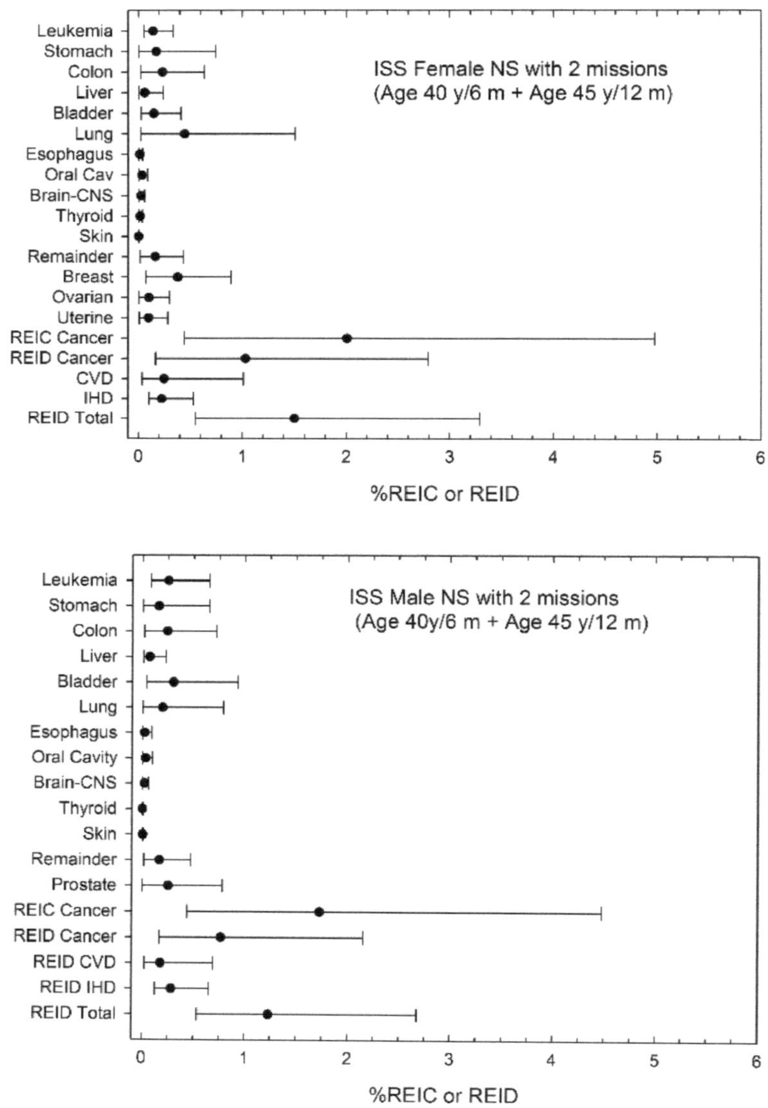

Figure 3. Predictions of tissue (disease) specific percent risk of exposure induced cancer (%REIC) or percent risk of exposure induced death (%REID) for participation in two ISS missions at age 40-y and age 45-y (6-months at solar median and 1-year near solar minimum) for F and M never-smoker populations.

Figure 4 shows a similar comparison as Figure 3 for astronauts participating in three ISS missions of total duration of 2-year with a 1-year mission near solar minimum at age 50-y. In this comparison upper 95% CIs exceed 3% for females and approach 3% for males for cancer alone. The inclusion of circulatory disease risk leads to a predictions where both males and females have upper 95% CIs above 3% with values close to 4% for females.

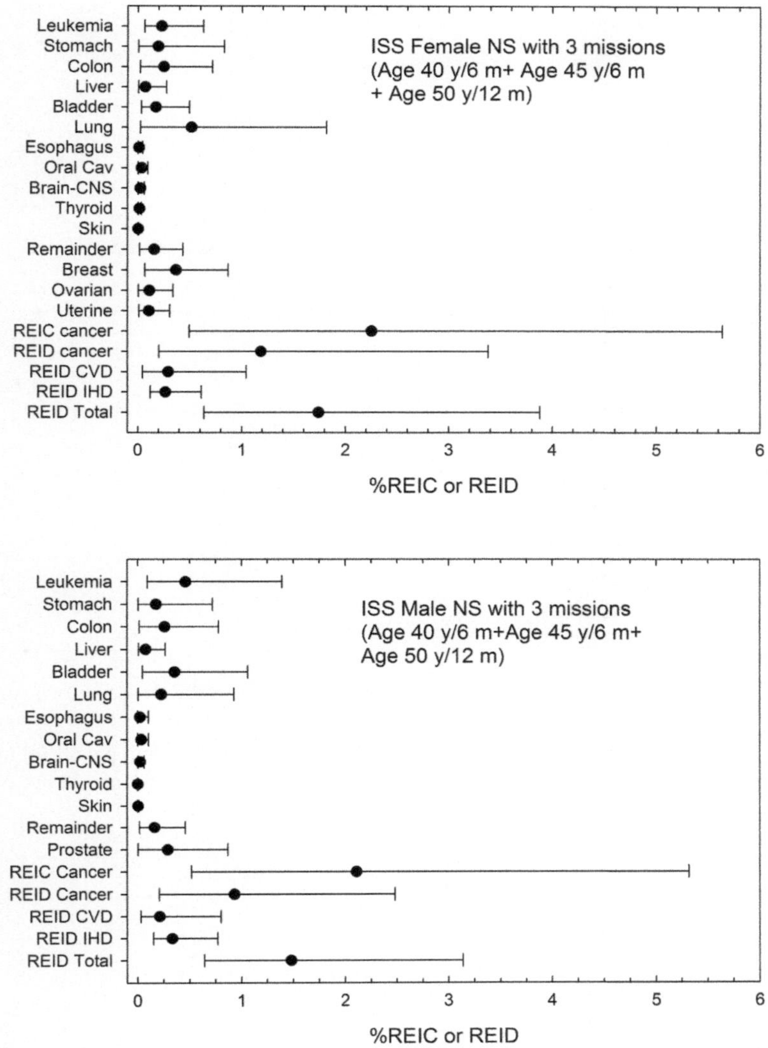

Figure 4. Predictions of tissue (disease) specific percent risk of exposure induced cancer (%REIC) or percent risk of exposure induced death (%REID) for participation in three ISS missions at age 40-, 45, and 50-y (6-month at solar median, 6-months near solar maximum, and 1-year near solar minimum) for F and M never-smoker populations.

Figure 5 shows predictions of the PC following participation in two ISS missions corresponding to the results of Figure 3. Results are shown for F and M NS with disease diagnosis of age 55-y and 65-y which correspond to 15- and 25-y after the first ISS mission, and 5- and 15-y after a 1-year ISS mission, respectively. By age 65-y, %PC at the upper 95% confidence interval exceed 20% for leukemia, stomach, colon, lung, esophageal and ovarian cancers. %PC for circulatory diseases are modest (<10%) because of the large background and longer latency that results from epidemiology analysis compared to radiation induced cancers. %PC for leukemia's decline at older ages while %PC for solid cancers, CVD and IVD increase modestly at older ages (>65 y) (result not shown). Similar results for 1-year missions with no other space exposures for mission age of 45-y and PC estimates at age 65-y are shown in Figure 6. These results suggest a 1-y mission near solar minimum would not exceed NASA radiation limits for astronauts with no prior occupational radiation exposures. Our predictions at solar minimum support that 1-year missions at any time in a solar cycle are below limits. However, other prior occupational exposures and changes to risk assessment models may alter this conclusion. Table 3 and 4 also show the average years of life-loss expectancy (LLE) if death from space radiation exposure would occur. Leukemia has a LLE of about 23-y, overall cancer 15-y, and specific solid cancers varying from 12- to 20-y of life-loss. The LLE for circulatory diseases is less than that of cancer with values between 9- and 10-y resulting from our analysis.

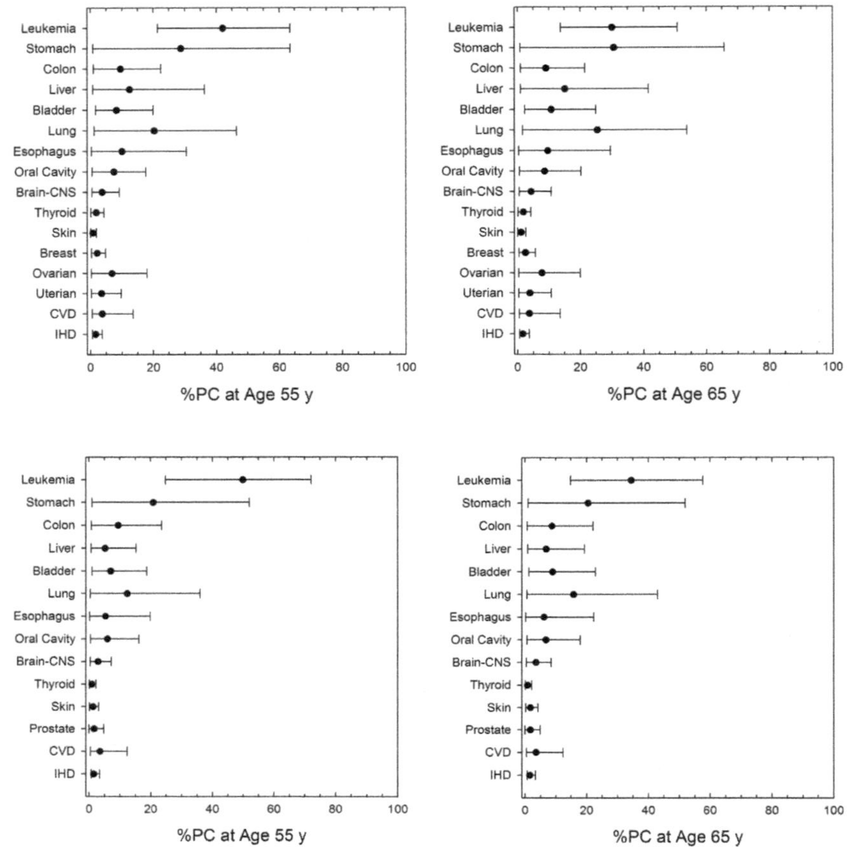

Figure 5. Predictions of tissue (disease) specific %PC at age 55-y (left panel) and age 65-y (right panel) following participation in two ISS missions at age 40-y and age 45-y (6-month at solar median, and 1-year near solar minimum) for F and M never-smoker populations.

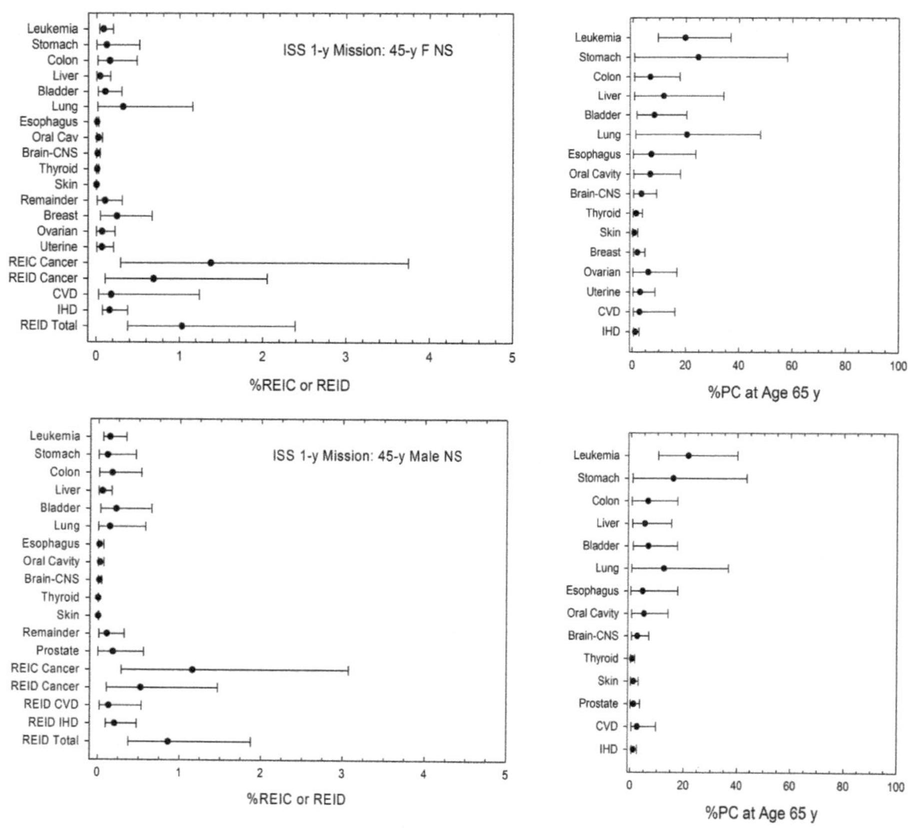

Figure 6. Predictions tissue (disease) specific percent risk of exposure induced cancer (%REIC) or percent risk of exposure induced death (%REID) or percent probability of causation (%PC) at age 65-y (right panels) following participation in1-y ISS missions at age 45-y for F and M never-smoker populations.

Table 3. Predictions for female never-smokers participating in multiple ISS missions of organ dose equivalents (H_T) and average loss of life expectancy (LLE) if radiation induced death occurs.

	Two ISS Missions for total duration of 18 m		Three ISS Missions for total duration of 24 m	
Tissue	H_T, Sv or Gy-Eq	LLE, y	H_T, Sv or Gy-Eq	LLE, y
Leukemia, Sv	0.151	23.1	0.179	24.9
Stomach	0.235	16.3	0.281	15.5
Colon	0.261	16.7	0.311	16.1
Liver	0.229	13.5	0.274	13.1
Bladder	0.231	11.2	0.276	11
Lung	0.264	13.2	0.314	12.8
Esophagus	0.249	15.1	0.297	14.6
Oral Cavity	0.308	15.3	0.365	14.6
Brain-CNS	0.286	18	0.339	17.2
Thyroid	0.308	22	0.365	20.8
Skin	0.282	11.8	0.336	11.7
Remainder	0.264	12	0.315	11.6
Breast	0.289	15.7	0.343	15.2
Ovarian	0.241	17.9	0.287	17.1
Uterine	0.241	17.1	0.287	16.4
Total Cancer	0.244	15	0.29	14.8
CVD, Gy-Eq	0.182	9.1	0.215	9.1
IHD	0.182	9.5	0.215	9.5

Results shown are for two missions at age 40, and 45 y of 180 d (at solar median), and 1-y (average solar minimum), respectively, or three missions at age 40, 45, and 50 y of 180 d (average solar maximum), 180 d (solar median), and 1-y (average solar minimum), respectively.
doi:10.1371/journal.pone.0096099.t003

Table 4. Predictions for male never-smokers participating in multiple ISS missions of organ dose equivalents (H_T) and average loss of life expectancy (LLE) if radiation induced death occurs.

	Two ISS Missions for total duration of 18 m		Three ISS Missions for total duration of 24 m	
Tissue	H_T, Sv or Gy-Eq	LLE, y	H_T, Sv or Gy-Eq	LLE, y
Leukemia, Sv	0.145	22.1	0.171	24.6
Stomach	0.227	15.6	0.272	14.9
Colon	0.251	16.4	0.299	15.7
Liver	0.235	14	0.281	13.5
Bladder	0.224	10.9	0.269	10.7
Lung	0.245	13.6	0.292	13.2
Esophagus	0.242	14.9	0.289	14.4
Oral Cavity	0.261	15.8	0.311	15.1
Brain-CNS	0.279	17	0.332	16.2
Thyroid	0.261	20.8	0.311	19.7
Skin	0.308	12	0.365	11.8
Remainder	0.253	11.7	0.302	11.3
Prostate	0.260	11.5	0.309	11.4
Total Cancer	0.228	15	0.272	15.6
CVD, Gy-Eq	0.174	9.8	0.205	9.8
IHD	0.174	10.6	0.205	10.6

Results shown are for two missions at age 40, and 45 y of 180 d (at solar median), and 1-y (average solar minimum), respectively, or three missions at age 40, 45, and 50 y of 180 d (average solar maximum), 180 d (solar median), and 1-y (average solar minimum), respectively.
doi:10.1371/journal.pone.0096099.t004

Figure 7 and Table 5 show comparisons from results of sensitivity analysis of the role of increased lethality from HZE particles and nuclear secondaries using the adjusted mortality rate of Eq. (11). Results for 1-year ISS missions and two missions consisting of a 1-year mission at age 45 and a previous mission at age 40-y with median solar cycle conditions of 6-months are shown. The PDF for cancer in the NSCR-2012 model, total REID for cancer and circulatory disease risks combined, and total REID with inclusion of the enhanced tumor lethality assumption for densely ionizing particles with F_{lethal}=1.5 are shown in Figure 7. These results suggest that an increase in tumor lethality of 25 to 50%, which are values suggested by animal studies with high LET radiation, would reduce the mission duration for ISS missions with 95% CIs to be below the acceptable risk limits to less than 18 months. The combination of increased tumor lethality and addition of fatal circulatory disease risks could possibly impact crew participation on a 1-year mission within NASA's radiation safety standards.

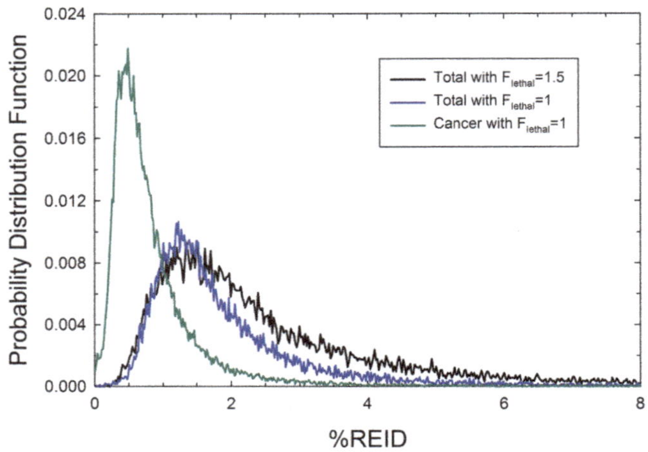

Figure 7. Predictions of the PDF for percent risk of exposure induced death (%REID) for cancer in NSCR-2012 model [2], and current results for the total (cancer and circulatory disease combined) and the modification of total %REID for the case of increased tumor lethality for highly densely ionizing particle.

Predictions are for participation in two ISS missions at age 40-y and age 45-y (6-month at solar median and 1-year near solar minimum) for F never-smoker population.

Table 5. Predictions of the increased percent risk of exposure induced death (%REID) for ISS missions due to potential qualitative difference leading to increases in tumor lethality for highly ionizing particles compared to tumors occurring in non-radiated populations or induced by low LET radiation. Results for F and M never-smokers are shown for cancer %REID and total %REID (cancer and circulatory diseases combined) assuming 20 g/cm^2 average aluminum shielding.

Uncertainty Model	%REID (F) Cancer	%REID (F) Total	%REID (M) Cancer	%REID (M) Total
1-y ISS mission at age 45 y				
NSCR-2012	0.69 [0.11, 2.07]	1.03 [0.38, 2.37]	0.52 [0.11, 1.49]	0.86 [0.38, 1.9]
F_{lethal} = 1.25	0.78 [0.13, 2.89]	1.12 [0.4, 3.12]	0.59 [0.12, 2.09]	0.93 [0.40, 2.45]
F_{lethal} = 1.5	0.87 [0.16, 3.9]	1.21 [0.43, 4.0]	0.65 [0.14, 2.84]	0.99 [0.43, 3.08]
6-m ISS mission at Age 40 y and 1-y ISS mission at age 45 y				
NSCR-2012	1.01 [0.16, 2.79]	1.52 [0.55, 3.29]	0.77 [0.17, 2.15]	1.26 [0.54, 2.69]
F_{lethal} = 1.25	1.12 [0.2, 4.13]	1.59 [0.58, 4.41]	0.87 [0.2, 3.03]	1.32 [0.58, 3.48]
F_{lethal} = 1.5	1.25 [0.22, 5.46]	1.71 [0.61, 5.61]	0.96 [0.23, 4.02]	1.41 [0.62, 4.35]

Increases in tumor lethality is considered with the parameter, F_{lethal} as described by Eq.(11). The NASA Space Cancer Risk model (NSCR-2012) assumes F_{lethal} = 1 with no uncertainty.
doi:10.1371/journal.pone.0096099.t005

DISCUSSION

Uncertainties in Risk Estimates

The detailed uncertainty analysis of radiation risks in this report lend support to the acceptable radiation risks for astronauts selected for 6-month or 1-year ISS missions. However because astronauts may have flown on prior ISS missions more detailed analysis was made for participation on multiple ISS missions. Any time spent on extra-vehicular activities (EVA) would marginally increase these results. However near solar maximum, the uncertainty in SPE occurrence is an important consideration, especially for EVAs if ISS orbits are within weak geomagnetic field locations or where trapped electron belt exposure occur, which could be increased by geomagnetic storms associated with SPEs. Other occupational exposures for astronauts, include possible participation in past space shuttle missions, medical diagnostic exposure related to fitness of duty and aviation exposures [40], [41]. The cumulative dose from these exposure increases with astronaut age. These exposures are not considered herein, but could raise estimates for individual crew members compared to the predictions described.

A major finding of our analysis is that female astronauts may exceed NASA radiation standards onward of 18 months in LEO and male astronauts onward of 24 months in LEO. Some variability in these times is expected due to solar cycle effects, other occupational radiation exposures, and the possibility of large solar particle events. Uncertainty reduction remains the most important area to improve risk predictions, extend allowable mission lengths, and ensure the safety of astronauts returning from long-term space missions. Improvements in the understanding of radiation quality and dose-rate effects could significantly reduce upper confidence intervals in the NSCR-2012 model. Improved information on specifying tissue specific transfer weights used in applying epidemiology data, and understanding differences in disease rates between model populations could also reduce uncertainties in risk estimates.

Human studies on circulatory disease risks are a more recent concern from epidemiology analysis of low dose radiation exposures [31], [42], [43]. For circulatory disease predictions the deterministic effects RBE model recommended by the International Commission on Radiological Protection (ICRP) is used as the central estimate [44], which as shown in Tables 2 and 3 leads to a lower GCR organ averaged equivalent dose compared to solid cancer risk and higher value compared to leukemia risk [3]. Uncertainty analysis for circulatory disease risk estimates were described in a recent report [3]. Concerns about a possible dose threshold for circulatory disease risks are an important consideration for ISS missions. Meta-analysis results that were based in-part to chronic exposures of radiation workers [31] suggests no dose threshold occurs. However, basic radiobiological understanding of how radiation increases circulatory disease risk at low dose and for highly ionizing radiation is lacking at this time. Life-style factors related to circulatory disease risk are expected to be larger compared to cancer risks, and also need to be considered in the understanding of possible radiation risks.

In the NSCR model a DDREF of 1.5 is used for solid cancers based on the BEIR VII report[34], and the recommendations of the NRC to NASA [11]. For circulatory disease risk predictions a DDREF is not applied because models were based on meta-analysis of several chronically exposed populations as described by Little et al. [31]. For cancer risks the low value for the DDREF of 1.5 leads to an uncertainty distribution that is skewed towards higher DDREF values and lower REID, which opposes the QF uncertainty estimate which is skewed to higher REID values [2].

Because of the lack of human data following exposure to high LET radiation, animal studies continue to be the main source of information for risk estimates. These studies [16]–[24]suggest that HZE particles and neutrons could produce more lethal tumors compared to tumors from low LET radiation or background tumors, which is a qualitative difference not accounted for in current risk estimates. For low LET radiation there is an implicit assumption made by epidemiology models that the tumors induced by radiation are similar to background tumors in a population. This assumption is consistent with the multiplicative risk model, and also based on lack of information to make an alternative assumption. I considered a sensitivity analysis of the role of increased tumor lethality by adjusting the cancer mortality rates of Eq. (11) for the portion of each particle radiation track that acts in a distinct mode compared to low LET radiation. Also considered is a model (result not shown) where this ratio was adjusted in a tissue specific manner. The lethality fractions in the U.S. population varies substantially with tissue type and such an alternative approach could be further investigated if more information were available. The results of **Table 5** suggests that increased tumor lethality for highly ionizing radiation compared to background or low LET induced tumors that is suggested by animal studies could substantially increase risk estimates and uncertainties estimates for ISS missions, and therefore warrants further study.

QFs are largely based on cellular studies of gene mutation and chromosomal aberrations and limited data on tumor induction in mice from the studies of Fry et al. [16] and Alpen et al. [17]for Harderian gland tumors with a variety of particles. The Harderian gland tumor studies used pituitary implants which acted as tumor promoters such that the effects of radiation exposure was largely on tumor initiation [16], [17]. Therefore information used to estimate radiation QFs are reflective of cancer initiation and provide no information on whether the probability of tumor metastasis is dependent on radiation quality. Alpen et al. [17] showed the tumor response of Fe particles was similar with or without the use of a promoter, which was distinct from the response found for gamma rays.

HZE particle tumor studies reported to date are dissimilar with limitations in particle types, dose and dose-rates, and animal models considered; however are consistent in supporting the hypothesis that HZE particles produce solid tumors in a qualitatively distinct manner compared to low LET radiation, and suggest that RBEs alone do not properly account for potential risks. For leukemia induction, HZE particles appear to be more similar to gamma rays with a low RBE reported [19]. Detailed studies of solid cancers for a variety of particle types and energies and tumor types, with time serial analysis of tumor occurrence and molecular analysis of tumor quality including metastatic potential are needed. These studies should include M and F mice of various strains, including genetically engineered mice, in order to follow-up on the information in studies reported to date [16]–[22].

Probability of Causation and Early Detection of Cancers

In the past uncertainty analyses of PC estimates have been developed by the National Institutes of Health [28], [29] and in the nuclear industry [30] for terrestrial radiation exposures to screen exposed persons for a potential causal relationship to an observed cancer, and in the determination if monetary compensation should be awarded. The PC predictions reported here suggest that a large portion of cancers that would be observed from astronauts that participated in multiple ISS missions could be attributed to GCR exposure. In contrast, PC predictions for single ISS missions of 6-months are not estimated to be significant. The majority of astronauts would be classified as "healthy workers" based on established evidence of optimal nutrition, exercise, medical care, and abstinence from use of tobacco products. It is well known that NS have lower rates of cancer, circulatory and pulmonary diseases, and longer life-span than former or current smokers [45], [46]. Because cancer risk estimates are made using a mixture of multiplicative and additive risk transfer models, the lower background cancer rates of a NS population reduce radiation risk estimates compared to estimates for the U.S. average population [2], [32]. This leads to the paradoxical result that radiation cancer risks are estimated to be significantly reduced for NS and healthy workers such as astronauts compared to the average U.S. population, while PC estimates for several cancer types are increased. Furthermore, the use of a NS population to represent astronauts may lead to an under-estimation of PC's, which is suggested by Kaplan-Meir survival analysis and standard mortality ratio (SMR) results reported previously [2]. Results suggest that adjustment for smoking effects relative to the U.S. population does not account for the entire increase in longevity found for astronauts at this time.

Family history and an individual's possible exposure to other carcinogens should be considered in an assessment of possible causality. The use of family history data should consider the possibility that genetic pre-disposition of specific cancer types [41] may also confer increased radiation sensitivity. Other factors to be considered include smoking history which effects lung, esophagus, oral cavity, bladder and several other cancers, and reproductive history which can impact the risk of breast and other cancers in women [29]. The collection of biodosimetry and biomarker data prior to flight and at multiple time points over several years post-flight [47] would aid in understanding of causation, especially for repeat ISS flyers.

Considerations on the potential role of early cancer detection as a mitigation measure to reduce REID from space radiation exposure lends further support for research studies of HZE particle tumor induction. Radiation has been shown to increase a large number of cancer types (>15) [33]–[35] possibly limiting the benefits from improvements in early detection, which are only available for a few cancer types. For example if ten tissues each contributed 10% to the cancer REID each of which had a background mortality to incidence ratio of 0.5, an improvement of 50% in cure rate through early detection in four cancer types would lead to a reduction in REID of only 20%. However, this result would only be true if space radiation induced tumors were similar to cancers in the general population. Information on HZE particle carcinogenesis is extremely sparse, however animal studies suggest important differences occur. Therefore determining whether or not the etiology of HZE particle and neutron induced tumors are distinct from cancers in the general population or induced by low LET radiation should be a major focus of space radiobiology research. This research not only supports improved risk assessments, but has large implications that could impact possible treatment approaches, studies of individual sensitivity, and considerations of mitigation approaches.

NCRP and NRC Reviews of Space Radiation Risks and Limits

NASA has been concerned for many years the potential health risks and limitations that could arise from long-term exposure to GCR and possible exposures to sporadic solar particle events. In developing approaches to acceptable risk levels and approaches to quantify and mitigate radiation risks, NASA has sought and received external guidance from the NCRP, and several bodies at the NRC, including the Institute of Medicine (IOM) [48] and Space Science Board (SSB) [49]. Key recommendations with respect to NASA's regulatory framework for radiation limits, levels of acceptable risk, and approaches to manage uncertainties in risks estimates.

In 1989 the NCRP [4] discussed three types of comparisons of space radiation risks to other risks to form the basis for an acceptable lifetime risk level for space radiation exposure: 1) to limits for ground-based radiation workers, 2) to accidental deaths in the "safe", "less-safe", and "hazardous" occupations, and 3) to other accidental fatality risks faced by crew-members. Ground-based radiation workers have lifetime radiation risks no greater than risks experienced on average in the "safe industries", which was estimated as 0.5% in 1989 [4]. However, the dose limits for ground-based radiation workers were similar to the accidental deaths probability in the "less-safe industries" were life-time risks of up to 3% were estimated at that time. The NCRP noted that because astronauts face other occupational fatality risks, comparison of radiation limits to life-time fatality risks in "hazardous industries" was not appropriate. Based on these observations, the NCRP recommended NASA use a 3% lifetime fatality risk as the basis for dose limits, and for the use of epidemiology based models to estimate age at exposure and sex specific dose limits for astronauts working in LEO [4]. NASA implemented the NCRP recommended sex and age-at-exposure specific dose limits in 1990.

Within a decade of the publication of NCRP Report No. 98, the NCRP reported that the comparison of space radiation risks to the "less-safe industries" no longer supports a 3% fatality risk as a basis for radiation dose limits, because of the improvements in safety leading to lower fatality rates in ground-based occupations [5], [6]. The comparison to less-safe industries would lead to a lower acceptable risk level and stated [5]: "The NCRP now considers the comparison with lifetime risk associated with the occupational exposure limits recommended for workers on the ground to be the most direct and the most valid. Consequently, the NCRP recommends that the excess lifetime fatal cancer risk due to the radiation exposure of space workers for missions in LEO be limited to three percent excess mortality and that this be the basis for career limits." Indeed improvements in ground-based occupational safety since 1989 have occurred with average lifetime fatality risks in most less-safe industries now below 1% [7]. In addition the risk for loss of crew from spaceflight is recently estimated by NASA as 1 in 270 with the NASA Aerospace Safety Advisory Panel (ASAP) suggesting technology investments to reduce this value to less than 1 in 750 [8]. In order to make a comparative risk basis of the 1 in 33 radiation limit to the lower risks for other safety areas, estimates of expected life-loss from radiation risks are needed. In this report we provide estimates of expected life-loss for radiation induced cancer and circulatory diseases following participation in multiple ISS missions.

The IOM noted in their 2001 Safe Passage report [48] and re-affirming an earlier SSB report[49], "Until the radiation hazards to astronauts can be controlled or otherwise mitigated by physical shielding, a 1998 National Research Council report states, 'long-duration space travel should be postponed (SSB and NRC, 1998)'. Even if an effective physical radiation shield is developed, it in no way diminishes the need for clinical study, including monitoring of crewmembers' exposures, long-term medical follow-up, and the development of preventive medical treatments to make astronauts more resistant to deep space-induced radiation damage". In reviewing the NASA PELs [1], which stated the career radiation limit of 3% Risk of Exposure Induced Death (%REID) at the 95% confidence level (CL), the NRC noted [10],"The committee strongly recommends that the permissible exposure limits specified in the current NASA radiation protection standards not be violated to meet engineering resources available at a particular level of funding." These external safety recommendations to NASA[10], [48], [49] were focused on deep space missions, however it is shown in this report that similar concerns hold for multiple or long-term (1 year or longer) ISS missions especially for missions near solar minimum were dose-rates dominated by GCR can approach 1 mSv/day and about 2-fold higher than missions near solar maximum for similar ISS altitudes.

CONCLUSIONS

The NSCR-2012 models predicts the upper 95% CL for space radiation risk for ISS missions near solar minimum could exceed the NASA REID limit for cancer fatality by 18 months or 24 months for females and males, respectively. Also, median PC and upper 95%-confidence intervals of PC values are predicted to exceed 50% for several cancers for participation in two or more ISS missions of 18-months or longer total duration near solar minimum, or for longer missions at other phases of the solar cycle. Radiation risk estimates will likely continue to be modified as new findings are reported from research studies, especially for highly ionizing radiation, and it is vital that uncertainty analysis be performed to anticipate how such information could modify safety considerations for space missions occurring in the future. The present report suggests that possible qualitative differences related to radiation quality and tumor lethality, and additional risks for circulatory disease from chronic low dose radiation are major issues for astronauts participating in multiple or 1-year ISS missions, as well as for exploration missions to Mars and other deep space destinations.

ACKNOWLEDGMENTS

I am grateful for discussions with Dr. Myung-Hee Kim on the ISS environment and Dr.'s Mary Helen Barcellos-Hoff and Michael Weil on tumor lethality after radiation exposures. The results of the NSCR-2012 model are available using a WEB based tool [50], and the NSCR-2014, which was described in-part in this report, will be available in the future at the University of Nevada, Las Vegas from the author.

AUTHOR CONTRIBUTIONS

Conceived and designed the experiments: FAC. Performed the experiments: FAC. Analyzed the data: FAC. Contributed reagents/materials/analysis tools: FAC. Wrote the paper: FAC.

REFERENCES

1. National Aeronautics and Space Administration (2007) NASA Space flight human system standard volume I; Crew health. NASA STD-3001.
2. Cucinotta FA, Kim MY, Chappell L (2013) Space radiation cancer risk projections and uncertainties- 2012. NASA TP 2013–217375.
3. Cucinotta FA, Kim MY, Chappell LJ, Huff JL (2013) How safe is safe enough: Radiation risks for a human mission to Mars. PLoS One 8: e74988. doi: 10. 1371/journal. pone. 0074988
4. National Council on Radiation Protection and Measurements (1989) Guidance on radiation received in space activities. NCRP Report 98: Bethesda, MD.
5. National Council on Radiation Protection and Measurements (2000) Recommendations of dose limits for low Earth orbit. NCRP Report 132: Bethesda MD.
6. National Council on Radiation Protection and Measurements (1997) Acceptability of risk from radiation- application to human space flight. NCRP Symposium Proceedings No. 3: Bethesda MD.
7. National Safety Council (2011) Injury facts 2011 edition. National Safety Council: Itasca IL.
8. Aerospace Safety Advisory Panel, Annual Report for 2010. 9. http://oiir. hq. nasa. gov/asap/documents/2010_ASAP_Annual_Report. pdf. Accessed 2013 June 1.
9. National Academy of Sciences Space Science Board (1996) Report of the task group on the biological effects of space radiation: Radiation hazards to crews on interplanetary missions. The National Academies Press: Washington DC.
10. National Research Council, Aeronautics and Engineering Board (2008) Managing space radiation risk in the new era of space exploration. The National Academies Press: Washington DC.
11. National Research Council (2013) Technical evaluation of the NASA model for cancer risk to astronauts due to space radiation. The National Academies Press: Washington DC.
12. National Council on Radiation Protection and Measurements (2006) Information needed to make radiation protection recommendations for space missions beyond low-Earth orbit. NCRP Report 153: Bethesda MD.
13. National Council on Radiation Protection and Measurements (1997) Uncertainties in fatal cancer risk estimates used in radiation protection. NCRP Report 126: Bethesda MD.
14. Cucinotta FA, Schimmerling W, Wilson JW, Badhwar GD, Dicello JF, et al. (2001) Space radiation cancer risks and uncertainties for Mars missions. Radiat Res 156: 682–688. doi: 10. 1667/0033-7587(2001)156[0682:srcrau]2. 0. co;2
15. Cucinotta FA, Kim MY, Ren L (2006) Evaluating shielding effectiveness for reducing space radiation cancer risks. Radiat Meas 41: 1173–1185. doi: 10. 1016/j. radmeas. 2006. 03. 011
16. Fry RJM, Powers-Risius P, Alpen EL, Ainsworth EJ (1985) High LET radiation carcinogenesis. Radiat Res 104: S188–S195. doi: 10. 2307/3576646
17. Alpen EL, Powers-Risius P, Curtis SB, DeGuzman R (1993) Tumorigenic potential of high-Z, high-LET charged particle radiations. Radiat Res 88: 132–143. doi: 10. 2307/3578551
18. Dicello JF, Christian A, Cucinotta FA, Gridley DS, Kathirithhamby R, et al. (2004) In vivo mammary tumorigenesis in the sprague-dawley rat and microdosimetric correlates. Phys Med Biol 49: 3817–3830. doi: 10. 1088/0031-9155/49/16/024
19. Weil MM, Bedford JS, Bielefeldt-Ohmann H, Ray AF, Gernik PC, et al. (2009) Incidence of acute myeloid leukemia and hepatocellular carcinoma in mice irradiated with 1 GeV/nucleon ^{56}Fe ions. Radiat Res 172: 213–219. doi: 10. 1667/rr1648. 1
20. Imaoka T, Nishimura, Kakinuma S, Hatano Y, Ohmachi Y, et al. (2007) High relative biological effectiveness of carbon ion irradiation on induction of rat mammary carcinoma and its lack of H-ras and Tp53 mutations. Inter J Radiat Oncol Biophys 69: 194–203. doi: 10. 1016/j. ijrobp. 2007. 05. 026
21. Trani D, Datta K, Doiron K, Kallakury B, Fornace Jr AJ (2010) Enhanced intestinal tumor multiplicity and grade

in vivo after HZE exposure: mouse models for space radiation risk estimates. Radiat Environ Biophys 49: 389–396. doi: 10. 1007/s00411-010-0292-2

22. Datta K, Suman S, Kallakury BV, Fornace Jr AJ (2013) Heavy ion radiation exposure triggered higher intestinal tumor frequency and greater β-catenin activation than γ radiation in APC $^{Min/+}$ mice. PLoS One 8 e59295.

23. Grahn D, Lombard LS, Carnes BA (1992) The comparative tumorigenic effects of fission neutrons and Cobalt-60 γ rays in B6CF$_1$ mouse. Radiat Res 129: 19–36. doi: 10. 2307/3577899

24. Wolfe C, Lafuma J, Masse R, Morin M, Kellerer A (2000) Neutron RBE for induction of tumors with high lethality in spraque-dawley rats. Radiat Res 154: 412–420. doi: 10. 1667/0033-7587(2000)154[0412:nrfiot]2. 0. co;2

25. Cucinotta FA, Chappell LJ (2010) Non-targeted effects and the dose response for heavy ion tumor formation. Mutat Res 687: 49–53. doi: 10. 1016/j. mrfmmm. 2010. 01. 012

26. Barcellos-Hoff MH, Nyugen DH (2009) Radiation carcinogenesis in context: how do irradiated tissues become tumors? Health Phys 97: 446–453. doi: 10. 1097/hp. 0b013e3181b08a10

27. Kadhim M, Salomaa S, Wright E, Hildenbrandt G, Belyakov OV, et al. (2013) Non-targeted effects of ionizing radiation- implications for low dose risk. Mutat Res 752: 84–98. doi: 10. 1016/j. mrrev. 2012. 12. 001

28. U. S. Department of Health and Human Services (2002). 42 CFR Part 81: 30. Guidelines for determining the probability of causation under the energy employees 31. occupational illness compensation program act of 2000, final rule, 67 FR 22296–22314. U. S. Government Printing Office: Washington DC.

29. National Institutes of Health (2003) Report of the NCI-CDC working group to revise the 1985 NIH radioepidemiological tables. NIH Publication No. 03–5387: Bethesda MD.

30. Leigh WJ, Wakeford R (2001) Radiation litigation and the nuclear industry - the experience in the United Kingdom. Health Phys 81: 646–654. doi: 10. 1097/00004032-200112000-00014

31. Little M, Azizova D, Bazyka S, Bouffler SD, Cardis E, et al. (2012) Meta-analysis of circulatory disease from exposure to low-level ionizing radiation and estimates of potential population risks. Environ Health Persp 120: 1503–1511. doi: 10. 1289/ehp. 1204982

32. Cucinotta FA, Chappell LJ, Kim MY, Wang M (2012) Radiation carcinogenesis risk assessments for never-smokers. Health Phys 103: 643–651. doi: 10. 1097/hp. 0b013e318267b3ad

33. United Nations Scientific Committee on the Effects of Atomic Radiation (2008) Sources and effects of ionizing radiation UNSCEAR 2006 Report to the general assembly, with scientific annexes. United Nations: New York NY.

34. National Academy of Sciences Committee on the Biological Effects of Radiation (2006) Health risks from exposure to low levels of ionizing radiation. National Academy of Sciences Press: Washington DC.

35. Preston DL, Ron E, Tokuoka S, Funamota S, Nishi N, et al. (2007) Solid cancer incidence in atomic bomb survivors: 1958–1998. Radiat Res 168: 1–64. doi: 10. 1667/rr0763. 1

36. Cucinotta FA, Kim MY, Willingham V, George KA (2008) Physical and biological organ dosimetry analysis for International Space Station astronauts. Radiat Res 170: 127–138. doi: 10. 1667/rr1330. 1

37. Zeitlin CJ, Hassler DM, Cucinotta FA, Ehresmann B, Wimmer-Schweingruber RF, et al. (2013) Measurements of energetic particle radiation in transit to Mars on the Mars Science Laboratory. Science 340: 1080–1084. doi: 10. 1126/science. 1235989

38. Badhwar GD, Cucinotta FA (2000) A comparison on depth dependence of dose and linear energy transfer spectra in aluminum and polyethylene. Radiat Res 153: 1–8. doi: 10. 1667/0033-7587(2000)153[0001:acoddo]2. 0. co;2

39. Barkas H. Nuclear Research Emulsions. Academic Press Inc, New York. Vol. 1, Chap. 9, p. 371, 1963.

40. Cucinotta FA, Wu H, Shavers MR, George K (2003) Radiation dosimetry and biophysical models of space radiation effects. Grav Space Biol Bull 16: 11–18.

41. National Council on Radiation Protection and Measurements (2011) Potential impact of individual genetic susceptibility and previous radiation exposure on radiation risks for astronauts. NCRP Report 167: Bethesda MD.

42. Shimizu Y, Kodama K, Nishi N, Kasagi F, Suyama A, et al. (2010) Radiation exposure and circulatory disease risk: Hiroshima and Nagasaki atomic bomb survivor data, 1950–2003. British Med J 340: b5349 doi:10. 1136/bmj. b5349.

43. Darby S, Ewertz M, McGale P, Bennet AM, Blom-Goldman U (2013) Risk of ischemic heart disease in women after radiotherapy for breast cancer. New Eng J Med 368: 986–998. doi: 10. 1056/nejmoa1209825

44. International Commission on Radiation Protection (2003) Relative biological effectiveness (RBE), Quality factor (Q), and radiation weighting factor (w_R). ICRP Publication 103: Pergamon.

45. Doll R, Peto R, Boreham J, Sutherland I (2004) Mortality in relation to smoking: 50 years' observations on male British doctors. British Med J. doi: 10. 1136/bmj. 38142. 554479.

46. Thun MJ, Day-Lally C, Calle E, Flanders W, Heath C (1995) Excess mortality among cigarette smokers: changes in a 20-year interval. Amer J Public Health 85: 1223–1230. doi: 10. 2105/ajph. 85. 9. 1223

47. George KA, Rhone J, Beitman A, Cucinotta FA (2013) Cytogenetic damage in the blood lymphocytes of astronauts: effects of repeat long-duration space missions. Mutat Res 756: 165–169. doi: 10. 1016/j. mrgentox. 2013. 04. 007

48. National Academy of Sciences Institute of Medicine (2001) Safe passage: astronaut care for exploration

missions. The National Academies Press: Washington DC.

49. National Research Council Space Science Board (1998) A strategy for research in space biology and medicine in the new century. The National Academy Press: Washington DC.

50. Cucinotta FA, Kim MY, Chappell LJ, O'Neill PM, Hu S, et al. . (2013) NASA Space cancer risk-2012 (NSCR-2012) V1. 0 web based computer tool. Available:http:// spaceradiation. usra. edu/irModels. Accessed 26 March 2014.

CHAPTER 9

THE PERILS OF ADAPTING TO DOSE ERRORS IN RADIATION THERAPY

Velibor V. Mišić and Timothy C. Y. Chan

INTRODUCTION

The treatment of lung cancer using intensity-modulated radiation therapy (IMRT) is challenging in part due to the uncertainty that arises from breathing motion during delivery and potential interfractional changes in the patient's breathing. In [1], the authors proposed the first method for lung cancer IMRT that combines robust optimization (RO) [2, 3] and adaptive radiation therapy (ART) [4]. In this adaptive robust method, the treatment planner specifies an uncertainty set of breathing patterns before the start of treatment. Prior to each fraction, an optimization problem is solved to determine the corresponding fluence map. During or after each fraction, the patient's breathing pattern is measured, and is used to update the uncertainty set for the next fraction. The process is then repeated until the end of the treatment. They showed that this adaptive robust method results in further improvements in both cumulative tumor coverage and healthy tissue dose relative to the non-adaptive robust approach of [3], which is already capable of providing tumor coverage comparable to a margin treatment but with significantly less dose to the healthy tissue. More recently, [5] showed that this approach is also able to account for drift in the patient's breathing pattern.

In this paper, we study a different paradigm for treatment planning, which we refer to as dose reaction. A dose-reactive method is a treatment planning method in which the target dose for the upcoming fraction is updated based on the dose delivered to date and the treatment is then re-optimized prior to the next fraction. In this way, the method is potentially able to correct errors in dose as the treatment progresses. However, due to the regular modification of the target dose, the daily doses that are delivered over the treatment may vary and deviate significantly from the daily prescribed dose. This is important clinically because the effect of deviating from the daily prescribed dose in a given fraction is compounded as the treatment progresses. This can potentially result in treatment failure, even when the final dose meets the prescribed requirements [6].

The purpose of this paper is not to develop a new dose-reactive method and to present the merits of this method relative to existing methods for lung cancer IMRT. Rather, our objective is to demonstrate the surprising negative finding that combining dose reaction with an existing adaptive robust framework is not necessarily advantageous. We make the following contributions:

1. We show computationally using real patient data that although dose reaction leads to improvements in the final cumulative dose, it may result in explosive growth in the daily underdose and daily overdose over the course of the treatment, and in increased spatial heterogeneity in the daily dose distribution.
2. We show that this growth in daily underdose and overdose in the presence of the dose-reactive element persists when robustness is used without uncertainty set adaptation, but can be substantially mitigated through regular adaptation of the uncertainty set.
3. We prove that uncertainty set adaptation without dose reaction guarantees diminishing daily underdose and overdose asymptotically and provide theoretical justification for why dose reaction will generally lead to growing daily underdose and overdose.

Since [4], there has been increasing interest in ART methods (e.g., [7], [8], [9], [10], [11], [12]). Dose-reactive methods for fractionated radiation therapy, outside of lung cancer IMRT, constitute a major subset of the ART literature (e.g., [13], [14], [15], [16], [17] and [18]). However, few studies in dose

Citation: Mišić VV, Chan TCY (2015) The Perils of Adapting to Dose Errors in Radiation Therapy. PLoS ONE, 10(5): e0125335. DOI:10.1371/journal.pone.0125335.ss reaction account for the daily dose. One example is [19], which builds on [20]. In [19], the authors consider an iterative IMRT optimization approach that adapts to interfraction changes in the tumor geometry and aims to satisfy both per-fraction and cumulative dose constraints. Their approach differs from ours in that it optimizes the number of fractions, which results in an integer programming problem, whereas ours keeps the number of fractions fixed and leads to a linear programming problem. Also, our approach considers both intrafraction and interfraction uncertainty through a robust optimization model with adaptation.

Another closely related paper is that of [21], who proposes a framework where, in each fraction i of an n-fraction treatment, one delivers $1/(n - i + 1)$ of the residual dose distribution—the difference of the dose delivered so far and the target dose distribution. Our work builds on [21] in three key aspects. First, our method uses RO, so that the fluence map delivered in each fraction is designed to deliver the target dose under many instances of the uncertainty; [21] assumes the tumor to be in a single position. Second, our method updates an estimate of the uncertainty by updating an uncertainty set, whereas [21] assumes the tumor to be in the same position from fraction to fraction. As stated in contribution #2, these two differences lead to important insights: the explosive growth in daily underdose and overdose that is alluded to in [21] occurs even in the presence of robustness, but it is possible to reduce its severity through uncertainty set adaptation. Lastly, the results of [21] do not actually show how the daily underdose and overdose increase, and their results pertain only to a stylized one-dimensional model.

METHOD

We begin by describing the two elements of our framework: a previously developed adaptive robust optimization model (the "Robust optimization model with adaptation" subsection) and the new dose reaction component (the "Dose reaction" subsection). For the benefit of the reader, Table 1 provides a summary of all of the mathematical notation used here and in the later section titled "Theoretical insight into daily dose performance" that presents our theoretical results.

Table 1. Summary of mathematical notation.

Symbol	Description
x	Breathing motion state (e.g., full inhale)
X	Set of breathing motion state
$p(x)$	Probability of breathing motion state x
$\mathbf{p}$	Breathing motion probability mass function (PMF); $\mathbf{p} = (p(x))_{x \in X}$
$\ell(x)$	Lower bound on $p(x)$
$\boldsymbol{\ell}$	Vector of lower bounds; $\boldsymbol{\ell} = (\ell(x))_{x \in X}$
$u(x)$	Upper bound on $p(x)$
$\mathbf{u}$	Vector of upper bounds; $\mathbf{u} = (u(x))_{x \in X}$
P	Uncertainty set (set of possible breathing motion PMFs)
$\mathcal{P}$	Set of all possible PMFs (the $(\|X\| - 1)$-dimensional unit simplex)
v	Voxel index
$\mathcal{V}$	Set of all voxels
$\mathcal{T}$	Set of tumor voxels
b	Beamlet index
β	Set of all beamlet indices
w_b	Intensity of beamlet b
$\mathbf{w}$	Beamlet intensity vector; $\mathbf{w} = (w_b)_{b \in \beta}$
$\Delta_{v,x,b}$	Dose deposition coefficient; dose delivered to voxel v by beamlet b at unit intensity when the motion state is x
θ_v	Minimum cumulative prescription dose for voxel v
γ	Dose multiplier for maximum prescription dose (i.e., $\gamma\theta_v$ is the maximum cumulative prescription dose for voxel v)
$\underline{\boldsymbol{\delta}}v$	Target minimum dose for voxel v
$\boldsymbol{\delta}_v^{i+1}$	Target minimum dose for voxel v for fractions $i + 1$ to n
$\boldsymbol{\delta}$	Vector of target minimum doses; $\boldsymbol{\delta} = (\boldsymbol{\delta}v)_{v \in \mathcal{T}}$
$\bar{\boldsymbol{\delta}}_v$	Target maximum dose for voxel v
$\bar{\boldsymbol{\delta}}_v^{i+1}$	Target maximum dose for voxel v for fractions $i + 1$ to n
$\bar{\boldsymbol{\delta}}$	Vector of target maximum doses; $\boldsymbol{\delta} = (\bar{\boldsymbol{\delta}}_v)_{v \in \mathcal{T}}$
n	Number of fractions in the treatment
i	Fraction index
$\mathbf{w}^*(\boldsymbol{\ell}, \mathbf{u})$	Set of optimal solutions $\mathbf{w}$ to problem (Eq 2) when $\bar{\boldsymbol{\delta}}_v = \theta_v$, $\bar{\boldsymbol{\delta}}_v = \gamma\theta_v$ for each $v \in \mathcal{T}$ and P is defined by $\boldsymbol{\ell}$ and $\mathbf{u}$
$\mathbf{p}^*$	Limiting breathing motion PMF
$\Delta\mathbf{p}\ \mathbf{w}$	Dose distribution (vector of doses) when patient breathes according to $\mathbf{p}$ and $\mathbf{w}$ is delivered; vth element, for $v \in \mathcal{V}$, is defined as $\sum_{x \in X} \sum_{b \in \beta} \Delta_{v,x,b}\, p(x) w_b$
$\mathbf{d}$	Dose distribution; $\mathbf{d} = (d_v)_{v \in \mathcal{V}}$
$\mathbf{D}$	Set of optimal dose distributions; $\mathbf{D} = \{\mathbf{d} \in \mathbb{R}^{\|\mathcal{V}\|} \mid \mathbf{d} = \Delta\mathbf{p}^*\ \mathbf{w}$ for some $\mathbf{w} \in \mathbf{w}^*(\mathbf{p}^*, \mathbf{p}^*)\}$
$U(\mathbf{D}, \epsilon)$	Epsilon neighborhood of $\mathbf{D}$; $U(\mathbf{D}, \epsilon) = \{\mathbf{d}' \in \mathbb{R}^{\|\mathcal{V}\|} \mid \|\mathbf{d} - \mathbf{d}'\|_1 < \epsilon$ for some $\mathbf{d} \in \mathbf{D}\}$

doi:10.1371/journal.pone.0125335.t001

Robust Optimization Model with Adaptation

Our framework builds on the adaptive robust framework of [1], which builds on the stylized robust model introduced in [3]. In this framework, the patient's breathing in a given fraction is modeled by a breathing motion probability mass function (PMF) [22], which gives the frequency of each breathing motion state x from a finite set of breathing motion states X. The robust optimization model is then built around an uncertainty set P, which is a set of breathing motion PMFs that we believe may be realized in a given fraction. An uncertainty set is defined by a lower bound vector $\ell \geq 0$ and an upper bound vector $u \leq 1$ as

$$P = \left\{ \mathbf{p} \in \mathbb{R}^{|X|} \;\middle|\; \forall x \in X,\ \ell(x) \leq p(x) \leq u(x);\ \sum_{x \in X} p(x) = 1 \right\}. \tag{1}$$

When $\ell = 0$ and $u = 1$, P is the set of all PMFs on X, which we denote by $\mathcal{P}$.

The robust optimization model is then defined as

$$\begin{aligned} \text{minimize} \quad & \sum_{v \in \mathcal{V}} \sum_{x \in X} \sum_{b \in \mathcal{B}} \Delta_{v,x,b} \bar{p}(x) w_b \\ \text{subject to} \quad & \sum_{x \in X} \sum_{b \in \mathcal{B}} \Delta_{v,x,b} p(x) w_b \geq \underline{\delta}_v, \quad \forall v \in \mathcal{T},\ \mathbf{p} \in P, \\ & \sum_{x \in X} \sum_{b \in \mathcal{B}} \Delta_{v,x,b} p(x) w_b \leq \bar{\delta}_v, \quad \forall v \in \mathcal{T},\ \mathbf{p} \in P, \\ & w_b \geq 0, \quad \forall b \in \mathcal{B}, \end{aligned} \tag{2}$$

where all notation follows [1] (see Section 3 of that paper for further details), with the exception of $\underline{\delta}_v$ and $\bar{\delta}_v$, which respectively denote the target minimum dose and target maximum dose for each voxel v. We remark that the optimal solution **w** of this problem is not the beamlet intensity vector that is actually delivered; it must be scaled by the number of fractions that $\underline{\delta}$ and $\bar{\delta}$ correspond to. In particular, if we are planning for fraction i, and thus $\underline{\delta}$ and $\bar{\delta}$ correspond to the dose that remains to be delivered over the remaining $n - i + 1$ fractions, then we will scale the intensity vector w by $1/(n - i + 1)$ and deliver $1/(n - i + 1) \cdot w$ to the patient in fraction i.

The adaptive element of our framework is the generation of a new uncertainty set from the current uncertainty set and the current breathing motion PMF, which is done by updating the lower bound vector ℓ and the upper bound vector u defining the uncertainty set. In this paper we use the exponential smoothing update described in [1]. This update is controlled by a parameter $\alpha \in [0, 1]$ that specifies how much weight is placed on the most recent PMF: lower values of α lead to slower rates of adaptation to new PMFs, while higher values lead to faster rates of adaptation.

Dose Reaction

The main element of our framework, which constitutes the new contribution of this paper to the existing adaptive and robust optimization framework, is dose reaction. We consider two methods for updating the target minimum vector $\underline{\delta}$ and the target maximum dose vector $\bar{\delta}$. In the non-reactive dose update method, we set $\underline{\delta}$ and $\bar{\delta}$ as

$$\underline{\delta}_v^{i+1} = \frac{n-i}{n} \theta_v, \tag{3}$$

$$\bar{\delta}_v^{i+1} = \frac{n-i}{n} \gamma \theta_v, \tag{4}$$

in each fraction $i + 1$, where θ_v is the prescribed minimum dose for voxel v and $\gamma\theta_v$ is the prescribed maximum dose for voxel v, with γ being a constant greater than or equal to 1. In this method, the initial minimum and maximum target dose are scaled by the number of remaining fractions, and are not updated using the delivered dose.

In the reactive$^{\pm}$ dose update method, after observing the PMF p^i in fraction i, we set $\underline{\delta}_v^{i+1}$ and $\bar{\delta}_v^{i+1}$ for fraction $i + 1$ as

$$\underline{\delta}_v^{i+1} = \max \left\{ 0,\ \underline{\delta}_v^i - \sum_{x \in X} \sum_{b \in \mathcal{B}} \Delta_{v,x,b} p^i(x) \frac{w_b^i}{n - i + 1} \right\}, \tag{5}$$

$$\bar{\delta}_v^{i+1} = \max \left\{ 0,\ \bar{\delta}_v^i - \sum_{x \in X} \sum_{b \in \mathcal{B}} \Delta_{v,x,b} p^i(x) \frac{w_b^i}{n - i + 1} \right\}, \tag{6}$$

for each voxel $v \in \mathcal{T}$. This update reduces the target minimum and maximum dose—the "dose-to-go"—for a given tumor voxel v by the dose delivered to that voxel in fraction i; the more dose a voxel v has accumulated up to and including fraction i, the smaller $\underline{\delta}_v^{i+1}$ and $\bar{\delta}_v^{i+1}$ will be, and the less dose will be delivered to voxel v over the remaining $n - i$ fractions. If a given voxel v has accumulated its prescribed minimum dose of θ_v, the use of $\max\{0, \cdot\}$ ensures that the target minimum dose is set to zero, so that subsequent beamlet intensity vectors are not forced to deliver any dose to that voxel.

In [23] we also describe two other methods for updating $\underline{\delta}$ and $\bar{\delta}$, the reactive^{-} method and the reactive^{+} method. These two update methods are "one-sided" update methods: the reactive^{-}method reacts to underdose only, while the reactive^{+} method reacts to overdose only. Appropriately regarded, these methods behave similarly to reactive$^{\pm}$; detailed results for them can be found in [23].

The complete sequence of steps involved in the dose-reactive method is displayed in Fig 1.

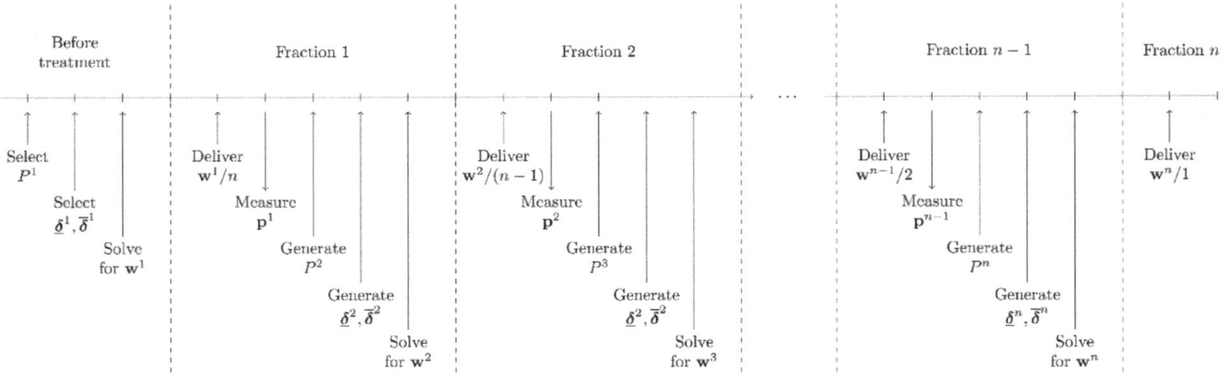

Figure 1. Schematic of dose-reactive method.

RESULTS

Computational Setup

We used the same data as in [3] and used the same computational setup as in [1]; for further details, the reader is referred to these papers. Two PMF sequences consisting of 30 PMFs were used to test the dose-reactive and non-reactive methods. The PMFs were obtained from RPM data using the method of [22]. The range of breathing motion was divided into five phases, resulting in a set X consisting of five breathing motion states.

Five equispaced coplanar beam directions were used, for a total of 1625 beamlets. The patient geometry was subdivided into 110,725 voxels of size 2.93 mm × 2.50 mm × 2.93 mm; the tumor voxel set $\mathcal{T}$ contained all clinical target volume (CTV) voxels, which numbered 5495. The normal tissues for this patient geometry consisted of the left lung (containing the tumor), heart, esophagus and spinal cord. The dose deposition coefficients were computed from pre-treatment 4D-CT images using the method of [24]; the anatomical voxels from the CT image from one reference phase (full inhale) were transformed to corresponding voxels in other phases using voxel-based affine and non-rigid registration [25]. The dose distribution for each fraction was computed by summing the delivered beamlet intensities weighted by the $\Delta_{v,x,b}$ values and the realized PMF; the final treatment dose was obtained by accumulating the individual daily dose distributions.

The prescribed minimum and maximum tumor doses θ_v and $\gamma\theta_v$ for each tumor voxel v were 72Gy and 79.2Gy (corresponding to $\gamma = 1.1$). The initial uncertainty sets used were the same as in [3]. Specifically, we considered a nominal uncertainty set (N) consisting of only the nominal PMF $(P = \{\bar{p}\})$; a margin uncertainty set (M) consisting of all PMFs $(P = \mathcal{P})$; and a robust uncertainty set (R) that is between the nominal and margin uncertainty set in size. We also evaluated two different daily prescient treatments (see [1]). Each of the daily prescient treatments incorporates one of the two target dose updates, thus resulting in non-reactive daily prescient and reactive$^{\pm}$ daily prescient treatments.

In the subsections that follow, we restrict our attention to results for the first PMF sequence, as the results obtained using the second PMF sequence were qualitatively similar. We restrict our focus to results corresponding to α values of 0 (no uncertainty set adaptation), 0.1 (slow adaptation), and 0.9 (fast adaptation). Complete results for both PMF sequences, as well as precise definitions of the dose metrics, can be found in [23]. To simplify the exposition, we will use the notation (·, ·) to represent each tested implementation. The first term in the parentheses indicates the method: static (S); exponential smoothing with smoothing constantα and the non-reactive target dose update (ES(α)); exponential smoothing with smoothing constant α and the reactive$^{\pm}$ target dose update (R$^{\pm}$ES(α)); and daily prescient with the reactive$^{\pm}$ target dose update (R$^{\pm}$DLYP). The second term in the parentheses, where provided, indicates the initial uncertainty set: nominal (N), robust (R) and margin (M), as defined in [3].

Cumulative Dose Results

Table 2 presents dose statistics for the final dose distribution obtained from the reactive$^{\pm}$ implementations. These results show that incorporating dose reaction into the adaptive robust framework leads to treatments that are acceptable with respect to the final dose distribution. With regard to the tumor dose, every reactive$^{\pm}$ implementation listed in Table 2 achieves a minimum tumor dose that is within 0.5% of 72Gy. With regard to healthy tissue dose, Table 2shows that when $\alpha > 0$ (i.e., the uncertainty set is updated on a daily basis), all of the reactive$^{\pm}$ implementations have mean left lung doses that are less than 90% and mean normal tissue doses that are less than 91% of their respective static margin treatment values.

Table 2. Dose statistics for the first PMF sequence under the non-reactive and reactive± methods.

Implementation	Min. tumor dose		Max. tumor dose		Mean lung dose		Mean n. tissue dose	
	Gy	%[1]	Gy	%[2]	Gy	%[3]	Gy	%[4]
(R±ES(0),N)	71.86	99.81	79.34	100.18	17.57	86.19	9.10	89.53
(R±ES(0),R)	71.94	99.91	79.22	100.03	17.76	87.08	9.19	90.46
(R±ES(0),M)	72.00	100.00	79.20	99.99	18.57	91.06	9.50	93.54
(R±ES(0.1),N)	72.00	100.00	79.20	100.00	17.55	86.08	9.06	89.17
(R±ES(0.1),R)	72.00	100.00	79.20	100.00	17.72	86.89	9.08	89.41
(R±ES(0.1),M)	72.00	100.00	79.20	100.00	17.92	87.89	9.18	90.32
(R±ES(0.9),N)	71.99	99.99	79.21	100.01	17.58	86.22	9.06	89.13
(R±ES(0.9),R)	71.99	99.99	79.21	100.01	17.59	86.27	9.06	89.17
(R±ES(0.9),M)	71.99	99.99	79.21	100.01	17.66	86.61	9.08	89.33
(R±DLYP)	72.00	100.00	79.20	100.00	17.59	86.25	9.06	89.12

[1] Percentage of the prescribed minimum dose (72Gy).
[2] Percentage of the prescribed maximum dose (79.2Gy).
[3] Percentage of the mean left lung dose delivered in the static margin treatment (implementation (S,M)).
[4] Percentage of the mean normal tissue dose delivered in the static margin treatment (implementation (S,M)).

doi:10.1371/journal.pone.0125335.t002

These results also indicate that the performance of the dose-reactive methods varies relative to the non-reactive methods (see Table 1 of [1] for cumulative dose results for the non-reactive static and exponential smoothing implementations). In some cases, the reactive± update leads to improvement in both tumor coverage and healthy tissue dose (for example, compare (R±ES(0.1),R) to (ES(0.1), R)). In other cases, the performance change brought about by dose reaction is mixed. For example, comparing the (R±ES(0.9,M)) with the (ES(0.9),M) treatment, we can see that the mean left lung dose was improved, but the maximum tumor dose increased slightly.

In addition to statistics such as minimum tumor dose and mean left lung dose, we examine the full dose distribution in the patient geometry through dose volume histograms (DVHs). Fig 2(d)shows the final DVHs for the (ES(0.1),M) and (R±ES(0.1),M) treatments. From this figure, we see that both the (R±ES(0.1),M) and (ES(0.1),M) treatment result in acceptable tumor doses, while the (R±ES(0.1),M) treatment results in slightly lower healthy tissue dose. Overall, though, the differences between the two families of DVHs are small, indicating that in this case dose reaction has a minimal effect on the final treatment dosimetry.

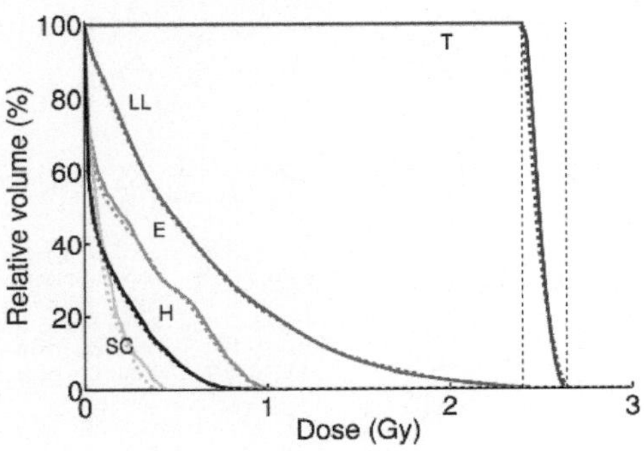

(a): Daily DVHs, fraction 10.

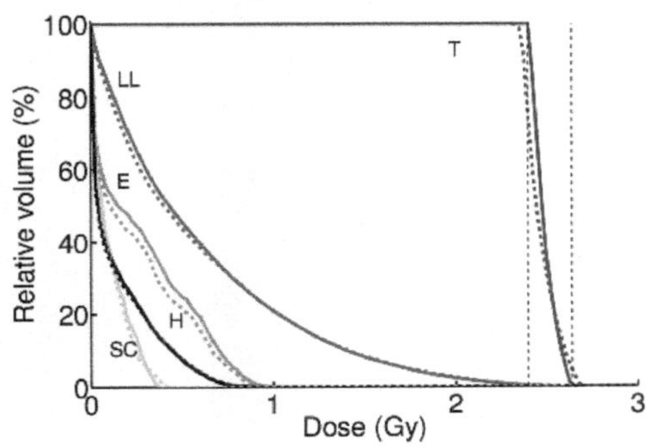

(b): Daily DVHs, fraction 20.

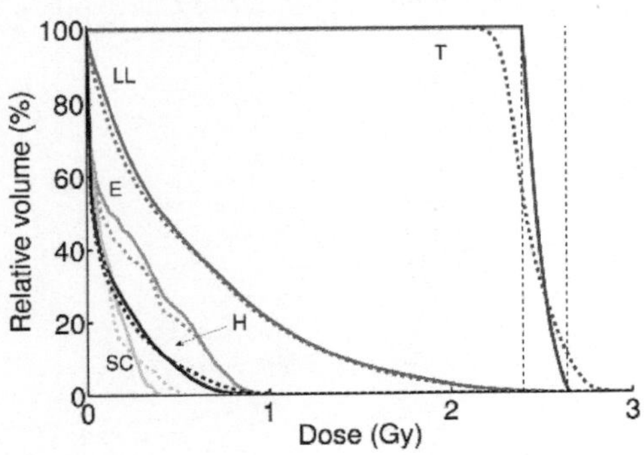

(c): Daily DVHs, fraction 30.

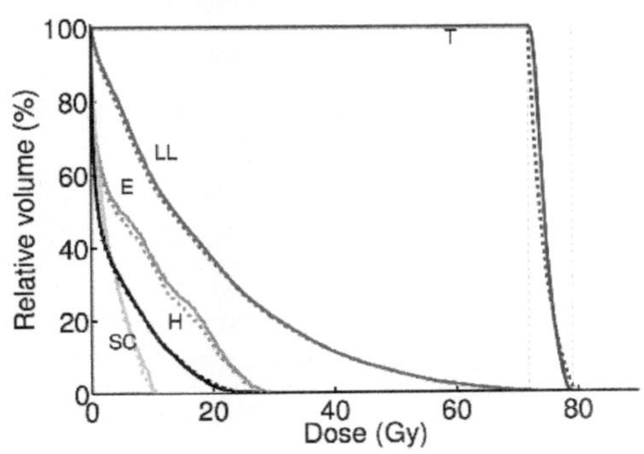

(d): Final DVHs.

Figure 2. Dose-volume histograms (DVHs) for the daily dose distribution at fractions 10, 20, 30 and the final cumulative dose distribution for (ES(0.1),M) (solid curves) and (R±ES(0.1),M) (dashed curves) for the first PMF sequence. Letters indicate DVHs for tumor (T), left lung (LL), esophagus (E), heart (H) and spinal cord (SC).

Daily Dose Results

Figs 3, 4 and 5 display the mean and maximum underdose and overdose by fraction for the non-reactive and reactive$^{\pm}$ implementations with α = 0,0.1,0.9, respectively, while Fig 6additionally displays the same metrics for the reactive$^{\pm}$ daily prescient treatment. The mean and maximum underdose values are given as percentages of the daily prescribed minimum dose of 2.4Gy (= 72Gy/30 fractions), while the mean and maximum overdose values are given as percentages of the daily prescribed maximum dose of 2.64Gy (= 79.2Gy/30 fractions). From the perspective of daily dose performance, the results shown in Figs 3, 4 and 5 indicate that the reactive$^{\pm}$ method does not perform as well as the non-reactive method. In particular, we can see that the reactive$^{\pm}$ method's daily underdose and overdose grow over the course of the treatment and exceed the levels of underdose and overdose exhibited by the non-reactive method. In the non-reactive case, when α = 0 (the uncertainty set is not adapted), Fig 3(a) and3(b) show that the daily underdose and overdose stay roughly constant. When α > 0, the daily underdose and overdose of the non-reactive method rapidly decrease to zero (e.g., see Fig5(a) and 5(b) for α = 0.9).

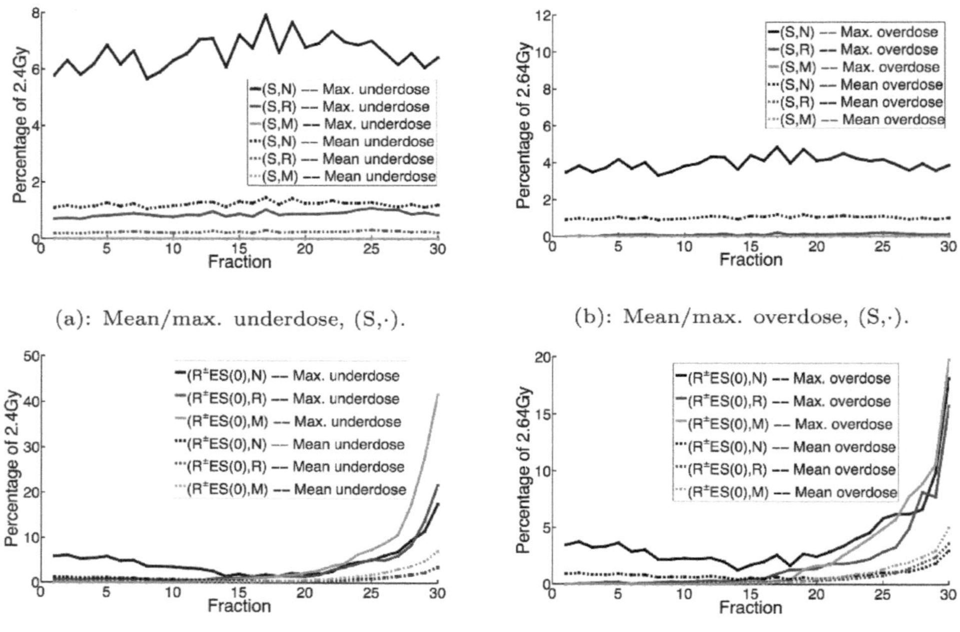

(a): Mean/max. underdose, (S,·).

(b): Mean/max. overdose, (S,·).

(c): Mean/max. underdose, (R$^{\pm}$ES(0),·).

(d): Mean/max. overdose, (R$^{\pm}$ES(0),·).

Figure 3. Mean and maximum underdose and overdose by fraction for S and R$^{\pm}$ES(0) implementations.

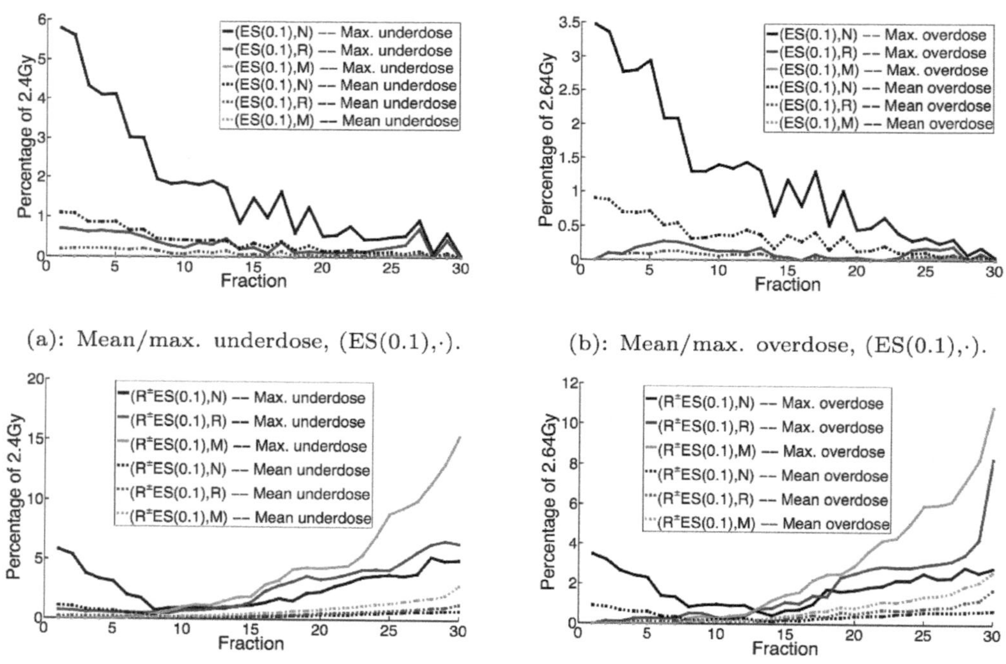

(a): Mean/max. underdose, (ES(0.1),·).

(b): Mean/max. overdose, (ES(0.1),·).

(c): Mean/max. underdose, (R$^{\pm}$ES(0.1),·).

(d): Mean/max. overdose, (R$^{\pm}$ES(0.1),·).

Figure 4. Mean and maximum underdose and overdose by fraction for ES(0.1) and R$^{\pm}$ES(0.1) implementations.

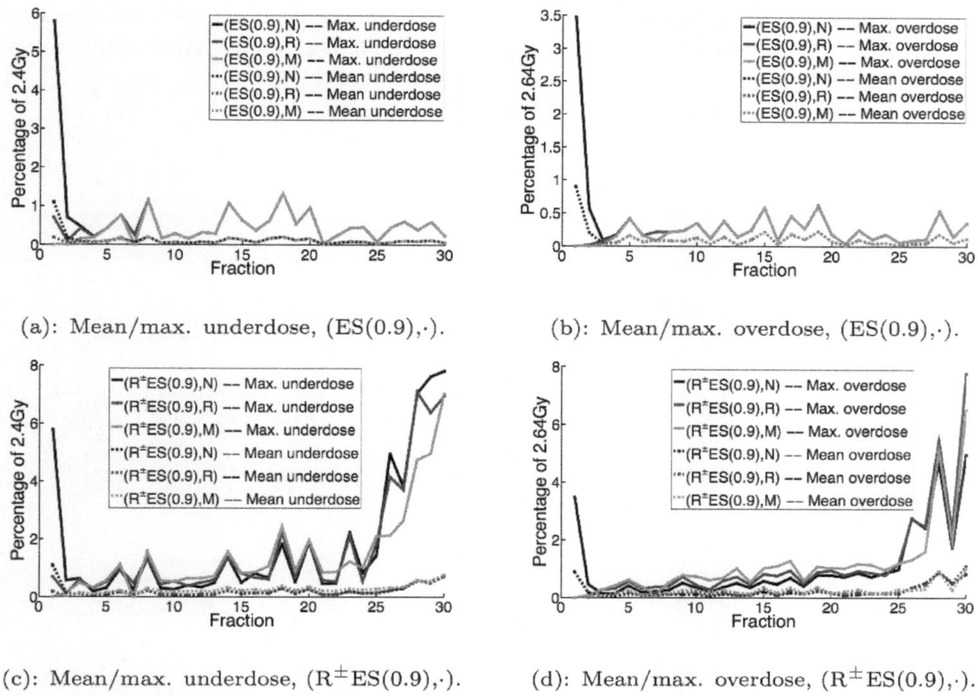

(a): Mean/max. underdose, (ES(0.9),·). (b): Mean/max. overdose, (ES(0.9),·).

(c): Mean/max. underdose, (R±ES(0.9),·). (d): Mean/max. overdose, (R±ES(0.9),·).

Figure 5. Mean and maximum underdose and overdose by fraction for ES(0.9) and R±ES(0.9) implementations.

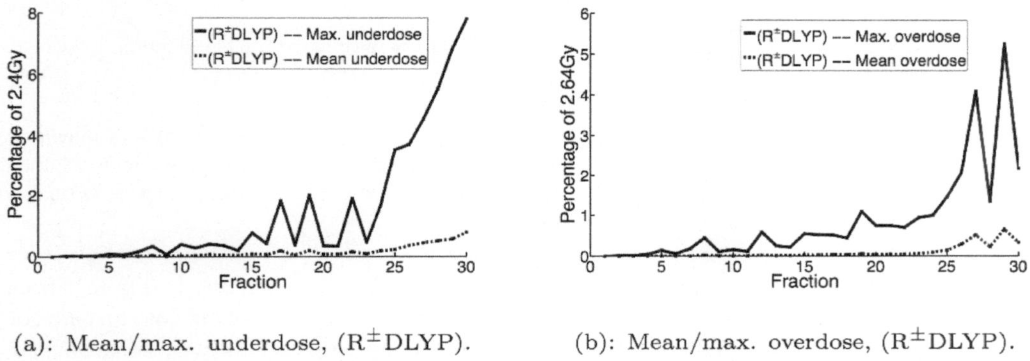

(a): Mean/max. underdose, (R±DLYP). (b): Mean/max. overdose, (R±DLYP).

Figure 6. Mean and maximum underdose and overdose by fraction for R±DLYP implementations.

We also examine the DVHs of the daily delivered dose distributions over the treatment course, at fraction 10 (Fig 2(a)), fraction 20 (Fig 2(b)) and fraction 30 (Fig 2(c)). At fraction 10, Fig 2(a)shows that there is little difference between (ES(0.1),M) and (R±ES(0.1),M). By fraction 30, however, approximately 40% of the tumor volume receives less than 2.4Gy and approximately 10% of the tumor volume receives more than 2.64Gy under (R±ES(0.1),M), while practically all of the tumor volume receives between 2.4Gy and 2.64Gy under (ES(0.1),M). Moreover, the tumor DVH drops from 100% to 0% at a much slower rate for (R±ES(0.1),M), indicating that the tumor dose for (R±ES(0.1),M) is less homogeneous than for (ES(0.1),M).

Cause of Daily Dose Performance of Dose-Reactive Methods

Given the difference between the non-reactive and dose-reactive methods in daily dose performance that is highlighted in the previous subsection, a fundamental question arises: what causes this difference? Our results provide us with an important insight towards understanding this question. Consider Fig 6(a) and 6(b), which display the daily underdose and overdose of the daily prescient implementations. These figures provide us with an interesting insight: even if we correctly anticipate the PMF in each fraction, performing a dose-reactive update to the target dose distribution can lead to both growing daily underdose and overdose. The reason this behavior occurs in the case of the reactive± daily prescient algorithms is because for a fixed PMF, it is in general not possible to deliver a completely uniform dose to the entire tumor. Therefore, in a given fraction there will be some heterogeneity in the delivered dose across the tumor, resulting in heterogeneity in the target minimum and maximum doses for the next fraction. The heterogeneity in the target dose requirements for the next fraction then leads to further heterogeneity in the dose delivered in the next fraction. As this process continues, it inevitably results in the daily dose for some voxels deviating below 2.4Gy and for some voxels deviating above 2.64Gy in the later fractions of the treatment.

This process is further exacerbated if the prescience is removed and the uncertainty set is updated according to exponential smoothing. For these methods (R±ES(α) with $\alpha > 0$), the daily PMF may fall outside the uncertainty set, and thus the delivered dose need not satisfy the target dose requirements. As a result, more underdose and overdose may be realized in each fraction, and the target dose requirements may grow more heterogeneous as the treatment progresses. A concrete demonstration of the growth in tumor dose heterogeneity and target minimum and maximum dose requirement heterogeneity is shown in Fig 7.

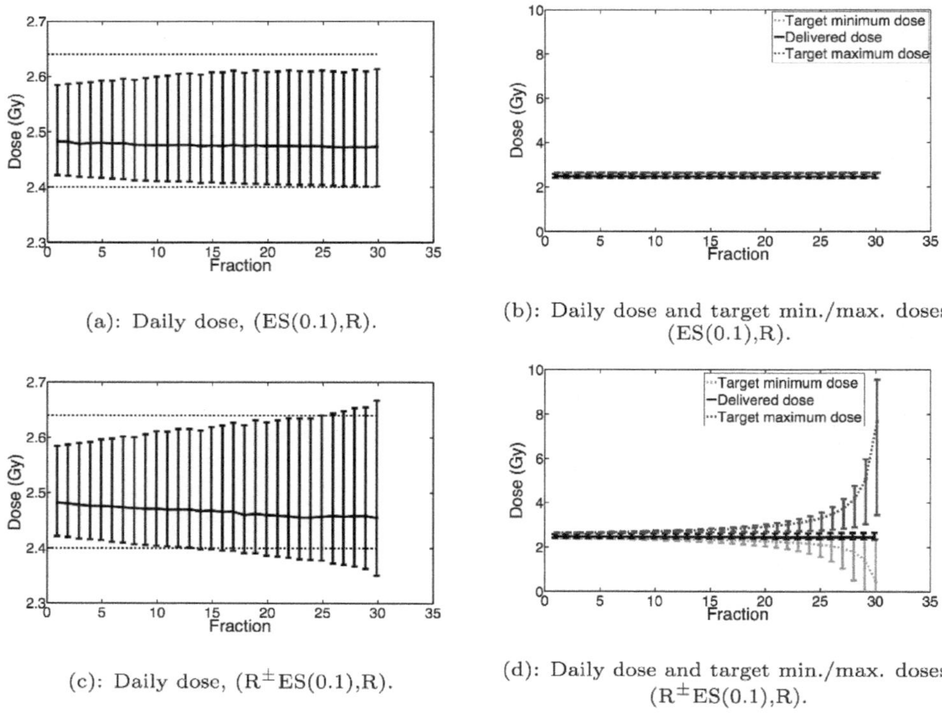

(a): Daily dose, (ES(0.1),R).

(b): Daily dose and target min./max. doses, (ES(0.1),R).

(c): Daily dose, ($R^{\pm}$ES(0.1),R).

(d): Daily dose and target min./max. doses, ($R^{\pm}$ES(0.1),R).

Figure 7. Daily delivered dose and target minimum/maximum doses for (ES(0.1),R) and ($R^{\pm}$ES(0.1),R). Where shown, the lower error bar, median and upper error bar for each fraction correspond to the 5th, 50th and 95th percentiles of the appropriate distribution, respectively. On the left-hand plots, the dashed horizontal lines correspond to 2.4Gy and 2.64Gy. The target dose requirements are normalized by $1/(n - i + 1)$ so as to be comparable to the actual delivered dose of that fraction.

As noted in the Introduction section, the outcome of a treatment depends not only on the cumulative tumor dose delivered at the end, but also on how that dose was delivered to the tumor. Indeed, it has been shown that an increase in the intrafraction dose variability leads to a decrease in tumor control probability and an increase in the probability of treatment failure [6]. We have shown that dose-reactive methods generally lead to increased heterogeneity in the daily dose distribution, as well as increased daily underdose and overdose, over the non-reactive method. Therefore, a dose-reactive treatment may be more likely to fail than a non-reactive treatment, even if both treatments achieve similar final dose distributions.

Sensitivity of Daily Dose Performance with Respect to Robustness and Uncertainty Set Adaptation

Given the growing daily underdose and overdose exhibited by dose-reactive methods, it is natural to ask how much this behavior is (1) dependent on the robust optimization component and (2) dependent on the uncertainty set adaptation component of the method. With regard to the effect of robustness, our results show that this behavior is relatively insensitive to the choice of uncertainty set. When $\alpha = 0$ and the initial uncertainty set is the nominal uncertainty set, Fig 3(c) and 3(d) show that the daily underdose and overdose grow as the treatment progresses. This makes sense because the actual PMF in each fraction is different from the anticipated PMF, which leads to errors in dose that are compounded as the treatment progresses. However, if that singleton is replaced by the robust uncertainty set, the daily underdose and overdose still grow. This is surprising because we would expect that with a larger uncertainty set, the error between the delivered dose distribution and the target lower and upper dose bounds should be smaller, which would reduce the rate at which the daily underdose and overdose grow.

With regard to the effect of uncertainty set adaptation, our results here and in [23] show that dose-reactive implementations that adaptively update the uncertainty set ($\alpha > 0$), generally result in slower growth in daily underdose and overdose than the dose-reactive implementations that do not modify the uncertainty set ($\alpha = 0$); compare, for instance, Fig 3(c)and 3(d) to Fig 5(c) and 5(d). This makes sense because as the uncertainty set is updated and becomes a more accurate representation of the patient's daily PMF, the error between the daily delivered dose distribution and the target lower and upper dose bounds should decrease, curbing how quickly the daily underdose and overdose grow. Given this last observation, our results indicate that by using dose reaction with uncertainty set adaptation—or more generally, planning the daily dose distribution with some updated estimate of the uncertainty—one can mitigate (though not fully eliminate) the growth in daily underdose and overdose.

THEORETICAL INSIGHT INTO DAILY DOSE PERFORMANCE

In addition to our computational results, we advance our understanding of the daily dose performance by building on the theory developed in [1]. There, the non-reactive adaptive robust method was analyzed by assuming that the sequence of breathing motion PMFs, as an infinite sequence, converges to a limiting PMF, and evaluating the dose distribution of an n-fraction treatment as n tends to infinity. The key result in the asymptotic analysis was that for a wide class of uncertainty set update algorithms, the final cumulative dose distribution approaches a set of optimal dose distributions that exhibit no tumor underdose or overdose and low healthy tissue dose. The same theoretical framework allows us to characterize the daily performance of the non-reactive and dose-reactive methods, which we now do.

Daily Dose Convergence under the Non-Reactive Method

The following result states that the daily dose distribution of the non-reactive adaptive robust method converges to the set of optimal dose distributions. Mathematically, the result assumes that the sequence of daily PMFs converges to a limiting PMF p^*. Under this assumption, the result asserts that when the lower and upper bound vectors ℓ and u are updated according to a convex-convergent update algorithm (such as exponential smoothing; see [1]), the daily dose distribution in fraction i, given by $\Delta p^i w^i$, can get arbitrarily close to a set D of dose distributions when i is sufficiently large. The set D is a set of optimal dose distributions that may be realized by delivering a treatment designed for $P = \{p^*\}$ when the patient breathes exactly according to p^*. In a sense, the dose distributions that are realized in this way are ideal because the treatment correctly anticipates the patient's breathing (i.e., $p^* \in P$), and does so in the least conservative way possible (since $P = \{p^*\}$). For further background, the reader is referred to Section 6 of [1].

Theorem 1 Let $(\mathbf{p}^i)_{i=1}^{\infty}$ be a sequence of PMFs that converges to p^*. Let $(\ell^i)_{i=1}^{\infty}$ and $(\mathbf{u}^i)_{i=1}^{\infty}$ be lower and upper bound sequences generated from $(\mathbf{p}^i)_{i=1}^{\infty}$ by any convex-convergent update algorithm. For each $i \in \mathbb{Z}_+$, let $w^i \in w^*(\ell^i,u^i)$. Then for every $\epsilon > 0$, there exists an $N \in \mathbb{Z}_+$ such that for all $i > N$,

$$\Delta \mathbf{p}^i \mathbf{w}^i \in U(\mathbf{D}, \epsilon). \tag{7}$$

Proof: See [23].

Note that in non-reactive treatments, the patient is treated with $(1/n)\cdot w^i$ and not w^i; therefore, the actual delivered dose distribution in fraction i is $(1/n)\cdot\Delta p^i w^i$. From Theorem 1, the actual daily delivered dose distribution $(1/n)\cdot\Delta p^i w^i$ therefore tends to $(1/n)\cdot d$ for some $d \in D$, and the dose distribution $(1/n)\cdot d$ is such that each tumor voxel v receives exactly between θ_v/n and $\gamma\theta_v/n$. We emphasize that this result is intended as a descriptive result rather than a prescriptive result: it is intended to show that if the breathing motion PMFs converge or stabilize, then the daily underdose and overdose of the adaptive robust method will tend toward zero in an asymptotic sense. This statement is relevant because indeed, in Fig 4(a) and 4(b), we see that the daily underdose and overdose diminish as the treatment progresses, in agreement with the theorem.

For the dose-reactive methods, Theorem 1 does not apply. We outline here the justification; for more details, the reader is referred to [23]. The proof of Theorem 1 relies on showing that the affine functions defining the feasible region of problem (Eq 2) converge to an affine function defining the feasible region with the uncertainty set $P = \{p^*\}$. The affine function in the ith fraction is dependent on the target dose requirements for the ith fraction. In the right-hand side plots of Fig 7 we showed how the normalized target dose requirements change as the treatment progresses for a given choice of exponential smoothing factor α and initial uncertainty set. From this figure, we see that the normalized target minimum and maximum dose requirements for all of the voxels do not converge to θ_v/n and $\gamma\theta_v/n$ by the end of the treatment. Since these normalized target dose requirements do not necessarily converge, the affine functions defining the feasible regions of the robust problem (Eq 2) do not converge. As a result, in the limit, the dose-reactive methods can exhibit underdose or overdose in certain tumor voxels with respect to the daily prescribed minimum and maximum doses θ_v/n and $\gamma\theta_v/n$, respectively.

Furthermore, it seems unlikely that the daily dose distribution under any of the dose-reactive methods will converge under a different set of assumptions. Our computational results show that even if we consider the daily prescient treatments, which perfectly anticipate the daily PMF in every fraction, the dose-reactive methods still grow in daily underdose and overdose (cf. Fig 6(a) and 6(b)). These results give us strong reason to believe that in general, the daily dose distribution under any of the dose-reactive methods will not converge, and will not exhibit daily underdose and overdose that diminishes in the limit.

CONCLUSIONS

In this paper, we compared the performance of methods that employ dose reaction with that of non-reactive methods using real patient data. We found that dose reaction may result in a modest improvement in both overall end-of-treatment tumor coverage and healthy tissue dose with respect to the non-reactive method. However, dose-reactive methods also result in growing daily underdose and overdose. In contrast, the non-reactive method performs well from a daily dose perspective, with daily underdose and overdose decreasing as the treatment progresses. We also proved theoretically that the daily dose distribution from the non-reactive method will converge to an ideal daily dose distribution that exhibits no tumor underdose or overdose. The same theoretical framework, together with our computational results, suggests that the dose-reactive methods will not exhibit the same convergence. The deterioration in daily dose performance we have shown has the potential to endanger the outcome of the treatment [6]. Thus, any clinical implementation of a dose-reactive strategy must account for and guard against this type of daily dose behavior to ensure a successful treatment. Overall, the key message of this paper is that reacting to dose errors—an adaptation strategy that is both simple and intuitively appealing—may backfire and lead to treatments that are clinically unacceptable.

Given the poor performance of dose-reactive methods with respect to daily dose performance, it is natural to ask how this performance can be improved. We have already highlighted the fact that uncertainty set adaptation reduces the degree of growth in daily underdose/overdose over the treatment course. An alternate avenue is to change how the dose requirements are modified. In particular, one may consider a modified dose-reactive update, where one takes a convex combination of the target minimum/maximum dose (after the normal dose-reactive update) with the corresponding non-reactive target minimum/maximum dose. More precisely, consider the following τ-reactive± update, where τ ∈ [0, 1], and we set δ—i+1vδ¯vi+1 for each fraction i + 1 as

$$\underline{\delta}_v^{i+1} = (1-\tau)\cdot\left(\frac{n-i}{n}\right)\theta_v + \tau\cdot\max\left\{0,\ \underline{\delta}_v^{i} - \sum_{x\in X}\sum_{b\in\mathcal{B}}\Delta_{v,x,b}\,p^i(x)\frac{w_b^i}{n-i+1}\right\}$$

and $\bar{\delta}_v^{i+1}$ for fraction i + 1 as

$$\bar{\delta}_v^{i+1} = (1-\tau)\cdot\left(\frac{n-i}{n}\right)\gamma\theta_v + \tau\cdot\max\left\{0,\ \bar{\delta}_v^{i} - \sum_{x\in X}\sum_{b\in\mathcal{B}}\Delta_{v,x,b}\,p^i(x)\frac{w_b^i}{n-i+1}\right\}.$$

In this way, the target minimum and maximum dose are not fully adjusted in response to the delivered dose and are less heterogeneous, potentially resulting in slower growth in daily underdose and overdose. Building on this idea, one may also consider a method where the constant τ in the formulae above is updated as the treatment progresses.

ACKNOWLEDGMENTS

The authors thank Thomas Bortfeld of Massachusetts General Hospital for providing the patient data used in the Results section. The authors thank Troy Long, H. Edwin Romeijn and Marina Epelman for insightful conversations that motivated our work on this topic.

AUTHOR CONTRIBUTIONS

Conceived and designed the experiments: TCYC VVM. Performed the experiments: VVM. Analyzed the data: VVM. Wrote the paper: TCYC VVM.

REFERENCES

1. Chan TCY, Mišić VV. Adaptive and robust radiation therapy optimization for lung cancer. Eur J Oper Res. 2013; 231: 745–756. doi: 10. 1016/j. ejor. 2013. 06. 003.
2. Chan T, Bortfeld T, Tsitsiklis J. A robust approach to IMRT optimization. Phys Med Biol. 2006; 51: 2567–2583. doi: 10. 1088/0031-9155/51/10/014. pmid:16675870
3. Bortfeld T, Chan T, Trofimov A, Tsitsiklis J Robust management of motion uncertainty in intensity-modulated radiation therapy. Oper Res. 2008; 56: 1461–1473. doi: 10. 1287/opre. 1070. 0484.
4. Yan D, Vicini F, Wong J, Martinez A. Adaptive radiation therapy. Phys Med Biol. 1997; 42: 123–132. doi: 10. 1088/0031-9155/42/1/008. pmid:9015813
5. Mar PA, Chan TCY. Adaptive and robust radiation therapy in the presence of drift. Phys Med Biol. 2015; in press. doi: 10. 1088/0031-9155/60/9/3599. pmid:25860509
6. Ebert M. Viability of the EUD and TCP concepts as reliable dose indicators. Phys Med Biol. 2000; 45: 441–457. doi: 10. 1088/0031-9155/45/2/313. pmid:10701514
7. Yan D, Wong J, Vicini F, Michalski J, Pan C, Frazier A, et al. Adaptive modification of treatment planning to minimize the deleterious effects of treatment setup errors. Int J Radiat Oncol Biol Phys. 1997; 38: 197–206. doi: 10. 1016/S0360-3016(97)00229-0. pmid:9212024
8. Yan D, Ziaja E, Jaffray D, Wong J, Brabbins D, Vicini F, et al. The use of adaptive radiation therapy to reduce setup error: a prospective clinical study. Int J Radiat Oncol Biol Phys. 1998; 41: 715–720. doi: 10. 1016/S0360-3016(97)00567-1. pmid:9635724
9. Löf J, Lind B, Brahme A. An adaptive control algorithm for optimization of intensity modulated radiotherapy considering uncertainties in beam profiles, patient set-up and internal organ motion. Phys Med Biol. 1998; 43: 1605–1628. doi: 10. 1088/0031-9155/43/6/018. pmid:9651029
10. Rehbinder H, Forsgren C, Löf J. Adaptive radiation therapy for compensation of errors in patient setup and treatment delivery. Med Phys. 2004; 31: 3363–3371. doi: 10. 1118/1. 1809768. pmid:15651619
11. Mohan R, Zhang X, Wang H, Kang Y, Wang X, Liu H, et al. Use of deformed intensity distributions for on-line modification of image-guided IMRT to account for interfractional anatomic changes. Int J Radiat Oncol Biol Phys. 2005; 61: 1258–1266. doi: 10. 1016/j. ijrobp. 2004. 11. 033. pmid:15752908
12. Lu W, Olivera G, Chen Q, Ruchala K, Haimerl J, Meeks SL, et al. Deformable registration of the planning image (kVCT) and the daily images (MVCT) for adaptive radiation therapy. Phys Med Biol. 2006; 51: 4357–4374. doi: 10. 1088/0031-9155/51/17/015. pmid:16912386
13. Ferris M, Voelker M. Fractionation in radiation treatment planning. Math Program. 2004; 101: 387–413. doi: 10. 1007/s10107-004-0530-y.
14. Deng G, Ferris M. Neuro-dynamic programming for fractionated radiotherapy planning. In: Alves C, Pardalos P, Vicente L, editors, Optimization in Medicine, Springer Verlag; 2008. pp. 47–70.
15. Sir M, Epelman M, Pollock S. Stochastic programming for off-line adaptive radiotherapy. Ann Oper Res. 2012; 196: 767–797. doi: 10. 1007/s10479-010-0779-x.
16. Birkner M, Yan D, Alber M, Liang J, Niisslin F. Adapting inverse planning to patient and organ geometrical variation: algorithm and implementation. Med Phys. 2003; 30: 2822–2831. doi: 10. 1118/1. 1610751. pmid:14596318

17. Wu Q, Liang J, Yan D. Application of dose compensation in image-guided radiotherapy of prostate cancer. Phys Med Biol. 2006; 51: 1405–1419. doi: 10. 1088/0031-9155/51/6/003. pmid:16510952

18. de la Zerda A, Armbruster B, Xing L. Formulating adaptive radiation therapy (ART) treatment planning into a closed-loop control framework. Phys Med Biol. 2007; 52: 4137–4153. doi: 10. 1088/0031-9155/52/14/008. pmid:17664599

19. Saka B, Rardin RL, Langer MP, Dink D. Adaptive intensity modulated radiation therapy planning optimization with changing tumor geometry and fraction size limits. HE Trans Health Sys Eng. 2011; 1: 247–263. doi: 10. 1080/19488300. 2011. 609871

20. Dink D, Langer M, Orcun S, Pekny J, Rardin R, Reklaitis G, et al. IMRT optimization with both fractionation and cumulative constraints. Amer J Oper Res. 2011; 1: 160–171. doi: 10. 4236/ajor. 2011. 13018.

21. Webb S. Adapting IMRT delivery fraction-by-fraction to cater for variable intrafraction motion. Phys Med Biol. 2008; 53: 1–21. doi: 10. 1088/0031-9155/53/21/B01. pmid:18182684

22. Lujan A, Larsen E, Balter J, Ten Haken R. A method for incorporating organ motion due to breathing into 3D dose calculations. Med Phys. 1999; 26: 715–720. doi: 10. 1118/1. 598577. pmid:10360531

23. Mišić VV. Adaptive and robust radiation therapy optimization for lung cancer. M. A. Sc. thesis, University of Toronto. 2012. Available:https://tspace. library. utoronto. ca/handle/1807/32485.

24. Bortfeld T, Schlegel W, Rhein B. Decomposition of pencil beam kernels for fast dose calculations in three-dimensional treatment planning. Med Phys. 1993; 20: 311–318. doi: 10. 1118/1. 597070. pmid:8497215

25. Trofimov A, Rietzel E, Lu H, Martin B, Jiang S, Chen GTY, et al. Temporo-spatial IMRT optimization: concepts, implementation and initial results. Phys Med Biol. 2005; 50: 2779–2798. doi: 10. 1088/0031-9155/50/12/004. pmid:15930602

CHAPTER 10

CELL TO CELL VARIABILITY OF RADIATION-INDUCED FOCI

Gaëtan Gruel, Carmen Villagrasa, Pascale Voisin, Isabelle Clairand, Marc Benderitter, Jean-François Bottollier-Depois, and Joan Francesc Barquinero

INTRODUCTION

DNA double-strand breaks (DSB) are critical lesions that produces a variety of radiobiological effects [1,2]. Understanding the interactions of different radiation qualities with DNA requires an accurate quantification of the yields of DNA DSBs. Among the techniques used to measure DSB yields in mammalian cells are: neutral sedimentation gradients, filter elution, pulsed field gel electrophoresis techniques (PFGE) [3], and more recently, immunofluorescence analysis of nuclear foci of DSB-signalling proteins, including phosphorylation of H2AX at Ser139 (alias gamma H2AX) [4], phosphorylation of ATM [5], or localization of MRE11 [6] or 53BP1 [7]. Specific antibodies enable the visualization of discrete nuclear foci (RIF for radiation induced foci) at DSB sites. Initial studies have shown a close correlation between the number of RIF and the number of DSBs expected after gamma-ray exposure and several have observed a linear relation between the mean per-cell RIF count and the mean macroscopic absorbed dose of photon radiation[8–10]. In general, these studies have assumed homogeneous cell irradiation, that is, that all cells receive the same amount of energy. The level of DNA lesions is therefore generally determined by averaging it over the entire population of exposed cells. Intercell variation in the number of RIF is used to measure a kind of uncertainty associated with biological and methodological phenomena, and the average level of damage is the value usually considered to be responsible for the final biological effect. Nevertheless, at the micrometric and nanometric (molecular) scales, the distribution of the energy deposited by ionizing radiation has a spread that is due to fluctuations in both the number of tracks passing the target and the energy deposition per track [11–14]. These fluctuations depend on the radiation quality and the target volume. Thus, the assessment of a stochastic phenomenon such as ionizing radiation by the measurement of an average effect cannot provide an adequate understanding of some aspects of the cellular response to this radiation. The RIF count variation among the cells implies that different quantities of damage have been signalled for these different cells, and hence that there exist cells for which the biological effect may be different from those with the mean level of damage. This point is important, both in the context of cancer treatment where the survival of just a few cells may induce relapse but also in analysing the processes underlying tissue response to low-dose exposures or low fluence. Accordingly, the evaluation of this RIF variance between cells appears to be as important as the mean number of RIF for assessing the biological significance of radiation exposure.

In this work, we accurately measured the variability of RIF counts in each nucleus in a population of cells exposed to three different macroscopic doses, in order to evaluate the portion of this variability associated with the microdosimetric variance calculated for the different target volumes and subvolumes in which RIF can be generated.

MATERIALS AND METHODS

Cell Culture and Irradiation

The human umbilical vein endothelial cells (HUVEC) we used were purchased from the Lonza Group (ref. C2519A, lot. 87758) and isolated by Lonza from human tissue (from 3 females and 1 male) donated after permission was obtained for its use in research applications by informed consent or legal authorization. Lonza holds donor consent and legal authorization that provides permission for all research

Citation: Gruel G, Villagrasa C, Voisin P, Clairand I, Benderitter M, Bottollier-Depois J-F, et al. (2016) Cell to Cell Variability of Radiation-Induced Foci, PLoS ONE, 11(1): e0145786. DOI:10.1371/journal.pone.0145786.

use. Hence, institutional review board or ethics committee approval was not necessary. The supplier states that it followed established ethical practices of United States donation and transplantation organizations. In addition, all experiments complied with French law (Act no. 2004–800) on bioethics. All cells tested negative for mycoplasma, bacteria, yeast and fungi. Cell lots and donors were tested and negative for HIV-1, hepatitis B and hepatitis C. The HUVEC were cultured at 37°C, with 95% humidity and 5% CO_2 in EGM-2 media optimized for the proliferation of endothelial cells and supplemented with 5% fetal bovine serum, hydrocortisone, hFGF-B, VEGF, R3-IGF-1, ascorbic acid, hEGF, gentamicin and amphotericin-B (EGM-2MV BulletKit, Lonza). For experiments, cells were seeded on glass in 1-well Nunc® Lab-Tek® II chamber slide systems (Thermo Fisher Scientific). The cells were grown until they formed a monolayer (approximately 75 to 85% confluent) and then exposed to gamma radiation from a 145817 GBq source (nominal activity 22/02/2002) of ^{60}Co radiation (ICO 4000 IRSN facility at Fontenay-aux-Roses, France), at a dose rate of 1.3 Gy.min^{-1}. The uncertainty for the delivered dose was estimated to be 6%. Two different platforms were used for the X-ray exposures to corroborate the results obtained with ^{60}Co: an Eleckta Synergy Platform (linac accelerator) was used to deliver radiation with a maximal energy of 4 MeV (X-rays 4 MVp) at a dose rate of 1.1 Gy.min^{-1} and with an uncertainty for the delivered dose estimated at 7%, and the X-RAD 320 X-ray system (XPI) delivered radiation with a maximal energy of 200 kVp, at a dose rate of 0.54 Gy.min^{-1}, and with an uncertainty for the delivered dose below 2%.

Immunostaining

HUVEC were immunostained after exposure to sham, 0.5 Gy, 1 Gy and 2 Gy of ^{60}Co irradiation. Briefly, 30 min after irradiation, cells were fixed with 4% paraformaldehyde in PBS for 15 min, washed with PBS (Life Technologies), permeabilized in 0.5% Triton X-100 solution (Sigma Aldrich) for 5 min, and then washed 3 more times with PBS. The cells were then incubated for 1 h with primary antibodies, either a mix of mouse IgG1 monoclonal anti-phospho-histone H2AX (Ser139) antibody (clone JBW301, Upstate) and/or rabbit polyclonal anti-KI67 (Life Technologies). Cells were then washed 3 more times and incubated for 1 h with a secondary antibody, i.e., a mix of goat anti-mouse IgG1 (γ1) coupled to Alexa Fluor® 488 (2 mg.mL^{-1}, Life Technologies) and/or goat anti-rabbit IgG (H+L) coupled to Texas Red®-X (2 mg.mL^{-1}, Life Technologies). Cells were washed as described above before applying ProLong® Gold Antifade mountant with DAPI (Life Technologies).

Image Acquisition and Analysis

Cell images were visualized with a ScanR platform (Olympus), which comprises an inverted microscope IX81 (Olympus) equipped with a motorized SCAN IM IX2 stage (Märzhäuser) and an MT20 fluorescence illumination system with a fast filter wheel. Images were acquired with a UPLSAPO 100XO oil immersion objective (Olympus) with an NA of 1.4 and an ORCA-R2 CCD camera (Hamamatsu). The image pixel size was 0.064 μm. The limit of resolution based on the NA of the objective in the Alexa Fluor® 488 channel was 0.2 μm (Rayleigh limit). Images were captured so that intensities for a given experiment were within the 12-bit linear range. Image analysis was performed with Scan^R analysis software. The edge-based segmentation algorithm implemented in the software was used to detect main objects (*i.e.*, nuclei) and subobjects (*i.e.*, foci). Different kinds of parameters were measured on each detected object and subobject. Those used for the data analysis were mainly the area, circularity, and integrated intensity of DAPI, Alexa Fluor® 488 and Texas Red®-X. Non-cycling cells were selected with a "flow cytometry like" analysis. A first selection based on areas and circularities of the nuclei was done through the definition of an adequate region on the corresponding scatter plot. This step allowed us to consider only isolated nuclei and to remove from the analysis objects corresponding to clusters of nuclei. A second region, based on the integrated intensity levels of DAPI and Alexa Fluor® 488, measured for each nucleus, was then done to isolate nuclei in the G0/G1 phase of the cell cycle. RIF in the objects within the gate formed by the intersection of the two regions were then analysed.

Specific Energy Distribution Calculation

Specific energy was calculated only for the ^{60}Co gamma radiation exposure. The energy absorbed by a specific target follows a frequency distribution $f(z)$ where z is a stochastic quantity corresponding to the energy ε imparted per mass m in the target of volume V. The macroscopic dose D corresponds to the expected value of the distribution $f(z)$ [11–14].

The probability of obtaining a specific energy z in the target is the result of two stochastic phenomena: the probability of ν tracks passing the target and the probability that these ν tracks deposit a specific energy equal to z.

$$f(z,D) = \sum_{\nu=0}^{\infty} p(\nu) \cdot f_\nu(z) \tag{1}$$

where, for small doses, the number of tracks is distributed following a Poisson distribution of mean value n,

$$p(\nu) = e^{-n}\frac{n^\nu}{\nu!}.$$

For n>20, the Poisson distribution can be approximated well by a normal distribution of mean value n and standard deviation √n [15]. This is true in this work because for ^{60}Co irradiation this condition is met in typical cell nucleus volumes for D> 0.2 Gy.

The function $f_\nu(z)$ can be calculated as the convolution of the single-track frequency distribution $f_1(z)$:

$$f_\nu(z) = \int_0^{z_{max}} f_{\nu-1}(z-z') \cdot f_1(z')\,dz' \quad . \tag{2}$$

This convolution rapidly converges to a normal distribution of the form:

$$N(\nu \cdot \bar{z}_1, \sqrt{\nu} \cdot SD_{z_1}),$$

wherez_1 and SDz_1 are respectively the mean value and the standard deviation of the single track frequency distribution. Thus, the convolution of both distributions in Eq 1 can be approximated to a normal distribution:

$$N(n \cdot \bar{z}_1; \sqrt{n \cdot (\bar{z}_1{}^2 + SD_{z_1}{}^2)})$$

Accordingly, and knowing thatz_1 and SDz_1 are both functions of the volume, we can calculate the parameters k_1 and k_2 needed to express the relative standard deviation of the specific energy distribution of the ^{60}Co irradiation as a function of the macroscopic dose D and the volume of the target V [15]:

$$SD_z^{rel} = \frac{k_1}{V^{k_2}\sqrt{D}} \quad (3)$$

In this work, we used this relation and the k_1 and k_2 values obtained by Villegas *et al.* [15] to calculate the specific energy distributions expected in different volumes related to the endothelial cell population irradiated with the ^{60}Co source at the IRSN facility.

RESULTS

Characterization of HUVEC Cells for RIF Analysis

The mean number of DSBs per cell induced by a given dose of gamma rays is proportional to the DNA content of the cells. Accordingly, it was necessary to use a cell population with a homogeneous DNA content, to be able to interpret the intercellular variability of RIF count per cell and be certain that intercellular variations in the initial DNA content were not the source of this post-exposure RIF variability. Preliminary analyses were conducted to characterize the HUVEC cells and ensure the robustness of this aspect of our experimental approach.

Because *in vitro* cell culture may induce genomic instability, HUVEC primary cells were used at low passage, and their cytogenetic state was evaluated by M-FISH during passages 2 (P2) and 4 (P4). Of the 78 cells analysed in P2, 51 were female (65%) and 27 male (35%), and only two were abnormal, both with trisomy ((47, XY, +12) and (47, XX, +18)). In P4, 105 cells were analysed, 80 female (76%) and 25 male (24%). Again, two abnormal cells were observed, one trisomy (47, XX, +11) and one cell with two non-reciprocal translocations and one double insertion (46, XY, t(14;5), t(14;Y), ins (2;22;3)). No clonal abnormality was observed, and the proportions of males and females obtained by cytogenetic analysis were consistent with the initial proportions of the pool of cells (3 females and 1 male).

Another factor influencing the amount of DNA in target cells is the cell cycle. It was therefore necessary to irradiate a maximum of cells in the G0/G1 phase of the cell cycle. Moreover, cells undergoing division (S, G2 and metaphase) have a very high gamma-H2AX background. Thus, non-dividing cells must be selected to analyse gamma-H2AX foci that are specifically due to ionizing radiation. The most effective method was to produce cell cultures at high confluence and to be able to characterize the cell cycle state of each nucleus during image acquisition and data treatment. This characterization was based on the measurement of integrated intensities of DAPI, corresponding to the DNA content of each nucleus, and Alexa 488, corresponding to the gamma-H2AX level in the whole nucleus. This representation can be used to define a subpopulation of nuclei with a low level of integrated intensity of both DAPI and Alexa 488 in both non-irradiated (Fig 1A) and irradiated (Fig 1B) conditions. This allowed us to select a well-defined population of nuclei, mainly out of the cell cycle. Remarkably, the integrated intensity associated with the gamma-H2AX background due to cell division was affected very slightly, if at all, by the fluorescence associated with RIF at the doses tested. As a control, we labelled KI67, a cell proliferation marker, to check the cell cycle state of the selected nuclei. As Fig 2 illustrates, the greater the KI67 labelling, the greater the gamma-H2AX background. On the contrary, non-irradiated nuclei with no or low KI67 detected also had no labelling for gamma-H2AX. This effect can be visualized at the scale of a cell population.Fig 3A and 3C plot the nucleus counts according to integrated DAPI intensity in a population of at least 1500 detected nuclei. The different phases of the cell cycle can be broadly distinguished in this representation and associated with the number of foci detected in the corresponding nuclei (Fig 3B and 3D respectively for 0 Gy and 0.5 Gy). Thus the unbiased selection of cells in the G0/G1 state is critical for studying the gamma-H2AX RIF.

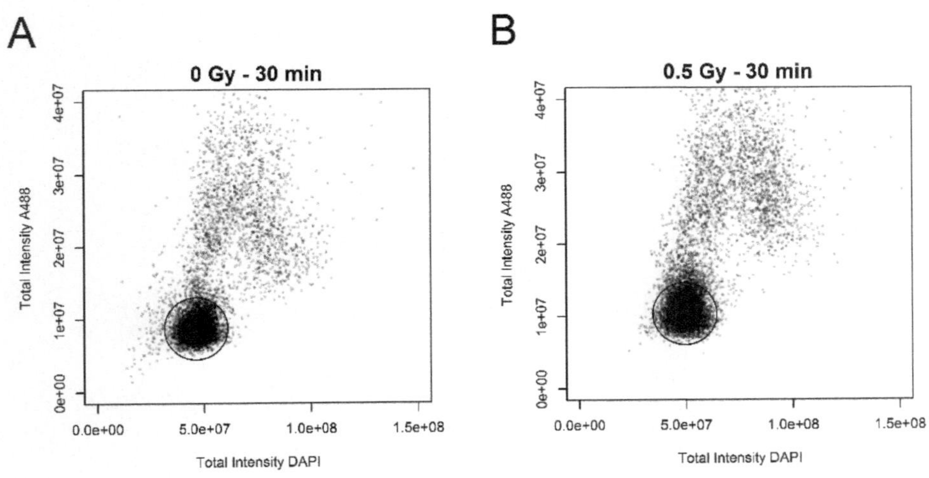

Figure 1. Scatter plots of the integrated intensities of DAPI and Alexa Fluor® 488. The integrated intensities of DAPI and Alexa Fluor® 488 correspond respectively to the DNA content and level of gamma-H2AX in the whole nucleus of each analysed cell. Black circles indicate a well-defined population of nuclei mainly in the G0/G1 phase of the cell cycle. (A) Non-irradiated condition. (B) Irradiated condition, 0.5 Gy.

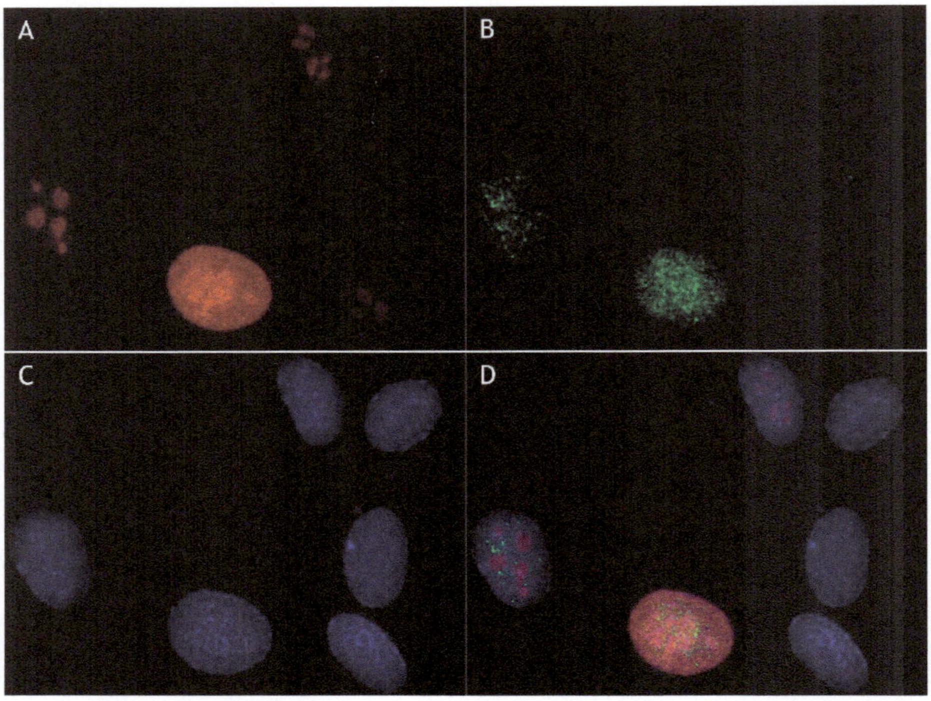

Figure 2. Co-labelling by immunofluorescence of gamma-H2AX and KI67 in non-irradiated HUVEC cells.

KI67 is a cellular proliferation marker. The greater the KI67 labelling, the greater the gamma-H2AX background. This confirms the relation between the global level of gamma-H2AX and the cell-cycle phase of each cell. (A) Photograph of Texas Red®-X fluorescence associated with KI67 immunodetection. (B) Photograph of Alexa Fluor® 488 fluorescence associated with gamma-H2AX immunodetection. (C) Photograph of DAPI fluorescence associated with DNA content. (D) Merge.

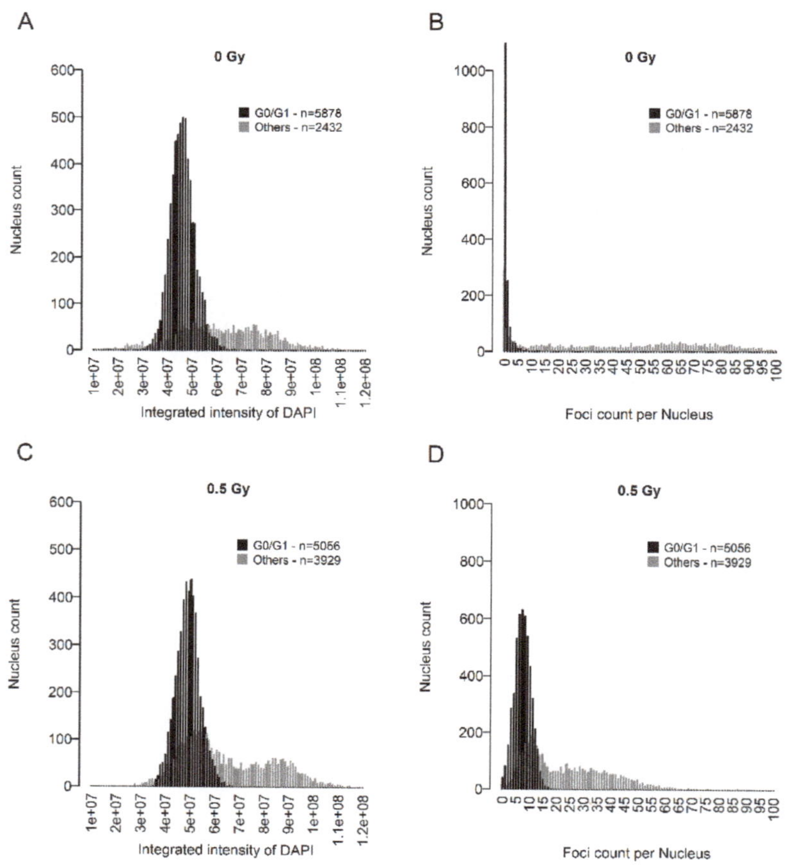

Figure 3. Histograms of nucleus count as a function of the integrated intensity of DAPI and number of gamma-H2AX foci. (A) and (C) correspond to histograms of the nucleus count as a function of their corresponding integrated DAPI intensities. (B) and (C) correspond to histograms of the nucleus count as a function of the corresponding number of gamma-H2AX foci. (A) and (B) Non-irradiated condition. (C) and (D) Irradiated condition, 0.5 Gy.

The second step of cell characterization was to evaluate the typical nucleus size of HUVEC in the G0/G1 state and thus define a concrete volume to be used for calculating specific energy distribution and for validating the use of conventional microscopy for analysing RIF in a large population of several thousand nuclei.

For these purposes, we used confocal microscopy to measure the mean dimensions of the nuclei and to analyse the distribution of foci through the entire cell nucleus volume. Fig 4Ashows gamma-H2AX foci viewed at the focal plane, as for conventional microscopy. Fig 4B and 4C show the foci for the same nucleus viewed after a 3D reconstruction with confocal microscopy. After confocal analysis of around 50 cells, the shape of nuclei was defined as an elliptic cylinder of dimensions 17±1.5 (major axis), 11±1.5 (minor axis) and 2±0.3 (thickness) μm ±SD. Given how thin the HUVEC nuclei are and the size of the RIF fluorescent volume (a sphere of 600 nm of diameter), it appears that all RIF detected with confocal microscopy can also be detected with a single focal plane with conventional microscopy. This statement is specific to our cells and culture conditions (monolayer on glass in Lab-Tek® chambers). It does not appear applicable to other cell types with differently shaped nuclei, for which z-stacks are mandatory.

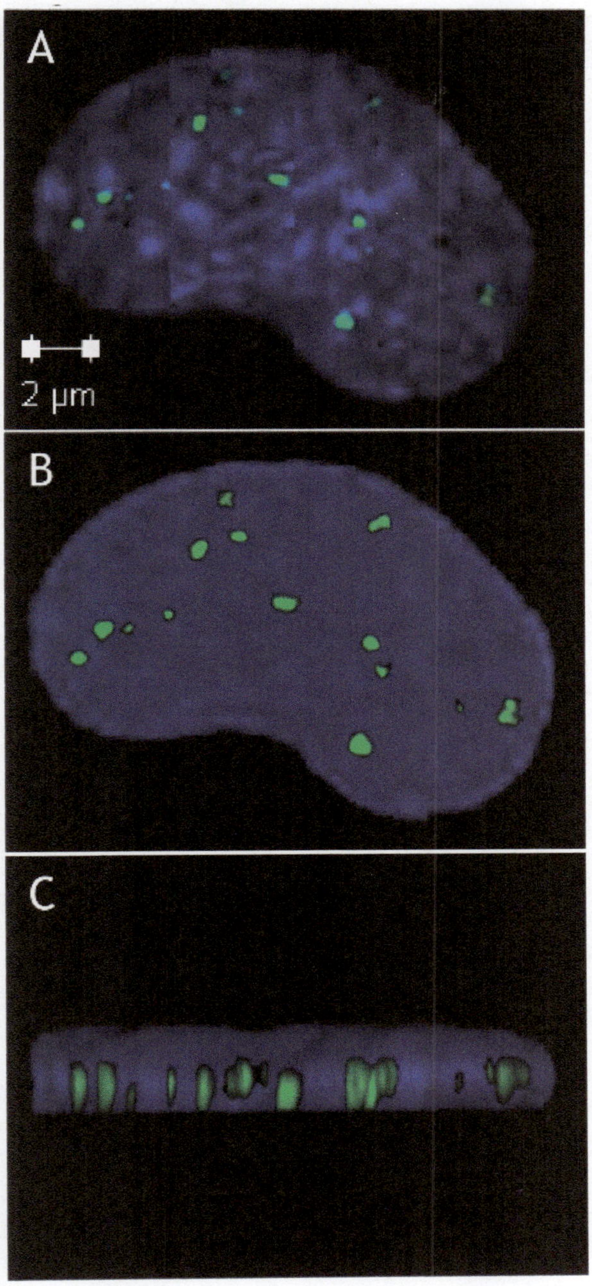

Figure 4. Labelling by immunofluorescence of gamma-H2AX acquired with confocal microscopy. This allows the study of the distribution of foci in the whole volume of irradiated endothelial cell nuclei, cultured as monolayers on glass in Lab-Tek® chambers. (A) Gamma-H2AX foci viewed at the focal plane, as for conventional microscopy. (B) Top view after 3D reconstruction, with confocal microscopy acquisition of 15 layers across the nucleus. The number of foci is identical to that observed at the focal plane. (C) Side view of the 3D reconstruction. In view of the size of the foci, the thickness of the endothelial nucleus and the depth of field of the x63 objective used, it appears that all foci that can be detected with confocal microscopy can also be detected at focal plane with conventional microscopy. The picture is representative of all the nuclei examined by confocal microscopy.

Dose Effect at the Macroscopic Scale

HUVEC samples were irradiated with ^{60}Co at two different macroscopic absorbed doses: 0.5, 1 and 2 Gy. Each experiment was independently replicated 3 times. Nine replicate experiments were performed for the non-irradiated condition. At least 1500 nuclei in G0/G1 were evaluated for each replication. The gamma-H2AX RIF were counted for each nucleus at 30 min after irradiation, because our preliminary analysis showed that this time point corresponded to the maximum RIF simultaneously observed per cell (data not shown). The boxplots in Fig 5A show the median RIF obtained for each condition and each replication. The mean RIF count per nucleus was 0.6±0.28 at 0 Gy, 9.1±0.66 at 0.5 Gy, 17.6±0.86 at 1 Gy and 30.7±0.60 at 2 Gy (Fig 5B). Errors were calculated as the standard deviation of the means obtained in each set of replications. These variations among replications appeared consistent with the uncertainty for the delivered dose, estimated at 6% for ^{60}Co irradiation. A linear relation was obtained for the dose-effect curve, as shown in Fig 5B. From the slope of the linear relation we can estimate a mean RIF count per gray of 15.5±0.33.

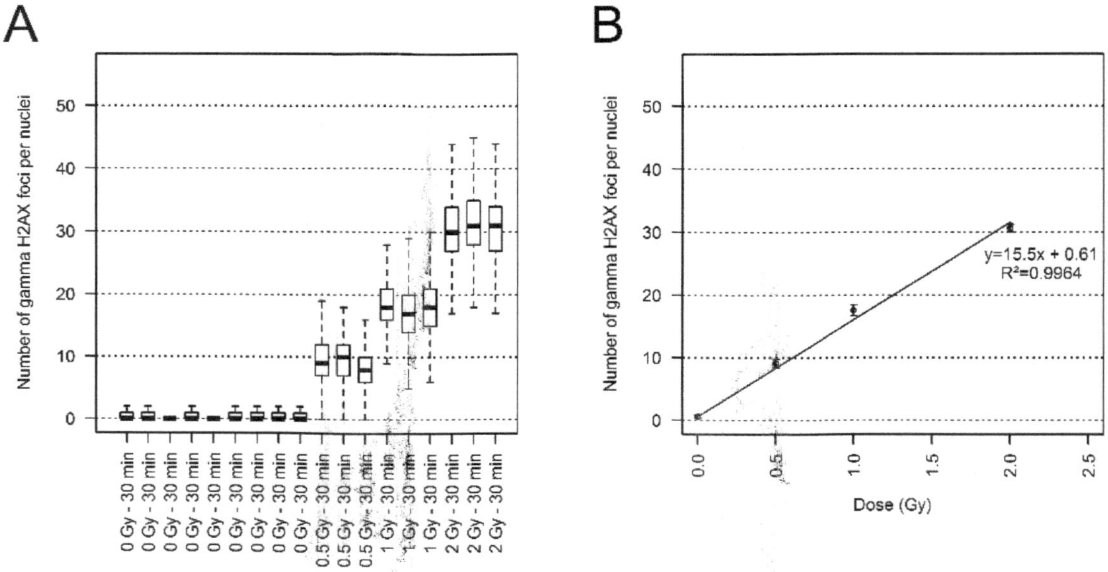

Figure 5. Dose-effect relations. (A) Box-and-whisker plot of the number of gamma H2AX foci per nucleus for each tested dose and their corresponding replications. Bold black bars of boxplots correspond to medians. The lower and upper borders of the box correspond to the first and third quartiles, respectively. The upper and lower whiskers correspond to 1.5 times the interquartile distance. (B) Linear regression based on mean values among replications performed for each tested dose. Error bars were calculated as the standard deviation between the average number of foci per nucleus obtained in each replication. Linear regression was done with the *lm* function of the *stats* package of R software.

RIF Distribution among the Nuclei

Given the absence of differences among each set of replications, the variability in the RIF count for each population of nuclei was evaluated with pooled data. The final sizes of each population were 8242, 8993 and 9010 nuclei, respectively, for doses of 0.5, 1 and 2 Gy; the mean RIF counts were 8.8±3.2, 17.6±4.4 and 30.6±5.6, and both medians and modes were very close to the corresponding means (Table 1). Standard deviations (SD) were computed as the square root of the variance calculated for each population. This value allowed us to quantify the cell-to-cell variability in terms of the number of RIF. The relative standard deviations (SD^{rel}, calculated as SD divided by the mean) for each dose population were 0.363, 0.253 and 0.182. Interestingly, the SD^{rel} was not constant and did not increase with the dose: the SD increased with dose, but the SD^{rel} decreased. The dose effect relation appeared to be linear: when the dose was multiplied by 2, the mean number of RIF per nucleus also doubled, but the corresponding SD did not. These results were confirmed with independent irradiations with two different X-ray sources. At each dose, the various parameters of the distributions were around the same, regardless of the type of radiation. More specifically, the variance of the distribution of the number of RIF per nucleus in the cell population appeared to be equal to the mean of the distribution. Table 1 summarizes all these descriptive statistics.

Table 1. Observed values for RIF.

Source	Dose[a]	nucleus number	Mean[b]	Median[b]	Mode[b]	Var	SD	SD^{rel}	Fold change SD^{rel}
	0	25114	0.6	0	0	2.1	1.5	2.558	
Cobalt 60	0.5	8242	8.8	9	8	10.2	3.2	0.363	0.696
	1	8993	17.6	18	17	19.7	4.4	0.253	0.719
	2	9010	30.6	31	31	30.9	5.6	0.182	
X rays 4 MV	0.5	7362	10.2	10	11	10.7	3.3	0.322	0.732
	1	8721	17.3	17	16	16.7	4.1	0.236	0.785
	2	5162	33.2	33	34	38.0	6.2	0.185	
X rays 200 kV	0.5	1555	8.8	9	9	9.81	3.1	0.357	0.710
	1	6796	17.6	18	18	19.76	4.4	0.253	0.759
	2	8149	30.2	30	31	33.73	5.8	0.192	

[a] gray
[b] Radiation induced foci per nucleus

doi:10.1371/journal.pone.0145786.t001

Distribution of Specific Energies Calculated in Nuclear and DNA Volumes

The main objective of these calculations was to obtain an evaluation of the dispersion of the energy deposition in the different target volumes and subvolumes in which RIF can be generated. Eq 3 was therefore used to calculate the relative standard deviations of the specific energy distributions for the ^{60}Co irradiations. Table 2 presents the descriptive statistics obtained for each of the absorbed doses in the biological experiments (0.5 Gy, 1 Gy and 2 Gy). These statistics were calculated from data generated assuming a normal distribution for the same number of events as in the biological experiments. Initially, two different target volumes were studied: 293.7 μm^3, the volume of the whole cell nucleus, and 8.5 μm^3, the volume of a 6-Gbp DNA molecule within the nucleus. The first volume was calculated from dimensions determined by the biological experiments, and the second on the assumption that a DNA molecule of 6 Gbp is a cylinder with a diameter of 2.3 nm and a height of 2.04 m. As expected, the standard deviation of the specific energy distribution within the population of targets increased as the target size decreased. For the DNA molecule, for example, the variance increased approximately 20-fold. Interestingly, for each of these two volumes, SD increased with dose while SD^{rel} decreased. It is important to note that both these volumes were calculated from mean sizes that were measured or estimated. Uncertainties and variability among the nuclei of each cell population are associated with these sizes. For a given target, however, a variation of about 15% around the mean volume did not significantly change the spread of the specific energy distributions that we calculated. Accordingly, considering this kind of variability for calculating these spreads was unnecessary because it did not significantly change the results of the calculation.

Table 2. Calculated values for specific energy.

Target volume	Dose[a]	Number of synthetic objects	Mean[a]	Median[a]	Var	SD	SD^{rel}	Fold change SD^{rel}
Calculation for whole nucleus (293.7 μm3)	0.5	8242	0.500	0.501	0.00047	0.022	0.043	0.708
	1	8993	1.000	1.001	0.00095	0.031	0.031	0.707
	2	9010	2.000	2.001	0.00190	0.044	0.022	
Calculation for DNA molecule (8.5 μm3)	0.5	8242	0.501	0.502	0.00867	0.093	0.186	0.709
	1	8993	1.001	1.003	0.01736	0.132	0.132	0.707
	2	9010	2.002	2.004	0.03473	0.186	0.093	
Calculation for a target volume of 1.6 μm3	0.5	8242	0.503	0.504	0.03400	0.184	0.367	0.710
	1	8993	1.002	1.005	0.06814	0.261	0.260	0.708
	2	9010	2.003	2.007	0.13627	0.369	0.184	

[a] gray

doi:10.1371/journal.pone.0145786.t002

Comparison between Distributions obtained for Specific Energy and for RIF

The results obtained experimentally and via specific energy calculation cannot be compared directly as they do not represent the same quantity (RIF per nucleus for the first, and Gy per target for the second). Nonetheless, some comparison can be made with the relative standard deviations for each (Table 1 and 2) as well as with Q-Q plots (Fig 6).

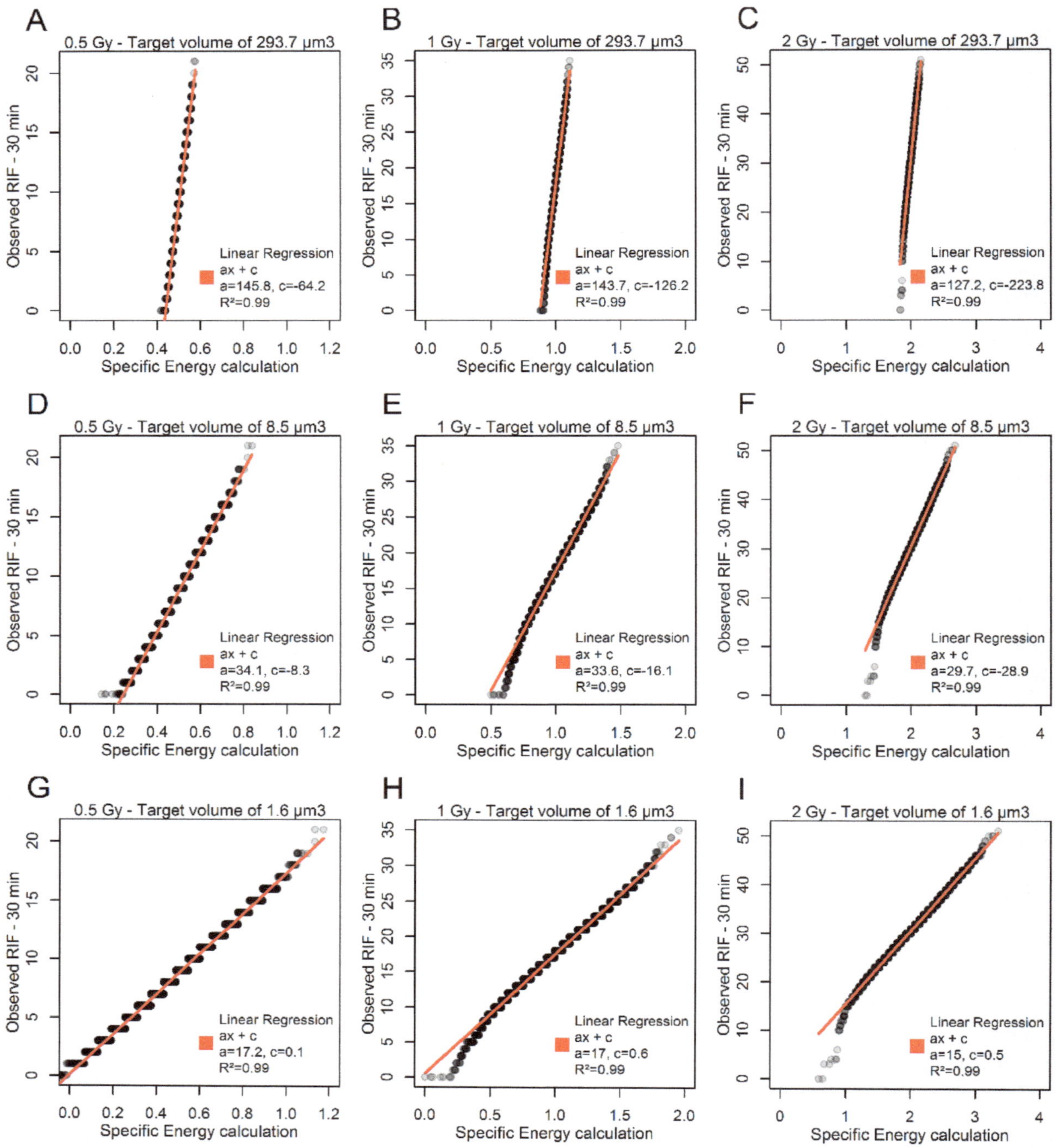

Figure 6. Q-Q plots for comparing probability distributions from experiments and simulations by plotting their quantiles against each other. Linear regression was done with the lm function of the stats package of R software. (A), (B), and (C) correspond to Q–Q plot of observation versus simulation for doses of 0.5, 1 and 2 Gy respectively considering a target volume of 293.7 μm³. (D), (E), and (F) correspond to Q–Q plot of observation versus simulation for the same doses, considering a target volume of 8.5 μm³. (G), (H), and (I) correspond to Q–Q plot of observation versus simulation for the same doses, considering a target volume of 1.6 μm³.

The SD^{rel} were not constant with dose changes for either RIF or specific energy distributions. SD increased with dose while SD^{rel} decreased with dose, and the rates of increase and decrease were approximately the same for the biological and physical measurements. For example, when the mean doubled between the doses 0.5 and 1 Gy, the corresponding fold change for the specific energy calculations and the RIF observation were the same: 1.4 for the SD and 0.7 for the SD^{rel}. This was observed for all irradiation sources tested and all target volumes considered. Nonetheless, the SD^{rel} of the specific energy distribution remained smaller than the SD^{rel} of the observed distribution of the number of RIF per nucleus: the latter was twice as large as the first for a volume corresponding to DNA molecule (8.5 μm³) and around 8 times larger than the first for the whole nucleus (293.7 μm³). Using Eq 3 and for ^{60}Co, we calculated a third target volume that might produce a SD^{rel} for specific energy similar to that observed for RIF. Hence for the SD^{rel} of 0.363, 0.253 and 0.182 (corresponding to 0.5, 1 and 2 Gy respectively) (Table 1), we calculated similar target volumes around 1.6 μm³ (Fig 7).

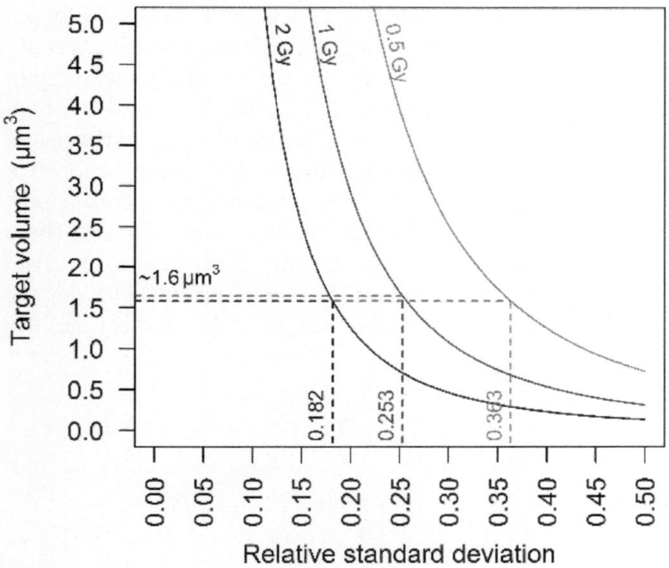

Figure 7. Graphic representation of the relation between the SD^{rel} of the specific energy distribution and the target volume. The relations were plotted with Eq 3, using k_1 and k_2 calculated by [15] for ^{60}Co. The relations for doses of 0.5, 1 and 2 Gy are represented by light grey, grey and dark grey curves respectively. A target volume of around 1.6 µm³ was calculated to explain the totality of the SD^{rel} of the RIF distribution by the spread of energy specific distribution, regardless of the dose considered.

The Q-Q plot method is used for comparing probability distributions from experiments and simulations by plotting their quantiles against each other. These probability plots and the associated linear regression analysis appear to show a good match between the quantiles obtained by calculations and those obtained by observation of RIF. Fig 6G, 6H and 6I show the Q-Q plots obtained for the smallest target volume (1.6 µm³). This volume produces the same SD^{rel} for the RIF and specific energy distributions at each dose tested. Note that, in this case, the slope of the regression line obtained for each dose corresponds to the observed mean number of RIF per gray.

DISCUSSION

This study accurately estimated the distribution of the number of RIF per cell in a large population of primary and "low passage" endothelial cells exposed to ^{60}Co. To be able to interpret the intercellular variability of RIF count per cell and be certain that intercellular variations in the initial DNA content were not the source of this post-exposure RIF variability, we developed an approach that combines the advantages of flow cytometry and microscopy. We demonstrated that this approach can sort a cell population according to the state of the cell cycle, as flow cytometry can. It also allows the accurate analysis of the number of RIF in each cell of a given subpopulation.

Other studies have used flow cytometry to investigate the level of DNA damage in large cell populations [16–19]; this technique can be used to measure the intensity of fluorescently tagged biomolecules within individual cells. By staining cells with propidium iodine or DAPI and a fluorescently labelled antibody conjugated to a DNA damage response phosphoprotein, several authors of flow cytometric studies have been able to determine both the cell cycle phase and the level of specific phospho-proteins in individual cells within a population [19]. This methodology has been successfully used to compare the effect of low LET and high LET radiation (photon vs Iron-Ion Exposure) and enabled the study of how radiation quality and cell cycle stage affect phospho-kinetics [17]. However, flow cytometry measures an absolute intensity of gamma H2AX antibody binding per cell. Although the dose–response relation between mean total gamma H2AX fluorescence levels and mean RIF numbers is similar after low-LET radiation exposures, the distributions of phosphorylation levels are strongly skewed [16,17]. Despite its simplicity and speed, this methodology does not appear sensitive enough to characterize accurately the intercellular RIF variability for a given dose of photon radiation. The methodology used in our study enabled us to estimate the RIF count variance accurately among a large population of cells exposed to ionizing radiation and thus to observe and quantify significant cell-to-cell variability in the number of gamma H2AX RIF. This observation is especially important for photon radiation because it underlies the likely variation in cell response and behaviour. Cell fate is indeed linked to its rate of DNA-induced damage. The analysis of the distribution of RIF per nucleus within the population of cells exposed to 1 Gy of^{60}Co gamma rays shows that 15% of the cell nuclei had from around 25% (the 85th centile of the distribution) to almost 200% (maximum of the distribution) more RIF than the median of the population. On the other hand, for a fraction used in standard radiation therapy (*i.e.*, 2 Gy), the DNA damage rate for around 15% of the cell population is 18% lower than the mean rate. Moreover, the damage rate for around 1% of the cells exposed to 2 Gy is lower than the mean rate observed for 1 Gy. This result should be taken into account in cancer cell treatment, where the survival of a few cells may be the source of relapse. This kind of heterogeneity is well characterized for high-LET radiations, because of the condensed distribution of the energy deposits along the particle track. It has been studied and described much less frequently for such low-LET radiation as photons. Most studies measuring modulations in, for example, gene expression or protein level in response to ionizing radiation must work at the level of whole cell population because minimum amounts of material are required for measurements. When a significant modulation is observed, two contrary explanations are possible: all the cells modulate expression around the measured mean value or only a subpopulation of cells modulates expression to a much higher level than the average value measured. When modulation is dose dependent, these two hypotheses lead to distinct conclusions: modification of the expression level in each cell with the dose, or change as a function of dose in the proportion of the subpopulation which responds. For high LET particles, when the fluency decreases, the probability that key components of a cell will be damaged decreases, so that the second alternative is most likely. In the case of photon radiation, the first alternative is generally preferred. However, our results show clearly that for this kind of exposure all cells do not signal the same amount of damage and that the variation among cells is far from negligible. Given that signalling DNA damage is one of the first steps in cellular response to ionizing radiation insults, our observation may imply a significant variation in each individual cell response, especially if there are threshold effects for some cellular responses. Moreover, this relative cell-to-cell variability increased as the dose decreased, contrary to the mean number of RIF per cell. This result underlines that the dose effect, in terms of the number of DNA lesions indicated by RIF is not as simple as a purely proportional relation in which relative SD is constant with dose.

For these reasons, it is interesting to analyse the different potential origins of the cell-to-cell variability we observed. Several parameters can contribute to the measured standard deviation of the number of RIF per cell within the cell population. Three sources can be identified: measurement errors, biological variability and the stochastic nature of energy deposition.

First, the error related to the measurements and a portion of the biological variability can be estimated from the standard error calculated with the different replications performed for each dose of ^{60}Co radiation (Fig 5B): 0.28 for 0 Gy, 0.67 for 0.5 Gy, 0.86 for 1 Gy and 0.60 for 2 Gy. These measured errors are significantly smaller than the standard deviations measured in the same population of nuclei (3.2, 4.4 and 5.6 for 0.5 Gy, 1 Gy and 2 Gy respectively, as shown in Table 1) and are consistent with the estimated uncertainty for the delivered dose for ^{60}Co irradiation: 6%. At the same time, no correlation seems to exist between the errors measured and the doses studied. These errors would therefore not contribute to the relation observed between doses and standard deviations calculated from the distributions of the number of RIF per cells (Table 1 and Fig 8A, 8B and 8C).

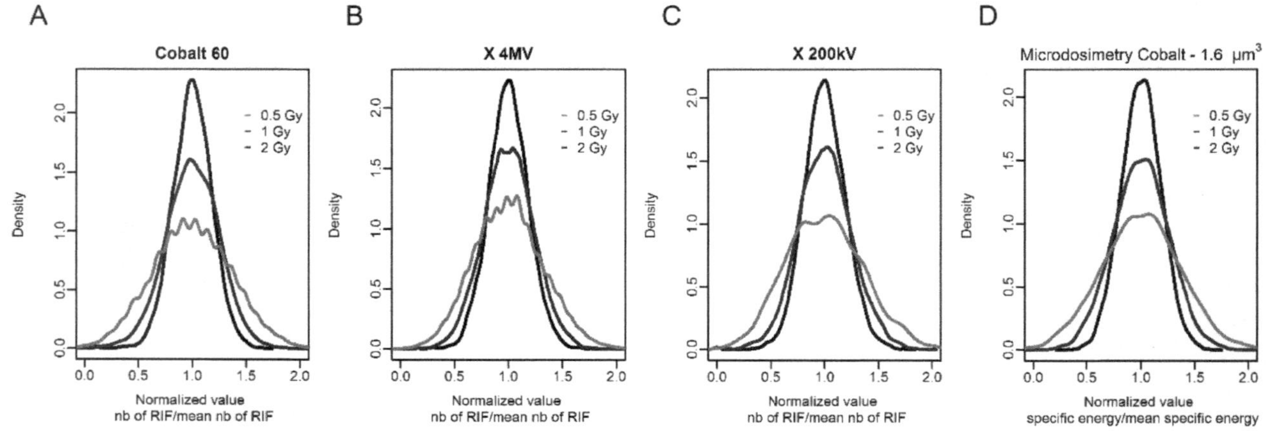

Figure 8. Density plot of normalized RIF count per nucleus and normalized computed specific energy per volume of 1.6 μm³. (A), (B) and (C) Density plot of normalized RIF count per nucleus measured after exposure of cells to macroscopic doses of 0.5 (light grey line), 1 (dark grey line) and 2 Gy (black line) for 3 different sources of radiation: ^{60}Co, 4 MVp X-rays and 200 kVp X-ray, respectively. (D) Density plot corresponding to the distribution of normalized computed specific energy per volume of 1.6 μm³. This was calculated from data generated with Eq 3, an assumption of a normal distribution, and the same number of events as in the ^{60}Co biological experiments. The light grey, dark grey and black lines correspond to macroscopic doses of 0.5, 1 and 2 Gy respectively.

Second, regarding the biological variability, the kinetics of signalling and repairing DNA damage is a critical parameter that may play a role in the dispersion of these RIF per nucleus distributions. As the work of Neumaier et al [20] illustrates, signalling and repair are dynamic processes that have, *a priori*, no reason to be perfectly synchronized from one cell to another, even in a population of cells simultaneously exposed to radiation. Thus, a portion of the cells with a low number of RIF could correspond to cells that have not yet completely signalled all their DNA damage or that have already repaired some of it. In Fig 6, we observe, for example, a deviation from the linear regression specifically for the nuclei with the fewest RIF per nucleus. This curvature corresponds to cells with fewer RIF detected than expected according to the linear relation between specific energy and RIF per nucleus. This deviation may thus illustrate the presence of cells asynchronous in signalling DNA damage.

The third phenomenon potentially involved in the variation observed in the number of RIF per nucleus is the stochastic nature of energy deposition. This number reflects a quantity of damage, generally assessed as DSBs, to the DNA molecule. At the scale of DNA, the initial number and position of DSBs should depend on the energy deposition structure at a micrometric scale—at which the energy deposition for photon radiation is not uniform [21]. For equivalent small volumes at the micrometric scale (target volumes and subvolumes in which RIF can be generated), the spread of the energy deposited by ionizing radiation is due to fluctuations in both the number of tracks passing the target and the energy deposition per track [11–14]. Thus the energy absorbed by a specific target follows a frequency distribution f(z) where z is a stochastic quantity corresponding to ε, the energy imparted per mass m, in the target of volume V. The macroscopic dose D corresponds to the expected value of the distribution f(z). Following F. Villegas et al. [22], we calculated variances, standard deviations and relative standard deviations for 3 target volumes and 3 doses of ^{60}Co and we observed that these values changed with the dose in the same way for the calculations and the observations (Tables 1 and 2, Fig 8). The similarity of this behaviour is an important argument in supporting the hypothesis of the conservation of the link between the two phenomena: number of RIF per nucleus and specific energy absorbed per target volume. More specifically, it appears that when the macroscopic dose doubles, the relative standard deviation is changed by a factor of around $\frac{1}{\sqrt{2}}$, both for RIF and calculated specific energy. This relation is independent of the target volume considered. The same relation was observed for the distribution of the number of RIF per nucleus for the other two radiation qualities tested (4 MVp or 200 kVp X-ray). This relation between mean and relative standard deviation is typical of distributions for which variance is equal to the mean, such as Poisson's distribution. Our data show that this relation was more or less present in all distributions of RIF counts per nucleus (Table 1). It is also accepted that there is a Poisson component in the calculation of the distribution of specific energy in a given volume, associated with the fluctuation of the number of electron tracks passing through the volume [11–14]. Consistent with these observations, we hypothesise that the number of DSBs on a target is associated with the number of electron tracks through the same target.

The volume of the target is interesting to analyse. If we consider the total volume of the endothelial cell nucleus as the target volume (293.7 µm^3), the variation of specific energy absorbed from one nucleus to another explains roughly 10% of the SD^{rel} measured for RIF. In this case, around 90% of the variation in the number of RIF from one nucleus to another could be attributed to measurement error and biological variability, as explained above. This assumption does not appear likely, given that the RIF reflect damage to a specific molecule, DNA, which occupies less than 3% of the volume of the nuclei of the endothelial cells we used. The total nuclear volume thus does not appear to be a relevant target volume. Energy deposition explains around 50% of the RIF count variation between nuclei when we consider the volume of the hydrated DNA molecule—8.5 µm^3 (including hydration shell water). We calculated that a target volume of 1.6 µm^3 would explain the totality of the SD^{rel} of the RIF distribution by the spread of specific energy distribution (Fig 7). This value is consistent with the order of magnitude of the volume occupied by the hydrated sugar-phosphate backbone of the DNA molecule, which is the part of the DNA molecule responsible for strand breaks. Moreover, following up this hypothesis, we observe a linear relation between the number of RIF per nucleus and the specific energy absorbed per sugar-phosphate backbone, regardless of the macroscopic dose (Fig 6G, 6H and 6I). It is important to note that the constants and slopes calculated from these different relations are consistent with the foci background and number of RIF per gray calculated in Fig 5 and measured in Table 1.

Although this hypothesis is not very intuitive, considering that the variance of observed RIF is completely explained by the variance of the specific energy distribution in the volume of the sugar-phosphate backbone of the DNA molecule might be consistent with the existence of indirect effects. This would require that the amount of scavengeable damage, as defined by Ward [23], is a constant percentage over the cell population of the amount of unscavengeable damage (also improperly called direct damage) produced in a given cell. In this case, the value of SD^{rel} of the distribution of the number of RIF per nucleus would be determined by the mean and variance of unscavengeable damage or lesions, which appear to be linked to the mean and variance of specific energy in a volume of 1.6 µm^3. Our laboratory is currently investigating the SD^{rel} of the number of RIF per nucleus in the presence of scavengers of reactive oxygen species.

An alternative hypothesis can also be applied to the result we obtained with our assumption of a target volume of 1.6 µm^3. Recent work by Lorat *et al* [24,25] suggests that that the RIF observed at 30 min after exposure by immunofluorescence detection of 53BP1 or gamma-H2AX could correspond to damage that occurs in a specific region of the chromatin. After using transmission electron microscopy to locate gold-labelled pKu70, 53BP1 and gamma-H2AX, they described different kinetics of resolution of DNA damage and different signalling partners, all varying according to the location of the damage. In sparse DNA regions (defined as euchromatin by the authors), they observed fast signalling kinetics (maximum at 5 min post-irradiation), with pKu70 dimers and neither 53BP1 nor phosphorylation of H2AX. In dense DNA regions (which they defined as heterochromatin), they described slower signalling kinetics (maximum at 30 min post-irradiation), with pKu dimers associated with 53BP1 or phosphorylation of H2AX. Although they did not control for the cell cycle state of the analysed cells, their results may suggest that the distribution of RIF number per nucleus observed in our study corresponds to damage occurring in dense DNA regions. Thus, the target volume of 1.6 µm^3 could reflect the volume of DNA in that specific state in our cells. Additionally, this assumption leads to two non-exclusive consequences. First, if the percentage of condensed DNA is constant in a population of a given cell type, then for a given dose and radiation quality, it should play a role in the variation of the mean and variance of the RIF distributions between two cell types showing a significant difference in that percentage. Second, the variability of the heterochromatin/euchromatin ratio among cells of a given cell type might also contribute to the variance of the RIF distribution. These two points are currently under investigation.

Microdosimetry showed that, for a given macroscopic absorbed dose, variations of microscopic specific energy could be measured in volumes of the order of magnitude of key molecules in the cell, such as the DNA molecule, even for photon irradiation [11–14,21,26]. As far as we know, our study is the first to report a putative biological consequence of this characteristic of energy deposition due to photon exposure at a submicrometric scale. The study of the relation between the fraction of cells with a rate of DNA damage significantly higher than the median of the population and their behaviour appears interesting. The reasons that only a fraction of cells die, for example, at a given macroscopic dose are not well understood. A combination of the variability of the initial biological state of cells and the stochastic production of critical damage has been generally hypothesized to explain the fate of a portion of the exposed cell population. However, in light of our results, it seems particularly interesting to study the contribution of the spatial distribution of energy deposition at the scale of key cell molecules, such as DNA, even for photon exposure. Preliminary Monte Carlo calculations using low energy photons show that the variance of absorbed dose in a population of DNA molecules is greater than that calculated for ^{60}Co irradiation (data not shown). Biological confirmation of the results of these simulations with low energy X-rays should be investigated.

In conclusion, this study demonstrates how biological observations and specific energy calculation can converge to improve understanding of the consequences of irradiation at the scale of a key cell component, such as DNA. The results presented here, based on the convergence of two approaches, could help to improve the evaluation of risk associated with the different types of radiation qualities. Heterogeneity of the response at the cell level might have consequences for the more integrated response of cell populations. We demonstrate that microdosimetric quantities might predict this heterogeneity. These quantities might then be usefully considered in several fields of radiation biology, including studies of non-targeted effects and low dose effects but also for clinical applications, such as improving treatment planning or evaluating or identifying adjuvants that might improve therapeutic effectiveness by increasing the homogeneity of energy deposition at the micrometric scale—the scale of the target molecules.

ACKNOWLEDGMENTS

The authors would like to thank S. Heinrich S. and F. Pouzoulet for performing the radiation exposure with the X-RAD 320 X-ray system and the related dosimetry. The authors would also like to thank M. Baumann, Y. Ristic and L. Van Ryckeghem for performing the radiation exposure with Elekta Synergy Platform and the related dosimetry.

AUTHOR CONTRIBUTIONS

Conceived and designed the experiments: GG CV. Performed the experiments: GG PV. Analyzed the data: GG CV PV JFB IC JFBD MB. Wrote the paper: GG CV JFB. Performed specific energy calculations: CV GG.

REFERENCES

1. Goodhead DT. Initial events in the cellular effects of ionizing radiations: clustered damage in DNA. Int J Radiat Biol. 1994;65: 7–17. Available:http://www. ncbi. nlm. nih. gov/pubmed/7905912 pmid:7905912
2. Olive PL. The role of DNA single- and double-strand breaks in cell killing by ionizing radiation. Radiat Res. 1998;150: S42–51. Available:http://www. ncbi. nlm. nih. gov/pubmed/9806608 pmid:9806608
3. Prise KM, Ahnström G, Belli M, Carlsson J, Frankenberg D, Kiefer J, et al. A review of dsb induction data for varying quality radiations. Int J Radiat Biol. 1998;74: 173–84. Available: http://www. ncbi. nlm. nih. gov/pubmed/9712547 pmid:9712547
4. Rogakou EP, Pilch DR, Orr H, Ivanova VS, Bonner WM. DNA double-stranded breaks induce histone H2AX phosphorylation on serine 139. J Biol Chem. 1998;273: 5858–68. Available: http://www. ncbi. nlm. nih. gov/pubmed/9488723 pmid:9488723
5. Bakkenist CJ, Kastan MB. DNA damage activates ATM through intermolecular autophosphorylation and dimer dissociation. Nature. 2003;421: 499–506. doi: 10. 1038/nature01368. pmid:12556884
6. Maser RS, Monsen KJ, Nelms BE, Petrini JH. hMre11 and hRad50 nuclear foci are induced during the normal cellular response to DNA double-strand breaks. Mol Cell Biol. 1997;17: 6087–96. Available: http://www. pubmedcentral. nih. gov/articlerender. fcgi?artid=232458&tool=pmcentrez&rendertype=abstract pmid:9315668
7. Schultz LB, Chehab NH, Malikzay A, Halazonetis TD. p53 binding protein 1 (53BP1) is an early participant in the cellular response to DNA double-strand breaks. J Cell Biol. 2000;151: 1381–90. Available: http://www. pubmedcentral. nih. gov/articlerender. fcgi?artid=2150674&tool=pmcentrez&rendertype=abstract pmid:11134068
8. Sedelnikova OA, Rogakou EP, Panyutin IG, Bonner WM. Quantitative detection of (125)IdU-induced DNA double-strand breaks with gamma-H2AX antibody. Radiat Res. 2002;158: 486–92. Available: http://www. ncbi. nlm. nih. gov/pubmed/12236816pmid:12236816
9. Rothkamm K, Löbrich M. Evidence for a lack of DNA double-strand break repair in human cells exposed to very low x-ray doses. Proc Natl Acad Sci U S A. 2003;100: 5057–62. doi: 10. 1073/pnas. 0830918100. pmid:12679524
10. Grudzenski S, Raths A, Conrad S, Rübe CE, Löbrich M. Inducible response required for repair of low-dose radiation damage in human fibroblasts. Proc Natl Acad Sci U S A. 2010;107: 14205–10. doi: 10. 1073/pnas. 1002213107. pmid:20660770
11. KellererAM, Chmelevsky D. Concepts of microdosimetry. I. Quantities. Radiat Environ Biophys. 1975;12: 61–9. doi: 10. 1007/BF02339810. pmid:1178822
12. KellererAM, Chmelevsky D. Concepts of microdosimetry II. Probability distributions of the microdosimetric variables. Radiat Environ Biophys. 1975;12: 205–16. doi: 10. 1007/BF01327348. pmid:1202555
13. Chmelevsky D, Kellerer AM. Computation of microdosimetric distributions for small sites. Radiat Environ Biophys. 1977;14: 123–36. doi: 10. 1007/BF01332148. pmid:897064
14. Kellerer AM, Chmelevsky D. Concepts of microdosimetry. III. Mean values of the microdosimetric distributions. Radiat Environ Biophys. 1975;12: 321–35. doi: 10. 1007/BF01323420. pmid:1202563
15. Villegas F, Tilly N, Ahnesjö A. Microdosimetric spread for cell-sized targets exposed to 60co, 192ir and 125i sources. Radiat Prot Dosimetry. 2015; 1–4. doi: 10. 1093/rpd/ncv200.
16. Whalen MK, Gurai SK, Zahed-Kargaran H, Pluth JM. Specific ATM-mediated phosphorylation dependent on radiation quality. Radiat Res. 2008;170: 353–64. doi: 10. 1667/RR1354. 1. pmid:18763865
17. Chappell LJ, Whalen MK, Gurai S, Ponomarev A, Cucinotta F, Pluth JM. Analysis of flow cytometry DNA damage response protein activation kinetics after exposure to x rays and high-energy iron nuclei. Radiat Res. 2010;174: 691–702. doi: 10. 1667/RR2204. 1. pmid:21128792
18. MacPhail SH, Banáth JP, Yu Y, Chu E, Olive PL. Cell cycle-dependent expression of phosphorylated histone H2AX: reduced expression in unirradiated but not X-irradiated G1-phase cells. Radiat Res. 2003;159: 759–67. Available:http://www. ncbi. nlm. nih. gov/pubmed/12751958 pmid:12751958
19. Olive PL. Detection of DNA damage in individual cells by analysis of histone H2AX phosphorylation. Methods Cell Biol. 2004;75: 355–73. Available:http://www. ncbi. nlm. nih. gov/pubmed/15603433 pmid:15603433
20. Neumaier T, Swenson J, Pham C, Polyzos A, Lo AT, Yang P, et al. Evidence for formation of DNA repair centers and dose-response nonlinearity in human cells. Proc Natl Acad Sci U S A. 2012;109: 443–8. doi: 10. 1073/pnas. 1117849108. pmid:22184222
21. Kliauga P, Dvorak R. Microdosimetric measurements of ionization by monoenergetic photons. Radiat Res. 1978;73: 1–20. Available:http://www. ncbi. nlm. nih.

gov/pubmed/622453 pmid:622453

22. Villegas F, Tilly N, Ahnesjö A. Monte Carlo calculated microdosimetric spread for cell nucleus-sized targets exposed to brachytherapy 125I and 192Ir sources and 60Co cell irradiation. Phys Med Biol. 2013;58: 6149–62. doi: 10. 1088/0031-9155/58/17/6149. pmid:23941885

23. Ward JF. Mechanisms of Radiation Action on DNA in Model Systems—Their Relevance to Cellular DNA. In: Fielden EM, O'Neill P, editors. The Early Effects of Radiation on DNA SE—1. Springer Berlin Heidelberg; 1991. pp. 1–16. doi: 10. 1007/978-3-642-75148-6_1.

24. Lorat Y, Brunner CU, Schanz S, Jakob B, Taucher-Scholz G, Rübe CE. Nanoscale analysis of clustered DNA damage after high-LET irradiation by quantitative electron microscopy—The heavy burden to repair. DNA Repair (Amst). Elsevier B. V. ; 2015;1: 1–14. doi: 10. 1016/j. dnarep. 2015. 01. 007.

25. Lorat Y, Schanz S, Schuler N, Wennemuth G, Rübe C, Rübe CE. Beyond repair foci: DNA double-strand break repair in euchromatic and heterochromatic compartments analyzed by transmission electron microscopy. PLoS One. 2012;7: e38165. doi: 10. 1371/journal. pone. 0038165. pmid:22666473

26. Kellerer AM. Electron spectra and the RBE of X rays. Radiat Res. 2002;158: 13–22. Available: http://www. ncbi. nlm. nih. gov/pubmed/12071799 pmid:12071799

CHAPTER 11

ELECTROMAGNETIC THERMOGRAPHY NONDESTRUCTIVE EVALUATION: PHYSICS-BASED MODELING AND PATTERN MINING

Bin Gao, Wai Lok Woo, and Gui Yun Tian

INTRODUCTION

Since 1960s, thermal testing has been successfully explored in NDT&E applications[1,2] to measure the surface temperature variations in response to induced energy. The energy generates a temperature contrast at material discontinuities that can be detected by an infrared (IR) camera. It was the development of the infrared camera in the late 1970s which made it possible to directly detect the temperature contrast over large inspection areas. The IR cameras detect radiation in the IR range of the electromagnetic spectrum and generate images of IR or thermal emission called thermograms, allowing very sensitive non-contact temperature measurement. Thermal testing is also used for defect characterization and material property evaluation and inspection since it is completely noncontact and offers for the rapid inspection over a large area within a short time. It can be used in a wide range of areas[3], such as in agriculture, civil engineering and architecture, diagnosing electrical equipments, automotive industry, medicine and biology, manufacturing industry, food quality control and protection of historic heritage. Thermal testing is generally divided into two main streams: passive infrared thermography (PIT) and active infrared thermography (AIT). Passive Thermography (PIT) is defined as measuring the temperature differences between the target materials and the surroundings under different ambient temperature conditions. AIT[4] was developed to provide more accurate information by considering the amount of thermal radiation and heat transfer. The common thermal stimulation techniques in AIT[5] are: pulsed thermography (e.g., flash thermography), step heating (long pulse), lock-in thermography, and vibrothermography (e.g., ultrasonic IR thermography). Traditional thermal radiation heating is the earliest and the simplest direct technique in AIT. The method employs a lighting source or radiative source to heat the surface of the test object. Flaws or suspicious response can be captured, according to the slow heat transfer, by an infrared (IR) camera inspecting system.

Electromagnetic thermography (EMT)[6,7,8,9,10,11,12,13,14,15] which combines eddy current (EC), magnetic and thermography, and involves the application for a short period of a high current electromagnetic pulse to the conductive material under inspection. In comparison with other thermography NDT&E techniques, the heat in EMT is not limited to the sample surface, rather it can reach a certain depth, which governed by the skin depth of eddy current. Furthermore, EMT focuses the heat on the defect due to friction or eddy current distortion, and subsequently increase the temperature contrast between the defective region and defect-free areas. From point of view of inspection depth, flash thermography is adaptable by changing the lock-in frequency for defects at different depths. From adaptability in terms of defect orientation, EMT can enhance specific excitation direction to optimize the directional evaluation along the defect orientation which is more effective for geometrically complex components and showed more crack indication. Furthermore, EMT allows area imaging of defects without scanning and enables the detection of both magnetic and non-magnetic metals with rich frequency

Citation: Bin Gao, Wai Lok Woo, and Gui Yun Tian. Electromagnetic Thermography Nondestructive Evaluation: Physics-based Modeling and Pattern Mining, DOI: 10.1038/srep25480 (2016).

components fabricated from excitation power. In addition, for optic-excited thermography, the disadvantage also includes the duration until the heat response of the crack reaches the surface is twice longer than with EMT testing. Since the test part is passing through the testing plant and the thermal wave just has a very short time to go through the material, this is not a practical testing method. EMT can only work with conductive material and it has already been applied in small defects detection for compressor blades[16], impact damage and delamination detection of composite[17,18], probability of detection (POD) estimation[10] of fatigue cracks and multiple cracks detection.

All above works require signal processing tools to enable defects or materials characterization analysis. Running temperature contrast method[19] uses the source temperature image which is replaced with the image of the defective thermal image divided by the non-defective thermal image where the process is independent of heating power. However, this method requires manually selection and it may enhance random noise as well. Differentiated contrast method[20] assumes that at earlier times, any sample behaves as a semi-infinite body where no human selection is necessary. It is only applicable for shallow defects and works for a sample that can be considered as a semi-infinite body. Deviation from these conditions rendered the method ineffective. Polynomial fitting method[21] attempts to fit noisy temperature signals with polynomial functions. IR image sequence of arbitrary length can be replaced with images of a few polynomial coefficients; however, the images of polynomial coefficients lose the physics of heat conduction. Neural networks[22] are proposed as universal technique that takes into consideration subtle variations in signal evolution. Each class of test objects requires special training of the network. In thermal testing, several thermal transient response features have been used as an indicator of defect status, which is critical for acceptance/rejection decisions for maintenance and lifetime prediction[23]. To enhance the flaw contrast and improve noise rejection qualities, pattern based image enhancement has been conducted by introducing the raw data upon a set of orthogonal basis functions. Fourier transform has been applied to pulsed thermography, and enhanced the flaw-contrast significantly using phase map[24] and image normalization[25]. Influence of non-uniform heating and surface emissivity variation was removed by using a Fourier transformation based image reconstruction algorithm[26]. Instead of a prescribed set of basis functions, empirical orthogonal functions were also employed to maximize the anomalous patterns of transient response. The efficiency of principal component analysis (PCA) and independent component analysis (ICA) has been compared on thermography features extraction by considering the initial sequence as either a set of images or a set of temporal profiles[27]. In reviewing the current defect detection methods for IT, two main challenges have been identified. Firstly, the lack of capability in automatically detecting and identifying the defects, and secondly, the need to enhance the detectability and resolution of different types of defects which is the key point to achieve Quantitative NDT&E. However, most recent methods are limited on manually selecting the proper contrast components and pattern extraction based methods are only employed as a signal processing tool. The mathematical justification as to why these algorithms can enhance an image and how these techniques are linked to physics models are not provided. The results are acceptable but generally not predictable. The proper contrast components have to be empirically selected. This ambiguous case prevents the use of thermal testing based NDT&E in automated environments.

From the physics viewpoint, in particular the NDT&E, physics-mathematical pattern modeling and mining (PPMM) has already started to push for a new frontier and led up to a new horizon of performance achievement that cannot be achieved using conventional methods. PPMM has given birth to a new statistical signal processing tools. In this review, we will concentrate on the thermal PPMM methods have enabled spatial-, time-, frequency-, and sparse-patterns to be extracted according to the whole transient response behavior without resorting to any fixed library patterns. In such study, the physics principles and the signal processing models must be linked up, and understood prior to applying PPMM methods. The proposed method directly benefits the industry not only in terms of automatic defect detection but also enhances the detectability and resolution of the defects especially for such challenge tasks of detecting natural complex geometric cracks as well as micro defects. However, the advantages gained by the proposed methods will be augmented by the increase of computational power and higher data storage requirements of the processors. In our implementation, a high specification computer with a PC with of Core i7 32 GB RAM is required to implement all the proposed algorithms.

METHOD

Electromagnetic Thermal Conduction

When an electromagnetic (EM) field is applied to a conductive material, the temperature increases owing to resistive heating from the induced electric current which is known as Joule heating. Joule heating is the coupling of the electromagnetic and thermal fields. According to Joule's Law:

$$Q^H = I^2 R t \tag{1}$$

where Q^H is the sum of the generated heat, I represents electric current, R is electrical resistance, and t is time. According to the definition of electrical resistance:

$$R = \frac{L}{\sigma S} \text{ where } \sigma = \frac{\sigma_0}{1 + \alpha(T - T_0)} \tag{2}$$

where L is the length of the conductor, S is the cross-sectional area of conductor, σ is the electrical conductivity which dependent on temperature T and σ_0 is the conductivity at the reference temperatureT_0 and α is the temperature coefficient of resistivity, which describes how resistivity varies with temperature. Since the relationship between the current and the induced current density $\vec{J_s}$ is:

$$I = \vec{J_s} \times S \tag{3}$$

The Eqs (2) and (3) are substituted into Eq. (1) to obtain Eq. (4):

$$Q^H = (\vec{J_s} \times S)^2 \times \frac{L}{\sigma S} \times t = \frac{1}{\sigma}(\vec{J_s})^2 \times V \times t \quad \text{where } V = L \times S \tag{4}$$

Consider the unit volume per unit time, thus Eq. (4) can be reduced to $Q^H = \frac{1}{\sigma}(\vec{J_s})^2$. Following the energy conservation and Fourier heat conduction, the inductive heat conduction equation can be expressed as:

$$\frac{\partial T}{\partial t} = \frac{k}{\rho C_p}\left(\frac{\partial^2 T}{\partial x^2} + \frac{\partial^2 T}{\partial y^2} + \frac{\partial^2 T}{\partial z^2}\right) + \frac{1}{\rho C_p} Q^H(x, y, z, t) \tag{5}$$

where T=T(x, y, z, t) is the temperature distribution, k is the thermal conductivity of the material (W/m K), which is dependent on temperature, ρ is the density (kg/m^3), C_p is specific heat (J/kg K), and$Q^H(x, y, z, t)$ is the internal heat generation function per unit volume, which is the result of the eddy current excitation. The variation of temporal temperature depends on the spatial temperature variation for heat conduction. According to Eq. (5), heat conduction is influenced byT(x, y, z, t), ξ, υ, σ, μ, and l. Here ξ denotes the sensor geometry factor; υdenotes the parameter of the excitation (frequency, amplitude, etc.) andl denotes the lift-off (distance between the sensor and sample). From the above analysis, it becomes clear that the variation of temperature spatially and its transient response recorded from the IR camera directly reveals the intrinsic properties variation of the conductive material. In addition, variation of surface emissivity introduces spurious temperature inhomogeneity, according to Stefan-Boltzmann law[28] the energy emitted by a black body per second per unit of area is proportional to the fourth power of its absolute temperature. This can be described as

$$j^* = \varepsilon \sigma_{sb} T^4 \tag{6}$$

where σ_{sb}=5.67×10−8W/(m2·k4) is the Stefan-Boltzmann constant andT is the absolute temperature. This difference can be described by the emissivity $0 \leq \varepsilon \leq 1$ which denotes the ratio of radiation of actual object with respect to the black body. When the temperature of the material changes slightly, the radiation power will cause a large change. The radiance of the actual object depends on the properties of the material and the surface preparation besides the temperature.

Interpretation of Electromagnetic Thermal Patterns

Figure 1 shows the diagram of Electromagnetic Thermography NDT&E system. The excitation signal generated by the excitation module is a short period of high frequency current. It is driven to the coil on the conductive material. The current in the coil will subsequently induce eddy currents and generate the resistive heat in the conductive material. The heat will diffuse in time until it reaches an equilibrium state in the material. If a defect (e.g., crack) is present in the conductive material, eddy current distribution or the heat diffusion process will vary (as be interpreted in Fig. 1 bottom panel). Consequently, the spatial distribution of temperature on the surface of the material and the temperature transient response will show the variation. This is captured by an infrared camera as it records both the spatial and the transient response of temperature variation on the specimen. Mathematically, this can be represented as a spatial-transient tensor $\overline{Y}$ which has dimensions $\underbrace{N_x \times N_y}_{spatial} \times \underbrace{N}_{Transient}$.

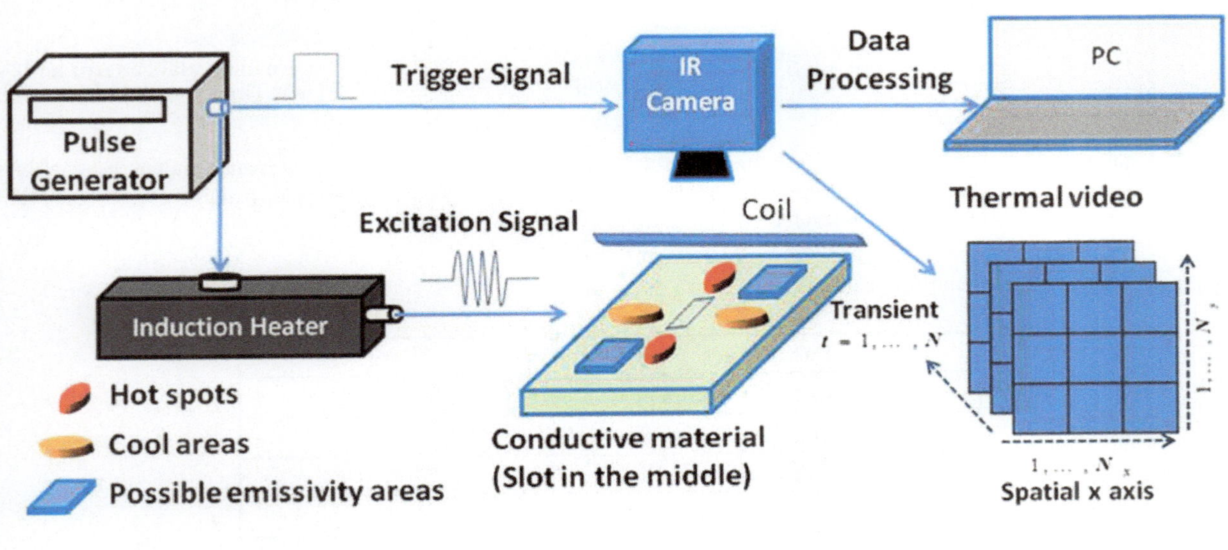

Figure 1: Electromagnetic thermal patterns. Electromagnetic Thermography and interpretation of thermal patterns.

To interpret the thermal patterns, a sample with penetrated slot is used as example for one type of fundamental defect. Specifically, when eddy current encounters a discontinuity, e.g., a slot or notch, they are forced to divert, leading to areas of increased and decreased eddy current density. Therefore, in the heating phase, different areas have different heat generation rates which subsequently lead to temperature spatial variation. Hot spots are observed around the slot tips while the cool areas are located at both sides of the slot. In the cooling phase, heat diffuses from high temperature area to low temperature area, and reduces the contrast, the illustration can be seen in Fig. 2a. Figure 2bshows the numerical simulations for fusion of Eddy current and temperature distribution which performed using COMSOL Multi-physics simulation software via the electro-thermal module which combines the application mode for induction currents and general heat transfer. The heat transfer process and the magnetic field propagation were solved simultaneously by this module for an accurate description of the heating mechanism around a particular defect. The slot defect for the simulation are modeled in a steel block measuring 110 × 76 × 6.4 mm. The electrical and thermal parameters for the steel used in these simulations are shown in Table 1. A square coil with an outer diameter of 100 mm and inner diameter of 87.3 mm was used in the simulation. The coil is positioned perpendicular to the sample and at 90° to the defect. The current input for the coil was set at 350ARMS with an excitation frequency of 256 kHz.

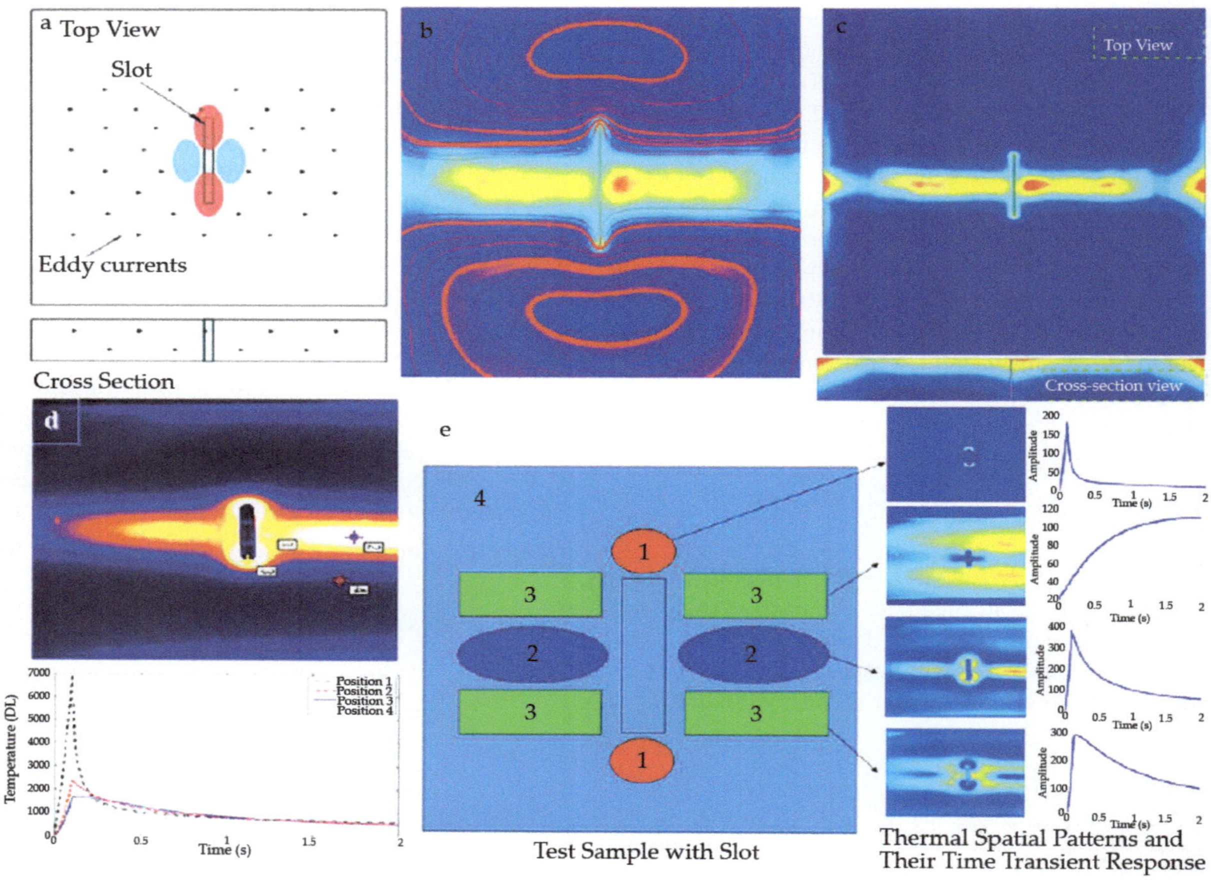

Figure 2: Illustration of Thermal- Electromagnetic patterns. (a) Schematic of theoretical EC distribution and resultant heating for slot. (b) Simulation of fused EC and heat distribution. (c) Simulation of heat. (d) Real test sample and its thermal spatial-transient signal. (e) Spatial-Transient pattern interpretation and separation results.

Table 1: Electrical and thermal parameters setting.

Parameters	Steel
Conductivity, σ (S/m)	4.0319×10^6
Relative permeability, μ	100
Temperature coefficient (K^{-1})	12.3×10^{-6}
Density, d (kg/m^3)	7850
Heat capacity, Cp (J/kg K)	475
Thermal conductivity, k (W/m K)	44.5

Figure 2b illustrates the simulation results for the slot after 200 ms of heating. The eddy current (EC) flow and thermal distribution for the defect is visualized by the streamline plot in Fig. 2b,c. In the presence of a defect, EC will divert to complete their closed loop path which leaves a unique EC distribution based on the defect geometry that can provide useful multi-physics information to identify a defect. It illustrates the situation where EC cannot flow underneath the defect, hence are forced to flow around the end of the defect, leading to regions of high EC density and resulting in hot areas at the tips of the defect. The regions at either side of the defect are characterized with EC forced to spread out resulting in comparable cooler areas. The real test sample and its thermal spatial image after heating 0.1s and four positions of thermal transient curves are shown in Fig. 2d as well.

The streamline plots illustrate the defects with the geometry and orientation, but different positions on the sample under inspection can interact with the induced EC in different ways and cause characteristic heat spatial-transient distributions. The defect region is influenced by hybrid two physics of electromagnetic and thermal conduction and these mainly refer to factors of thermal conductivity k and generated heat due to eddy current density $Q^H(x, y, z, t)$. Thus, the thermal-transient pattern separation results (detailed description to be presented in next section) for slot tips (region 1 as shown in Fig. 2e) are seen with high induced current density and the temperature distribution according to Eq. (5) can be simply referred as $T^{tip}(x,y,z,t) - T^{tip}(k^{tip}, Q^H_{tip})$, where k^{tip} is the thermal conductivity influenced by temperature of the defect (W/m K) and Q^H_{tip} is the generated heat influenced by current density at slot tips. This happens as a result of high temperature rising rate generated in the heating phase. Fourier's law of heat conduction states that the time rate of heat transfer through a material is proportional to the negative gradient in the temperature and to the cross section area of the material. Due to the singular areas around the slot tips, a high temperature gradient is generated at the end of heating phase. Therefore, a high falling rate is observed at the early stage of the cooling phase (transient curve of region 1 as shown in Fig. 2e). The cool area (region 2 as shown in Fig. 2e) with comparable lower induced current density, the temperature distribution can be referred as $T^c(x,y,z,t) - T^c(k^c, Q^H_c)$ where k^c is the thermal conductivity influenced by temperature of defect (W/m K) and Q^H_c is the generated heat influenced by current density at side of slot. Compared to the area around crack tips, the area underneath the coil has a continual material distribution; compare to the area located at the side of the slots, the area underneath the coil has a higher eddy current density. Consequently, a moderate rising and cooling rate of transient in the heating phase and cooling phase are generated (transient curve of region 2 as shown in Fig. 2e). For non-directly heating region (region 4 as shown in Fig. 2e) with rare induced current density, the temperature distribution can be approximately considered as $T^{NH}(x, y, z, t) - T^{NH}(k^{NH})$ where k^{NH} is the thermal conductivity influenced by temperature of material after induced heating procedure. As a result, the temperature rising rate in the heating phase is lower than the area underneath the coil, the slowest falling rate appears at region 4 while the temperature continuously rises at the beginning of the cooling phase (transient curve of region 4 as shown in Fig. 2e). For others, such as region 3 as shown in Fig. 2e, while high eddy current density appears around the slot tips, they are forced to spread out and result in lower density at either side of the slot. As a result, the temperature rising rate in the heating phase is lower than the area underneath the coil in which the slowest falling rate appears at region 3 while the temperature continually rises at the beginning of the cooling phase (transient curve of region 3 as shown in Fig. 2e). Therefore, the spatial-transient thermal distribution of tested sample T can be approximated as

$$T = T^{tip}(k^{tip}, Q^H_{tip}) + T^c(k^c, Q^H_c) + T^{NH}(k^{NH}) + \sum_{i=1}^{N_o} T^i(k^i, Q^H_i) \quad (7)$$

where $\sum_{i=1}^{N_0} T^i(k^i, q^H_i)$ denotes other possible characteristic thermal spatial-transient pattern region and N_o denotes the number. For example, the samples under test possibly have oil, oxide and other stains on the surface. Oil and oxide can drastically increase the thermal radiation, and results in their own characteristic spurious high temperature in the infrared images. Thus, all these characteristic thermal-transient regions can be considered as the pattern regions since each of them share similar transient responses in the sample. The infrared camera functions as an image capturing device which records the mixture contributed by each thermal pattern. To avoid the influences of arbitrary selection of image frame from the transient thermal videos, extraction of abnormal patterns has become ever more crucial. Therefore, the task of the proposed method is to separate the IR camera recorded image sequence into thermal pattern images as well as to automatically identify the one pattern image that relates directly to the defect. Specifically, $\mathbf{X}_i(t)$, where $t=0, \ldots, N$ are defined as thermal-transient patterns which have specific thermal region and characteristics in both spatial, transient and frequency domain. As an example, consider slot tips (region 1 as shown in Fig. 2e) with high induced current density, the temperature distribution according to Eq. (5) can be simply referred as $T^{tip}(x,y,z,t) - T^{tip}(k^{tip}, Q^H_{tip})$. The Fourier's law of heat conduction states that the rate of heat transfer through a material is proportional to the negative gradient in the temperature and to the cross section area of the material. For a uniform thickness plate used in this study, the cross section area is constant. Due to the singular areas around the slot tips, a high temperature gradient is generated at the end of heating phase. Therefore, a high falling rate is observed at the early stage of the cooling phase (transient curve of region 1 as shown in Fig. 2e). The thermal camera captures both the spatial and the transient response of temperature variation on the specimen which consist of thermal patterns $\mathbf{X}_1(t)$, where t=0, ..., N that corresponds to $T^{tip}\left(k^{tip}, Q_{tip}^{H}\right)$. Similarly, Fig. 2e region 2 represents a cool area $\mathbf{X}_2(t)$ with moderate rising and falling rate; region 3 represents a non-defect region $\mathbf{X}_3(t)$ with high rising rate followed by a continually low speed rising and then drop down; and region 4 represents a non-excitation area $\mathbf{X}_4(t)$ with continually temperature increasing. Mathematically, the thermography image captured by the infrared camera is considered as a mixing observation image $\mathbf{Y}(t)$. The term m_i is the mixing parameter which describes the contribution of the i^{th}position to the induced recorded thermography image in Fig. 1. In real applications, the number N_s is not necessary limited to 4 where $N_s$denotes the number of thermal patterns.

Physics-based Modeling and Mining of Thermal Patterns in Spatial-Time, Frequency and Sparse domain

As there is only one infrared camera, this leads to the single channel signal separation problem. The mathematical model[29] can be described as:

$$\mathbf{Y}(t) = \sum_{i=1}^{N_s} m_i \mathbf{X}_i(t) \tag{8}$$

The visual representation of Eq. (8) is shown in Fig. 3.

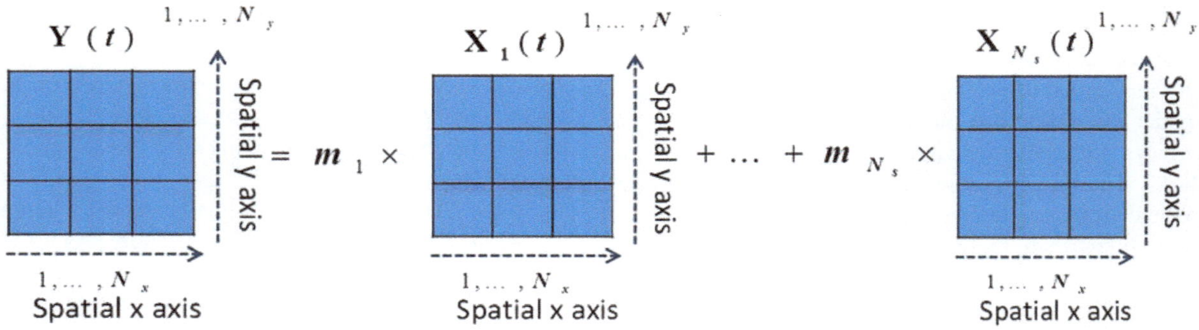

Figure 3: Mixing modeling. Mathematical representation of mixing process of ECPT.

In Fig. 3, $\mathbf{Y}(t)$ and $\mathbf{X}_i(t)$ denote the recorded image and the independent image generated by the area of position i at time t with dimensional $N_x \times N_y$, respectively. The task is automatically estimate $\mathbf{X}_i(t)$ given only$\mathbf{Y}(t)$. To solve the above ill-posed problem, we adopt a decomposition-based approach The approach is used for analyzing non-stationary signals[30] by expressing a fixed-length segment drawn from transient response, such that continuous transient slices of length N can be chopped out of a set of image sequences from t to t+N−1, and the subsequent segment is denoted as equivalent as image sequences captured by N observations $\mathbf{Y}'=[\text{vec}(\mathbf{Y}(t)), \text{vec}(\mathbf{Y}(t+1)), \ldots, \text{vec}(\mathbf{Y}(t+N-1))]^T$ where 'T' denotes transpose operator and 'vec' denotes the vectorize operator. The constructed image sequences is then expressed as a linear combination of different thermal patterns such that

$$\mathbf{Y}' = M\mathbf{X}' \tag{9}$$

where $M = \left[m_1, \ldots, m N_s\right]$ is the mixing matrix, $\mathbf{m}_i$ is the ith mixing vector and $X' = \left[vec\left(X_1(t)\right), vec\left(X_2(t)\right) \ldots, vec\left(X_N(t)\right)\right]^T$. Assuming that$N_s$=N and **M** has full rank so that the transforms between $\mathbf{Y}'$ and $\mathbf{X}'$ be reversible in both directions such that we can find the inverse matrix $\mathbf{W}=\mathbf{M}^{-1}$ which refers to the BSS method. The purpose of this decomposition is to model the multivariate distribution of $\mathbf{Y}'$ in a statistically efficient manner.

The phase information of thermography has been proved to offer deeper thickness of probing under the surface, less sensitivity to optical and infrared specimen surface features, better defect shape resolution, non-necessity to know a priori position of a non-defect area in the field of view to compute contrast image, ability to inspect high thermal conductivity specimens. In particular, the magnitude thermal image is proportional to local optical and infrared surface features. Of significant interest then is the phase image which being related to the propagation time delay, is independent of optical or surface features. Besides the spatial-time thermal pattern modeling, the spatial-frequency thermal pattern modeling is also investigated by computing the Discrete Fourier Transform (DFT) for each transient response:

$$\overline{\mathbf{Y}}_{xy}(f) = \Delta t \sum_{n=0}^{N-1} \overline{\mathbf{Y}}_{xy}(n\Delta t) e^{-i2\pi fn\Delta t} = R_{xy}(f) + iI_{xy}(f) \tag{10}$$

where, Δt is the sampling time step, R(f) and I(f) are the real and imaginary components of $\overline{Y}_{xy}(f)$, respectively. The subscript x, y are the coordinate index of spatial x and spatial y, respectively. This gives complex-valued tensor $\overline{Yf}$ as shown in Fig. 4.

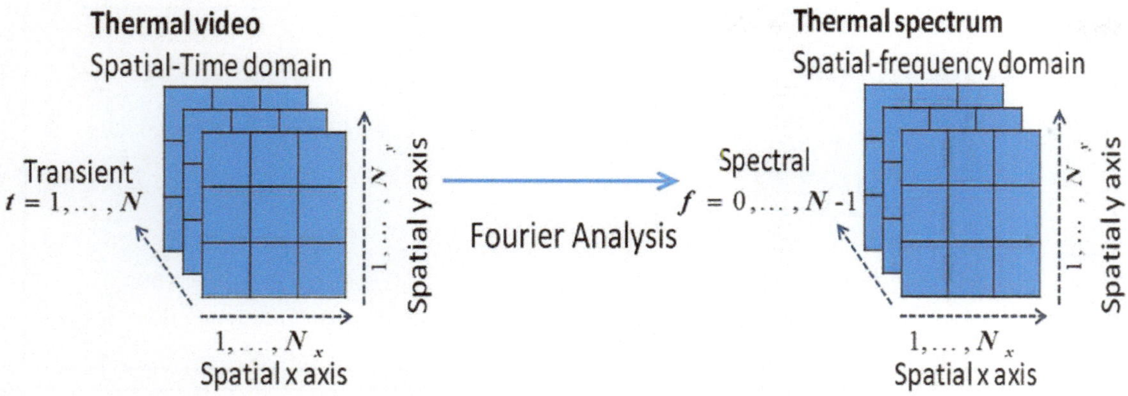

Figure 4: Time frequency transform. (a) Thermal spatial-transient domain and (b) Thermal spatial-frequency domain.

The spatial-phase spectrum from the pulse phase thermography system can be calculated as $\Phi_{xy}(f) = \tan^{-1}\left(R_{xy}(f)/I_{xy}(f)\right)$ across the x- and y-axes. The observed spatial-phase spectrum is a sum of contribution from thermal events given by $\Phi_{xy}(f) = \sum_{i=1}^{N_s} m_i X_i(f)$ Similar to time domain analysis, thermography spatial-phase image $\mathbf{\Phi}_{xy}$ is a 3-D tensor representation when taking in all (x, y, f) elements. Nonetheless, we can form a 2-D matrix format of the spatial-phase spectrum as $\Phi' = \left[vec(\Phi_{xy}(0)),\ vec(\Phi_{xy}(1))...,\ vec(\Phi_{xy}(N-1))\right]^T$. The aim of pattern separation is to factorize the spatial-phase matrix $\mathbf{\Phi}'$ into a product of two matrices as

$$\mathbf{\Phi}' = \mathbf{M}^f \mathbf{X}^f \tag{11}$$

Not with standing above, the sparse factors enforce the solution to consider only the significant region where the defect may lie within the surrounding background. This is shown in Fig. 1. For data with sparse outliers or partially contaminated by noise of overwhelming magnitude, sheer low-rank assumption cannot fully capture its complex structure. Therefore, (9) and (11) can be considered as a model of combination of sparse pattern (e.g. hot spots) and non-sparse patterns

$$\mathbf{Y}' = \underbrace{[M\mathbf{X}']_{i=1,\ldots,N_s, i\neq j}}_{\mathbf{L}} + \underbrace{\mathbf{M}_j\mathbf{X}'_j}_{\mathbf{S}} + \mathbf{G} \tag{12}$$

In reality, they play an important role in enhancing the defect detectability of IT system. A general assumption of Eq. (12) can be denoted as $\mathbf{Y}'=\mathbf{L}+\mathbf{S}+\mathbf{G}$, i.e., the pattern matrix $\mathbf{Y}'$ can be decomposed as the sum of a low-rank matrix **L** (e.g. for position 2, 3 and 4 reflected patterns in Fig. 1), a sparse pattern **S** (e.g. hot spots) which contains the spiky anomalies that are rarely shared by different instances, and **G** which is the noise term. When the algorithm optimizes the sparse patterns **S**, it finds the joint sparse estimation of $\mathbf{M}_j$ and $\mathbf{X}'_j$ (not just $\mathbf{X}'_j$). The sparse estimation of $\mathbf{X}'_j$ is required to obtain the correct shape of the pattern while the sparse estimation of $\mathbf{M}_j$ is to enable the user to determine the exact time when the target pattern takes place. In addition, the constraint of sparse factor f(**S**) can be selected optionally to satisfy different applications, where this could be selected as L_1-norm (e.g. $f(S) = \lambda\|S\|_1$ λ is sparse control parameter), L_2-norm, Gaussian priors, Bernoulli sparse prior and so on. Similar to time domain analysis, thermography spatial-phase model can also be emphasized with sparse domain.

Thermal Pattern Mining

To avoid the influences of arbitrary selection of image frame from the transient thermal videos, the task of the pattern mining is to blind separate the observed $\mathbf{Y}'$ and $\mathbf{\Phi}'$ into different characteristic patterns $\mathbf{X}'$, $\mathbf{X}^f$ and automatically identify the one which relates to defect. There exists several criteria for mining purpose such as principal component analysis which emphasize the decorrelation of separated patterns or independent component analysis where the separated patterns are said to be statistically independent[31]. The part-based patterns separation can be achieved by using nonnegative matrix factorization[32] as well as sparse factorization[33]. The brief steps of pattern mining procedure have been summarized in Fig. 5.

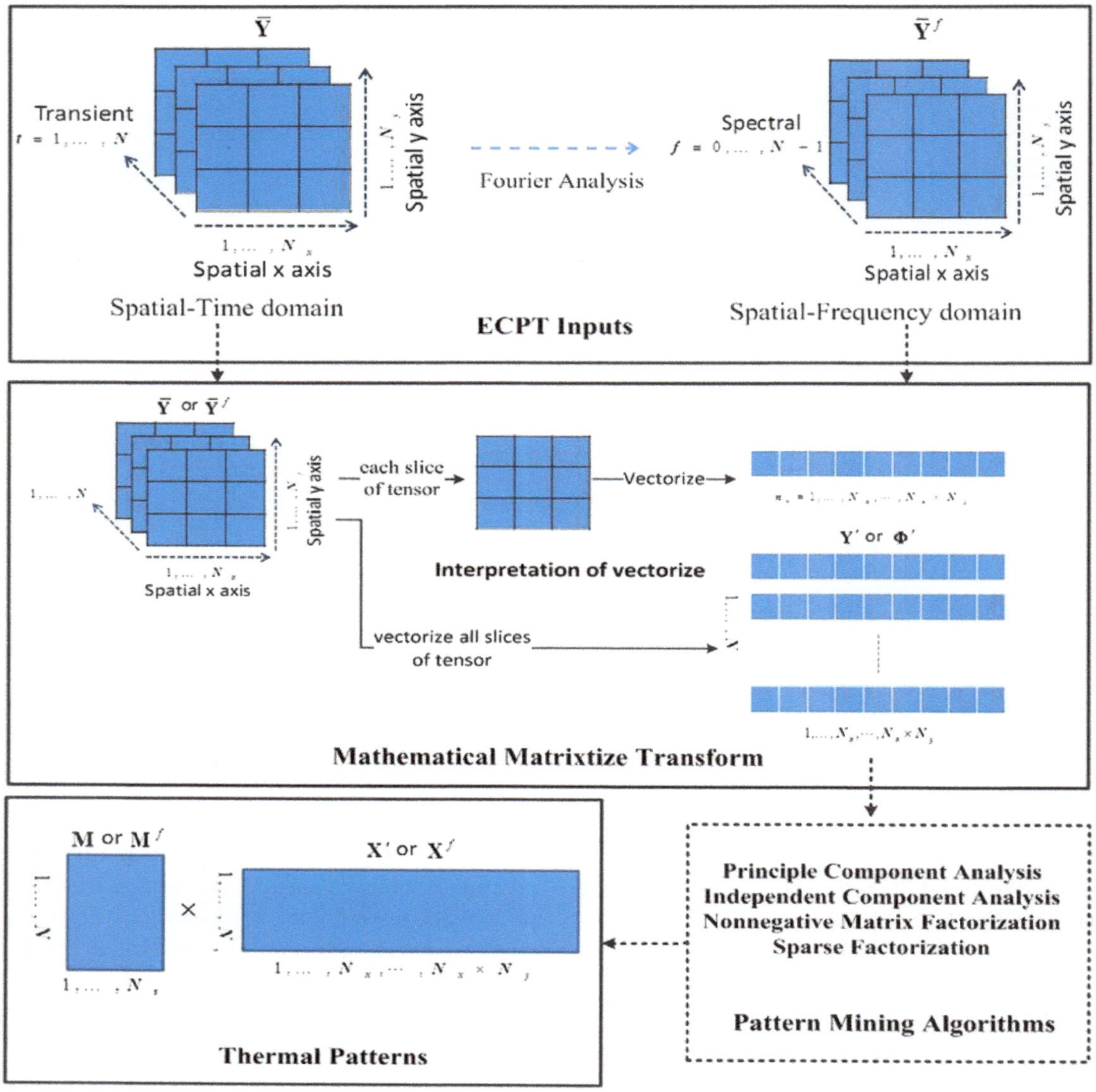

Figure 5: Procedure for thermal pattern mining. Schematic illustration of the spatial, time, frequency and sparse thermal pattern mining.

RESULTS

The experimental setup is shown in Fig. 6a. An Easyheat 224 from Cheltenham Induction Heating is used for coil excitation. The Easyheat has a maximum excitation power of 2.4 kW, a maximum current of 400 A_{rms} and an excitation frequency range of 150–400 kHz (380 A_{rms} and 256 kHz are used in this study). The system has a quoted rise time (from the start of the heating period to full power) of 5ms, which was verified experimentally. Water cooling of coil is implemented to counteract direct heating of the coil. The IR camera, SC7500 is a Stirling cooled camera with a 320 × 256 array of 1.5–5 μm InSb detectors. This camera has a sensitivity of <20 mK and a maximum full frame rate of 383 Hz, with the option to increase frame rate with windowing of the image. In this study, 2s videos are recorded in the experiments. A rectangular coil is constructed to apply directional excitation. This coil is made of 6.35 mm high conductivity hollow copper tube. A steel sample (0.24 × 45 × 100 mm³) with a slot of 10 mm length, 2mm width was prepared, as shown in Fig. 6a. Thermal conductivity of the stainless steel is 14 $Wm^{-1}K^{-1}$. There are equally spaced shinning and black stripes with 5 mm width on the sample surface. The bare strips are polished areas and the black strips were created by spraying the area with black paint to illustrate different emissivity (The emissivity of the black region is 1, which is the same for a blackbody. While, the emissivity of the shinning stainless steel surface is about 0.16). Therefore, the recording in thermal camera is the result of mixture of several complex thermal patterns (such as hot spots, cool area, emissivity area, non excitation area). This brings challenge task of the pattern mining methods. Thus, the validation of different automatic pattern mining methods is necessary. Of significant interest is the ability to accurately and automatically extract patterns that are directly related to defects. In the experiments, coil and IR camera were placed on the opposite side, presenting transmission mode. The coil was perpendicular to the slot and across the slot centre. Only one edge of the rectangular coil was used to stimulate eddy current in the sample, as shown in Fig. 6b.

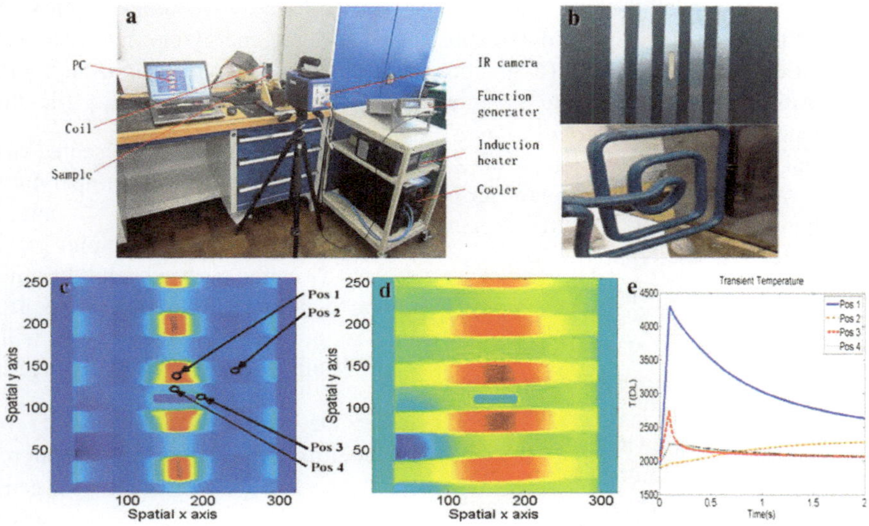

Figure 6: Experiment set up. (a) ECPT platform (b) Test sample (c) Original recorded infrared image at 0.1s (the end of heating phase) (d) Original recorded infrared image at 1.6s (the cooling phase) (e) Transient responses of different positions.

Figure 6c shows the temperature distribution at the end of heating (0.1s). Due to the high emissivity of the black area, there is no obvious high temperature region around the slot tips. The high temperature can only be observed at the black area above the coil. In addition, Fig. 6dshows the temperature distribution at the cooling phase (1.6s). The high temperature still can only be observed at the black strip area because of both high emissivity and heat diffusion. The transient temperature behavior at different positions is shown in Fig. 4e. Pos 1 is at the crack side with black strip (high emissivity), Pos 2 is at the black strip where the area is far away from the excitation, Pos 3 is at the crack tip with the shinning strip, Pos 4 is at the crack side with shinning strip above the coil. As can be seen in Fig. 4e, different position behaves with different temperature transient characteristics. However, Pos 1 as well as other similar black strip area (above the coil) exhibits extreme high temperature transient in both heating and cooling phases in which other thermal patterns have been over-shadowed and therefore, they cannot be distinguished. Both transient and frequency domain are difficult to tackle in defect detection using the inductive thermography method where the hot spot around defect tips cannot be taken as an indicator of defects especially for small cracks. Notwithstanding this, it will lead to error when both black stain and cracks are present on the surface of the test sample. In order to solve this issue, the thermal pattern separation method is conducted. The thermal pattern separation methods are tested on recorded Thermal image sequences as described in Fig. 7. All methods are conducted using a PC with Intel Core i7 8GB RAM and the program platform is based on MATLAB. The experiments consist of three case studies: thermal-transient domain pattern mining, thermal-frequency domain pattern mining and thermal-sparse domain pattern mining.

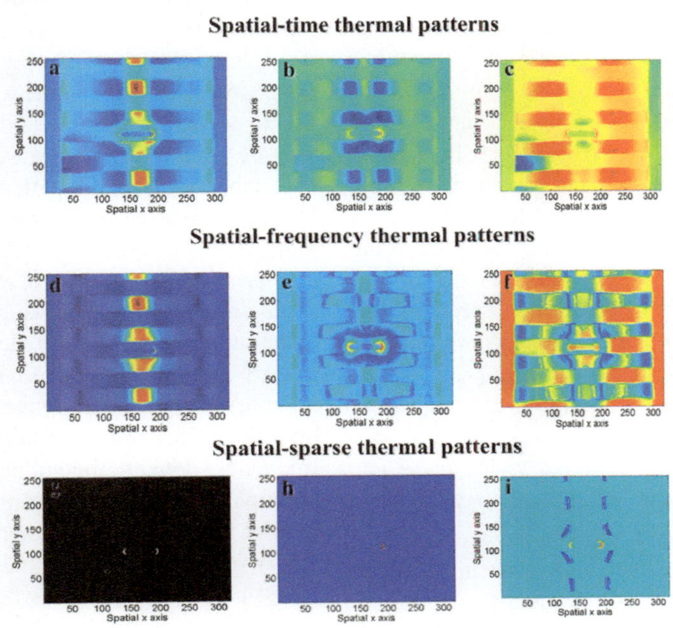

Figure 7: Thermal patterns. Mining thermal patterns using spatial-time domain pattern separation (a–c), spatial-frequency domain pattern separation (d–g) artificially annotation results of defect edgy, (h) sparse thermal pattern mining in spatial-time domain, (i) sparse thermal pattern mining in spatial-frequency domain.

Case (i): In order to validate the efficiency of spatial-time domain pattern mining methods, Principal Component Analysis (PCA), Independent Component Analysis (ICA) and Nonnegative Matrix Factorization (NMF) are tested to separate original thermal image sequences recorded by thermal camera. The number of initial thermal patterns N_s is varied as $N_s=2$, 3, …, 10. Each method is validated by using Monte-Carlo repeated experiment involving more than 20 independent trials to get robust separation results. The optimal selection of method as well as N_s are based on subjective human judgement and cognitive control has been set in place to deal with any inter- judgement reliability issues. Finally, $N_s=3$ and ICA are selected where three separated patterns directly indicating the specific thermal-transient characteristics. Figure 7a highlights the cool area with black strip (emissivity) where black region has spatial high emissivity and causes higher temperature. The transient characteristic of highlighted region pattern is similar to Pos 1 which can be seen in Fig. 6e. This pattern area underneath the coil has a continuous material distribution where the behavior of the transient response is independent of the emissivity. In order to prove this, Stefan-Boltzmann law states the energy emitted by a black body per second per unit of area is proportional to the fourth power of its absolute temperature. According to Eq. (6), the transient response of spatial pixel (x, y) can be presented as $j^*_{x,y}(t)=\varepsilon_{x,y}\sigma_{sb}T^4_{x,y}(t)$ where $T_{x,y}(t)$ denotes the temperature response of the area corresponding to pixel (x, y), and is independent of the emissivity $\varepsilon_{x,y}$. At the beginning of the heating phase, the sample is at the thermal equilibrium state $T_{x,y}(t_0)=T_0$, T_0 is equal to the ambient temperature. If the cooling time after this is long enough, the sample will reach a new thermal equilibrium state, $T_{x,y}(t_1)=T_1$ where t_1 denotes the elapsed time. Define $J_e=j^*_{x,y}(t_1)-j^*_{x,y}(t_0)=\varepsilon_{x,y}\sigma_{sb}\left[T_1^4-T_0^4\right]$ as the coefficient which is proportional to the surface emissivity. As the sample absorbs Joule heat generated by eddy current, $T_1>T_0$, the transient response rise $j^*_{x,y}(t)=j^*_{x,y}(t)-j^*_{x,y}(t_0)$ is divided by J_e, namely

$$j^*_{x,y}(t)=\frac{j^*_{x,y}(t)-j^*_{x,y}(t_0)}{J_e}=\frac{\varepsilon_{x,y}\sigma_{sb}\left[T^4_{x,y}(t)-T_0^4\right]}{\varepsilon_{x,y}\sigma_{sb}\left[T_1^4-T_0^4\right]}=\frac{\left[T^4_{x,y}(t)-T_0^4\right]}{\left[T_1^4-T_0^4\right]} \tag{13}$$

where $T_1^4-T_0^4$ is the coefficient corresponding to heating power, time and the sample property, such as density, specific heat capacity, and quality. It is constant in each test. Therefore $j^*_{x,y}(t)$ is independent of the emissivity, and characteristic of transient patterns does not be influenced by emissivity[37]. However, compared with separation, the time domain separated pattern of cool area still retains the mixing of hot spots around the right side of tips. Figure 7b highlights the hot spots where the transient characteristic of this thermal pattern is similar to Pos 3 as can be seen in Fig. 6e. Ideally, the extracted thermal-transient patterns should only highlight slot tips while the behavior of the transient response is the same as the curve with high rising and falling rate. However, the time domain separation recovers both sides of a hot spot but still mixes with stronger interference. Figure 7chighlights the region besides the excitation coil. The transient characteristic of this thermal pattern is similar to Pos 2 as can be seen in Fig. 6e. Ideally, the extracted thermal-transient patterns should only highlight non excitation region besides the coil and slot while the behavior of the transient response is the same as the curve which continuously rises. The separated results indicate that time domain separation does not completely separate this pattern and still mixes the patterns of both coil and slot.

Case (ii): In order to validate the efficiency of spatial-frequency domain pattern mining methods, similar to Case (i), PCA, ICA and NMF are tested and similar selection steps are conducted. Finally, $N_s=3$ and ICA are selected. Figure 7d highlights the cool area with black strip (emissivity). Compared with the time domain separation, the thermal-phase pattern separation performs better since the interference interface from other source has been maximally suppressed. Similar better results are shown in Fig. 7e where thermal-phase pattern separation has fully recovered both sides of the hot spots and reduced the interference interface contrast. The reason is attributed to the feature of phase information that it is less sensitive to the optical and infrared specimen surface and better shape resolution. However, the extraction pattern of non excitation region besides the coil and slot has not been completely separated due to the interference interfaced from both coil and slot. This could be the reason that the phase image is highly related to the propagation time delay, is independent of optical or surface features.

Case (iii): In this case study both Thermal-sparse-spatial-time domain and Thermal-sparse-spatial-frequency domain pattern mining methods are conducted. The tested sparse pattern methods include: greedy sparse decomposition method[33], variational Bayesian sparse decomposition with Gaussian sparse prior[34] and Bayesian sparse decomposition based on Monte Carlo Markov Chain[35]. $N_s=2$ is chosen since the sparse pattern separation only considers the pattern is either sparse or non-sparse. After test is conducted, the greedy sparse decomposition method is selected and more discussion will be found in the next section. In order to validate the detectability of sparse pattern, Fig. 7g shows the results of human annotation where the crack edge region (slot tips) is marked as "1" and the rest denoted as "0". In Fig. 7h,i, by emphasizing the sparseness of solution, the edge of the hot spots on crack tips can be quantified and has benefitted the quantitative sizing of the defect. Both time and frequency domain spatial-sparse pattern mining methods has successfully accentuate the expected sparse locations which indicate the hot spots of the slot tips and suppressing the interference. The frequency domain method obtains better contrast between slot tips and others while it mixes interference from cool area besides the coil. On the other hand, the time domain method nearly completely extract the slot tips, however, the level of sparseness is not optimum where it loses information of the left side of tip. In order to quantitatively characterize the error rate of the separated pattern, the following section on Discussion will summarize the error rate of the proposed thermal pattern separation system.

DISCUSSION

In addition, it is found that emphasizing the sparseness of pattern extraction takes an important role in quantitatively analyzing the defect. In order to clarify this, the quantitative rate (QR)[36] is introduced as

$$QR = \frac{TP}{TP + FN} \tag{14}$$

where TP refers to true positive which represent the situation where the sample contains a defect and the method indicates a defect is present as well as quantitative size of the defect, and FN refers to false negative which represents the situation where the sample does not contain a defect and the method does not indicate a defect is present as well as error quantitative size of the defect. The tested samples for validation study are set of steel samples ($0.24\times45\times100\,mm^3$) with variation slot size $L_j \times W_j$ where $L_j = \{10\,mm, 9\,mm, 8\,mm\}$ and $W_j = \{2\,mm, 1.5\,mm, 1\,mm\}$ width were prepared. The QR study is the comparison results between the referenced annotation with the pattern mining algorithms in spatial-time and spatial-frequency (phase) as well as sparse domain, respectively. The referenced human annotation defect region is shown in Fig. 7g. For Case (i) and (ii), only defect related thermal patterns are chosen for calculating QR, e.g. Fig. 7b,e.

Figure 8 shows the quantitative rate comparison results for defect pattern analysis by using the different domain pattern mining methods with human annotation results: Spatial-Time Pattern Mining (STPM) with 0.75 ± 0.06, Spatial-Frequency Pattern Mining (SFPM) with 0.85 ± 0.05, Sparse Spatial-Time Pattern Mining (SSTPM) with 0.89 ± 0.1, Sparse Spatial-Frequency Pattern Mining (SSFPM) with 0.87 ± 0.1. The standard deviation is given by using Monte-Carlo repeated experiment involving more than 20 independent trials of different pattern mining algorithms such as PCA, ICA, NMF and et al. A higher performance is attained by emphasizing sparseness for both time and frequency domain pattern mining methods with an average accuracy of approximately 90%. However, the standard deviation varies significantly where the sparseness level is difficult to be controlled. The sparse pattern extraction method is highly reliant on λ. Thus to determine λ, model order selection is used where experiment is repeated by progressively increasing λ or using Bayesian strategy to estimate the λ. Although the update parameters has advantages to bypass human intervention, it brings the drawbacks of incorrect selection of prior distribution for the model parameters and results in convergence to local minima. This brings about sub-optimum performance.

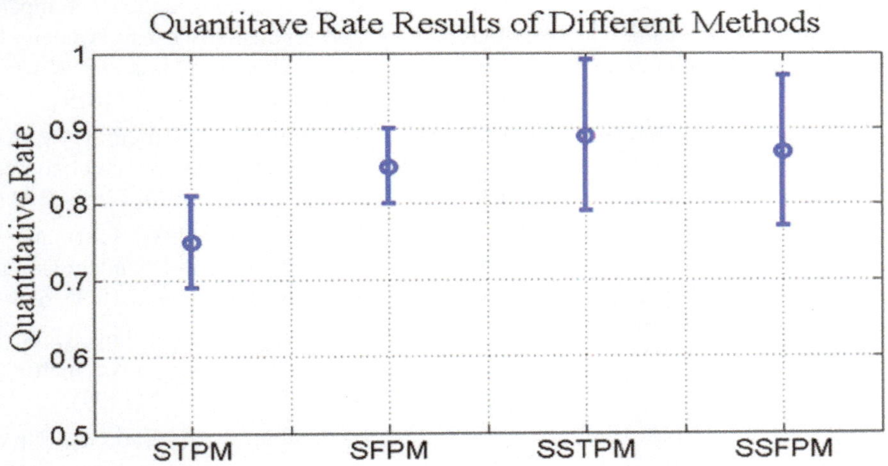

Figure 8: Comparison results. Quantitative rate comparison results of defect pattern mining by using different methods.

In this paper, a thermal physics-based pattern modelling and mining based imaging methods have been proposed for NDT&E. The inductive thermography-based NDT methods have been tested to validate the method. The pattern modelling and mining methods allows thermal defects patterns to be extracted automatically for flaw contrast enhancement. The methods have been tested on man-made defects. Future work will focus on samples with complex surface condition, e.g. roughness and geometry variation. Complexity defects thermal pattern separation, e.g. subsurface defects, impact damage and delamination in composite structures will also be investigated.

ACKNOWLEDGEMENTS

This research is supported by National Natural Science Foundation of China (Grant Nos 51377015, 61401071 and 61527803), NSAF (Grant No. U1430115), FP7 HEMOW IRSES project 269202, and the Fundamental Research Funds for the Central Universities (Grant No. ZYGX2014J068).

REFERENCES

1. 1. Ibarra-Castanedo, C. & Maldague, X. P. Infrared thermography Handbook of Technical Diagnostics: Fundamentals and Application to Structures and Systems. ed Czichos, H. (Berlin, Springer), 175–220 (2013).
2. 2. Watmough, D. J. & Oliver, R. Variation of Effective Surface Emissivity with Angle and Implications for Clinical Thermography. Nature 222, 472–473 (1969).
3. 3. Maldague, X. Theory and Practice of Infrared Technology for Nondestructive Testing. 1st ed., Wiley Interscience (2001).
4. 4. Lahiri, B. B. et al. Quantification of defects in composites and rubber materials using active thermography. Infrared Phys. Technol. 55 191–199 (2012).
5. 5. Meola, C. & Carlomagno, G. M. Recent advances in the use of infrared thermography. Meas. Sci. Technol. 15, R27–R58 (2004).

6. 6. He, Y., Tian, G. Y., Pan, M. & Chen, D. Eddy current pulsed phase thermography and feature extraction. Appl. Phys. Lett. 103, 084104 (2013).

7. 7. Oswald-Tranta, B. Thermo-inductive crack detection,Nondestruct. Test. Eval. 22, 137–153 (2007).

8. 8. Zenzinger, G., Bamberg, J., Satzger, W. & Carl, V. Thermographic crack detection by eddy current excitation. Nondestruct. Test. Eval. 22, 101–111 (2007).

9. 9. Noethen, M., Jia, Y. & Meyendorf, N. Simulation of the surface crack detection using inductive heated thermography.Nondestruct. Test. Eval. 27, 139–149 (2012).

10. 10. Weekes, B., Almond, D. P., Cawley, P. & Barden, T. Eddy-current induced thermography—probability of detection study of small fatigue cracks in steel, titanium and nickel-based superalloy.NDT&E Int. 49, 47–56 (2012).

11. 11. Louaayou, M., Nait-Said, N. & Louai, F. Z. 2D finite element method study of the stimulation induction heating in synchronic thermography NDT. NDT&E Int. 41, 577–581 (2008).

12. 12. Wilson, J. et al. Modelling and evaluation of eddy current stimulated thermography. Nondestruct. Test. Eval. 25, 205–218 (2010).

13. 13. Abidin, I. Z. et al. Quantitative evaluation of angular defects by pulsed eddy current thermography. NDT&E Int. 43, 537–546 (2010).

14. 14. Biju, N., Ganesan, N., Krishnamurthy, C. V. & Balasubramaniam, K.Frequency optimization for eddy current thermography. NDT&E Int. 42, 415–420 (2009).

15. 15. Kumar, C. N. K., Krishnamurthy, C. V. & Balasubramaniam, K.Comparison between tone burst eddy-current thermography (TBET) and flash thermography using numerical simulation studies. J. Nondestruct. Test. Eval. 8, 23–28 (2009).

16. 16. Gao, B. et al. Automatic Defect Identification of Eddy Current Pulsed Thermography Using Single Channel Blind Source Separation. IEEE Trans. Instrumentation and Measurement. 63(4), 913–922 (2014).

17. 17. Cheng, L. & Tian, G. Y. Surface crack detection for carbon fiber reinforced plastic (CFRP) materials using pulsed eddy current thermography. IEEE Sensors Journal 11(12), 3261–3268 (2011).

18. 18. Bui, H. K., Wasselynck, G., Trichet, D. & Ramdane, B. 3-D Modeling of Thermo Inductive Non Destructive Testing Method Applied to Multilayer Composite. IEEE Trans. Magnetics 49(5), 1949–1952 (2013).

19. 19. Vavilov, V. P. Pulsed thermal NDT of materials: back to basics.Nondestr Test Eval 22(2–3), 177–97 (2007).

20. 20. Shepard, S. Advances in pulsed thermography. Proceedings of SPIE "Thermo-sense-XXIII" 4360, 511–5 (2001).

21. 21. Shepard, S. Inventors; Temporal noise reduction, compression and analysis of thermo-graphic image data sequences, United States patent US 6516084, 2003 Feb 4.

22. 22. Ciliberto, A. et al. Porosity detection in composite aeronautical structures. Infrared Phys. Technol. 43, 139–43 (2002).

23. 23. Lahiri, B. B. et al. Infrared thermography based defect detection in ferromagnetic specimens using a low frequency alternating magnetic field. Infrared Phys. Technol. 64, 125–133 (2014).

24. 24. Maldague, X. & Marinetti, S. Pulse phase infrared thermography. J Appl Phys 79(5), 2694–8 (1996).

25. 25. Ibarra-Castanedo, C. et al. Infrared image processing and data analysis. Infrared Phys. Technol. 46(1–2), 75–83 (2004).

26. 26. Chatterjee, K. & Tuli, S. Image enhancement in transient lock-in thermography through time series reconstruction and spatial slope correction. IEEE Trans. Instrument and Measurement 61(4), 1079–1089 (2012).

27. 27. Marinetti, S. et al. Statistical analysis of IR thermographic sequences by PCA. Infrared Phys. Technol. 46, 85–91 (2004).

28. 28. Yin, A., Gao, B. & Tian, G. Y. Physical interpretation and separation of eddy current pulsed thermography. J Appl Phys. 113, 064101 (2013).

29. 29. Stefan, J. Über die Beziehung zwischen der Wärmestrahlung und der Temperatur. Sitzungsberichte der mathematisch-naturwissenschaftlichen Classe der kaiserlichen Akademie der Wissenschaften (in German) (Vienna) 79, 391–428 (1879).

30. 30. Jang, G. J. & Lee, T. W. A maximum likelihood approach to single channel source separation. J. Mach. Learn. Res. 4(40732), 1365–1392 (2003).

31. 31. Hyvarinen, A. Fast and Robust Fixed-Point Algorithms for Independent Component Analysis. IEEE Trans. Neural Network10(3), 626–634 (1999).

32. 32. Lee, D. D. & Seung, H. S. Learning the parts of objects by non-negative matrix factorization. Nature 401(6755), 788–791 (1999).

33. 33. Zhou, T. & Tao, D. Greedy bilateral sketch, completion & smoothing. In Proc. of 2013 JMLR Workshop and Conference 31, 650–658 (2013).

34. 34. Babacan, S. D., Luessi, M., Molina, R. & Katsaggelos, A. K. Sparse Bayesian Methods for Low-Rank Matrix Estimation, IEEE Trans. Signal Processing 60(8), 3964–3977 (2012).

35. 35. Ding, X., He, L. & Carin, L. Bayesian robust principal component analysis, IEEE Trans. Image Processing 20, 3419–3430 (2011).

36. 36. Powers, D. M. W. Evaluation: From Precision, Recall and F-Measure to ROC, Informedness, Markedness & Correlation.Journal of Machine Learning Technologies 2(1), 37–63 (2011).

37. 37. Libing, Bai, et al. Reducing the Effect of Surface Emissivity Variation in Eddy Current Pulsed Thermography. IEEE Sensors 14(4), 1137–1142 (2013).

CHAPTER 12 RADIATION INDUCED CHROMATIN CONFORMATION CHANGES ANALYSED BY FLUORESCENT LOCALIZATION MICROSCOPY, STATISTICAL PHYSICS, AND GRAPH THEORY

Yang Zhang, Gabriell Máté, Patrick Müller, Sabina Hillebrandt, Matthias Krufczik, Margund Bach, Rainer Kaufmann, Michael Hausmann, and Dieter W. Heermann

INTRODUCTION

A major goal of ongoing research in biophysics is to understand the potential interaction of nuclear architecture ("structuromics") and nuclear functions ("genomics") in order to elucidate the mechanistic principles behind spatial organisation of chromatin and chromatin re-arrangements during intra-nuclear processes like DNA repair after exposure of ionizing radiation ("radiomics") [1,2]. It is well known that individual chromosomes occupy distinct sub-volumes of a cell nucleus called chromosome territories [3,4,5]. These territories are sub-divided into domains of different compaction levels correlated to functional activities [6,7, 8,9]. One example of such domains is the distinction between decondensed, transcriptionally active euchromatin and tightly compacted heterochromatin generally to be assumed to be inactive [10, 11,12,13,14]. Gene-rich regions tend to be located towards the nuclear interior whereas gene-poor regions are generally found towards the periphery [15,16,17,18]. Up-regulation of genes during tumour genesis or DNA radiation damage response as well as DNA double strand break repair mechanisms were shown to be associated with re-organisation of chromosome territories [19, 20,21,22,23,24,25]. Chromatin on the nano-scale seems to have a dynamic structure [1,26] that allows re-arrangements with high flexibility in order to ensure appropriate functioning or damage response. Chromatin architecture appears to have an influence on the sensitivity to DNA radiation damage [27] and consequently the following repair behaviour [28,29]. Thus, chromatin arrangement reflects genome activities [30] and may correlate to radiation caused damage. Repair processes on the other hand should show systematic re-arrangements due to heterochromatin de-compaction for repair [26,27,31] or sub-diffusive movement of chromatin break ends [32].

In conclusion, many investigations have shown that the detailed study of the genome architecture would offer parameters directly correlated to the damaging process during irradiation and the following repair. This, however, requires global insights in conformation changes of chromatin and appropriate methods of quantification.

Recent technological advances allow the study of the nucleosome positions [histone proteins] in the 3D space and the chromatin arrangement not only on the micro- but also on the nano-scale [33,1] indicating that, besides the organisation of chromosome territories, the chromatin conformation below dimensions of 100 nm, independently of the cell type, is also not random. In order to obtain nanoscopic insights into 3D-conserved intact cell nuclei, light microscopic techniques are required that surpass the diffraction dependent resolution limit described by Abbe and Rayleigh more than hundred years ago [34,35]. In modern microscopes with high numerical aperture objective lenses, this resolution limit is still valid and is about 200 nm laterally and 600 nm axially.

Novel approaches in light microscopy circumventing the Abbe-Rayleigh boundary conditions enable effective optical resolutions down to the order of 10 nm or even better

Citation: Zhang Y, Máté G, Müller P, Hillebrandt S, Krufczik M, Bach M, et al. (2015) Radiation Induced Chromatin Conformation Changes Analysed by Fluorescent Localization Microscopy, Statistical Physics, and Graph Theory. PLoS ONE, 10(6): e0128555. DOI:10.1371/journal.pone.0128555.

[36,37,38]. One of these techniques is localization microscopy [39,40] which is based on the fundamental concept of optical isolation of objects by different spectral signatures, e.g. by using constant differences in the absorption/emission spectrum (see for instance SPDM [41]); or by using differences in the time domain, for example fluorescence life times [42], or fluorophores/fluorescent proteins that can be switched between two different spectral states (see for instance PALM [43], (F) PALM [44], STORM [45], SPDM [46,47], GSDIM [48] etc.) to achieve a temporal isolation and thus a spatial separation of single signals. This allows the determination of object positions and their spatial distances even if they are very close together, i.e., closer than the Abbe-Rayleigh resolution limit. All acquired positions of fluorescent molecules can be merged into one "pointillist", super-resolution image, in which the effective resolution is only depending on the localization accuracy and the density of the detected molecule positions.

A certain embodiment of localization microscopy used in the experiments described here is SPDM (Spectral Position Determination Microscopy; [49,46,47]) which has the advantage of using conventional fluorescent proteins or fluorescent fluorophores which are switched to a "dark" state by laser light-induced reversible photo bleaching [50,51]. From this dark state the fluorescent molecules randomly fall back into the emission state and emit their photons when irradiated. Each of the emitting fluorophores is represented by an Airy disc in the microscopic image. The centre-of-mass [barycentre] of such a disc approximates the location of the emitting molecule with high accuracy. So far, the resolution power of SPDM has been demonstrated in 2D-analyses of different applications, e.g. analyses of chromatin in cell nuclei, of proteins in cytoplasm and membranes, of antibody arrangements on cell surfaces and in cell nuclei, etc. [33,39,1,52,53,54].

Although in cellular specimens the typical localization precision and the point-to-point distance resolution of SPDM images presently is in the order of 10–20 nm, pointillist images locally differing in point densities are not obvious to be interpreted considering the complete structural information [53]. Visualization techniques have been developed considering localization accuracy and point density [55,56]. Images showing solely the detected molecule positions (or the positions blurred with the individual localization accuracy) give a better idea of the scattering of the detected points but make it harder to recognise the (correct) underlying structures by the human visual system especially if they represent the result of a dynamic process like chromatin re-arrangements during DNA damage repair after ionizing radiation exposure.

Therefore, we present novel evaluation procedures of SPDM images based on statistical physics and graph theory to provide a quantitative description of structural changes of chromatin after ^{137}Cs irradiation and during the following repair processes. Histones labelled with fluorescent proteins by transfection [56] or fluorescent antibodies specific for heterochromatin or euchromatin mark the point positions of individual histone proteins or individual labelling sites in heterochromatic or euchromatic regions, respectively, and are detected by SPDM in a 2D optical section through the cell nucleus. Statistical analyses of specimens exposed to different doses and fixed at different time points post irradiation will allow the investigation of the chromatin conformation changes during the repair process.

MATERIALS AND METHODS

Cell Culture and Irradiation

In all experiments stably transfected HeLa cell lines, originally developed by Tobias A. Knoch [57], expressing either green fluorescent protein (GFP) labelled histone H2B or yellow fluorescent protein (YFP) labelled histone H2A [58,59], were cultured in an incubator at 37°C and 5% CO_2 according to standard cell culture protocols. The used RPMI 1640 medium (Life technologies GmbH, Darmstadt, Germany) was composed of 10% fetal bovine serum (FBS) (Biochrom AG, Berlin, Germany), 1% penicillin (stock: 5000 units/ml) / streptomycin (stock: 5000 µg/ml) (Life technologies GmbH, Darmstadt, Germany) and 1% L-glutamine (stock: 200 mM) (Life technologies GmbH, Darmstadt, Germany). Additionally 10 mM N-2-hydroxyethylpiperazine-N-2-ethane sulfonic acid (HEPES) (Carl Roth GmbH, Karlsruhe, Germany) was added to provide an extra buffering capacity for cells which has an extended period outside the $C0_2$ incubator (e.g. irradiation process). The cells were passaged in T75 culture flasks over 2–3 days with a dilution of 1:10. For each radiation experiments approx. 75.000 cells were seeded in Lab-Tek Flaskette Slide/ Flask (VWR International GmbH, Darmstadt, Germany) and incubated for 2 days (until 70%–80% confluency).

Afterwards the cells were irradiated with γ-rays of two opposing ^{137}Cs sources. The dose rate of both sources was 0.5 Gy / min. The cells received a total dose of 0.5 Gy, 2 Gy or 3.5 Gy / 4 Gy. From each of these samples aliquots were fixed with 4% formaldehyde 30 minutes, respectively up to 48 hours after irradiation. In addition non-irradiated specimens were prepared as control (see also [33]). Samples prepared for the study of the nucleosomal positions were not immunostained.

Immunostaining of Heterochromatic and Euchromatic Regions

Immunostaining of heterochromatic and euchromatic regions was performed according to a standard protocol on separate cell samples. The cells were permeabilized with 0,2% Triton X-100 (Merck KGaA, Darmstadt, Germany) diluted in 1 x PBS (Life technologies GmbH, Darmstadt, Germany). After blocking with 2% bovine serum albumin (BSA) (Carl Roth GmbH, Karlsruhe, Germany) in 1x PBS the antibodies were diluted in 2% BSA blocking solution. The used primary antibodies were either directed against H3K4me3 (= mainly euchromatin regions) or H4K20me3 (= mainly constitutive heterochromatin regions) (Abcam, Cambridge, Great Britain). Secondary antibodies (Life technologies GmbH, Darmstadt, Germany) labelled with Alexa568 ($\lambda_{ex/em}$ = 560 nm / 610 nm) were used for the fluorescence imaging. All samples were counterstained using DAPI ($\lambda_{ex/em}$ = 364 nm / 454nm) and embedded in Prolong Gold (Life technologies GmbH, Darmstadt, Germany) before SPDM imaging.

Localizaton Microscopy

The following parameters refer to the SPDM setup. For the excitation of the fluorescent proteins GFP (green) or YFP (yellow), a laser with an excitation wavelength of 488 nm was used (Coherent (Deutschland) GmbH, Dieburg, Germany). The antibody fluorescence of Alexa568 was excited by a laser with the wavelength of 568 nm (Coherent (Deutschland) GmbH, Dieburg, Germany). The laser intensity was about 13 kW / cm^2 (488nm) and 25 kW / cm^2 (568nm). For each SPDM image further evaluated, a time stack of about 1000 images was acquired with an integration time of 55 ms (GFP/YFP) or 150 ms (Alexa568). The detection-off time between single images of these time stacks was 1 ms.

Optical isolation of signals was achieved utilizing a light-induced reversibly bleached state of GFP, YFP or Alexa568. By illuminating the sample some fluorescent proteins or dye molecules are bleached irreversibly while another amount is transferred to a reversibly bleached state. The stochastic recovery of these molecules to the fluorescent state can be used for optical isolation of the detected single molecule signals.

The laser beam was expanded by a factor of 2.5 before being focused into the back focal plane of an oil immersion objective lens (HCX PL APO, 63×, NA = 0.7–1.4, Leica, Wetzlar, Germany). The emitted fluorescent light passed a dichroic mirror (AHF Analysetechnik, Tübingen, Germany) and an appropriate blocking filter before being focused onto the charge-coupled device camera (SensiCam QE, PCO Imaging, Kehlheim, Germany). An additional lens was mounted in the excitation pathway for increasing the laser intensity in the object plane to obtain appropriate conditions for the reversible photo bleaching (for details see [49]).

Segmentation of IMAGES

In order to detect the regions of interest, a segmentation of the image is performed in the first step of the analysis. In this process the areas that have a considerably lower than average number of localized fluorophores are excluded. This includes the area that is on the outside of the cell nucleus but also areas inside the nucleus, e.g. at the site of nucleoli.

In the image, the fluorophores represent a set of points in the two-dimensional plane. To perform the segmentation a density distribution for the fluorophores on the entire image was calculated by applying a Gaussian kernel density estimation [60]. This means that each point on the image is replaced with a two-dimensional Gaussian probability distribution with a mean value corresponding to the coordinates of the point. Radially symmetric Gaussian distributions are chosen by setting the bandwidth matrix to a multiple of the unit matrix. The multiplier is a parameter in the model which defines a correspondence between the standard normal distribution and the physical scales in the experiment, and it is set to 40 nm. The sum of all the Gaussian probability distributions is then renormalized yielding a probability distribution for the points of the image. Since the values of the probability distribution are proportional to the density of points, the described procedure yields an accurate density distribution of the points on the complete image.

Using the density distribution, a mask is calculated that accepts all areas with a density that is above 25% relative to the lowest value, and blanks out all other areas. In order to make sure that also the low density regions at the border of the cell nucleus are excluded from the analysis, the boundary of the masked areas are further reduced by another 150 nm. Thus areas that are outside of the cell nucleus and areas which have a low marker density (e.g. sites of nucleoli) are efficiently excluded.

Radial Distribution Function

The radial pair correlation function $g(\mathbf{r}_1,\mathbf{r}_2))$ is a measure of structure for many particle systems such as liquids. It is the probability distribution function that two particles are at the positions$\mathbf{r}_1$ and $\mathbf{r}_2$. Since absolute positions are not important, the correlation function is in fact only dependent on the directed distance between the two positions $\mathbf{r} = \mathbf{r}_{12} = \mathbf{r}_2 - \mathbf{r}_1$. Thus the radial distribution function can be simply written as $g(\mathbf{r})$ and is given by

$$g(\mathbf{r}) = \frac{1}{N}\langle\sum_{i=1}^{N}\sum_{j=1}^{N}\delta(\mathbf{r} - \mathbf{r}_{ij})\rangle$$

The probability to find a second particle in the directed distance $\mathbf{r}$ of the first particle is $g(\mathbf{r})d\mathbf{r}$. Assuming an isotropic system, the pair correlation function only depends on the undirected distance $r = |\mathbf{r}|$, and the probability to find a second particle in the distance r of the first particle is given by $4\pi g(r)dr$.

For each image the pair correlation function is determined by calculating all pair distances between points inside of the masked regions of interest. Due to the finite system size, not all points can be used for the calculation of g(r). Points that are close to the border of the masked image have a different surrounding than the ones in the bulk, therefore including these points in the calculation of g(r) would distort the results. To take this into account, first the masked image was isotropically reduced from the border by a distance d_{shrink}, thus yielding a second masked image that is considerably smaller than the first one. All points in the second mask have then equal environments for distances up to d_{shrink}. Then, for each of the points in the second mask the distances to all other points that lie in the original mask were calculated. The normalized distribution of these distances then yields the radial distribution function g(r) for the image.

To observe the generic behaviour, the radial distributions obtained for the different images were averaged. The standard deviation of the mean value is then used as a measure for the uncertainty of the averaged g(r) at each distance r.

Analysis by Graph Topological Approach

Another possibility to gain insight in the structure presented by the localization data is to build a graph on the skeleton defined by the localized points. This graph then can be investigated by means of graph theoretical methods and the topological or relational properties of the underlying structure can be concluded.

Graphs [61] are abstract mathematical objects designed to capture interdependencies of certain entities. Entities are represented by nodes (or vertices) while the connections are encoded by edges between nodes. A graph is usually denoted by G(E,V), where V is the set of nodes and $E = \{(a,b)|a \in V, b \in V\}$ is the set of edges. Graphs have been used to study a variety of structures and phenomena [62, 63, 64, 65, 66], most of these studies relying on the mathematical field called graph-theory.

In the present study, the main interest is the observation of local properties of the geometric arrangements formed by the points. Therefore, the chosen graph building procedure must construct graphs that emphasize the local relations among the fluorophores. In other words, a nearest-neighbour graph (NNG) must be built, in which each node is connected with its first-order neighbours.

There are many possible ways to build the NNG for a given set of points. The most widely used approach is the construction of the Delaunay triangulation [67]. In order to have an intuitive understanding of this method, let us first introduce the dual of this triangulation, the Voronoi tessellation [68]. By definition, the Voronoi tessellation of a set of points S is a tessellation in which each Voronoi cell V_i corresponding to the site S_i consists of all the points of the space closer to S_i than any other site. The faces of the Voronoi diagram consist of all the points in the space that are equidistant to sites corresponding to touching Voronoi cells. Thus the Voronoi cell V_i defines the space dominated by the site S_i. The Voronoi tessellation can be transformed into the Delaunay triangulation by connecting the sites of the neighbouring Voronoi cells. Two points will be considered neighbours if they are directly connected by an edge of the Delaunay triangulation or equivalently, if their corresponding Voronoi cells are touching. Fig 1 illustrates the Voronoi tessellation and the Delaunay triangulation for a given set of points. Through the Delaunay triangulation, the NNG is constructed for each experiment and two properties of the obtained graphs are calculated: the rescaled probability density f(r) of the edge lengths and the conditional probability p(r|r′) of the edge lengths.

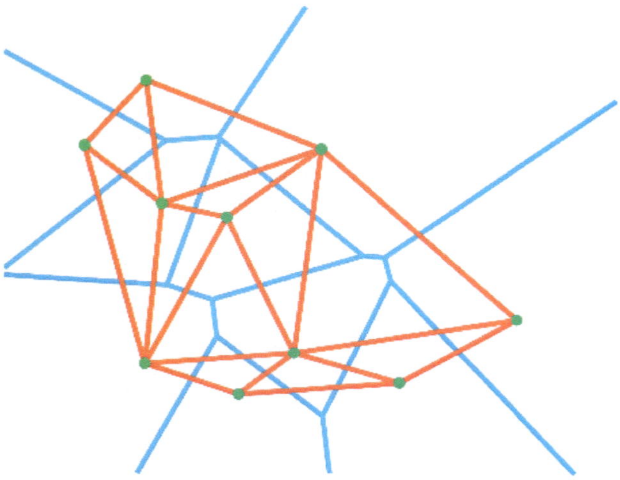

Figure 1. Sketch of a Delaunay Triangulation. The Delaunay triangulation and its dual, the Voronoi tessellation for a random set of points. The blue lines are the segments of the Voronoi tessellation, the red ones are the edges of the Delaunay graph (triangulation).

Let us denote the probability distribution of the length of the edges in a given graph G(E,V) obtained by the Delaunay triangulation of a point-set corresponding to one of the localization images by $\bar{f}(r)$. For different experiments different $\bar{f}(r)$ distributions are expected. The differences may stem either from different underlying structures or from different experimental conditions as these can vary from experiment to experiment (slightly different concentration of stains or different microscope gain). Provided that different experimental conditions have a liner effect on the density ρ of marked sites, variations $\bar{f}(r)$ can be eliminated. This is achieved by rescaling the distributions to a reference density ρ_0. For this, the following procedure is applied: Since the $\bar{f}(r)$ functions are probability distributions, the edge lengths, in fact, are treated in a probabilistic manner, that is, r is considered a random variable.

Thus, the rescaling of the distributions to a reference density ρ_0 is in fact a probability transformation over r. To see this, let $d_{ij} = d[(x_i,y_i),(x_j,y_j)]$ denote the length of the edge between vertexes i and j. If the coordinates (x,y) of all the points are multiplied with a positive real number $\alpha = \rho_0/\rho$ the following relation holds:

$$d[(\alpha x_i, \alpha y_i), (\alpha x_j, \alpha y_j)] = \alpha d[(x_i, y_i), (x_j, y_j)].$$

On the other hand, this multiplication corresponds to a uniform dilation (or contraction) of the system, that is, a uniform scaling of the density. Therefore, to calculate the scaled probability density, a probability transformation defined by

$$t(r) = \alpha r$$

must be applied. Using basic probability theory, the rescaled probability density

$$f(r) = \frac{1}{\alpha}\bar{f}\left(\frac{1}{\alpha}r\right)$$

is obtained.

The reference density ρ_0 can be, for instance, arbitrarily defined and the corresponding transformations for the different experiments can be carried out. Alternatively, the probability densities can be fit to each other, using α as a fitting parameter.

Certain local properties are averaged out both by the g(r) and the f(r). For instance, non-regular density variations are not captured by these measures. Another example is a situation when certain regular structures appears multiple times but the size of the structures varies.

In order to detect these situations, the conditional probability p(r|r′) of the edge lengths of the nearest neighbour graph is calculated. This conditional probability is the probability of finding an edge with length r attached to a node which for sure has an edge with length r′. The conditional probability can numerically be represented in a matrix structure P where each row corresponds to a condition for a given interval over r′ and each column represents an interval over r. The matrix entry P_{ij} corresponding to a given row i and a column j will give the probability of finding an edge with a length between r_j and r_j + dr attached to a node which has at least one edge with a length between r_i' and $r_i'+dr$. In case the localization points are arranged according to a specific structure, the P matrix will indicate a preferential attachment. For instance, in a long chain which has constant link-lengths over larger domains, but different domains have different link lengths, the P matrix will be almost diagonal. Fig 2 shows the Pmatrix for two randomly generated data-sets, one set containing points with coordinates distributed uniformly while the other set has additional Gaussian clusters. As the figure illustrates, uniformly distributed points will produce a rather uniform matrix, while point-sets with clusters will have a more emphasised diagonal.

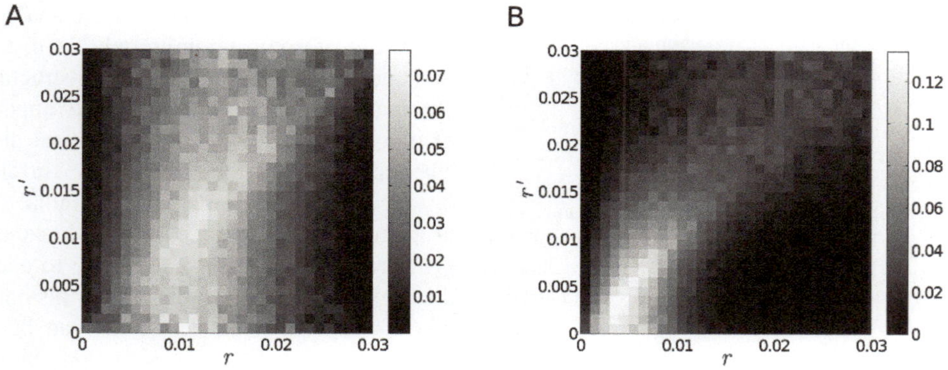

Figure 2. Conditional Probabilities of Edge Lengths for Random Data. The figures illustrate how the p(r|r') conditional probability looks for randomly generated point positions. Panel A. Conditional probability of points with coordinates generated according to a uniform distribution. Panel B. Conditional probability of points with coordinates generated according to a mixture of uniform distribution and clusters of Gaussian distributions. In the latter example an emphasized diagonal is observed which the result of the Gaussian clusters is. Tightly packed points tend to produce short edges, while points from the edges of the clusters mostly have longer edges.

RESULTS

Stably transfected HeLa cells expressing either GFP labelled histone H2B or YFP labelled histone H2A were fixed and embedded in antifade media for SPDM imaging. The cell nuclei were selected before SPDM imaging by visual inspection of wide-field images. A focus section of a depth of about 600 nm was chosen through the centre of each nucleus. About 1000 images of the same section were acquired and merged. The stochastic blinking of the fluorescent proteins was registered during the image stack and resulted in a localization map for all molecules detected. Typically about 70,000 fluorescent points were registered in the given optical section of a nucleus.

Exposure to Ionizing Radiation Cause Local but No Global Changes of the Genomic Organisation

From the experimental performance it can be assumed that the radiation damage sites were distributed all over the whole cell nucleus. Since they were not labelled specifically, the first approach was to globally study the distribution of nucleosomes represented by the blinking fluorescent proteins and their spatial variations after irradiation and during repair. The following processes describe the image analysis procedures:

At first a segmentation of each of the images is performed to cut out those areas in the image that do not belong to the cell nucleus. Additionally, areas inside the nucleus that have a very low density of markers are neglected since these areas are indicative for nucleoli. The segmentation is based on the calculation of the density distribution of markers in the image. Only the areas with a density of more than 25% of the largest density are taken into consideration. Fig 3 shows an example of an image with the localized H2B histones and their density distribution and the final segmented image in comparison to a widefield image as usually obtained by standard microscopy. To assess how the overall organization of chromatin changes induced by ionizing radiation compared to non-irradiated cells, the pair correlation function g(r) for localized H2B histones in non-irradiated cells and cells that were exposed to ionizing radiation is calculated. The pair correlation function is a measure for the positional correlation of points in a many-particle system. At this, $2\pi r g(r) dr$ denotes the probability of finding two points separated by a distance between r and r + dr for infinitesimal dr.

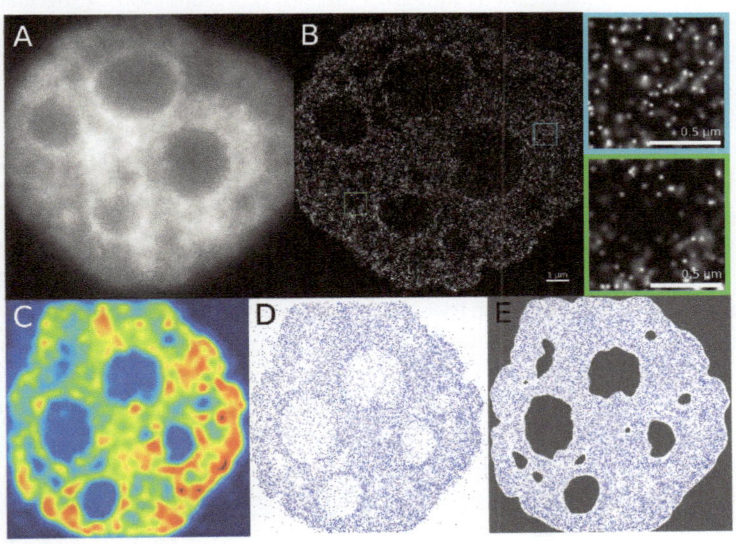

Figure 3. Localization Microscopy Images. Panel A. Widefield image of a cell nucleus, as usually obtained by standard microscopy. Panel B. Pointilist image obtained after merging the acquired time series of SPDM images. Each point represents a detected blinking process during

image acquisition. The green insert shows an area with a low average density, which could correspond to euchromatin and the blue area corresponds to an area with high point density, possibly belonging to heterochromatin. Panel C. This panel shows the calculated density distribution of the localized markers using a Gaussian kernel density estimation with a uniform Gaussian kernels. Panel D. The figure shows the localized points of the image. From the points, areas with very low point density, possibly corresponding to nucleoli, can clearly be made out visually. Panel E. Shown is the segmented image where only the area of interest is kept for the analysis. The segmentation was based on the density distribution; areas below a threshold density were discarded for analysis.

Typical results for the radial pair correlation function of H2B markers in non-irradiated and irradiated cells are shown in Fig 4 panel A. Images of non-irradiated cells and cells fixed 30 minutes respectively 48 hours after exposing them to 0.5 Gy, 2 Gy and 4 Gy of γ-irradiation were analysed. For all setups a deviations of g(r) from unity only for distances up to 300 nm were detectable. It thus shows that structured organisation of chromatin in the cell nucleus is only apparent up to distances of roughly 300 nm. Below this critical distance, locations of labelled histones H2B are visibly correlated. However, on distances larger than 300 nm the radial correlation function drops to unity and the locations of histones can be viewed as being randomly distributed relative to each other. The radial distribution functions for the H2B histones are lying on top of each other and no deviations can be seen for cells that were exposed to ionizing radiation. Since static chromatin architecture is in contrast to all findings so far, it seemed to be obvious that such results could be interpreted as the result of averaging distance distributions over the complete cell nucleus.

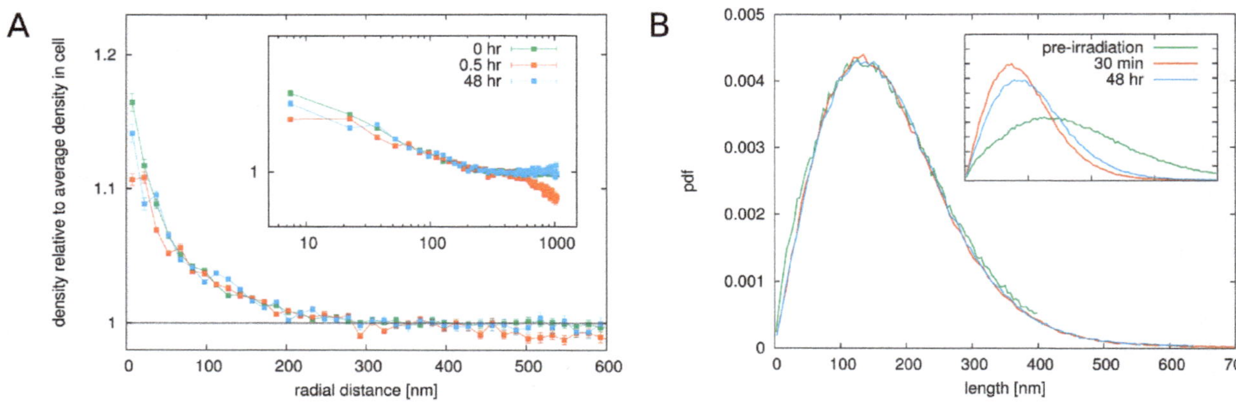

Figure 4. Results for cells exposed to 0.5 Gy radiation. Panel A. Radial pair correlation functions determined at different repair times after exposure to 0.5 Gy radiation dose. The radial pair correlation function g(r) shows that correlations between the positions of labeled H2B histones exist up to a distance of roughly 300 nm. Marker and thus chromatin densities in the surroundings of each marker are elevated compared to the average density of markers in the cell nucleus. Above 300 nm, however, histone positions are uncorrelated and the marked histones can be viewed as being positioned randomly relative to each other. Furthermore, the radial pair correlation function for cells exposed to 0.5 Gy γ-irradiation apparently does not differ from the one of untreated cells, regardless of the time passed after irradiation. Panel B. Rescaled distribution of the length of edges in a Delaunay triangulation of the H2B marker positions after different repair times post 0.5 Gy irradiation. The inset shows the original distributions for the different images. The differences in the edge length distributions are due to the different marker densities in the images. Therefore a rescaling of the distributions was performed with respect to the point density to clear out this effect. The rescaled distributions can be seen in the main panel and show that the distributions belong to the same family.

In order to assess the local positional correlations that are apparent up to a length of 300 nm a graph theoretical approach was pursued. First of all, the nearest neighbour distance distribution of the localized fluorophores was calculated. For this, a Delaunay triangulation was performed to obtain graphs for all points in the segmented images and then the length distribution of the edges of the graph was calculated. Results for H2B markers for non-irradiated cells and cells fixed 30 minutes and 48 hours, respectively, after exposure to ionizing radiation are shown inFig 4B. A significant difference between them can be observed (see inset). However, the distributions belong to the same family since the rescaled distributions f(r) are exactly the same. Therefore we can state that the observed differences may stem from different experimental conditions such as different overall recorded marker densities. This example demonstrates that it is necessary for comparison to rescale detected images to a comparable amount of points since labelling efficiency as well as detection efficiency of the microscope may vary between different series of experiments.

Additionally, a calculation of the p(r|r′) conditional probability for the localized H2B markers was performed. The matrix representations P of the conditional probabilities are plotted in Fig 5, the three panels A, B and C corresponding to pre-irradiation configuration and to configurations fixed 30 minutes and 48 hours post-irradiation, respectively. While the plots resemble a mixture of the plots from Fig 2, they do not exhibit obvious big discrepancies amongst each other. Panels D, E and F in Fig 5 present the differences between the three panels A, B and C. These plots show that for samples imaged shortly after irradiation, the diagonal of the conditional probability is more prominent but for samples recorded after a longer healing time the diagonal recedes. This means that, while upon irradiation the system appears to change towards a less uniform structure, that is towards a less homogeneous P matrix, with longer healing time the changes are reverted. These results indicate that after irradiation a formation of nucleosome clusters seem to increase whereas in the later repair phase this effect decreases.

In all cases the results of YFP-labelled H2A did not differ from GFP-labelled H2B (data not shown).

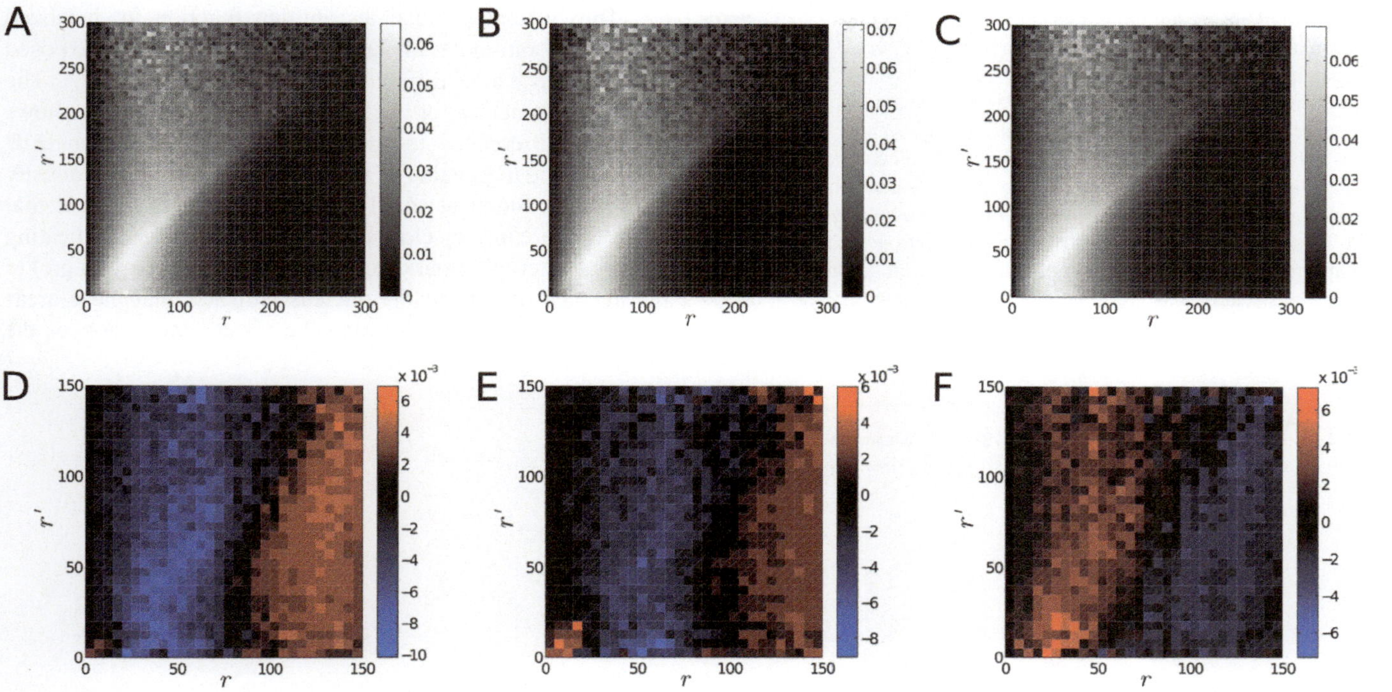

Figure 5. Conditional Probability Distribution of the Edge Lengths. Panel A. The panel shows the conditional probability distribution p(r|r′) of the edge lengths for the H2B markers before irradiation. The relatively prominent diagonal indicates locally a varying density. Panel B. The panel shows the conditional probability for the H2B markers 30 minutes after irradiation. Panel C. The panel shows the conditional probability for the H2B markers 48 h after irradiation. Panel D. The panel shows the difference of the conditional probabilities p(r|r′) measured for structures recorded before irradiation and for structures registered 30 min after irradiation. Shades towards red indicate values which are larger in the samples before irradiation, while values towards the shades of blue indicate probabilities which are larger in images registered 30 min after irradiation. The plot indicates slightly increased values along the diagonal after irradiation. This might mean a slightly increased clustering of the points. Panel E. The panel shows the differences of the conditional probability before irradiation and 48 h after irradiation. Entries in shades of red are larger in samples recorded before irradiation, while entries in shades of blue are larger in the samples recorded 48 h after irradiation. The trend is similar to that observed in panel D, however differences are less prominent. Panel F. The panel shows the differences if the conditional probability measured 30 min and 48 h after irradiation respectively. The red shades indicate larger probabilities in samples recorded 30 min after irradiation while blue shades indicate larger probabilities in samples registered 48 h after irradiation. Here a reversed trend compared to panel D was observed.

Heterochromatic Regions Show a Decondensation upon Exposure to γ-radiation

In addition to the stably nucleosome labelling by fluorescent proteins, antibodies for H4K20me3 were used as markers for heterochromatic regions. These experiments were carried out independently from the ones that focus on the positions of the nucleosomes, and a separate set of cells was prepared and immunolabeled according to the procedure introduced in the Methods section. Images were processed and segmented with the same methods described above and in the Methods section. In Fig 6 the density distribution of the heterochromatin antibody markers on panel A and the segmented image on panel B is shown. The density distribution shows clearly how heterochromatic regions can be seen as coarse structures located within the nucleus. These areas are visible as bright spots in the density distribution. All localized H4K20me3 antibodies, which were not discharged by the segmentation step, were considered in the calculations. That is, the presented results characterize post-irradiation heterochromatic regions on average, and not only domains where double-strand breaks occurred.

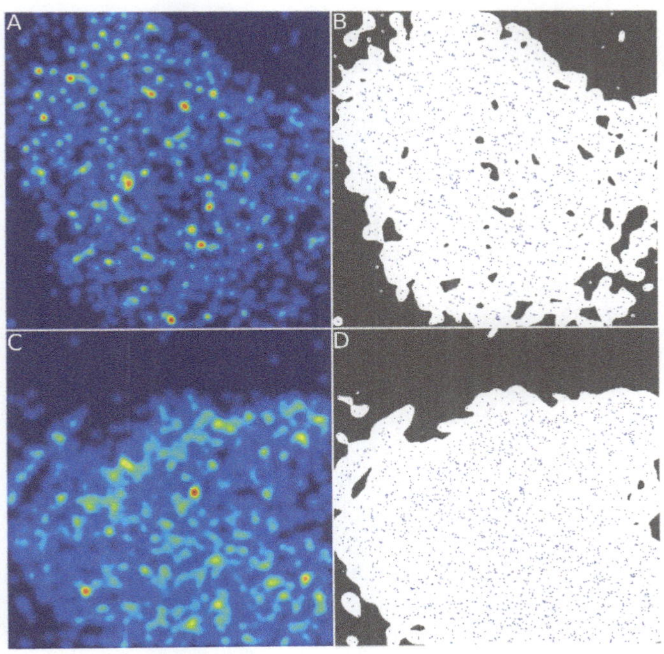

Figure 6. Examples of Localization Microscopy Images of Heterochromatin Markers. Panel A. Shown is the density distribution of the localized markers in a cell prior to irradiation. Small, very bright spots

where markers are agglomerated can be seen. This means that heterochromatin is mainly organized in coarse areas. Panel B. Shown is the segmented image of the not irradiated cell that is used for subsequent analysis of the marker distribution. Panel C. The density distribution of a cell at 30 min after irradiation with 0.5 Gy is shown here. Differences between this cell and the not irradiated cell can be made out by visual inspection. We observe that the density has much less agglomerated and bright spots and is instead much more homogeneous. Panel D. This effect can also be seen by visual inspection of the heterochromatin markers directly. Marker positions are visibly more spread out and less strongly clustered together. Heterochromatin clearly undergoes structural changes upon irradiation.

The calculated radial distribution function for localized H4K20me3 antibodies in non-irradiated cells and cells exposed to 0.5 Gy dose after different times are shown in Fig 7A. The correlation function for the heterochromatin antibodies shows apparent differences to the correlation function for H2B histones. The high value of up to 20 times the average density that can be found at small distances r reflects the fact that antibodies are in very close proximity of each other, indicating compact heterochromatic domains. The quick decay of g(r) to the average density in the nucleus indicates that these areas are relatively small confirming the visual impression of the images.

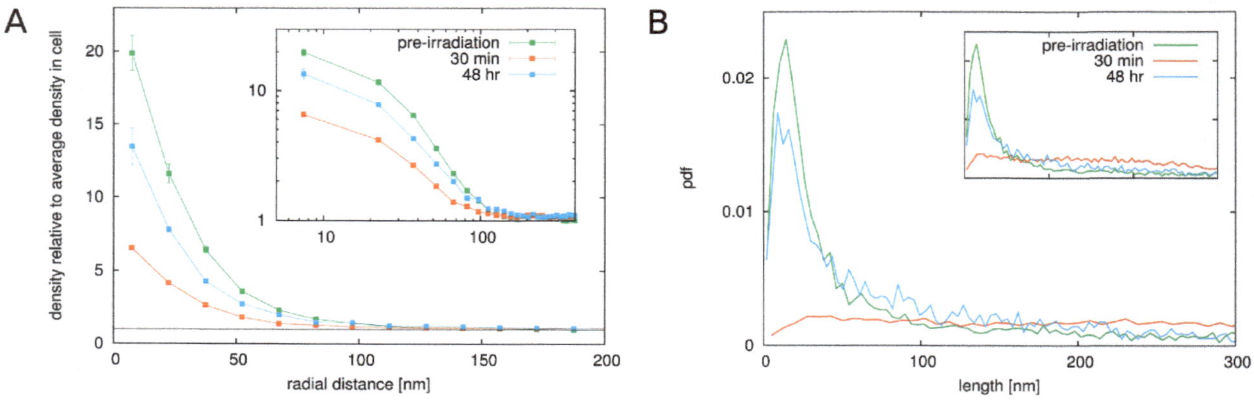

Figure 7. Results for cells exposed to 0.5 Gy radiation. Panel A. The figure shows the radial radial distribution function for H4K20 antibodies representing heterochromatin (methylated histone variants) for non-irradiated and irradiated cells. Error bars represent the standard deviation of the mean value after averaging over the sample of cells. The value for g(r) at small distances goes up to around 20, indicating the high marker densities in regions where heterochromatin is located. The rapid drop off of the radial distribution function within a distance of less than 100 nm shows that heterochromatin forms small clustered areas that are spread throughout the cell nucleus. Upon exposure to 0.5 Gy γ-irradiation, a dramatic change in the correlation function can be observed in cells that were imaged after 30 min. The value at small radial distances drops to around 6, or around 70% smaller than in non-irradiated cells. This indicates that the density in the heterochromatic regions becomes on average much lower in irradiated cells. In cells measured 48 h after irradiation, the correlation function have recovered again and the value at small r is at around 14, only 30% less than in unirradiated cells. Panel B. The distribution of edge lengths in the Delaunay triangulation of the markers confirms these observations. A sharp peak in the distribution at around 30 nm can be seen in untreated cells. In 30 min post-irradiation cells the peak vanishes and a spread distribution can be seen. In 48 h post-irradiation cells however, the peak reappears again but less pronounced than in untreated cells.

Upon irradiation, the value of the correlation function drops for small distances r. This means that the average density of antibodies in the surrounding of each antibody is lower during the first repair phase. It indicates that the overall chromatin density becomes smaller in the heterochromatic areas. This could be verified within the nucleosomal pattern 5 min after radiation exposure if the analysed regions of interest were locally reduced to areas only highlighted by heterochromatic antibody accumulation (data not shown).

It can be concluded that regions of constitutive heterochromatic chromatin on average become less compact, i.e., the strongly compacted organisation opens up and adopts a more loose structure. An average drop of 70% of the mean antibody density in a sphere with a radius of 30 nm around an antibody for cells irradiated with 0.5 Gy γ-irradiation after 30 minutes was observed. Therefore, DNA double-strand breaks caused by irradiation in heterochromatin seems to require a drastic decrease of the chromatin density and a strong relaxation of the compact organisation of the chromatin fibre in order to make the damaged sites accessible for repair. 48 h after irradiation, this value is only at around 30% which indicates that structures seem to have recovered after successful repair of DNA damages.

The conclusions drawn from the radial distribution function are verified by the graph theoretical analysis. In Fig 7B the length distribution of the edges in the Delaunay triangulation of the marked H4K20 antibodies is shown. The distribution for non-irradiated cells shows a very characteristic peak at small distances centred at around 30 nm. This emphasizes that there is a characteristic nearest-neighbour distance for the H4K20 markers thus meaning a preference of them to form compact areas. In cells at 30 min after exposure to ionizing radiation, the sharp peak in the edge length distributions vanishes. Instead, the distribution becomes a uniform distribution up to large lengths. The disappearance of the peak is a clear indicator that the heterochromatic regions are no longer organized as compact areas in the nucleus. This difference can be seen visually in Fig 6C. Compared to the non-irradiated cell nucleus shown inFig 6A, it can be observed that the very bright spots have mostly vanished and the heterochromatic regions in the irradiated cell are much more smeared out. The graph theoretical analysis therefore verifies the observations of the behaviour of the radial distribution function. The heterochromatic regions undergo a decondensation upon exposure to ionizing radiation. At 48 h after irradiation, the peak in the edge length distribution emerges again. Just as the pair correlation function is again very similar to that of non-irradiated cells, the edge length distribution has also the same shape as in the case of non-irradiated cells.

The calculation of the conditional probability p(r|r′) shows that the corresponding matrix-representations are strongly diagonal (Fig 8). This is due to the tight clusters of the antibodies marking heterochromatic regions. The structure of the conditional probability matrices supports the previous conclusions. Upon irradiation, the conditional probability (panel B in Fig 8) becomes more homogeneous, indicating a more uniform structure. 48 h after irradiation the conditional probability is again diagonal (panel C in Fig 8). Note that in this case the colour-map has a wider range and values on the diagonal are in fact very close to values from panel A, except for very small radii.

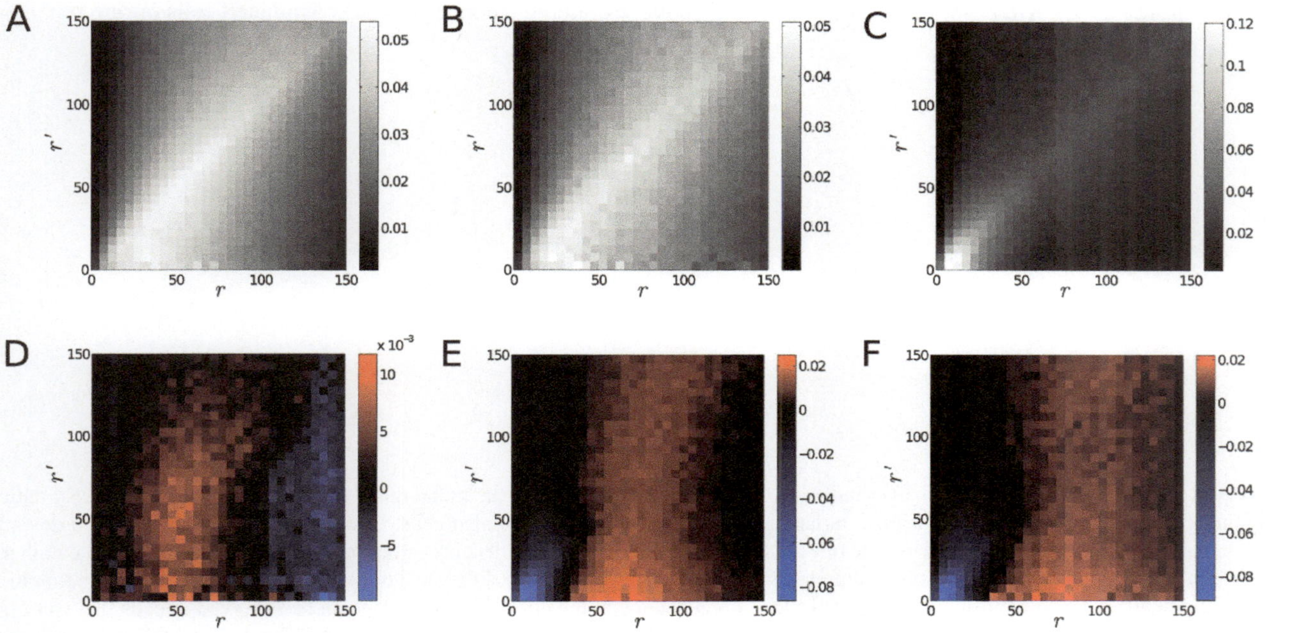

Figure 8. Conditional Probability Distribution of the Edge Lengths for Heterochromatin Markers. Panel A. The panel shows the conditional probability distribution p(r|r′) of the edge lengths calculated for the positions of the antibodies marking heterochromatic regions before irradiation. Panel B. The panel shows the conditional probability for the heterochromatin markers 30 min after irradiation. Panel C. The panel shows the conditional probability for the heterochromatin markers 48 h after irradiation. In all three cases the diagonal is emphasized indicating preferential spatial distribution of the edges. This may stem from the clustering of the heterochromatin markers. Note that although shades along the diagonal are darker in panel C, the value of the corresponding probabilities are very close to the probabilities along the diagonal of panel A except for small radii. Panel D. The panel shows the difference in the conditional probability distribution p(r|r′) before irradiation and 30 min after irradiation. A red shade of the color-map means that the probability is higher before irradiation while a blue shade means that it is higher after irradiation. The panel indicates a slightly stronger change along the diagonal indicating a more homogeneous system after irradiation. However, the change is almost independent of the value of the condition r′. Panel E. The panel shows the difference of the conditional probability distribution calculated for samples before and 48 h after irradiation. Shades of red indicate higher probabilities for the samples recorded before irradiation while shades of blue indicate higher probabilities in samples recorded after irradiation. Panel F. The panel illustrates the difference of the conditional probability distribution 30 min and 48 h after irradiation. Red shades correspond to higher probabilities 30 min post-irradiation while shades of blue indicate larger values 48 h after irradiation. The difference between structures observed 30 min after irradiation and 48 h after irradiation indicate a reversed trend compared to panel D.

The differences of the conditional probabilities are plotted in Fig 8C–8E. While the changes upon irradiation barely depend on the condition (the value of r′), smaller radii were observed to be more abundant before irradiation (red colour in panel C). The difference between the structure 30 min after irradiation and the structure 48 h after irradiation (in panel D, E) indicates an almost uniform and unconditioned increase in the probabilities of the short edges, just as in the case of the unconditioned edge length distribution.

Our results here show that heterochromatic domains undergo structural reorganizations after exposure to ionizing radiation. At 30 min after irradiation the previously very compact and densely organized domains open up and adopt a more loose organization. After 48 h the structures are rehabilitated and the organization approaches again the initial configuration of the non-irradiated cells. In case of 4 Gy irradiation the detected effects were compatible but less pronounced which may be due to a higher amount of double-strand breaks and consequently more repair activity requiring additional space for recruited repair proteins. Moreover, it has to be considered that the percentage of repair activity may be shifted from homologous recombination repair to non-homologous end-joining.

Euchromatic Regions React Complementary to Heterochromatic Regions upon Exposure to γ-radiation

Our results for antibodies that are specific for euchromatic regions show that euchromatin responds very differently to irradiation than heterochromatin. The radial distribution function for euchromatic markers is shown in Fig 9 panel A. As for the heterochromatin markers, we obtain high values for the radial distribution function at distances up to 50 nm which means that the markers are also concentrated in small regions. This is expected, since euchromatic regions within the chromosome are organized in specific domains. In cells at 30 minutes after exposure to 0.5 Gy or 4 Gy of ionizing radiation, the value for the radial distribution function is increased compared to non-irradiated cells. Euchromatin appears to show a complementary behaviour to heterochromatin, which was observed to expand. The euchromatic regions seem to condense upon irradiation, possibly due to the expansion of the heterochromatic regions that relocate damage sites into euchromatin [28, 29]. After 48 hours, the structures have slightly recovered. The results of the graph theoretical analysis (Fig 9B) confirm these observations. Upon irradiation, the value of the first peak in the distribution becomes even larger compared to the first minimum indicating a condensation of the euchromatic regions. After 48 hours, the structure of the markers is still not the same as in the beginning. Above all, in contrast to the heterochromatin markers, where the peak was observed to have completely vanished, euchromatin domains undergo a condensation in irradiated cells during repair.

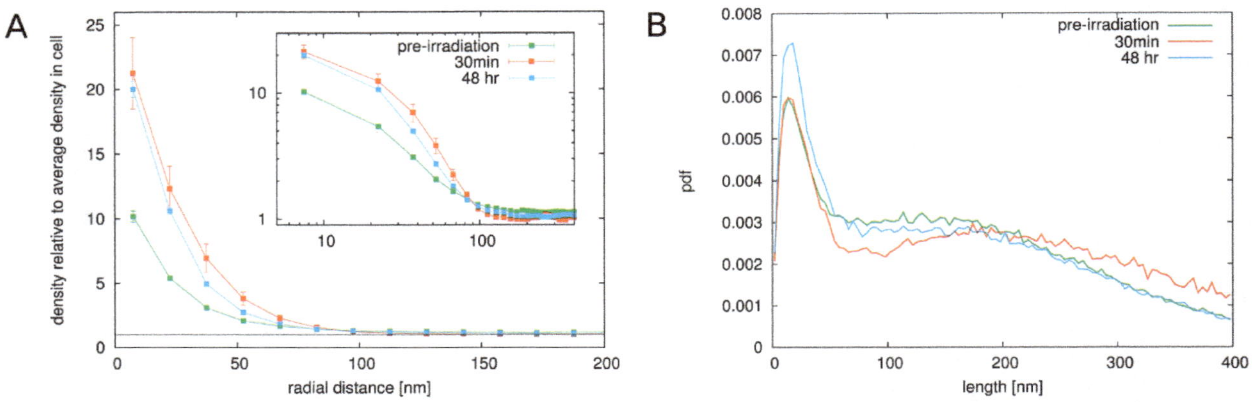

Figure 9. Results for cells exposed to 0.5 Gy radiation. Panel A. The figure shows the radial radial distribution function for H3K4 antibodies representing euchromatin (methylated histone variants) for non-irradiated and irradiated cells. Error bars represent the standard deviation of the mean value after averaging over the sample of cells. The value for g(r) at small distances goes up to around 20, indicating the high marker densities during repair. The rapid drop off of the radial distribution function within a distance of about 50 nm shows that euchromatin forms small clustered areas. Upon exposure to 0.5 Gy γ-irradiation, a change in the correlation function can be observed in cells that were imaged after 30 min and 48 hrs. The value at small radial distances increases compared to non-irradiated cells. This indicates that the density in the euchromatic regions becomes on average higher in irradiated cells. Panel B. The distribution of edge lengths in the Delaunay triangulation of the markers confirms these observations. A sharp peak in the distribution at around 30 nm can be seen in untreated cells. In 48 h post-irradiation cells, the peak spreads slightly.

Cluster Analysis Independently Supports the Presented Findings

To double-check our observations, we further investigated the behaviour of antibody-position clusters. Two additional sets of cells were prepared and immunolabaled with antibodies for heterochromatin and euchromatin separately. Groups of cells were irradiated using the same radiation source with doses of 0.5 Gy and 3.5 Gy, and 0.5 h, 6 h and 24 h repair times were considered. The data obtained this way was investigated with a simple cluster analysis. Clusters were defined based on the proximity of the localization markers: a point is considered to belong to a given cluster if it has at least three neighbours within a distance of 40 nm. Then, the overall percentage of points in such cluster, compared to the total number of points in a cell, is a good measure of the condensation of the chromatin fibre for the considered markers (for details see [1]).

Fig 10 shows the results for this analysis. Panel A presents the results for heterochromatin. This shows how the relative number of points in dense clusters decreases 6 h after irradiation and increases again close to the original value 24 h after irradiation. The drop in the number of such points after 6h indicates an opening up of the structure (decondensation), while the increase observed after 24 h corresponds to a recondensation.

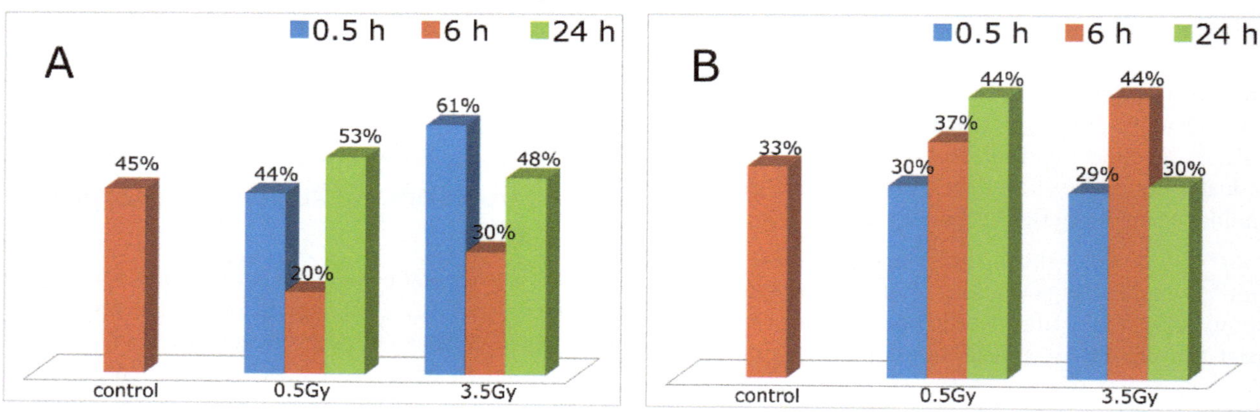

Figure 10. Cluster analysis of the spatial distribution of heterochromatin and euchromatin after irradiation with 0.5 Gy and 3.5 Gy. The analysis was performed on non-irradiated samples, and on samples fixed 6 h and 24 h post irradiation, respectively. Panel A present the behaviour of heterochromatic regions irradiated with 0.5 Gy and 3.5 Gy. We observe a decrease in the ratio of the clustered points 6 h after irradia-

tion for both doses. 24 h after irradiation these changes are reverted. This means that a few hours after irradiation the heterochromatin decondenses and after one day the decondensation is reverted. Panel B shows the cluster analysis result for euchromatin. These regions behave differently, compared to heterochromatin. For 0.5 Gy, the number of clustered points is increased after 6 h, and the trend continues at the 24 h timestamp. However, for 3.5 Gy, after the initial increase in the percentage of clustered points at 6 h, the ratio drops again in the 24 h measurements. The interpretation of the increase/decrease in the number of clustered points is similar in this case: when the ratio increases, the studied domains condense, when the ratio decreases, the domains relax. This means, that heterochromatin and euchromatin react to irradiation in an opposite way: This analysis, in accordance with the other results, indicates that while heterochromatin opens up soon after irradiation, euchromatin condensates. Given enough time, these processes are reverted in both cases.

For euchromatin, in turn (Panel B), the relative number of such points increases after irradiation. While for 0.5 Gy, the trend continues also after 24 h, for 3.5 Gy the changes observed after 6h are reverted after 24 h. The increase in the number of points in dense clusters at the 6 h timestamp, indicates a condensation of the euchromatin. Similarly, the decrease of the number of such points after 24 h (compared to the 6 h situation) corresponds to a relaxation of the euchromatin domains. In conclusion, the cluster formation in heterochromatin and euchromatin is behaving complementarily.

This separate experiment analysed with a completely different method fully supports our previous observations and result detailed in the sections above.

DISCUSSION

Many investigations have shown that the detailed study of the genome architecture would offer parameters directly correlated to the chromatin damaging process during irradiation and the following repair [1,2]. Since often all chromatin damage sites cannot be visualized simultaneously, alternative procedures leading to global insights into conformation changes of chromatin are useful but require appropriate methods of quantification. Here we have systematically studied effects obtained from localization microscopy investigations of the nano-architecture of chromatin.

Such studies apply novel approaches in fluorescent light microscopy to circumvent the diffraction limit of light microscopy based on optical separation of individual fluorescent molecules and the determination of their spatial positions. Such techniques are called localization microscopy (for review see [36,37,39]) and have been realized in several slightly different embodiments from which SPDM is one having demonstrated its usefulness in many applications in cell biophysics (for review see [54]). The clear advantages of SPDM are on hand: the use of standard microscopic components, standard preparation techniques and dyes or fluorescent proteins as well as the simultaneous acquisition of wide-field fluorescence images and localization images of the same object without changing the microscopic setup.

Although the typical localization precision and the point-to-point distance resolution of SPDM and other localization microscopy techniques presently is in the order of 10–20 nm especially in biological specimens, the images result in a pointillist presentation which may be incomplete due to limited labelling and detection efficiencies [59]. In addition pointillist images may represent visual local differences of point densities but usually omit any quantitative structural information of the cellular or nuclear environment. This might not be a serious shortcoming in cases where labelled molecules are spatially concentrated to sub-cellular structures which can be clearly separated. In the case of chromatin radiation response we intended to find a global measure over the cell nucleus indicating all architectural changes during the repair process. Since the detected point density appeared to be similar over the entire distribution of nucleosomes, local density fluctuations had to be figured out by advanced techniques of image analysis and calculation. Therefore we applied a novel approach based on statistical physics and graph for the structural non-random chromatin arrangement below 300 nm dimensions. While certain approaches focus on determining the absolute number of nucleosomes [59], we develop a methodology which is independent of the density of these. Nevertheless, the raw data present a reasonable compatibility with the results of Weidemann et al. [59] indicating that the transfection efficiency was still maintained over further cultivation procedures.

The calculation of the distance dependent pair correlation function as well as the application of the graph topological approach of Delaunay triangulation revealed a significant measure for the behaviour of heterochromatin and euchromatin after irradiation and during 48 hours of repair. It indicates that the overall density of antibody positions against heterochromatin becomes smaller in the first fast repair phase (30 min post irradiation) and increases again during the longer repair phase of 48 hours whereas euchromatin behaves complementarily. From these data it can be concluded that heterochromatic regions on average become less compact and the strongly compacted organisation opens up and adopts a more loose structure upon exposure to ionizing radiation. An average drop of 70% of the mean antibody density in a sphere with a radius of 30 nm around an antibody for cells irradiated with 0.5 Gy irradiation after 30 min was observed. Therefore, initial repair of DNA double-strand breaks caused by irradiation in heterochromatin seems to require a drastic decrease of the chromatin density and a strong relaxation of the compact organisation of the chromatin support recent results. 48 h after irradiation, this value is only at around 30% which indicates that structures seem to have recovered after successful repair of the broken DNA strands. Although so far the repair foci (e.g. γH2AX foci) were not analysed (being subject of future investigations), these data support recent findings of others who describe a transfer of break-point foci after X-ray or heavy ion exposure to the border of heterochromatic regions or into euchromatic regions for further repair [2,20,28, 29,69,70]. These findings are also supported by computer simulations of double-strand breaks [71]. However, further effort has to be spent in the systematic analysis of heterochromatin and also euchromatin behaviour after ionizing radiation exposure [Krufczik et al., manuscript in preparation]. Using the same cell line as in our studies, a decondensation of the heterochromatin was observed also in histone acetylation processes on length scales of chromosome territories from 200 nm up to the micrometre scale [58]. These regulatory processes without DNA-breakage, however, are different in nature from the effects of ionizing radiation, which, as our results showed it, appear below 300 nm. Thus, it can be concluded that heterochromatin conformation changes are occurring on different size scales but recover after a certain time of cell activity. This indicates that the architecture on the micro- as well as on the nano-scale remains "ordered in randomness" [72].

The goal of this publication presented here is to demonstrate the power of the applied analysis techniques and to validate them on data sets typical for radiation research. Further investigations will study not only different doses but also different photon spectra at more time points during repair. In addition dynamics of molecular repair foci conformation will be studied. Since the detected effects are not correlated to the kind of damage induced, such data may be useful not only to describe global behaviour of heterochromatin and euchromatin after irradiation but also to obtain a sensitive measure for biological dosimetry at least in the so far difficult to access low dose range.

In this context it may argued that the selection of a 2D image section through the cell nucleus covering only about 1/10 of the nuclear volume may be an incomplete description of the radiation induced re-arrangements in a cell nucleus. From the microscopic side of view this shortcoming could be overcome by the application of 3D-SPDM [49,52]. Although the principle feasibility of this approach using a combination of SPDM and standing wave-field illumination has been demonstrated for cellular imaging, it is very time consuming and extremely data loaded. However, present approaches of large scale data management [73] may improve data handling. On the other hand the data presented here indicate that a 2D section contains enough information for an approach of comparison even if the analyses are restricted to an arbitrary selected part of the nucleus′ volume.

In contrast to the results obtained for heterochromatin, the results of pair correlation functions and Delaunay triangulation for the spatial nucleosomal distribution seem to be rather insensitive either for dose difference or for repair time. At a first glimpse this would not have been expected from all experimental evidence of chromatin re-arrangements and functional cellular activities during repair. On the other hand considering the results of heterochromatin and euchromatin there may be complementary trends in the compaction behaviour of heterochromatin and euchromatin during the repair process so that on average it looks like a compensation of heterochromatin de-compaction and euchromatin increase of compaction. If one would accept this principle behaviour our results could be seen as a validation for this effect.

As recently shown [53] SPDM pointillist images of molecular processes and cellular structures offer differently structured regions by visual inspection which however averages by calculation of density and distance frequency distributions. Therefore more detailed evaluations of sub-regions may be advantageous and/or further sophisticated procedures should be applied. Here the calculation of the conditional probability of the edge lengths of the nearest neighbour graph was tested for the analyses of nucleosomal pattern after radiation exposure.

SPDM imaging as well as many other techniques of localization microscopy [36,37] offer fascinating novel insights into the nano-cosmos of cells and cell nuclei [54,74] and may become key tools for investigations of molecular cellular dynamics and mechanisms behind epigenetic functions. The pointillist highly resolved images contain huge amount of individual information of molecules. The interpretation of the "nicely looking" images in terms of biological relevance and functional mechanisms challenges image analysis and bio-informatics. Depending on the scientific questions sophisticated approaches of quantitative image evaluation and interpretation beyond "nice" visualization have to be tested and validated against optical insufficiencies [37]. Under this perspective our work combining experimental and theoretical biophysics contributes to the elucidation of the so far insufficiently understood repair mechanisms depending on the nano-architecture of chromatin and its dynamics. Further investigations are in progress.

ACKNOWLEDGMENTS

MH, PM, SH and MB gratefully acknowledge the financial support of the German Federal Ministry for the Environment, Nature Conservation, Building and Nuclear Safety (FKZ: SR/StSch/INT 3610S30015). Furthermore the authors thank Christoph Cremer, Institute for Molecular Biology, Mainz, for his continuous support and the accessibility to the SPDM instrumentation. Data curation and archiving has been supported to M.H. by the Helmholtz Portfolio Extension Large Scale Data Management and Analysis with contributions from the Data Life Cycle Lab Key Technologies and the Data Services Integration Team. GM gratefully acknowledges support from the German Science Foundation (DFG) as member of the Research Training Group "Spatio/Temporal Probabilistic Graphical Models and Applications in Image Analysis", grant GRK 1653. YZ was funded by the German National Academic Foundation (Studienstiftung des Deutschen Volkes). GM and YZ acknowledge support by the Heidelberg Graduate School of Mathematical and Computational Methods for the Sciences (HGS MathComp) and the Institute for Theoretical Physics of the Heidelberg University.

AUTHOR CONTRIBUTIONS

Conceived and designed the experiments: MH PM RK MB. Performed the experiments: SH PM MB RK MK MH. Analyzed the data: YZ GM DH MK. Contributed reagents/materials/analysis tools: YZ GM MK. Wrote the paper: YZ GM MH PM DH.

REFERENCES

1. Falk M, Hausmann M, Lukášová E, Biswas A, Hildenbrand G, Davídková M, et al. (2014) Giving OMICS spatiotemporal dimensions by challenging microscopy: From functional networks to structural organization of cell nuclei elucidating mechanisms of complex radiation damage response and chromatin repair–PART B (Structuromics). rit. Rev. Eukaryot. Gene Express. 24: 225–247. doi: 10. 1615/critreveukaryotgeneexpr. v24. i3. 40
2. Falk M, Lukášová E, Hausmann M, Biswas A, Hildenbrand G, Davídková M, et al. (2014) Giving OMICS spatiotemporal dimensions by challenging microscopy: From functional networks to structural organization of cell nuclei elucidating mechanisms of complex radiation damage response and chromatin repair–PART A (Radiomics). Crit. Rev. Eukaryot. Gene Express. 24: 205–223. pmid:25072147 doi: 10. 1615/critreveukaryotgeneexpr. 2014010313

3. Bolzer A, Kreth G, Solovei I, Koehler D, Saracoglu K, Fauth C, et al. (2005) Three-dimensional maps of all chromosomes in human male fibroblast nuclei and prometaphase rosettes. PlosBiol 3: e157. pmid:15839726 doi: 10. 1371/journal. pbio. 0030157

4. Cremer T, Cremer C (2001) Chromosome territories, nuclear architecture and gene regulation in mammalian cells. Nat Rev Genet 2: 292–301. pmid:11283701 doi: 10. 1038/35066075

5. Cremer T, Cremer M, Dietzel S, Müller S, Solovei I, Fakan S (2006) Chromosome territories—a functional nuclear landscape. Curr. Opin. Cell Biol. 18: 307–316. pmid:16687245 doi: 10. 1016/j. ceb. 2006. 04. 007

6. Albiez H, Cremer M, Tiberi C, Vecchio L, Schermelleh L, Dittrich S, et al. (2006) Chromatin domains and the interchromatin compartment form structurally defined and functionally interacting nuclear networks. Chromos. Res. 14: 707–713. doi: 10. 1007/s10577-006-1086-x

7. Cavalli G, Misteli T (2013) Functional implications of genome topology. Nat. Struct. Mol. Biol. 20: 290–299. doi: 10. 1038/nsmb. 2474. pmid:23463314

8. Lanctôt C, Cheutin T, Cremer M, Cavalli G, Cremer T (2007) Dynamic genome architecture in the nuclear space: regulation of gene expression in three dimensions. Nat. Rev. Genet. 8: 104–115. pmid:17230197 doi: 10. 1038/nrg2041

9. Postberg J, Lipps HJ, Cremer T (2010) Evolutionary origin of the cell nucleus and its functional architecture. Essays Biochem. 48: 1–24 doi: 10. 1042/bse0480001. pmid:20822483

10. Craig JM (2004) Haterochromatin-many flavours, common themes. BioEssays 27: 17–28. doi: 10. 1002/bies. 20145

11. Dimitri P, Caizzi R, Giordano E, Accardo MC, Lattanzi G, Biamonti G (2009) Constitutive heterochromatin: a surprising variety of expressed sequences. Chromosoma 118: 419–435 doi: 10. 1007/s00412-009-0211-y. pmid:19412619

12. Dimitri P, Corradini N, Rossi F, Verni F (2004) The paradox of functional heterochromatin. BioEssays 27: 29–41 doi: 10. 1002/bies. 20158

13. Du Toit A (2012) Chromatin: Defining heterochromatin. Nat Rev Mol Cell Biol 13: 684–685 doi: 10. 1038/nrm3452. pmid:23034452

14. Eissenberg JC, Elgin SCR (2014) Heterochromatin and Euchromatin. In: eLS. John Wiley & Sons Ltd, Chichester. http://www. els. net. doi: 10. 1002/9780470015902. a0001164. pub3.

15. Foster HA, Bridger JM (2005) The genome and the nucleus: a marriage made by evolution. Genome organisation and nuclear architecture. Chromosoma 114: 212–229. pmid:16133352 doi: 10. 1007/s00412-005-0016-6

16. Küpper K, Kölbl A, Biener D, Dittrich S, von Hase J, Thormeyer T, et al. (2007) Radial chromatin positioning is shaped by local gene density, not by gene expression. Chromosoma 116: 285–306. pmid:17333233 doi: 10. 1007/s00412-007-0098-4

17. Lukásová E, Kozubek S, Kozubek M, Falk M, Amrichová J (2002) The 3D structure of human chromosomes in cell nuclei. Chromosome Res 10: 535–548. pmid:12498343 doi: 10. 1023/a:1020958517788

18. Parada LA, McQueen PG, Munson PJ, Misteli T (2002) Conservation of relative chromosome positioning in normal and cancer cells. Curr Biol 12: 1692–1697. pmid:12361574 doi: 10. 1016/s0960-9822(02)01166-1

19. Bekker-Jensen S, Lukas C, Kitagawa R, Melander F, Kastan MB, Bartek J, et al. (2006) Spatial organization of the mammalian genome surveillance machinery in response to DNA strand breaks. J. Cell Biol. 173: 195–206. pmid:16618811 doi: 10. 1083/jcb. 200510130

20. Falk M, Lukasova E, Kozubek S (2010) Higher order chromatin structure in DSB induction, repair and misrepair. Mutat Res 704: 88–100. doi: 10. 1016/j. mrrev. 2010. 01. 013. pmid:20144732

21. Jerabek H, Heermann DW (2012), Expression-Dependent Folding of Interphase Chromatin, PLoS One 7: e37525 doi: 10. 1371/journal. pone. 0037525. pmid:22649534

22. Monajembashi S, Rapp A, Schmitt E, Dittmar H, Greulich KO, Hausmann M (2005) Spatial association of homologous pericentric regions in human lymphocyte nuclei during repair. Biophys. J. 88: 2309–2322 pmid:15626712 doi: 10. 1529/biophysj. 104. 048728

23. Schwarz-Finsterle J, Scherthan H, Huna A, González P, Müller P, Schmitt E, et al. (2013) Volume increase and spatial shifts of chromosome territories in nuclei of radiation-induced polyploidizing tumour cells. Mutat. Res. : Genet. Toxicol. Environ. Mutagen. 756: 56–65 doi: 10. 1016/j. mrgentox. 2013. 05. 004

24. Skalníková M, Kozubek S, Lukásová E, Bártová E, Jirsová P, Cafourková A, et al. (2000) Spatial arrangement of genes, centromeres and chromosomes in human blood cell nuclei and its changes during the cell cycle, differentiation and after irradiation. Chromos. Res. 8: 487–499.

25. Wiech T, Stein S, Lachenmaier V, Schmitt E, Schwarz-Finsterle J, Wiech E, et al. (2009) Spatial allelic imbalance of BCL2 genes and chromosome 18 territories in nonneoplastic and neoplastic cervical squamous epithelium. Eur. Biophys. J. 38: 793–806 doi: 10. 1007/s00249-009-0474-5. pmid:19495739

26. Falk M, Lukasova E, Gabrielova B, Ondrej V, Kozubek S (2007) Chromatin dynamics during DSB repair. Biochim Biophys Acta 1773: 1534–1545. pmid:17850903 doi: 10. 1016/j. bbamcr. 2007. 07. 002

27. Falk M, Lukasova E, Kozubek S (2008) Chromatin structure influences the sensitivity of DNA to γ-radiation. Biochim Biophys Acta 1783: 2398–2414. doi: 10. 1016/j. bbamcr. 2008. 07. 010. pmid:18706456

28. Falk M, Lukášová E, Stefančíková L, Baranová E, Falková I, et al. (2013) Heterochromatinization associated with cell differentiation as a model to study DNA double strand break induction and repair in the context of higher-order chromatin structure. Appl. Radiat. Isot. : doi: 10. 1016/j. apradiso. 2013. 01. 029.

29. Jakob B, Splinter J, Conrad S, Voss KO, Zink D, et al. (2011) DNA double-strand breaks in heterochromatin

elicit fast repair protein recruitment, histone H2AX phosphorylation and relocation to euchromatin. Nucleic Acids Res 39: 6489–6499. doi: 10. 1093/nar/gkr230. pmid:21511815

30. Rouquette J, Cremer C, Cremer T, Fakan S (2010) Functional nuclear architecture studied by microscopy: present and future. Int Rev Cell Mol Biol 282: 1–90. doi: 10. 1016/S1937-6448(10)82001-5. pmid:20630466

31. Ježková L, Falk M, Falková I, Davídková M, Bačíková A, Štefančíková L, et al. (2014) Function of chromatin structure and dynamics in DNA damage, repair and misrepair: γ-rays and protons in action. Appl. Radiat. Isot. : doi: 10. 1016/j. apradiso. 2013. 01. 022.

32. Girst S, Hable V, Drexler GA, Greubel C, Siebenwirth C, et al. (2013) Subdiffusion supports joining of correct ends during repair of DNA double-strand breaks. Scientific reports 3: 2511. doi: 10. 1038/srep02511. pmid:23979012

33. Bohn M, Diesinger P, Kaufmann R, Weiland Y, Müller P, Gunkel M, et al. (2010) Localization microscopy reveals expression-dependent parameters of chromatin nanostructure. Biophys. J. 99: 1358–1367 doi: 10. 1016/j. bpj. 2010. 05. 043. pmid:20816047

34. Abbe E (1873) Beiträge zur Theorie des Mikroskops und der mikroskopischen Wahrnehmung (Contributions to the theory of the microscope and microscopic observation). Archiv f. mikroskopische Anatomie 9: 411–468. doi: 10. 1007/bf02956176

35. Rayleigh L (1896) On the theory of optical images, with special reference to the microscope. Philos Mag 42: 167–195. doi: 10. 1080/14786449608620902

36. Cremer C, Masters BR (2013) Resolution enhancement techniques in microscopy. Eur Phys J H38: 281–344. doi: 10. 1140/epjh/e2012-20060-1

37. Deschout H, Zanacchi FC, Mlodzianoski M, Diaspro A, Bewersdorf J, Hess ST, et al. (2014) Precisely and accurately localizing single emitters in fluorescence microscopy. Nat Meth 11: 253–266. doi: 10. 1038/ nmeth. 2843

38. Schermelleh L, Heintzmann R, Leonhardt H (2010) A guide to super-resolution fluorescence microscopy. J Cell Biol 190: 165–175. doi: 10. 1083/jcb. 201002018. pmid:20643879

39. Cremer C, Kaufmann R, Gunkel M, Pres S, Weiland Y, Müller P, et al. (2011) Superresolution imaging of biological nanostructures by spectral precision distance microscopy. Biotechnol J 6:1037–1051. doi: 10. 1002/ biot. 201100031. pmid:21910256

40. Huang B, Wang W, Bates M, Zhuang X (2008) Three-Dimensional Super-Resolution Imaging by Stochastic Optical Reconstruction Microscopy. Science 319: 810–813. doi: 10. 1126/science. 1153529. pmid:18174397

41. Esa A, Edelmann P, Kreth G, Trakhtenbrot L, Amariglio N, Rechavi G, et al. (2000) Three-dimensional spectral precision distance microscopy of chromatin nanostructures after triple-colour DNA labelling: a study of the BCR region on chromosome 22 and the Philadelphia chromosome. J Microsc 199: 96–105. pmid:10947902 doi: 10. 1046/j. 1365-2818. 2000. 00707. x

42. Heilemann M, Herten DP, Heintzmann R, Cremer C, Mueller C, Tinnefeld P, et al. (2002) High-resolution colocalization of single dye molecules by fluorescence lifetime imaging microscopy. Analyt Chem 74: 3511–3517. pmid:12139062 doi: 10. 1021/ac025576g

43. Betzig E, Patterson GH, Sougrat R, Lindwasser OW, Olenych S, Bonifacino J, et al. (2006) Imaging intracellular fluorescent proteins at nanometer resolution. Science 313:1642–1645. pmid:16902090 doi: 10. 1126/ science. 1127344

44. Hess ST, Girirajan TP, Mason MD (2006) Ultra-high resolution imaging by fluorescence photoactivation localization microscopy. Biophys J 91:4258–4272. pmid:16980368 doi: 10. 1529/biophysj. 106. 091116

45. Rust MJ, Bates M, Zhuang X (2006) Sub-diffraction-limit imaging by stochastic optical reconstruction microscopy (STORM). Nature Meth 3: 793–795. doi: 10. 1038/nmeth929

46. Lemmer P, Gunkel M, Baddeley D, Kaufmann R, Urich A, Weiland Y, et al. (2008) SPDM–light microscopy with single molecule resolution at the nanoscale. Appl Phys B 93: 1–12. doi: 10. 1007/s00340-008-3152-x

47. Lemmer P, Gunkel M, Weiland Y, Müller P, Baddeley D, Kaufmann R, et al. (2009) Using conventional fluorescent markers for far-field fluorescence localization nanoscopy allows resolution in the 10 nm range. J Microsc 235: 163–171. doi: 10. 1111/j. 1365-2818. 2009. 03196. x. pmid:19659910

48. Fölling J, Bossi M, Bock H, Medda R, Wurm C, Hein B, et al. (2008) Fluorescence nanoscopy by ground-state depletion and single-molecule return. Nature Methods 5: 943–945. doi: 10. 1038/nmeth. 1257. pmid:18794861

49. Kaufmann R, Lemmer P, Gunkel M, Weiland Y, Müller P, Hausmann M, et al. (2009) SPDM–Single molecule superresolution of cellular nanostructures. Proc. SPIE 7185: 71850J1–71850J19 doi: 10. 1117/12. 809109.

50. Hendrix J, Flors C, Dedecker P, Hofkens J, Engelborghs Y (2008) Dark states in monomeric red fluorescent proteins studied by fluorescence correlation and single molecule spectroscopy. Biophys J 94: 4103–4113. doi: 10. 1529/biophysj. 107. 123596. pmid:18234806

51. Sinnecker D, Voigt P, Hellwig N, Schaefer M (2005) Reversible photobleaching of enhanced green fluorescent proteins. Biochemistry 44: 7085–7094. pmid:15865453 doi: 10. 1021/bi047881x

52. Kaufmann R, Müller P, Hildenbrand G, Hausmann M, Cremer C (2011) Analysis of Her2/neu membrane protein clusters in different types of breast cancer cells using localization microscopy. J Microsc 242: 46–54. doi: 10. 1111/j. 1365-2818. 2010. 03436. x. pmid:21118230

53. Müller P, Lemmermann NA, Kaufmann R, Gunkel M, Paech D, Hildenbrand G, et al. (2014) Spatial distribution and structural arrangement of a murine cytomegalovirus glycoprotein detected by SPDM localization microscopy. Histochem. Cell Biol. 142: 61–67. doi: 10. 1007/s00418-014-1185-2. pmid:24504601

54. Müller P, Weiland Y, Kaufmann R, Gunkel M, Hillebrandt S, Cremer C, et al. (2012) Analysis of fluorescent nanostructures in biological systems by

means of Spectral Position Determination Microscopy (SPDM). In: "Current microscopy contributions to advances in science and technology" (Méndez-Vilas A, ed.), Vol. 1: 3–12.

55. Baddeley D, Cannell MB, Soeller C (2010) Visualization of localization microscopy data. Microsc Microanal 16: 64–72. doi: 10. 1017/S143192760999122X. pmid:20082730

56. Kaufmann R, Piontek J, Grüll F, Kirchgessner M, Rossa J, Wolburg H, et al. (2012) Visualization and quantitative analysis of reconstituted tight junctions using localization microscopy. PLoS One 7: e31128. doi: 10. 1371/journal. pone. 0031128. pmid:22319608

57. Knoch TA (2002) Approaching the Three-Dimensional Organization of the Human Genome. Heidelberg, TAK Press, 3-00-009959-X.

58. Fejes-Toth KF, Knoch TA, Wachsuth M, Frank-Stohr M, Stohr M, Bacher CP, et al. (2004) Trichostatin A-induced histone acetylation causes decondensation of interphase chromatin. Cell Sci. 117: 4277–87. pmid:15292402 doi: 10. 1242/jcs. 01293

59. Weidemann T, Wachsmuth M, Knoch TA, Mueller G, Waldeck W, Langowski J (2003) Counting Nucleosomes in Living Cells with a Combinaiton of Fluorescence Correlation Spectroscopy and Confocal Imaging. J. Mol. Biol, 334, s. l. : pp. 229–240. pmid:14607115 doi: 10. 1016/j. jmb. 2003. 08. 063

60. Scott DW (1992) Multivariate densitz estimation, Wiley, New York, ISBN 0471547700

61. West DB (2000) Introduction to Graph Theory, Prentice Hall, ISBN 0130144002

62. Bajardi P, Poletto C, Ramasco JJ, Tizzoni M, Colizza V, Vespignani A (2011) Human mobility networks, travel restrictions, and the global spread of 2009 h1n1 pandemic. PLoS ONE, 6(1):e16591. doi: 10. 1371/journal. pone. 0016591. pmid:21304943

63. Buldyrev SV, Parshani R, Paul G, Stanley HE, Havlin S (2010) Catastrophic cascade of failures in interdependent networks. Nature, 464(7291):1025–1028. doi: 10. 1038/nature08932. pmid:20393559

64. O'Roak BJ, Vives L, Girirajan S, Karakoc E, Krumm N, Coe BP, et al. (2012) Sporadic autism exomes reveal a highly interconnected protein network of de novo mutations. Nature, 485(7397):246–250. doi: 10. 1038/nature10989. pmid:22495309

65. Vespignani A (2012) Modelling dynamical processes in complex sociotechnical systems. Nat Phys, 8(1):32–39 doi: 10. 1038/nphys2160

66. Vinayagam A, Stelzl U, Foulle R, Plassmann S, Zenkner M, Timm J, et al. (2011) A directed protein interaction network for investigating intracellular signal transduction. Science Signaling, 4(189):rs8. doi: 10. 1126/scisignal. 2001699. pmid:21900206

67. Delaunay B (1934) Sur la sphere vide. Izvestia Akademii Nauk SSSR, Otdelenie Matematicheskikh i Estestvennykh Nauk, 6: 793–800.

68. Aurenhammer F (1991) Voronoi diagrams–a survey of a fundamental geometric data structure. Acm Computing Surveys, 23(3):345–405 doi: 10. 1145/116873. 116880

69. Jakob B, Splinter J, Durante M, Taucher-Scholz G (2009) Live cell microscopy analysis of radiation-induced DNA double-strand break motion. Proc Natl Acad Sci U S A 106: 3172–3177. doi: 10. 1073/pnas. 0810987106. pmid:19221031

70. Jakob B, Splinter J, Taucher-Scholz G (2009) Positional stability of damaged chromatin domains along radiation tracks in mammalian cells. Radiat Res 171: 405–418. doi: 10. 1667/RR1520. 1. pmid:19397441

71. Zhang Y, Heermann DW (2014) DNA Double-Strand Breaks: Linking Gene Expression to Chromosome Morphology and Mobility. Chromosoma, 123(1–2): 103–15 doi: 10. 1007/s00412-014-0480-y. pmid:25106753

72. Kozubek S, Lukásová E, Jirsová P, Koutná I, Kozubek M, et al. (2002) 3D Structure of the human genome: order in randomness. Chromosoma 111: 321–331. pmid:12474061 doi: 10. 1007/s00412-002-0210-8

73. Grunzke R, Hesser J, Starek J, Kepper N, Gesing S, Hardt M, et al. (2014) Device-driven metadate management solution for scientific big data use cases. 22nd Euromicro Int. Conf. Parallel, Distributed, and Network-Based Processing (PDP 2014), February 2014, Turin, Italy. IEEE Comp. Soc. Proc. PDP 2014: 317–321 (doi: 10. 1109/PDP. 2014. 119)

74. Hausmann M, Müller P, Kaufmann R, Cremer C (2013) Entering the nano-cosmos of the cell by means of spatial position determination microscopy (SPDM): Implications for medical diagnostics and radiation research. IFMBE Proc 38: 93–95. doi: 10. 1007/978-3-642-34197-7_24

CHAPTER 13 THERAPEUTIC APPLICATION OF CCK2R-TARGETING PP-F11

Mark W. Konijnenberg, Wout A. P. Breeman, Erik de Blois, Ho Sze Chan, Otto C. Boerman, Peter Laverman, Petra Kolenc-Peitl, Marleen Melis, and Marion de Jong

Keywords: Preclinical radionuclide dosimetry, Radiobiology, Tumour cure model, Specific activityCCK2 peptide receptor saturation, Y-90, Lu-177, Bi-213, Minigastrin

BACKGROUND

PP-F11, a minigastrin analogue, was identified to be one of the most promising cholecystokinin 2 (CCK2) receptor-binding peptides to target medullary thyroid cancer (MTC) and small cell lung cancer lesions in a comparative search by the EU COST Action BM0607 [1]. Low retention in the kidneys by PP-F11 could be achieved by replacement of the gastrin pentaglutamic acid sequence in minigastrins with five d-glutamic acid residues. Indeed in nude mice, ^{111}In-PP-F11 showed low retention in the kidneys in combination with a high uptake in A431 xenografts transfected with the CCK2 receptor in comparison with other minigastrin analogues. The tumour and physiological organ uptake was measured at 1 and 4 h after injection of 370 kBq/0.03 nmol ^{111}In-labelled PP-F11. Moreover, in vitro cell uptake experiments showed a high affinity of PP-F11 for the CCK2 receptor and a high internalisation rate into CCK2 receptor-transfected A431 cells [2]. The next step towards clinical application of peptide receptor radionuclide therapy (PRRT) using this compound is a PRRT study in mice.

Preclinical PRRT studies are typically being performed in mice with tumours bearing an initial size of 8 to 9 mm in diameter, which corresponds to a spherical volume of 270 to 380 mm^3, but due to different growth patterns, tumours in different animals may show large variation in size.

Low-energy beta-emitting radionuclides, such as ^{177}Lu and ^{131}I, are considered favourable to maximise the absorbed dose in tumours of this small size. For pragmatic reasons, the choice for a therapeutic radionuclide is often between the beta-emitters ^{90}Y and ^{177}Lu, as both are readily available. The latter choice (^{177}Lu) seems to be optimal, as the mean beta-energy of 0.133 MeV yields a high probability of cure in the 1- to 3-mm (0.5 to 14 mm^3) size range [3]. The high-energy beta-emitter ^{90}Y (0.933 MeV) shows optimal tumour control in the 28- to 42-mm range. Neither ^{213}Bi nor any other α-emitter was evaluated in the paper by O›Donoghue et al., but with the availability of ^{225}Ac generators [4] the short-range emitter ^{213}Bi has become a very interesting radionuclide for PRRT as well.

The theoretical prediction of [3] was confirmed in preclinical studies of somatostatin receptor-mediated PRRT comparing the therapeutic effects of ^{177}Lu-DOTA,Tyr^3-octreotate (DOTAtate) and ^{90}Y-DOTA,Tyr^3-octreotide (DOTAtoc) in large and small tumours implanted in rats [5],[6]. With ^{90}Y, the ideal tumour size for cure was found to be 3 to 9 cm^2 (length × width, product of the two largest perpendicular diameters), which corresponds to spherical tumours with diameters between 20 and 34 mm and masses between 4 and 20 g. The absorbed dose to these tumours was between 48 and 60 Gy. With ^{177}Lu, a more favourable response rate was found in rats bearing smaller tumours (size <1 cm or mass <0.5 g) compared with those bearing larger tumour masses. The absorbed dose to these small tumours was about 58 Gy.

Citation: Mark W. Konijnenberg, Wout A. P. Breeman, Erik de Blois, Ho Sze Chan, Otto C. Boerman, Peter Laverman, Petra Kolenc-Peitl, Marleen Melis, and Marion de Jong. Therapeutic application of CCK2R-targeting PP-F11, EJNMMI Research, (2014); 4: 47. DOI:10.1186/s13550-014-0047-1.

We reasoned for the PRRT study that the ideal β-emitting radionuclide for labelling PP-F11 should be selected taking into account not only the absorbed radiation dose, but also the relation between the uptake kinetics in various sizes of tumours and the peptide amount to be injected. The specific activity achievable for each radionuclide dictates the peptide amount to be injected for a tumour radiation dose of 60 Gy; tumour cure is not always possible with the same peptide amount of 0.03 nmol (corresponding to 0.1 μg) as was used in the biodistribution study. Especially, neutron capture reactor-produced radionuclides show a limitation in the maximum achievable specific activity [7]. The specific activity of the peptide should be optimized to achieve the highest possible absorbed dose to the tumour taking both the peptide mass with maximum receptor-mediated uptake and the maximum achievable specific activity into account. It is well known that unlabelled peptide will compete with the labelled peptide for the limited number of receptors and thereby reduce the uptake in target tissue [8]-[11].

Estimation of the optimal therapy setting has been performed in this study for preclinical testing of PP-F11, assumed to be labelled with either ^{90}Y, ^{177}Lu or ^{213}Bi. The absorbed dose in small tumours was determined, assuming the same biodistribution profile for all radiolabelled analogues and taking the influence of peptide amount on its pharmacokinetics into account as well as the radiation transport of the emitted spectra. The aim of this study was to determine which radionuclide is capable of reaching tumour-sterilizing absorbed radiation doses to the tumour of at least 60 Gy, as such a dose is expected to lead to a high probability of tumour cure over a wide range of tumour sizes according to the linear-quadratic (LQ) model (from 1 to 500 mm^3) [3],[6]. For this purpose, the most important parameters influencing the dose-effect relation for curing tumours have to be determined. In this study, only the mean absorbed dose to the tumour was taken into account, without correction for possible microdosimetry induced enhancements of the absorbed dose effects by high linear energy transfer (LET) spectra and/or bystander effects.

METHODS

Peptide Synthesis

The synthesis of the peptide PP-F11 has been described before by Kolenc-Peitl et al. [1],[12]. In summary, PP-F11 was synthesized using standard Fmoc-based solid-phase peptide synthesis and conjugated with 1,4,7,10-tetraazacyclododecane-1,4,7,10-tetraacetic acid (DOTA), using one of the carboxylic groups of DOTA. The peptide structure was confirmed by mass spectrometry and NMR. The amino acid sequence of PP-F11 is DOTA-DGlu-DGlu-DGlu-DGlu-DGlu-DGlu-Ala-Tyr-Gly-Trp-Met-Asp-Phe-NH2, and its molecular weight is 2,049 g/mol.

Radiolabelling

DOTA-conjugated peptides were radiolabelled with ^{111}In by incubation with $^{111}InCl_3$ (Covidien, Petten, The Netherlands) in 0.25 M ammonium acetate buffer, pH 5.0 under strict metal-free conditions. To reduce oxidation of the peptides during radiolabelling, 100 μg (10 μl) selenomethionine was added. The labelling mixture was incubated for 30 min at 95°C. After incubation, 50 mM EDTA was added to a final concentration of 5 mM. Radiochemical purity and the presence of oxidized peptide were checked on an HPLC system (1200 series LC system; Agilent Technologies, Palo Alto, CA, USA) equipped with an Alltima RP-C18 column (5 μm, 4.6 × 250 mm; Alltech, Deerfield, IL, USA) and an in-line NaI radiodetector (Raytest, Straubenhardt, Germany). A gradient from 0.1% trifluoroacetic acid in water to 0.1% trifluoroacetic acid in acetonitrile was used. The maximum specific activity of the peptide was 11 GBq/μmol.

Biodistribution Studies

Biodistribution and tumour targeting of the ^{111}In-labelled PP-F11 were studied in female athymic BALB/c mice with subcutaneous tumours induced by inoculation of A431 cells. Mice were inoculated with 2 × 10^6 A431-CCK2R cells (0.2 ml) in the left flank and with A431 mock-transfected cells in the right flank. After approximately 10 days, when the tumours had reached a weight of approximately 100 to 200 mg, the mice were randomly divided into groups of five mice. The mice were injected intravenously with 370 kBq (0.03 nmol) of ^{111}In-labelled peptide via the lateral tail vein. In an additional experiment, six groups of mice were injected with 370 kBq/0.05 nmol ^{111}In-PP-F11 supplemented with an increasing amount (range: 3, 10, 30, 100, and 300 times) of molar excess of the unlabelled PP-F11 to determine the receptor saturation effect as well as the non-receptor specific uptake in CCK2 receptor-expressing tissues. Mice were killed by CO_2 asphyxiation at 1 and 4 h after administration in the biodistribution study and after 2 h in the receptor saturation study. A blood sample was drawn, and organs of interest and the tumour were dissected, weighed and counted in a gamma counter. The animal experiments were approved by the local animal welfare committee and performed according to national regulations.

Dosimetry

Tumour Absorbed Dose Rate S-factors

Absorbed fractions of energy emitted from ^{90}Y, ^{111}In, ^{177}Lu, ^{213}Bi and its daughters were determined in a spherical geometry using the Monte Carlo code MCNP5 (version 1.4 [13]). The mean absorbed energies were calculated for spherical tumours of 1, 10, 100, 200, 300 and 500 mg containing ICRU-44 tissue [14] assuming an average tissue mass density of 1 g/ml. The emission spectra were taken from the Medical Internal Radiation Dose (MIRD) radionuclide data and decay schemes book [15]. The main characteristics of the emissions by ^{90}Y, ^{111}In, ^{177}Lu,^{213}Bi and its daughters ^{213}Po, ^{209}Pb and ^{209}Tl are listed in Table 1. Electrons and photons with an energy below 1 keV were assumed to be absorbed at the site of emission. The total energy emitted by electrons below 1 keV in the spectra from ^{111}In and ^{177}Lu is added to the absorbed energy by the higher energy electrons. The default settings for electron and photon physics within MCNP were used, with the exception of the electron energy straggling logic, where the option `DBCN 17J 2' was used to be independent of pre-set energy boundaries [16],[17]. For each component in the emission spectra, 10 million histories were calculated to keep the statistical variance below 5%.

Table 1. Emission spectra and decay half-lives of ^{90}Y, ^{111}In, ^{177}Lu and ^{213}Bi and its daughters

Radionuclide	Decay $T_{1/2}$	Radiation	Yield (/decay)	$E_{av.}$ (MeV)	E_{max} (MeV)
^{90}Y	64.1 h	β^-	1	0.9329	2.2801
^{111}In	67.3 h	γ	0.906	0.1713	
		γ	0.941	0.2454	
		Auger e$^-$ <1 keV	6.26	0.000159	
		Electrons >1 keV	1.33	0.0255	
		X-rays <1 keV	8.60	0.000017	
		X-rays >1 keV	0.901	0.0220	
^{177}Lu	159.5 h	β^-	1	0.1333	0.4978
		γ	0.064	0.1129	
		γ	0.11	0.2084	
		Auger e$^-$ <1 keV	0.819	0.000138	
		Electrons >1 keV	0.452	0.0322	
^{213}Bi	45.59 min	α	0.00155	5.55187	
		α	0.01935	5.86959	
		β^-	0.9791	0.4339	1.4220
		γ	0.261	0.44046	
		Auger e$^-$ <1 keV	0.474	0.000113	
		Electrons >1 keV	0.152	0.1261	
^{213}Po	4.2 µs	α	1	8.38	
^{209}Pb	3.253 h	β^-	1	0.1974	0.6444
^{209}Tl	2.161 min	γ	0.998	1.57	
		γ	0.969	0.465	
		γ	0.843	0.117	
		Auger e$^-$ <1 keV	2.64	0.000108	
		Electrons >1 keV	0.830	0.0384	

Energies are indicated for the beta ray (mean and maximum), Auger electrons, low-energy electrons and X-ray spectra. Below the cut-off value of 1 keV, all energy is assumed to be absorbed at the site of emission. Only gamma rays with an emission yield of more than 0.01/decay are indicated.

The absorbed energy distribution was determined in each spherical tumour by using 25 equal-volume concentric spherical shells within the source volume and 25 equal-volume spherical shells around the tumour extending to a radial distance of 1 cm as a consistency check of the electron transport model used. Absorbed dose rate per unit activity S-factors was calculated according to the equation: $S = k\frac{\sum_i y_i E_i \phi_i}{m}$, where k is a conversion factor to dose, ϕ_i is the absorbed fraction of emitted energy E_i that is emitted with yield y_i, and m is the mass of the spherical shell part. The dose to the tumour is calculated according to the MIRD scheme by the product of the cumulated activity Ã and the absorbed dose S-factor D = Ã × S = A_0 × Ã × S, where A_0 is the administered activity and Ã is the time-integrated activity coefficient (TIAC; formerly indicated by residence time τ) of the radioactivity in the tumour [18].

Influence of Peptide Kinetics and Receptor Saturation on Dosimetry

The cumulated activity in the tumour Ã is based on the ^{111}In-PP-F11 biodistribution data at 1 and 4 h for a peptide mass of 0.03 nmol (0.1 µg) (Figure 1A) [5]. In mice with s.c. CCK2 receptor-expressing A431 tumours, the radiolabelled PP-F11 showed a high tumour uptake and retention (9.7 × 1.8 and 6.3 × 2.8%ID/g, 1 and 4 h p.i.), which was among the highest of the 12 CCK2 analogues considered [1]. Based on the two time points, two possible biodistribution patterns were applied to evaluate the consequence of different kinetic profiles. The first approach was a mono-exponential curve with a biological clearance half-life of 4.9 × 2.3 h (Figure 1B). For the second approach, an additional slower clearance compartment was assumed with a clearance half-life of 150 h, being the median curve between the single exponential and the situation with just physical decay after 4 h, indicated in Figure 1C. As not only the clearance kinetics, but also the uptake kinetics will influence the cumulated activity, especially for the shortest half-life radionuclide ^{213}Bi (Figure 1B), additionally the effect of both slow and fast uptake kinetics was considered.

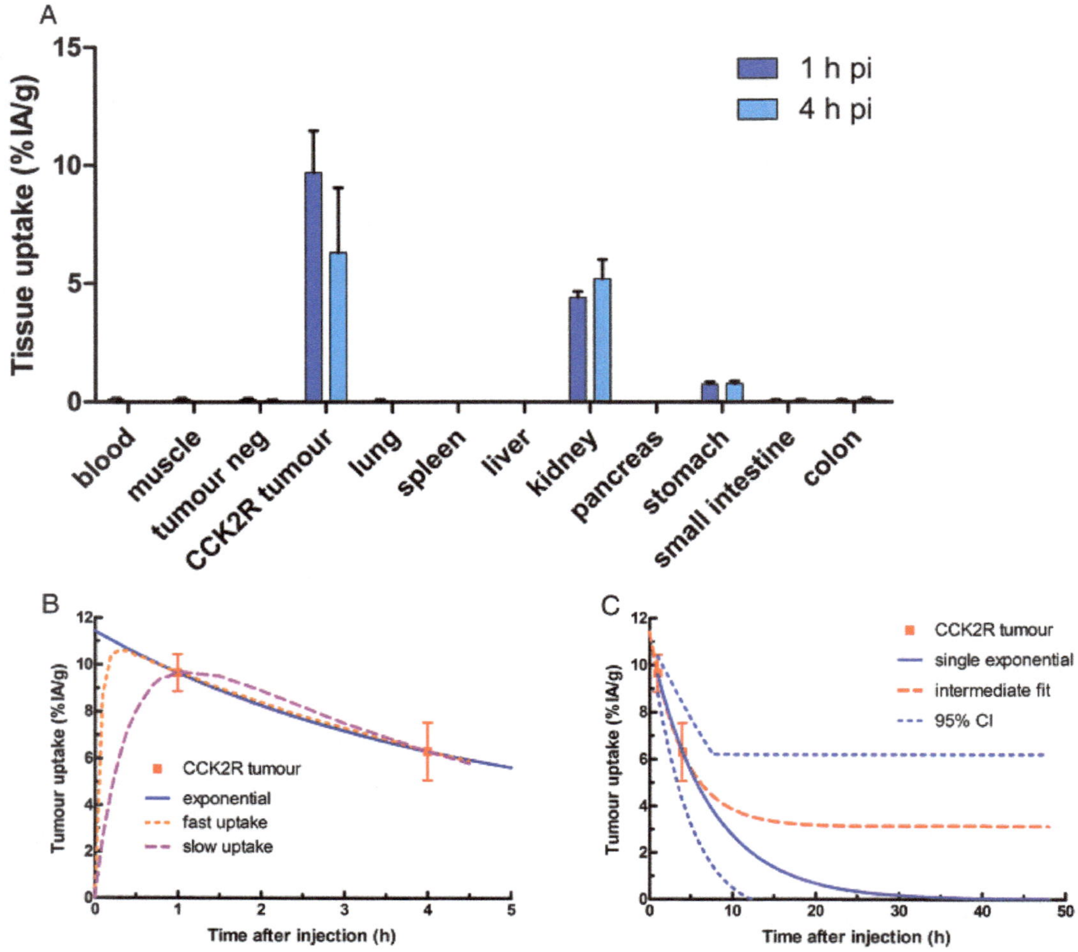

Figure 1. Biodistribution and kinetic profile. (A) Biodistribution of 0.03 nmol ^{111}In-labelled PP-F11 in nude mice with CCK2R-transfected A431 tumour xenografts at 1 and at 4 h (reproduced from [1]). (B) Kinetic profile of radioactivity uptake in the CCK2 receptor-positive tumour xenograft with three options that are considered for the uptake phase: single-exponential, fast uptake with $T_{1/2}$ of 2.7 min and slow uptake with $T_{1/2}$ of 17 min.(C) Variance in kinetic profile of the radioactivity clearance from the tumour: the solid blue curve shows the single exponential with $T_{1/2}$ of 4.9 h, the middle dashed red curve shows the double exponential with final clearance $T_{1/2}$ of 150 h and the blue dotted curves show the 95% confidence interval for the tumour clearance.

The in vivo behaviour of PP-F11 labelled with ^{90}Y, ^{177}Lu or ^{213}Bi was assumed to be equivalent to that of ^{111}In-labelled PP-F11.

The tumour uptake concentration data ([B]) as a function of peptide mass (M_p) was fitted to the sigmoid-shaped one-site competition curve:

$$[B(M_p)] = [B_{unsp}] + \frac{[B_{spec}]}{1 + \frac{M_p}{ED_{50}}}, \tag{1}$$

where $[B_{unsp}]$ is the unspecific-bound concentration asymptote at high peptide mass, $[B_{spec}]$ is the receptor-bound concentration, and ED_{50} is the peptide mass that lowers the tumour concentration by 50%. This curve gives an indication of the limited number of receptors available.

Activity for 60-Gy Tumour Dose

The amount of activity needed with each radionuclide to obtain a radiation dose of 60 Gy in a 300-mg tumour is derived for the dosimetry according to the 0.03 nmol peptide mass biodistribution. The dosimetry is adjusted according to the peptide mass needed to label the peptide at a practically achievable specific activity using the logarithmic receptor saturation function. Traditionally, the activity $A_0(M_p)$ needed to obtain an absorbed dose D in a tumour with mass m and using the biodistribution for a peptide mass of $M_p = 0.03$ nmol is obtained by:

$$A_0(0.03) = \frac{D}{\tilde{a}_m S(m \leftarrow m).} \tag{2}$$

The relation for $A_0(M_p)$ as a function of the peptide mass M_p changes for the maximum (achievable) specific activity A_{sp} at both sides of the equation:

$$A_0(M_p) = M_p \times A_{sp} = \frac{[B(0.03)]D}{[B(M_p)]\tilde{a}_m S(m \leftarrow m).} \tag{3}$$

This equation can be solved to obtain the amount of peptide mass M_p needed with specific activity A_{sp} that will deliver a dose D in a tumour with mass m. Not only the absorbed dose but also the amount of peptide, the specific activity used and the total number of receptor binding sites available are of importance. It is assumed the shape of the kinetics does not change with peptide mass, just the uptake value itself. The maximum and practically achievable specific activities for labelling peptides with ^{111}In, ^{90}Y and ^{177}Lu are indicated in Table 2, as obtained from Breeman et al. [7]. Maximum specific activity is reached when 1 nmol of DOTA incorporates 1 nmol of radionuclide. In practice, the specific activity is severely hampered by the reaction kinetics and challenged uptake by contaminants in the radionuclide solution, either from target material or from radioactive decay products. The highest practically achievable specific activity is obtained with ^{111}In, and ^{90}Y shows an almost four times higher specific activity (SA) than ^{177}Lu. The administered amount of peptide per injection was maximised at 0.5 nmol (1.02 µg) to stay within practically feasible limits in both volume and radioactivity. The practical limit in specific activity of ^{213}Bi-labelled peptides was obtained at our institute with a 220 MBq ^{225}Ac generator.

Table 2. Production methods and specific activities (SA) of ^{90}Y, ^{111}In, ^{177}Lu and ^{213}Bi, both per nmol PP-F11 with 2,049 g/mol

	^{90}Y	^{111}In	^{177}Lu	^{213}Bi
Production route	Elution from ^{90}Sr generator	Cyclotron $^{112}Cd(p,2n)^{111}In$	Reactor $^{176}Lu(n,\gamma)^{177}Lu$	Elution from ^{225}Ac generator
Maximum SA (GBq/nmol)	1.8	1.7	0.73	153
Practical SA (MBq/nmol)	400	800	120	40

The practical achievable SA of ^{213}Bi with peptide is much lower than after labelling with ^{90}Y, ^{111}In or ^{177}Lu, due to the at least twice higher reaction volume with ^{213}Bi. The elution volume of the generator is fixed at approximately 600 µl, dependent on the generator bed volume in the preclinical setting using a 220 MBq ^{225}Ac generator. Generators containing higher amount of ^{225}Ac activity have larger bed volumes and higher elution volumes [4],[19]. High labelling volume or low concentration of the labelled compounds results in poor reaction kinetics of the labelling, which can be solved by increasing the temperature or taking a longer reaction time. However, at a very high temperature, denaturation of biological materials might occur, and in the case of ^{213}Bi, a longer reaction time will result in decay of activity. By reducing the elution volume and reaction time of ^{213}Bi labelling, a higher SA can be achieved. Presently, the time between elution and injection in the animal is in the order of 30 min, by which already 36% of the initial ^{213}Bi radioactivity has decayed.

Tumour Control Probability Model

The suitability of the radionuclide for treating a tumour xenograft is investigated by constraining the tumour control probability (TCP) to at least 90% according to [3],[20],[21]:

$$\text{TCP} = \exp\left(-N_{\text{clonogens}}S(D)\right), \tag{4}$$

$$\text{with } S(D) = \exp\left(-\alpha D\left(1+\frac{G}{\left(\frac{\alpha}{\beta}\right)}\times\frac{D}{N}\right)\right), \tag{4a}$$

$$\text{with } G = \begin{cases} \dfrac{T_\mu}{T_\mu + T_{\text{eff}}} \\ \dfrac{\dfrac{T_\mu}{T_\mu+T_1}(T_1A_1)^2 + 2\dfrac{T_\mu T_1 T_2(T_\mu T_1 + T_\mu T_2 + T_1T_2)}{(T_\mu+T_1)(T_\mu+T_2)(T_1+T_2)}A_1A_2 + \dfrac{T_\mu}{T_\mu+T_2}(T_2A_2)^2}{(T_1A_1+T_2A_2)^2} \end{cases} \tag{4b}$$

The survival S of clonogenic cells as a function of dose D in the tumour is described by the linear-quadratic model. The dose per fraction D/N is used in the quadratic term to allow correction for fractionation of the therapy. The dose prolongation or Lea-Catcheside factor G is used to adjust the quadratic part of the LQ model for radionuclide-induced dose rates. During the exposure with effective half-life T_{eff}, sub-lethal damage is being repaired according to an exponential function with repair half-life T_μ. The single-exponential clearance with effective half-life T_{eff} is indicated in Equation 4a for G. Equation 4b is for a bi-exponential clearance curve with effective half-lives T_1 and T_2 and amplitudes A_1 and A_2. The second expression for G(4b) can be modified to take the uptake kinetics into account, with $A_2 = -A_1$ and $A(t) = A_1\left(e^{-\lambda_1 t} - e^{-\lambda_2 t}\right)$, which leads to

$$G = \frac{T_\mu(T_1T_\mu + T_2T_\mu + T_1T_2)}{(T_1+T_2)(T_1+T_\mu)(T_2+T_\mu)}. \tag{5}$$

In this work, the clonogenic cell density is assumed to be 10% of the total cell density of 10^9/g. The following LQ model parameters were considered: $\alpha = 0.27\ Gy^{-1}$, $\alpha/\beta = 6$ Gy and $T_\mu = 0.5$ h (squamous cells, see [22]). The repair half-life of 0.5 h is in the lower range for tumour sub-lethal repair half-lives [23].

Effect of Tumour Growth on TCP

Correction of TCP for tumour growth with doubling time T_D during the dose accumulation was made by including the tumour growth in the LQ model equation for cell survival:

$$S(D,T) = \exp\left(-\alpha D(T)\left(1+\frac{G}{\alpha/\beta}\times\frac{D(T)}{N}\right)+\gamma T\right), \tag{6}$$

where $\gamma = \ln(2)/T_D$ and T is the irradiation time. Overall, the TCP is adjusted by taking the power with $e^{\gamma T_{irr}}$ the growth of the tumour during the effective irradiation time T_{irr} when the slope, or derivative, of the cell survival curve remains positive, as the radiation effect outweighs the tumour growth [24]. The tumour doubling time for the A431-CCK2R cells was determined to be 4 days [25]. Only the absorbed dose delivered to the tumour before the irradiation timeT_{irr} has passed can be considered effective in cell kill. Therefore, both the absorbed dose and the TCP were corrected for the efficacious dose D_{eff} and the tumour growth during the irradiation time, with:

$$D_{\text{eff}} = S(m \leftarrow m) \int_{T_0}^{T_{\text{irr}}} A(t)dt. \tag{7}$$

In the case that it was impossible to give curative doses with the radionuclide in one administration, a treatment interval of 24 h between subsequent injections was assumed with unaltered growth in the treatment gap in between.

RESULTS

Biodistribution Studies

In mice with s.c. CCK2 receptor-expressing A431 tumours, the radiolabelled PP-F11 showed a high tumour uptake and retention (9.7 × 1.8 and 6.3 × 2.8%ID/g, 1 and 4 h p.i.) [1]. The mono-exponential curve with a biological clearance half-life of 4.9 × 2.3 h (Figure 1B) leads to higher cumulative activities for the shorter half-life radionuclides such as ^{90}Y and ^{213}Bi in comparison to ^{177}Lu. An additional clearance compartment was assumed with a clearance half-life of 150 h, being a median curve between the single exponential and the situation with just physical decay after 4 h, indicated in Figure 1C. Not only the clearance kinetics but also the uptake kinetics will influence the cumulated activity, especially for the shortest half-life radionuclide ^{213}Bi (Figure1B). The effect of both slow and fast uptake on the cumulated activity was considered.

The effect of increasing PP-F11 peptide mass on the uptake of the radiolabelled peptide in the tumour and the normal tissues is shown in Figure 2A. In the CCK2R-expressing tumour and stomach, the radioactivity uptake decreased with increasing peptide dose injected. This decrease was fitted with one-site dissociation curves (Equation 1) shown in Figures 2B,C.

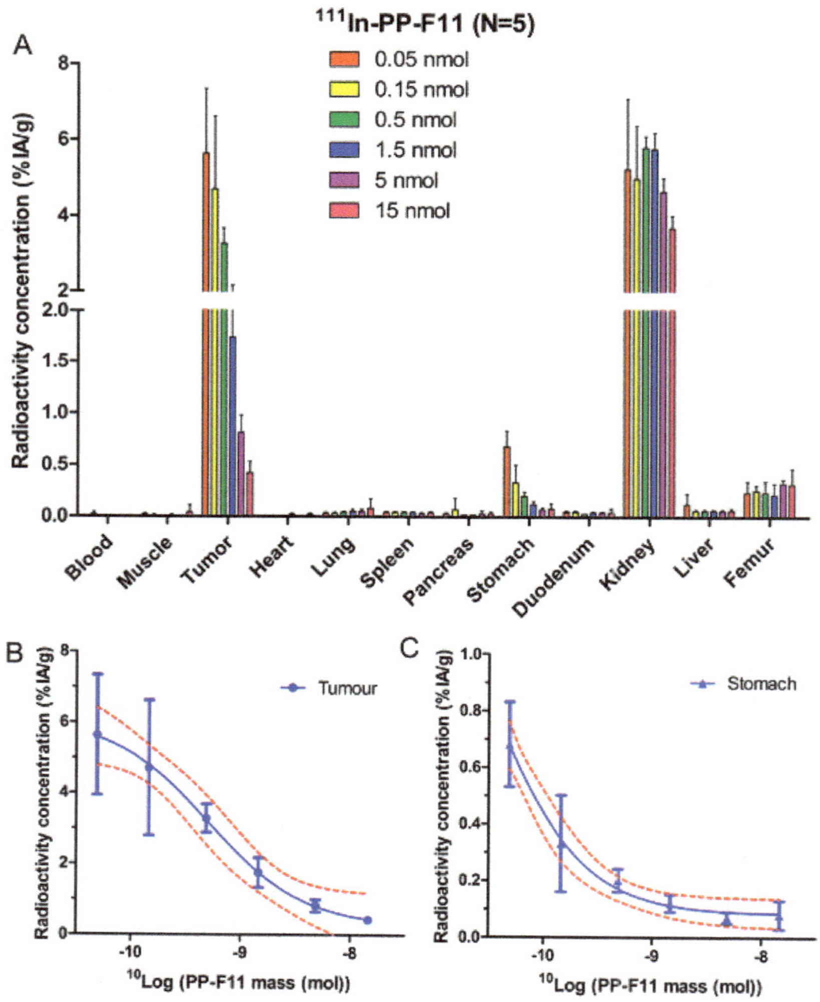

Figure 2. Biodistribution and fit of displacement curve. (A) Biodistribution of ^{111}In-labelled PP-F11 with increasing excess unlabelled peptide in nude mice (N = 5) with CCK2R-transfected A431 tumour xenografts at 2 h after injection, showing saturation of uptake in the CCK2R tumours and stomach. (B) Fit of displacement radioactivity curve to the CCK2R tumour xenograft data with $\log(ED_{50}) = -9.30 \times 0.19$ (ED_{50} = 0.51 nmol (95% CI: 0.2 to 1.2), correlation $R^2 = 0.80$). **(C)** Fit of displacement curve to stomach uptake data with $\log(ED_{50}) = -10.54 \times 0.38$ (ED_{50} = 0.03 nmol (0.005 to 0.17), $R^2 = 0.85$). Error bars indicate standard deviations of the mean values.

Dosimetry

Absorbed Dose in Tumours

Absorbed dose rates per MBq activity (S-values) were calculated for ^{90}Y, ^{111}In, ^{177}Lu, ^{213}Bi, ^{213}Po, ^{209}Pb and ^{209}Tl in small spherical tumours and are indicated in Table 3. For ^{111}In and ^{177}Lu, almost the complete emitted internal conversion electron and beta-energy are absorbed in the largest sphere, whereas for ^{90}Y, only 61% of the emitted energy is absorbed. In the 1-mg sphere the energy absorption ϕ = 10% for ^{90}Y and ϕ = 80% and 69% for ^{111}In and ^{177}Lu, respectively. The absorbed energy fractions by the β-particles from ^{213}Bi and ^{213}Po are more than 95% in the smallest sphere and reach 100% in the 100-mg spheres.

Table 3. S-values for ^{90}Y, ^{111}In, ^{177}Lu and ^{213}Bi with its daughters, in spheres with masses between 1 and 500 mg

Mass (mg)	Absorbed dose rate per radioactivity *S*-value (mGy/MBq s)						
	^{90}Y	^{111}In	^{177}Lu	^{213}Bi	^{213}Po	^{209}Pb	^{209}Tl
1	15.4	4.66	17.0	37.6	1273	17.4	19.4
5	5.21	1.04	3.92	9.55	260	4.48	6.14
10	3.26	0.539	2.05	5.28	131	2.41	3.72
50	1.06	0.112	0.436	1.30	26.5	0.545	1.08
100	0.643	0.0576	0.222	0.695	13.3	0.281	0.643
200	0.381	0.0295	0.113	0.367	6.65	0.144	0.364
300	0.278	0.0200	0.0756	0.252	4.44	0.0971	0.258
500	0.184	0.0123	0.0457	0.156	2.67	0.0591	0.166

The radioactivity was homogeneously distributed in the tissue-like material spheres within the calculation model set up with MCNP5 v1.4 [13].

The TIACs per gram of tumour, listed in Table 4, were obtained by integration of the time-activity curves of Figure 1B,C. Non-instantaneous uptake kinetics has the most influence on the TIAC for ^{213}Bi and ^{213}Po, e.g. 19% difference between the single exponential and slow uptake values. Slower uptake kinetics will influence the other radionuclides by maximally 6% in single-exponential clearance and by less than 3% for the double-exponential clearance pattern, assuming linear scaling of the uptake with tumour mass delivers the mean absorbed tumour doses per administered activity as listed in Table 5. These absorbed doses, however, are only valid for 0.03 nmol PP-F11. When this amount of peptide is used, the maximum absorbed doses with the β-emitting radionuclides for both types of clearance rates are obtained with ^{90}Y, e.g. for an injected activity of 12 MBq ^{90}Y which can be labelled to 0.03 nmol PP-F11, the dose to a 300-mg tumour is 3 to 9 Gy for the single and the double exponential clearance rate, respectively. The absorbed doses using the other radionuclides are much lower, around 1 Gy. Therefore, multiple injections with more peptide amounts are needed to achieve 60 Gy.

Table 4. Tumour time-integrated activity coefficients (TIAC) per mass for ^{90}Y, ^{111}In, ^{177}Lu and ^{213}Bi with its daughters

Kinetics	TIAC per tumour mass [in s/g]						
	^{90}Y	^{111}In	^{177}Lu	^{213}Bi	^{213}Po	^{209}Pb	^{209}Tl
1 – Exponential	261	262	272	380	372	228	8
+ Fast uptake	258	259	269	361	353	230	8
+ Slow uptake	245	246	256	309	303	238	7
2 – Exponential	928	956	1,523	388	380	256	8

The clearance kinetics was modeled by a single-exponential (1-Exp) or by double (2-Exp) clearance (see Figure 1B,C). The uptake kinetics in the case of single-exponential clearance was either instantaneous (1-Exp) or according to the fast or slow uptake curves indicated in Figure 1B. All values are for a peptide amount of 0.03 nmol PP-F11.

Table 5. Mean absorbed doses per administered activity for ^{90}Y, ^{111}In, ^{177}Lu and ^{213}Bi (including daughters) labelled to 0.03 nmol PP-F11

Mass (mg)	Absorbed dose per administered activity (mGy/MBq)							
	^{90}Y		^{111}In		^{177}Lu		^{213}Bi + daughters	
	1-Exp	2-Exp	1-Exp	2-Exp	1-Exp	2-Exp	1-Exp	2-Exp
1	40	143	12	45	46	259	492	503

5	68	242	14	50	53	299	508	519
10	85	302	14	52	56	311	514	525
50	139	493	15	54	59	332	524	536
100	168	597	15	55	60	338	527	539
200	199	708	15	57	61	343	530	542
300	217	773	16	57	62	345	532	544
500	240	853	16	59	62	348	533	545

Tumour spheres vary in mass between 1 and 500 mg. Single-exponential (1-Exp) clearance proceeds with $T_{1/2}$ = 4.8 h and double-exponential (2-Exp) clearance with $T_{1/2}$ = 2.7 h (60%) and 150 h (40%).

Effect of Peptide Mass

Higher amounts of peptide are needed to guide higher amounts of radioactivity and higher absorbed doses to the tumour. However, increasing the amount of peptide will at the same time reduce the tumour TIAC, according to the saturation curve shown in Figure 2. We postulated that the kinetics of the peptide clearance were not influenced by the saturation effect, but only the final uptake at each time-point, expressed as %IA/g.

Taking the single-exponential clearance rate into account, an absorbed dose of 60 Gy in a 300-mg tumour can only be achieved by administering 5 nmol of PP-F11 peptide labelled with 2 GBq of ^{90}Y or with 123 MBq ^{213}Bi labelled to 0.081 nmol of PP-F11. In Table 6, an overview is listed of activities and peptide mass needed to reach an absorbed dose of 60 Gy in a 300-mg tumour for the double-exponential clearance pattern, either by single or multiple (N) injections with ^{90}Y, ^{111}In, ^{177}Lu and ^{213}Bi labelled to PP-F11, together with the absorbed doses in other tumour sizes, varying from 1 to 500 mg.

Table 6. Activities and peptide mass needed for an absorbed dose of 60 Gy in a 300-mg tumour

	^{90}Y - PP-F11		**^{111}In - PP-F11**	**^{177}Lu - PP-F11**	**^{213}Bi - PP-F11**
N × activity (MBq)	1 × 111	4 × 20	8 × 174	6 × 47	10 × 19
N × peptide (nmol)	0.28	4 × 0.05	8 × 0.21	6 × 0.39	10 × 0.47
Relative uptake (%)	70	97	75	62	57
Tumour mass (mg)	Mean absorbed dose to tumour (Gy)				
1	11		47	45	55
5	19		52	52	57
10	23		54	54	58
50	38		56	58	59
100	46		57	59	59
200	55		59	60	60
300	60		60	60	60
500	68		61	38	60

Multiple (N) injections were considered; only ^{90}Y could attain 60 Gy by a single injection. The relative uptake reduction factor by the higher peptide mass is indicated. The mean absorbed doses are given for tumour spheres varying in mass between 1 and 500 mg according to the mentioned activity and assuming the double-exponential clearance with $T_{1/2}$ = 2.7 h (60%) and 150 h (40%) without tumour growth. The absorbed dose for ^{213}Bi was not corrected for its relative effectiveness (RBE = 1).

The TCPs for absorbed doses of 60 Gy in a 300-mg tumour are 77% for ^{90}Y, 74% for ^{111}In, and 48% for ^{177}Lu when given in one fraction, according to Equation 4. With fractionated therapy, the TCP drops to 21% (^{90}Y), 16% (^{111}In) and 12% (^{177}Lu), despite the same dose of 60 Gy. Both reductions in TCP are caused by the lower dose rates, either by the radionuclides' half-lives or by the fractionation scheme. The TCP for ^{213}Bi PP-F11 depends on the relative biological effectiveness (RBE) of its α-radiation (93% of the absorbed dose), which is not clear yet. A RBE higher than 1.2 will already result in a TCP of more than 90% in all tumours below 300 mg. Previously, the RBE for cell killing by ^{213}Bi-DOTA-octreotate has been shown to be 3.4 [26]. If this would also be the case for ^{213}Bi-PP-F11, 90% TCP will already be reached with 4 × 17 MBq (0.41 nmol).

When single-exponential clearance is assumed with consequently higher initial dose rate, the G-factor shows a rise: 60 Gy yields higher TCPs of 99% (^{90}Y), 32% (^{111}In) and 20% (^{177}Lu) vs. double-exponential clearance kinetics (Figure 3). The absorbed dose needed for a TCP of 90% is 42 Gy with a single-exponential curve and single-fraction administration. For both clearance patterns, only ^{90}Y and ^{213}Bi are capable of delivering these curable doses, as shown in Figure 3for the situation which does not take tumour growth into account, ^{213}Bi to the whole range and^{90}Y only to the larger size tumours. Both ^{111}In and ^{177}Lu show the maximum TCP at small tumour size: 76% to 81% in 1 mg with ^{111}In and 72% to 76% in 5 mg with ^{177}Lu. The absorbed dose needed for a TCP of 90% in a 300-mg tumour with ^{177}Lu is 70 Gy. The quadratic term is determinant for the TCP for the low-LET radiation, leading to higher TCPs for the single-exponential clearance pattern and to TCPs of 0 when the quadratic LQ model term β is neglected. The high amounts of total radioactivity needed to obtain cure with the α-emitters for the single-exponential clearance are not practically achievable.

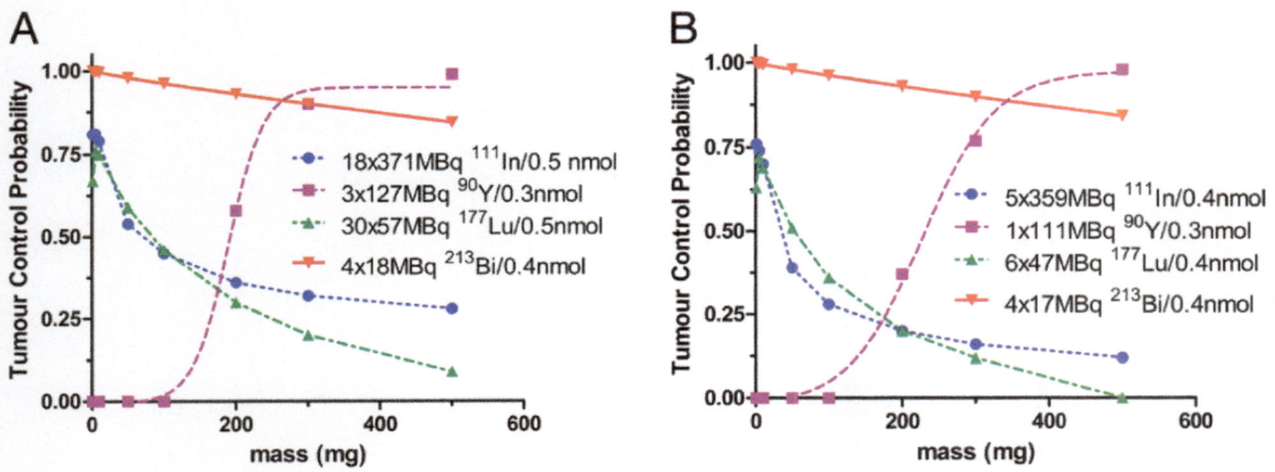

Figure 3. Tumour control probability. TCP as a function of tumour mass at activities producing a TCP of 90% in a static 300-mg tumour, or an absorbed dose of 60 Gy when lower. The clonogenic tumour cell density was 10^8/g and the LQ model parameters wereα = 0.27 Gy^{-1}, α/β = 6 Gy and T_μ = 0.5 h. For the alpha-particle part of the dose by ^{213}Bi, RBE = 3.4. (A) Single-exponential clearance kinetics and (B) double-exponential clearance kinetics.

The dose effect by ^{213}Bi is not influenced by the quadratic term of the LQ model due to the fact that 95% of its absorbed dose is caused by high LET α-radiation without repairable damage. Because of the short half-life, the uptake kinetics, however, do show a large influence on the cure possibilities with ^{213}Bi (Figure 2A). When the slow uptake kinetics ($T_{1/2}$ = 16 min) are applied, the absorbed dose will be reduced by 18%, whereas for the fast uptake ($T_{1/2}$ = 7 min), only a 4.2% reduction in dose is observed in comparison to the absorbed dose for instantaneous uptake. Compensation for this possible dose reduction can be obtained by administering either one additional therapy cycle or 9% more radioactivity per cycle.

Influence of Tumour Growth Rate

The tumour doubling time influences the tumour cure possibilities in therapies which need the double-exponential clearance kinetics to reach therapeutic doses. The irradiation time T_{irr}indicates the time until the radiation cell kill outnumbers the tumour growth. With 111 MBq ^{90}Y (sufficient to cure a static 300-mg tumour), T_{irr} can vary between 184 h ($T_{doubling}$ of 2 days) and 354 h ($T_{doubling}$ of 28 days). When ^{90}Y is given in 4 × 20 MBq with 24-h interval, T_{irr} ranges between 218 and 389 h. The irradiation times for 5 × 359 MBq ^{111}In are comparable to those of^{90}Y: 237 and 414 h. With 6 × 47 MBq ^{177}Lu, the tumour growth takes over at later times: its irradiation times vary between 317 h ($T_{doubling}$ of 2 days) and 611 h ($T_{doubling}$ of 28 days). For therapy with ^{213}Bi, the influence of the tumour doubling time is much less (16.8 MBq ^{213}Bi: 6.7 h (for $T_{doubling}$ of 2 days) and 11 h (for $T_{doubling}$ of 28 days)). The build-up of the dose over this irradiation time is reduced in comparison to the build-up to infinity; for ^{213}Bi, the reduction is below 0.5% and negligible like the maximal 5% reduction with ^{90}Y, but with ^{177}Lu, it is 18% at$T_{doubling}$ of 2 days and 5% at $T_{doubling}$ of 28 days. Both the effects by reduction in dose and tumour growth during the irradiation have influence on the tumour cure probabilities, as shown in Figure 4 for the double-exponential clearance.

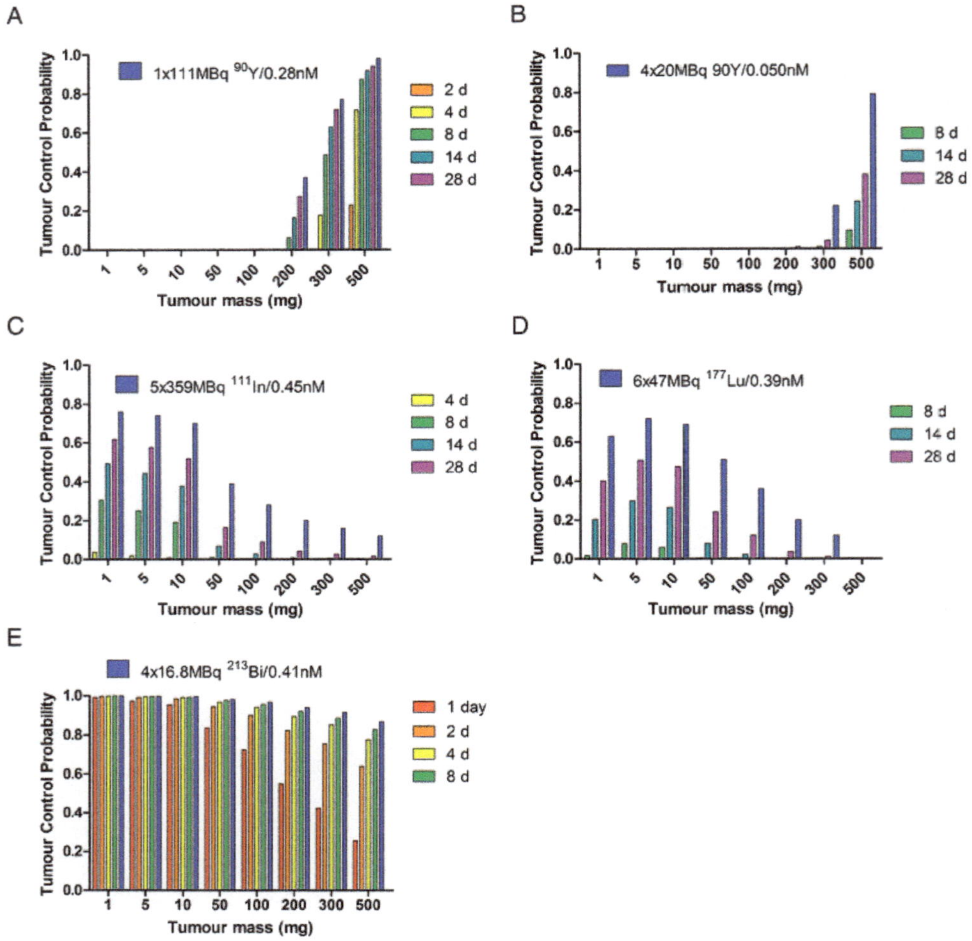

Figure 4. Tumour control probability vs tumour mass. TCP versus tumour mass for a single 111 MBq ^{90}Y (A), multiple administrations 4 × 20 MBq ^{90}Y (B), 5 × 359 MBq ^{111}In (C), 6 × 47 MBq ^{177}Lu (D) and 4 × 16.8 MBq ^{213}Bi (E) for tumour doubling times varying between 1 and 28 days, and for the static tumour, as shown in Figure 3. Only bars for TCP > 0.05 are shown, except for ^{213}Bi where the 14- and 18-day doubling time results were almost equal to the static (without tumour growth) TCP shown with the blue bars.

The reduction in tumour size as a function of time is shown in Figure 5 during a time period of 60 days. None of the tumours with a doubling time of more than 4 days grow back to their original size within this time period. The reduction in size is proportional to the radionuclide half-life and intervals (here 24 h) between the injections.

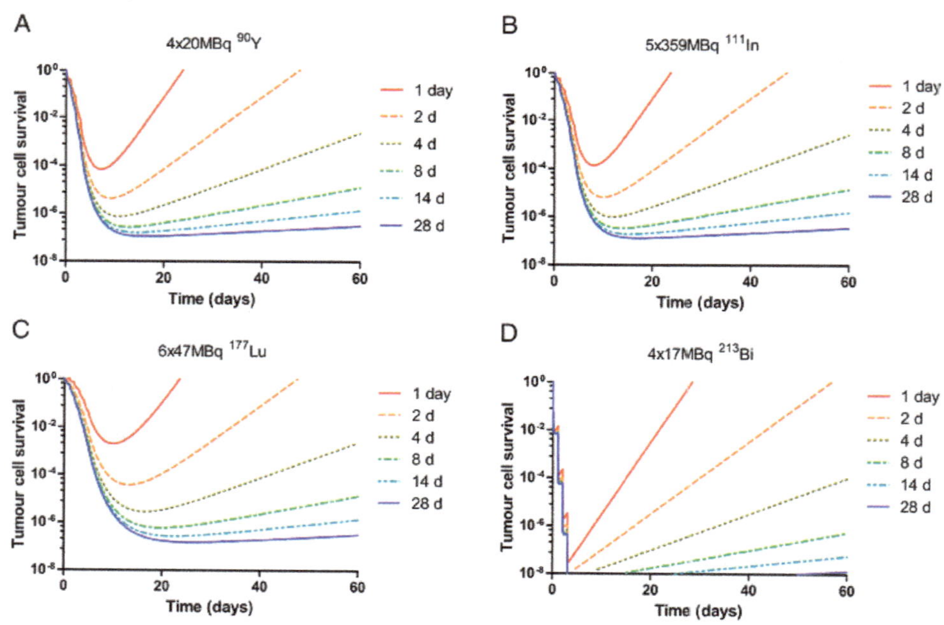

Figure 5. Models for tumour growth curves. After multiple administration of (A)^{90}Y,(B)^{111}In, (C)^{177}Lu or (D)^{213}Bi to a 300-mg tumour for different tumour doubling times. The same amount of peptide was used as indicated in Figure 4.

DISCUSSION

Based on studies with 12 CCK2 receptor-binding analogues, the biodistribution of the CCK2 analogue PP-F11 shows a very favourable uptake in CCK2 receptor-expressing tumours and relatively low renal retention, which makes it potentially suitable for therapeutic application. This study aimed to investigate its possibilities and hurdles for successful radionuclide therapy with this peptide analogue in mice with s.c. CCK2 receptor-expressing tumours. The particle range of the selected radionuclides has an important impact on the cure capability of the radioloabelled peptide for various sizes of tumours [3]. Since the receptor-mediated tumour uptake of radiolabelled PP-F11 shows a saturable relation with peptide mass, the maximum achievable specific activity is an important parameter in this respect. Furthermore, it has to be taken into account that the production method of radionuclides determines the amount that can be labelled to peptides. Therefore, the higher specific activities reachable with ^{90}Y and ^{213}Bi make both radionuclides very suitable for therapy of 200- to 300-mg tumours, using lower peptide mass and thus higher tumour uptake. Yttrium (^{90}Y) is capable of controlling larger-sized (>200 mg) tumours, whereas ^{213}Bi is capable of curing over the whole range of masses considered, but most optimal in the smallest sizes.

This receptor saturation effect has been observed previously with somatostatin receptor-targeted peptides, both in preclinical biodistribution studies [9], as in clinical use [27],[28], and has also been observed even more prominently with bombesin analogues [29]. The limited number of receptors influences the tumour uptake of the peptide at escalating peptide doses. Pharmacokinetic compartment modelling can be used to correct for the molar concentration and receptor binding [11]. In this study, we used the one-site dissociation curve to describe the saturable uptake in the tumour and stomach. Saturation of tumour uptake in humans after PRRT with ^{177}Lu-DOTA-octreotate has not been observed, whereas the receptor-mediated uptake in the liver and spleen did show a decrease by the therapeutic amount of peptide [30].

The α-emitter ^{213}Bi shows ideal properties to cure small lesions, with most of its absorbed dose coming from its short half-life daughter ^{213}Po. The RBE of ^{213}Bi-PP-F11 is not known, but when the effects are comparable to the RBE found for ^{213}Bi-DOTA-octreotate of 3.4 [26], its effect is tremendous. The absorbed dose to the normal organs such as the kidneys and stomach wall has not been considered in this evaluation, as kidney protection by blocking reuptake of the peptide can reduce the renal dose [31],[32]. For all radionuclides, radiation-induced toxicity in normal organs will form the limiting amount of radioactivity. Late kidney damage will occur after cumulative doses of >27 Gy with ^{90}Y-DOTA-octreotide [33]. Renal uptake of the PP-F11 peptide is hardly influenced by the injected peptide mass, contrary to the tumour uptake. Consequently, using a higher amount of peptides to increase the amount of radioactivity will lead to higher absorbed doses to the kidneys while the tumour absorbed doses are decreased due to receptor saturation. The stomach wall will show radiation-induced ulceration after 45-Gy fractionated external beam exposure [34]. For that reason, it is most probably not realistic to administer the huge amounts of radioactivity as suggested for ^{111}In and ^{177}Lu in the case of single-exponential clearance (Figure 3A).

Fractionation of the therapy is necessary for the practically achievable specific activities of the radionuclides considered. Fractionation will lead to higher cumulative absorbed doses in tumours and has been shown to lead to lower probability of renal toxicity in clinical application of radionuclide therapy [35]. Fractionation of therapy with ^{177}Lu-DOTA-octreotate in rats with CA20948 tumours has been shown to reduce renal toxicity while maintaining the same tumour response as for the single fraction therapy [36]. This reduction in renal toxicity was also influenced by the time interval between the fractions; renal toxicity was significantly reduced for intervals of a week or longer compared to a 1-day interval. This inter-fraction recovery of renal damage is not fully explained by the repair mechanism within the LQ model [37]. In clinical practice, ^{177}Lu-DOTA-octreotate is given in four fractions of 7.4 GBq with a 6-week interval, also in order to allow the bone marrow to recover [38].

The tumour growth rate has a large influence on the cure options using the longer half-life radionuclides. Tumours with a doubling time of less than 8 days show >50% reduction of the TCP for treatment using ^{90}Y or ^{111}In, and with ^{177}Lu, this reduction sets in at doubling times below 14 days. Due to its short half-life, ^{213}Bi is capable of controlling also fast-growing tumours. This growth effect is only of concern in preclinical studies with fast-growing tumour xenografts and hardly in the clinical setting in which tumour doubling times most often are longer than 14 days. Selective control of slower growing tumour subtypes could however induce a more aggressive type in any tumour regrowth. The concept of TCP may be a too strict criterion for cure, as for slower growing tumours, the regrowth may not be visible within the typical observation period of 2 to 3 months. A lag time without tumour growth and subsequent accelerated repopulation as observed in prolonged radiotherapy sessions has not been modelled [39]. The effect of repopulation after radionuclide therapy needs to be investigated further as it will strongly influence the cure rates for fast-growing tumours, e.g. with a lag time of 7 to 8 days, all growth effects would diminish when the therapy is completed within 1 week. The size of the tumour may not be completely representative for the number of viable cells within this volume. Doomed cells can form a part of the tumour volume in response to the radiation therapy, waiting to be cleared or encapsulated [40].

The basis for the radiobiological considerations is formed by the linear-quadratic model, which assumes that the tumour cells behave as cells in culture in response to radiation. The main LQ model parameters α and β are determined from external beam experiments. Response to radionuclide-induced doses is also very dependent on the repair process of sub-lethal damage. In external beam exposure, this repair takes place immediately after the dose given in a short time. With radionuclide-induced exposure, the repair is induced during the dose delivery and therefore the half-time value with which sub-lethally damaged lesions are repaired is very critical. In this work, this repair half-time was taken as 0.5 h, which is considered to be valid in general for tumours. Changing the repair half-time to 1 h increases the TCP by 10% to 20% for the beta-emitting radionuclides. Future work on radiobiological modeling for radionuclide therapy should focus on the repair mechanism and the influence of kinetics. The clearance kinetics is a dominant factor not only in the absorbed dose to the tumour, but also in the TCP by the projected dose rate. It is therefore of great importance to determine the kinetic pattern with more detail than just the two time points as taken in this study. Fractionation of radionuclide therapy should be studied on the basis of the absorbed doses given, taking the radiation sensitivity, the repair of sub-lethal damage and recovery by repopulation into account.

CONCLUSIONS

Receptor-mediated uptake of the CCK2 compound PP-F11 in tumours shows a steep saturation effect with increasing amounts of peptide.

The specific activities achievable for radiolabelling peptides limit the absorbed dose in tumours, as higher activities go parallel with higher peptide amounts, which might considerably reduce the tumour uptake.

Multiple injections are preferred to obtain an absorbed tumour dose in the order of 60 Gy.

For the larger xenografts (>200 mg), ^{90}Y is the preferable radionuclide, as its high specific activity allows the use of low peptide amounts, although it lacks the capability of curing smaller-sized tumours.

For tumour xenografts in almost the whole size range (<500 mg), ^{213}Bi shows high TCPs, taking an enhancement by increased RBE from its α-radiation into account.

The influence of the clearance kinetics is the largest with ^{177}Lu, whereas ^{213}Bi is most strongly influenced by the uptake kinetics.

Ongoing growth of the tumour during the absorbed dose build-up reduces the TCP for longer half-life radionuclides and has hardly any influence on the cure options for ^{213}Bi.

AUTHORS' CONTRIBUTIONS

MK designed the study, did the calculations including the statistics and wrote the article. WAPB, EdeB and HSC did the chemical analyses on labelling conditions. OB, PL and PKP did the animal experiments and chemical synthesis, and OB and MdeJ came up with the original question and set up the study design. All authors read the article and contributed their part. MM helped out with editing, and at the end, all authors approved the final manuscript.

ACKNOWLEDGEMENTS

This work was part of COST Action BM0607 within Framework 7 of the European Union. Lieke Joosten is acknowledged for performing the animal experiments.

REFERENCES

1. Laverman P, Joosten L, Eek A, Roosenburg S, Peitl PK, Maina T, Macke H, Aloj L, von Guggenberg E, Sosabowski JK, de Jong M, Reubi JC, Oyen WJ, Boerman OC: Comparative biodistribution of 12 (1)(1)(1)In-labelled gastrin/CCK2 receptor-targeting peptides. Eur J Nucl Med Mol Imaging 2011, 38: 1410–1416. 10.1007/s00259-011-1806-0
2. Aloj L, Aurilio M, Rinaldi V, D'Ambrosio L, Tesauro D, Peitl PK, Maina T, Mansi R, von Guggenberg E, Joosten L, Breeman WA, De Blois E, Koelewijn S, Melis M, Waser B, Beetschen K, Reubi JC, de Jong M: Comparison of the binding and internalization properties of 12 DOTA-coupled and (1)(1)(1)In-labelled CCK2/gastrin receptor binding peptides: a collaborative project under COST Action BM0607. Eur J Nucl Med Mol Imaging 2011, 38: 1417–1425. 10.1007/s00259-011-1816-y
3. O'Donoghue JA, Bardiés M, Wheldon TE: Relationships between tumor size and curability for uniformly targeted therapy with beta-emitting radionuclides. J Nucl Med 1995, 36: 1902–1909.
4. Morgenstern A, Bruchertseifer F, Apostolidis C: Bismuth-213 and actinium-225-generator performance and evolving therapeutic applications of two generator-derived alpha-emitting radioisotopes. Curr Radiopharm 2012, 5: 221–227. 10.2174/1874471011205030221
5. de Jong M, Breeman W, Bernard B, Bakker W, Visser T, Kooij P, van Gameren A, Krenning E: Tumor response after [(90)Y-DOTA(0), Tyr(3)]octreotide radionuclide therapy in a transplantable rat tumor model is dependent on tumor size. J Nucl Med 2001, 42: 1841–1846.
6. de Jong M, Breeman WAP, Bernard BF, Bakker WH, Schaar M, van Gameren A, Bugaj JE, Erion J, Schmidt M, Srinivasan A, Krenning EP: [177Lu-DOTA(0), Tyr3] octreotate for somatostatin receptor-targeted radionuclide therapy. Int J Cancer 2001, 92: 628–633. 10.1002/1097-0215(20010601)92:5<628::AID-IJC1244>3.0.CO;2-L
7. Breeman WA, De Jong M, Visser TJ, Erion JL, Krenning EP: Optimising conditions for radiolabelling of DOTA-peptides with ^{90}Y, ^{111}In and ^{177}Lu at high specific activities. Eur J Nucl Med Mol Imaging 2003, 30: 917-920.
8. Breeman WA, Kwekkeboom DJ, Kooij PP, Bakker WH, Hofland LJ, Visser TJ, Ensing GJ, Lamberts SW, Krenning EP: Effect of dose and specific activity on tissue distribution of indium-111-pentetreotide in rats. J Nucl Med 1995, 36: 623–627.
9. de Jong M, Breeman WA, Bernard BF, van Gameren A, de Bruin E, Bakker WH, van der Pluijm ME, Visser TJ, Macke HR, Krenning EP: Tumour uptake of the radiolabelled somatostatin analogue [DOTA0, TYR3] octreotide is dependent on the peptide amount. Eur J Nucl Med 1999, 26: 693–698. 10.1007/s002590050439
10. Bernhardt P, Kolby L, Johanson V, Nilsson O, Ahlman H, Forssell-Aronsson E: Biodistribution of ^{111}In-DTPA-D-Phe1-octreotide in tumor-bearing nude mice: influence of amount injected and route of administration. Nucl Med Biol 2003, 30: 253-260.
11. Kletting P, Muller B, Erentok B, Schmaljohann J, Behrendt FF, Reske SN, Mottaghy FM, Glatting G: Differences in predicted and actually absorbed doses in peptide receptor radionuclide therapy. Med Phys 2012, 39: 5708–5717. 10.1118/1.4747266
12. Kolenc-Peitl P, Mansi R, Tamma M, Gmeiner-Stopar T, Sollner-Dolenc M, Waser B, Baum RP, Reubi JC, Maecke HR: Highly improved metabolic stability and pharmacokinetics of indium-111-DOTA-gastrin conjugates for targeting of the gastrin receptor. J Med Chem2011, 54: 2602–2609. 10.1021/jm101279a

13. MCNP - a general Monte Carlo N-particle transport code, version 5 vol. I: Overview and theory Los Alamos National Lab Report: LA-UR-03–1987 2003. [https://laws.lanl.gov/vhosts/mcnp.lanl.gov/references.shtml#mcnp5_refs] https://laws.lanl.gov/vhosts/mcnp.lanl.gov/references.shtml#mcnp5_refs

14. Wambersie A: ICRU Report 44: Tissue Substitutes in Radiation Dosimetry and Measurement. International Commission on Radiation Units and measurements, Bethesda (US); 1989.

15. Eckerman K, Endo A: MIRD: Radionuclide Data and Decay Schemes. Society of Nuclear Medicine and Molecular Imaging, Reston (US); 2008.

16. Koivunoro H, Siiskonen T, Kotiluoto P, Auterinen I, Hippelainen E, Savolainen S: Accuracy of the electron transport in mcnp5 and its suitability for ionization chamber response simulations: a comparison with the egsnrc and penelope codes. Med Phys 2012, 39: 1335–1344. 10.1118/1.3685446

17. Schaart DR: The scaling method applied to beta particle line sources with a finite diameter.Med Phys 2002, 29: 2682–2686. 10.1118/1.1513567

18. Bolch WE, Eckerman KF, Sgouros G, Thomas SR: MIRD pamphlet no. 21: a generalized schema for radiopharmaceutical dosimetry-standardization of nomenclature. J Nucl Med2009, 50: 477–484. 10.2967/jnumed.108.056036

19. Morgenstern A, Bruchertseifer F, Apostolidis C, Giesel F, Mier W, Haberkorn U, Kratochwil C: Synthesis of^{213}Bi-DOTATOC for peptide receptor alpha-therapy of GEP-NET patients refractory to beta therapy. J Nucl Med 2012, 53(Supplement 1):455.

20. Joiner M, van der Kogel A: Basic clinical radiobiology. Hodder Arnold, London; 2009.

21. Dale RG: Dose-rate effects in targeted radiotherapy. Phys Med Biol 1996, 41: 1871–1884. 10.1088/0031-9155/41/10/001

22. Malaise EP, Fertil B, Chavaudra N, Guichard M: Distribution of radiation sensitivities for human tumor cells of specific histological types: comparison of in vitro to in vivo data. Int J Radiat Oncol Biol Phys 1986, 12: 617–624. 10.1016/0360-3016(86)90071-4

23. Ling CC, Gerweck LE, Zaider M, Yorke E: Dose-rate effects in external beam radiotherapy redux. Radiother Oncol 2010, 95: 261–268. 10.1016/j.radonc.2010.03.014

24. Wang JZ, Li XA: Impact of tumor repopulation on radiotherapy planning. Int J Radiat Oncol Biol Phys 2005, 61: 220–227. 10.1016/j.ijrobp.2004.09.043

25. Solomon B, Hagekyriakou J, Trivett MK, Stacker SA, McArthur GA, Cullinane C: EGFR blockade with ZD1839 ("Iressa") potentiates the antitumor effects of single and multiple fractions of ionizing radiation in human A431 squamous cell carcinoma. Epidermal growth factor receptor. Int J Radiat Oncol Biol Phys 2003, 55: 713–723. 10.1016/S0360-3016(02)04357-2

26. Nayak TK, Norenberg JP, Anderson TL, Prossnitz ER, Stabin MG, Atcher RW: Somatostatin-receptor-targeted alpha-emitting^{213}Bi is therapeutically more effective than beta(-)-emitting^{177}Lu in human pancreatic adenocarcinoma cells. Nucl Med Biol 2007, 34: 185-193.

27. Velikyan I, Sundin A, Eriksson B, Lundqvist H, Sorensen J, Bergstrom M, Langstrom B: In vivo binding of [^{68}Ga]-DOTATOC to somatostatin receptors in neuroendocrine tumours-impact of peptide mass. Nucl Med Biol 2010, 37: 265-275.

28. Beauregard JM, Hofman MS, Kong G, Hicks RJ: The tumour sink effect on the biodistribution of^{68}Ga-DOTA-octreotate: implications for peptide receptor radionuclide therapy. Eur J Nucl Med Mol Imaging 2012, 39: 50-56.

29. Breeman WA, Hofland LJ, de Jong M, Bernard BF, Srinivasan A, Kwekkeboom DJ, Visser TJ, Krenning EP: Evaluation of radiolabelled bombesin analogues for receptor-targeted scintigraphy and radiotherapy. Int J Cancer 1999, 81: 658–665. 10.1002/(SICI)1097-0215(19990517)81:4<658::AID-IJC24>3.0.CO;2-P

30. Sabet A, Nagarajah J, Dogan AS, Biersack HJ, Sabet A, Guhlke S, Ezziddin S: Does PRRT with standard activities of^{177}Lu-octreotate really achieve relevant somatostatin receptor saturation in target tumor lesions?: insights from intra-therapeutic receptor imaging in patients with metastatic gastroenteropancreatic neuroendocrine tumors. EJNMMI Res2013, 3: 82.

31. Behe M, Kluge G, Becker W, Gotthardt M, Behr TM: Use of polyglutamic acids to reduce uptake of radiometal-labeled minigastrin in the kidneys. J Nucl Med 2005, 46: 1012–1015.

32. Vegt E, Melis M, Eek A, de Visser M, Brom M, Oyen WJ, Gotthardt M, de Jong M, Boerman OC: Renal uptake of different radiolabelled peptides is mediated by megalin: SPECT and biodistribution studies in megalin-deficient mice. Eur J Nucl Med Mol Imaging 2011, 38: 623–632. 10.1007/s00259-010-1685-9

33. Barone R, Borson-Chazot F, Valkema R, Walrand S, Chauvin F, Gogou L, Kvols LK, Krenning EP, Jamar F, Pauwels S: Patient-specific dosimetry in predicting renal toxicity with (90)Y-DOTATOC: relevance of kidney volume and dose rate in finding a dose-effect relationship. J Nucl Med 2005, 46(Suppl 1):99S-106S.

34. Marks LB, Yorke ED, Jackson A, Ten Haken RK, Constine LS, Eisbruch A, Bentzen SM, Nam J, Deasy JO: Use of normal tissue complication probability models in the clinic. Int J Radiat Oncol Biol Phys 2010, 76: S10–19. 10.1016/j.ijrobp.2009.07.1754

35. Wessels BW, Konijnenberg MW, Dale RG, Breitz HB, Cremonesi M, Meredith RF, Green AJ, Bouchet LG, Brill AB, Bolch WE, Sgouros G, Thomas SR: MIRD pamphlet no. 20: the effect of model assumptions on kidney dosimetry and response-implications for radionuclide therapy. J Nucl Med 2008, 49: 1884–1899. 10.2967/jnumed.108.053173

36. Rolleman EJ, Krenning EP, Bernard BF, de Visser M, Bijster M, Visser TJ, Vermeij M, Lindemans J, de Jong M: Long-term toxicity of [(177)Lu-DOTA (0), Tyr (3)] octreotate in rats. Eur J Nucl Med Mol Imaging 2007, 34: 219–227. 10.1007/s00259-006-0232-1

37. Stewart FA, Oussoren Y, Van Tinteren H, Bentzen SM: Loss of reirradiation tolerance in the kidney with

increasing time after single or fractionated partial tolerance doses. Int J Radiat Biol 1994, 66: 169–179. 10.1080/09553009414551071

38. Kwekkeboom DJ, de Herder WW, Kam BL, van Eijck CH, van Essen M, Kooij PP, Feelders RA, van Aken MO, Krenning EP: Treatment with the radiolabeled somatostatin analog [177 Lu-DOTA 0, Tyr3]octreotate: toxicity, efficacy, and survival. J Clin Oncol 2008, 26: 2124–2130. 10.1200/JCO.2007.15.2553

39. Pedicini P, Strigari L, Benassi M: Estimation of a self-consistent set of radiobiological parameters from hypofractionated versus standard radiation therapy of prostate cancer. Int J Radiat Oncol Biol Phys 2013, 85: e231–237. 10.1016/j.ijrobp.2012.11.033

40. O'Donoghue JA, Sgouros G, Divgi CR, Humm JL: Single-dose versus fractionated radioimmunotherapy: model comparisons for uniform tumor dosimetry. J Nucl Med 2000, 41: 538–547.

CHAPTER
14

EARLY REDUCTION IN TUMOUR [18F]FLUOROTHYMIDINE (FLT) UPTAKE IN PATIENTS WITH NON-SMALL CELL LUNG CANCER (NSCLC) TREATED WITH RADIOTHERAPY ALONE

Ioannis Trigonis, Pek Keng Koh, Ben Taylor, Mahbubunnabi Tamal, David Ryder, Mark Earl, Jose Anton-Rodriguez, Kate Haslett, Helen Young, Corinne Faivre-Finn, Fiona Blackhall, Alan Jackson, and Marie-Claude Asselin

Keywords: [^{18}F] Fluorothymidine PET, Non-small cell lung cancer, Radiotherapy, Early response monitoring

INTRODUCTION

Lung cancer is the most common cause of cancer-related mortality worldwide [1]. Radiotherapy (RT) plays a major therapeutic role in patients with non-small cell lung cancer (NSCLC). RT is given with radical intent in patients with early-stage disease who are medically unfit for resection and in locally advanced inoperable disease [2]. Patients with locally advanced (stage III) NSCLC are generally treated with a combination of chemotherapy and RT delivered sequentially or concurrently [3]. Although concurrent chemo-RT has been shown to be associated with improved outcomes this is at a cost of added toxicity and utilized in empirically selected patients, underlining the need for robust efficacy and toxicity biomarkers in both approaches [4].

Further improvements in outcome will require the use of minimally invasive response biomarkers in two distinct but interdependent settings: Firstly, in the preclinical and early-phase clinical trial setting where the inclusion of surrogate pharmacodynamic end points, measured at the population level, may facilitate the rational selection and optimization of novel RT-based regimens [5, 6] and secondly, in late-phase clinical trials and, potentially, in routine clinical practice where response stratification across individual subjects and/or lesions may enable spatially and/or temporally adaptive radiotherapeutic approaches [7, 8]. As a prerequisite step further technical validation and qualification of candidate biomarkers is required [9].

Intrinsic radiosensitivity and tumour repopulation are (along with cell **r**epair, **r**e-oxygenation and cell cycle **r**edistribution) two of the five "R's" determining RT efficacy according to classical radiobiology [10]. As both are intimately linked to changes of tumour proliferation, it is reasonable to hypothesize that monitoring changes of tumour proliferation during RT may provide surrogate information on response and patient outcome.

3′-deoxy-3′-[^{18}F]Fluorothymidine (FLT) positron emission tomography (PET) allows non-invasive evaluation of tumour proliferation. FLT uptake primarily depends on phosphorylation mediated by thymidine kinase 1 (TK1). TK1 is up-regulated 10- to 20-fold during S phase; therefore, FLT uptake parameters provide a surrogate measurement for S-phase fraction and proliferation rate [11]. Validation studies have demonstrated significant correlations between baseline lung tumour FLT uptake parameters and the proliferation index Ki-67 [12–16].

Citation: Ioannis Trigonis, Pek Keng Koh, Ben Taylor, Mahbubunnabi Tamal, David Ryder, Mark Earl, Jose Anton-Rodriguez, Kate Haslett, Helen Young, Corinne Faivre-Finn, Fiona Blackhall, Alan Jackson, and Marie-Claude Asselin. Early reduction in tumour [18F]fluorothymidine (FLT) uptake in patients with non-small cell lung cancer (NSCLC) treated with radiotherapy alone, European Journal of Nuclear Medicine and Molecular Imaging, April 2014; Volume 41, Issue 4, pp 682–693. DOI: 10.1007/s00259-013-2632-3.

In xenograft models, irradiation induced early decreases of tumour FLT uptake, generally preceding [^{18}F] fluorodeoxyglucose (FDG) changes [17–20]. Two pilot studies have reported changes of tumour FLT uptake at variable time points during the course of concurrent/sequential chemo-RT, each including five patients with NSCLC [21, 22]. In the two patients who were studied after 2 days of treatment, primary tumour maximum standardized uptake value (SUV_{max}) exhibited changes of +22 and −27 %. After 8 days larger decreases of 39 and 40 % were measured in two patients [21]. The remaining patients were studied in the fifth week of treatment and large variable decreases were reported in primary tumour SUV_{max}, ranging from 25 to 71 %, after 44–48 Gy [22]. Although the first study reported "a disparity in the anatomical and metabolic response of primary tumour and lymph nodes" [21], no statistically significant differences were found in FLT responses between the two lesion types in the second [22]. As most patients studied received concurrent chemo-RT, the relative contribution of the two treatment components to the observed changes is unclear. To date there are no data available relating to FLT uptake changes in response to RT alone.

We conducted a prospective study aiming to investigate the magnitude, significance and variability of tumour FLT uptake changes after 1–2 weeks of radical RT without concurrent chemotherapy. This work was performed as a sub-study of RADAR (Radiation Damage And Resistance in lung cancer), a Manchester Lung Cancer Group multimodality study aiming to discover, evaluate and validate novel blood and imaging biomarkers of RT response and toxicity in lung cancer.

MATERIALS AND METHODS

Patients

We recruited patients with a histological or cytological diagnosis of NSCLC scheduled to receive radical RT as per standard of care. Patients who had received induction chemotherapy prior to RT were eligible; however, those planned to have concurrent chemo-RT were excluded. Other eligibility criteria included Eastern Cooperative Oncology Group (ECOG) performance status 0 or 1, presence of a primary tumour exceeding 2 cm in maximum diameter and written, informed consent. In women of childbearing potential, pregnancy was excluded by measurement of urine beta human chorionic gonadotropin (β-HCG). The study protocol was approved by the local Research Ethics Committee (REC, 09/H1011/55) and Administration of Radioactive Substances Advisory Committees (ARSAC, 595-3742/25138) and has therefore been performed in accordance with the ethical standards laid down in the 1964 Declaration of Helsinki and its later amendments.

Patients were treated on a linear accelerator using 6-MV photons with a total dose of 50–55 Gy in 20 once-daily fractions or 60–66 Gy in 30–33 fractions. Consenting patients underwent one or two (optional) baseline FLT PET/CT scans (Scan1/Scan2) followed by a further scan during the second week of treatment (Scan3). Therefore, patients were evaluable for either baseline reproducibility of FLT PET parameters, RT response or both.

The individual time intervals between scans and treatments are tabulated in Table 1. Patients who had received induction chemotherapy underwent the first baseline scan 11–49 days (median 26 days) after the last cycle. In reproducibility-evaluable patients, baseline scans were performed within 2–6 days (median 4.0 days) of each other. In response-evaluable patients, RT was initiated 1–13 days after the latest/single baseline scan (median 5.0 days). Response assessment scans were performed after 6–15 calendar days on treatment (median 8.5 days), corresponding to 5–11 RT fractions (median 7.5 fractions).

Table 1. Patient (Pt) characteristics. TNM tumour, node, metastasis staging, Adeno Ca adenocarcinoma, LUL left upper lobe, RLL right lower lobe, RML right middle lobe, LLL left lower lobe, RUL right upper lobe, PR partial response, SD stable disease, BED biologically effective dose, na, non-applicable, Cis cisplatin, Pem pemetrexed, Carbo carboplatin, Gem gemcitabine. Reproducibility-evaluable patients are highlighted in grey and response-evaluable patients are encompassed within redborder

Demographics			Histology	TNM			Induction chemotherapy		Scan intervals (days)			Radiotherapy delivered at response scan[d]	
Pt	Gender	Age (y)		Stage	Primary	Nodes[a]	Regimen[b]	Response	Last chemo[c]-1st baseline scan	Test-retest scans	Last baseline scan - RT start	Dose (Gy) / fractions	BED (Gy)
1	M	72	Large Cell	II	LUL	3A, 7	na	na	na	5	2	na	na
2	M	66	AdenoCa	IIIA	RLL	7, 4R, 10, 5	Cis-Pemx4	PR	33	4	2	na	na
3	M	74	Squamous	IIIA	RML	7	Carbo-Gemx4	PR	15	2	3	22.0 / 8	28.0
4	M	77	AdenoCa	IIIA	RUL	4R	Cis/Carbo-Pemx4	PR	49	na	5	30.2 /11	38.5
5	M	71	Squamous	IIIA	RML	4R	Carbo-Gemx3	PR	26	na	6	16.5 / 6	21.0
6	F	75	Squamous	IIIA	LUL	ne	Carbo-Gemx4	PR	23	na	4	22.0 / 8	28.1
7	F	73	Squamous	IIIA	LUL	7, 4R	na	na	na	na	10	22.0 / 8	28.1
8	F	72	Squamous	IIIB	LUL	7	Carbo-Gemx3	SD	17	na	12	16.5 / 6	21.0
9	M	82	Squamous	IIIA	RML	4R	na	na	na	na	8	13.7 / 5	17.5
10	M	68	Squamous	IIIA	LLL	7, 4R	Cis-Gemx4	PR	18	6	13	22.0 / 8	28.1
11	F	64	AdenoCa	IIIA	RLL	10, 4, 3A, 10	Cis-Pemx4	PR	32	na	5	27.5 /10	35.1
12	M	47	AdenoCa	IIIA	RLung	7	Cis-Pemx4	SD	44	na	1	19.2 / 7	24.5
13	M	58	Squamous	III/IV	RUL	10, 7, 4R	Cis/Carbo-Gemx4	PR	39	na	1	14.0 / 7	16.8
14	M	66	AdenoCa	III/IV	RLung	7	Cis/Carbo-Pemx4	PR	18	4	2	12.5 / 5	15.6
15	M	60	Squamous	IIIA	RUL	ne	Carbo-Gemx4	PR	11	2	3	na	na
16	F	75	Squamous	IIIA	RML	3A	Carbo-Gemx3	PR	30	2	4	na	na

[a] International Association for the Study of Lung Cancer lymph node map (2009). [b] / indicates drug switch, - denotes drug combination and x precedes number of chemotherapy cycles. [c] Date of last chemotherapy administration. [d] All patients in the response cohort were treated with a total dose of 50-55 Gy in 20 once-daily fractions except one patient (13) who was given 66 Gy in 33 fractions.

Clinical follow-up included medical history and physical examination 1, 3 and 6 months following completion of RT and subsequently as per local practice. Imaging follow-up included contrast-enhanced CT of thorax and abdomen at 4 weeks, 6 months and 12 months following completion of RT and subsequently as required at the discretion of the treating physician. Overall survival (OS) was defined as time from RT initiation to death, irrespective of cause. Locoregional control (LRC) was defined as time from RT initiation to local disease progression according to RECIST 1.1 criteria [23]. For patients that are still alive and/or local progression had not been detected at the time of death, LRC and OS were calculated relative to the date of last follow-up.

PET Data Acquisition

FLT was either synthesized in-house as described in [24] or externally supplied (PETNET Solutions Inc., Nottingham, UK or Wolfson Brain Imaging Centre, University of Cambridge, Cambridge, UK).

All PET scans were performed at the Wolfson Molecular Imaging Centre (WMIC, Manchester, UK) using the Biograph 6 Truepoint TrueV scanner (Siemens Molecular Imaging Inc., Knoxville, TN, USA). This is a four-ring lutetium oxyorthosilicate (LSO)-based 3D PET scanner with an axial field of view (FOV) of 21.6 cm coupled with a six-slice helical CT scanner. FLT was injected as a 30-s bolus of 254–361 MBq (mean 311 MBq), and each emission scan was performed at a single bed position without respiratory gating. The PET scan was followed by a non-breath-hold, non-contrast-enhanced CT scan according to manufacturer recommendations (peak energy 130 keV, 70 mAs). CT data were reconstructed at high and low spatial resolutions for volumes of interest (VOI) delineation and for attenuation and scatter correction purposes, respectively. PET data acquired 45–60 min post-injection were reconstructed as a single frame using 3D ordered subset expectation maximization (OSEM) with 4 iterations and 21 subsets to a $256 \times 256 \times 109$ matrix, corresponding to voxel size of $2.67 \times 2.67 \times 2.00$ mm^3. PET images were smoothed using a 3D 4-mm Gaussian filter post-reconstruction.

Image Analysis

PET images were decay-corrected and normalized for injected dose and patient body weight using Eq. 1 to generate parametric SUV maps:

$$SUV\left(\frac{g}{ml}\right) = Tissue\,radioactivity\left(\frac{kBq}{ml}\right) \times \frac{Weight(kg)}{Injected\,dose(MBq)} \quad (1)$$

Primary tumours and metastatic lymph nodes were manually delineated slice by slice transaxially by an experienced oncological radiologist (B.T.) to generate 3D VOIs on the baseline and response scans using Analyze image analysis software (Biomedical Imaging Resource, Mayo Foundation, Rochester, MN, USA). Lesion delineation aimed to include entire malignant lesions as whole, potentially heterogeneous anatomical entities and was not limited to FLT-avid areas. Hence VOI delineation was primarily CT-based and co-registered PET images were only considered as required, for example to aid in the delineation of tumour from consolidated lung or to more accurately determine the margins of masses which abutted the mediastinum. Standardized CT window settings were used to delineate tumour from adjacent lung (lung windows; level −500 HU, width 1,500 HU) or from adjacent soft tissues (soft tissue windows; level 0 HU, width 400 HU). A fixed visualization window between 0 and 4 was used for the smoothed SUV maps. Enlarged mediastinal nodes or nodes of normal size showing increased FLT uptake were included in the analysis and delineated on CT with soft tissue windows. Representative CT and PET SUV images of patient 11 are shown in Fig. 1 at baseline and after 10 RT fractions. Contamination of tumour VOIs by normal proliferating bone marrow signal may cause substantial errors such that in tumours adjacent to the skeleton particular care was taken to ensure a margin between the delineated VOI and bone. The quality of PET/CT co-registration, which can be compromised by patient movement, was visually assessed and VOIs were manually adjusted as required.

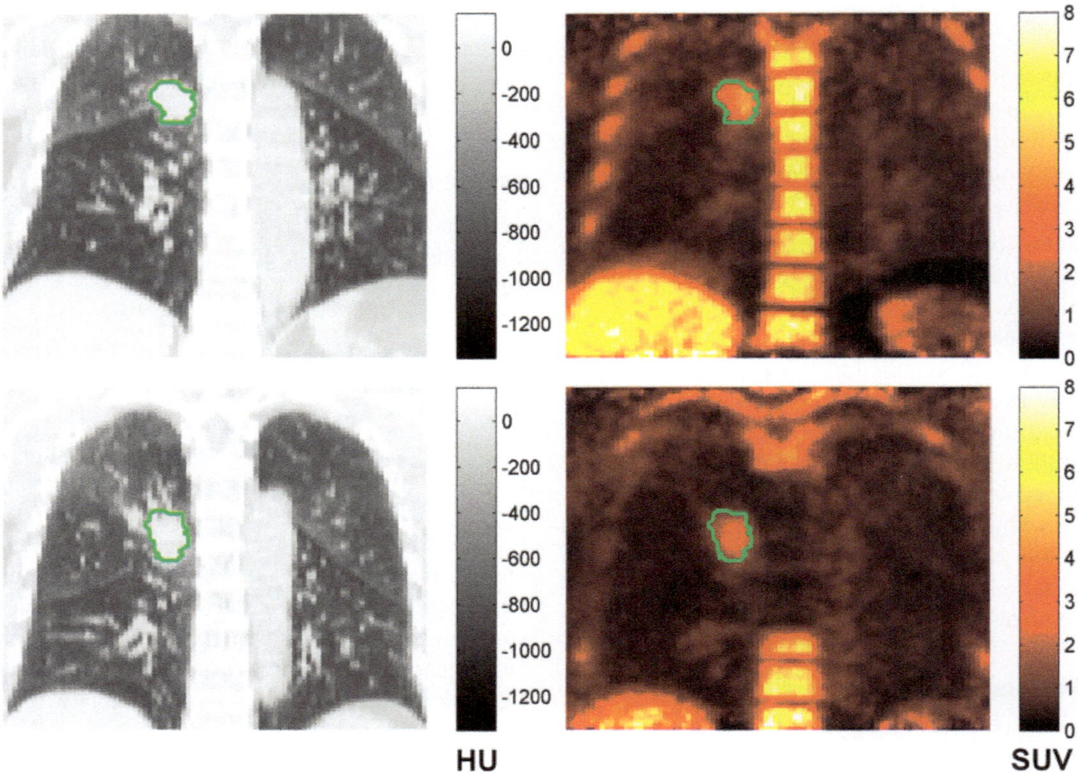

Figure 1. Representative CT (left) and PET (right, SUV 45–60 min) images of patient 11 acquired at baseline (top) and after delivery of 27.5 Gy (bottom). Primary tumour is manually delineated within green outline. Note sharply demarcated dramatic reduction in bone marrow uptake and modest reduction of tumour uptake after RT, as previously reported [21].

Statistical Analysis

For each evaluable VOI (primary tumour or metastatic lymph node), three parameters were extracted: volume in cm^3, SUV_{mean} and SUV_{max}. Individual test-retest difference and RT-induced response were calculated using Eqs. 2 and 3, respectively:

$$Test\text{–}retest\ difference\ (\%) = \frac{Scan2 - Scan1}{Scan1 + Scan2} \times 200 \tag{2}$$

$$Response\ (\%) = \frac{Scan3 - Baseline}{Baseline} \times 100 \tag{3}$$

where Baseline is the latest/single baseline parameter value for Scan1 or Scan2. Reproducibility was estimated as the standard deviation (SD) of the mean test-retest differences across patients and as the average of the absolute test-retest differences across patients (absolute reproducibility).

To allow comparison of the effects of different fractionation regimens, we calculated the biologically effective dose (BED) at the time of the response scan (Scan3) using Eq. 4:

$$BED = n \times D \times \left(1 + D \Big/ \left(\frac{a}{\beta}\right)\right) \tag{4}$$

where n is the number of RT fractions, D (in Gy) is the administered dose per fraction and α/βwas set to 10 for both primary and nodal lesions [25].

Descriptive Statistics

Descriptive summary statistics of the difference between Scan1 and Scan2 for each parameter including mean and SD were calculated. The repeatability coefficient (RC = 1.96 × SD) was also calculated to support comparison with previously published reproducibility values for FLT [26,27]. Differences between lesion volume and SUV before and during RT were tested using the Wilcoxon rank sum test. Potential correlations amongst baseline parameters and between baseline parameter values and reproducibility values were assessed using Spearman's rho coefficient test (two-sided). No correction for multiple testing was used in this exploratory analysis.

Mixed-effects Models

As most patients had more than one evaluable lesion, the SUV_{mean}, SUV_{max} and volume values, transformed to a common (base 10) logarithmic scale for the purpose of this analysis, were each fitted separately to two linear mixed-effects models using analysis of covariance (ANCOVA): The first model (A) pertains to the reproducibility-evaluable patients and was implemented on the duplicate baseline values with the Scan2 value representing the dependent variable. Covariates included the Scan1 value and type of lesion (primary vs node) as fixed-effect terms. The second model pertains to the response-evaluable patients and was implemented with the Scan3 value representing the dependent variable. Covariates included the latter/single baseline value (Scan1/2) and type of lesion (primary vs node) as fixed-effect terms. BED was also assessed as an additional covariate. To account for patients having more than one evaluable lesion, a random effect term was included in both models to account for potential nested effects within patients, i.e. heterogeneity across patients. The models are described in more details with the results presented in Table 3.

Analysis of Outcome Data

Median times for LRC and OS were calculated using the Kaplan-Meier method. Potential associations of both outcome end points with primary tumour continuous PET parameters (baseline, on-RT and response values for SUV_{mean} and SUV_{max}) were investigated using univariate Cox regression without correction for multiple testing.

Statistical tests were performed using SPSS version 19 (SPSS Inc., Chicago, IL, USA) or the statistical software R. A p value below 5 % was considered to be statistically significant.

RESULTS

Between June 2010 and August 2012, 19 patients were recruited into the study. Three patients withdrew after the first baseline scan and were therefore not evaluable. Of the remaining 16 patients, 3 underwent 2 baseline and 1 on-treatment scans and were evaluable for both reproducibility and response. Four patients underwent two baseline scans and were evaluable for reproducibility only. Nine patients underwent a single baseline and an on-treatment scan and were evaluable for response only. Overall, 7 patients with a total of 7 primary and 11 lymph node lesions were evaluable for reproducibility and 12 patients with a total of 12 primary and 18 lymph node lesions were evaluable for response.

Clinical characteristics of evaluable patients and information on the timing of FLT PET scans are summarized in Table 1. Most subjects had stage III disease (13 of 16) and most (13 of 16) received induction chemotherapy; of the latter, the majority (11 of 13) demonstrated partial response to treatment. Baseline volume, SUV_{mean} and SUV_{max} of all evaluable lesions are shown in Fig. 2. Respective summary statistics of baseline, reproducibility and response values for primary tumours and lymph nodes from the PET/CT images are given in Table 2. The primary tumour volumes were significantly larger (5.0–210.7 cm³) than nodal volumes (1.3–21.4 cm³) at baseline ($p<0.001$). Review of lesion SUVs reveals substantial variability of baseline uptake between patients, e.g. primary tumour SUV_{mean} ranged from 0.9 to 3.4 with similar variability observed in nodes (0.9–3.1). In several cases, substantial uptake differences were observed within subject: In 13/16, subjects' primary tumour uptake was higher than or similar to that of metastatic nodes, whereas in 3 subjects (patients 2, 10 and 16), nodal uptake was greater than the primary tumour.

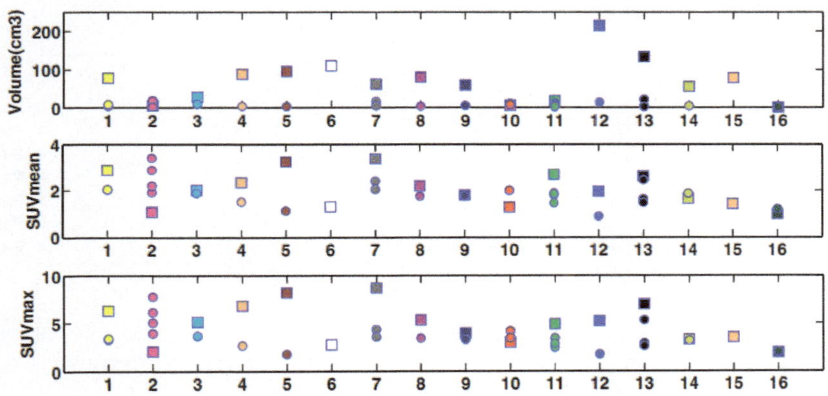

Figure 2. Baseline (single/average) volume (top), SUV_{mean} (middle) and SUV_{max} (bottom) of primary tumours (squares) and metastatic nodal lesions (circles) of 16 patients.

Table 2. Summary statistics of lesion imaging parameters (SUV_{mean}, SUV_{max} and volume) with reproducibility and response 1–2 weeks after RT initiation. Values are presented as mean±SD. For the reproducibility cohort, 7 primaries and 11 nodes are averaged. For the response cohort, 12 primaries and 18 nodes are averaged

Lesion	Reproducibility cohort		Response cohort		Test-retest differences (%)[b]	Responses (%)
	1st baseline values	2nd baseline values	Baseline values[a]	Response values		
Volume (cm³)						
Primaries	38±31	40±31	78±56	85±63	9.5±**12.8(9.8)**	**6.0**±19.1
Nodes	7.5±4.0	8.6±6.3	7.4±5.3	5.9±5.5	8.4±**22.5(19.3)**	**−16.9**±57.0
All	19±24	21±25	36±49	38±56	8.8±**18.9(15.6)**	**−7.7**±46.7
SUV_{mean}						
Primaries	1.6±0.7	1.6±0.6	2.2±0.7	1.6±0.4	−2.9±**8.9(6.8)**	**−24.3**±13.9
Nodes	2.1±0.5	2.2±0.7	1.7±0.4	1.1±0.4	0.6±**18.0(11.9)**	**−39.7**±14.6
All	1.9±0.6	1.9±0.7	1.9±0.6	1.3±0.5	−0.8±**14.9(9.9)**	**−33.5**±16.0
SUV_{max}						

Primaries	3.5±1.7	3.6±1.5	5.3±2.0	4.1±1.4	5.7±**12.6(9.5)**	**−22.9**±13.6
Nodes	4.0±1.3	4.3±1.9	3.2±0.9	1.8±0.7	3.1±**17.2(14.0)**	**−44.4**±15.9
All	3.8±1.5	4.1±1.8	4.1±1.7	2.7±1.5	4.1±**15.3(12.3)**	**−35.8**±18.2

[a]The second baseline scan was used for patients with two baseline scans

[b]Reproducibility given by the SD of the mean test-retest differences. Average of the individual absolute test-retest differences added in parentheses. Both estimates and mean responses highlighted in bold

Across all lesions, there was a strong significant correlation between baseline SUV_{max} and SUV_{mean} (Spearman's rho 0.91, $p<0.001$) and a modest but also significant correlation between SUV_{max} and volume (rho 0.58, $p<0.001$), whereas a weak significant correlation was found between SUV_{mean} and volume (rho 0.36, $p=0.020$). When primary tumours were examined separately from nodes, SUV_{max} correlated significantly with SUV_{mean} for both lesion types (primary tumours rho 0.93, $p<0.001$; nodes rho 0.92, $p<0.001$). Likewise, SUV_{max} correlated significantly with volume (primary tumours rho 0.59, $p=0.016$; nodes rho 0.53, $p=0.006$), but SUV_{mean} correlated significantly with volume only for the nodes (primary tumours rho 0.35, $p=0.19$; nodes rho 0.46, $p=0.020$).

Reproducibility of individual patients is plotted in relation to baseline values in Fig. 3a. Across all lesions, the absolute SUV test-retest differences did not correlate with average baseline lesion SUV_{max} (rho −0.10, $p=0.70$) or SUV_{mean} (rho −0.10, $p=0.69$). In contrast, we found a significant negative correlation between absolute volume test-retest differences and average lesion volume (rho −0.57, $p=0.015$). Accordingly, primary tumour volume reproducibility (SD 12.8) was substantially better compared to nodal lesions (SD 22.5). Consequently, volume RCs were estimated separately for these lesion types, whilst the SUV RC was estimated jointly for primary tumour and nodal lesions and was similar for SUV_{mean} (SD 14.9 %) and SUV_{max} (SD 15.3 %).

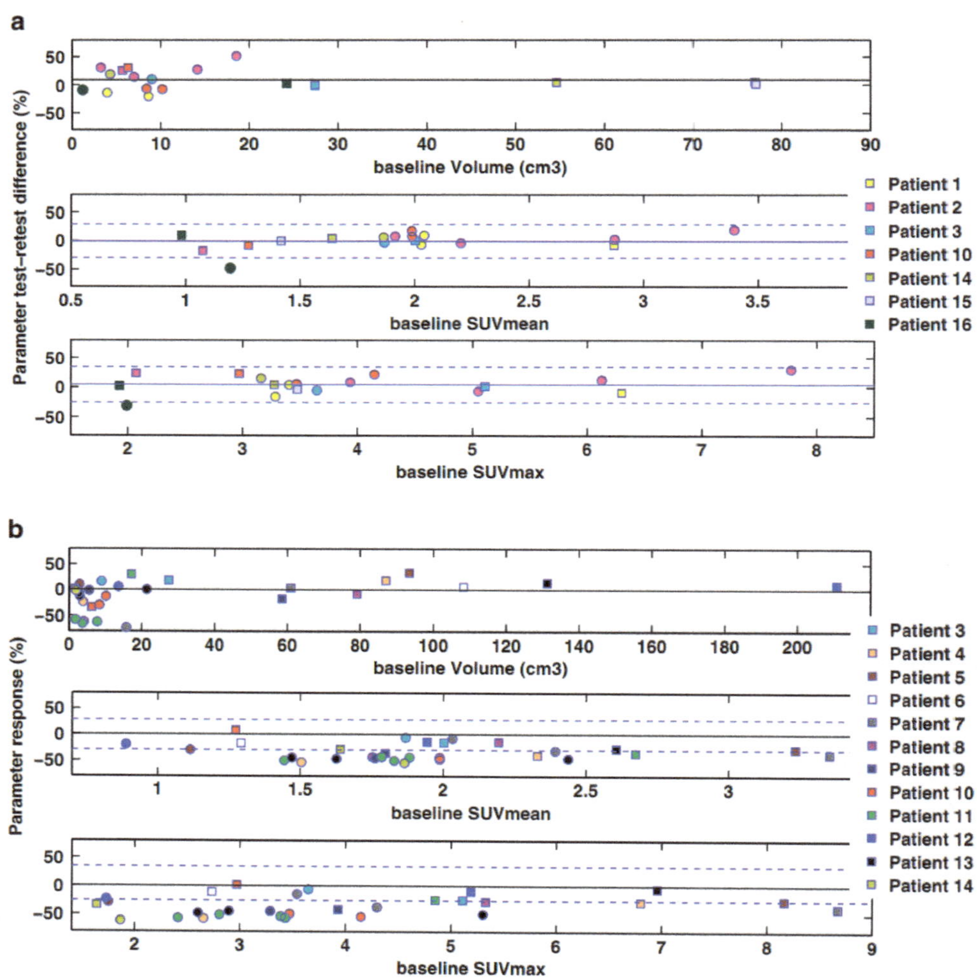

Figure 3. **a** Lesion reproducibilities (%) plotted against mean baseline lesion values for volumes (top), SUV_{mean} (middle) and SUV_{max} (bottom). **b** RT-induced responses (%) plotted against baseline parameter values (second baseline scan if two baseline scans acquired).Dashed lines in SUV graphs set at mean test-retest difference ± RC=1.96×SD, where SD is standard deviation of respective parameter reproducibility. In volume graphs dashed lines not displayed as absolute volume reproducibility correlated with baseline average volume. Primary tumours represented by squares and metastatic nodes by circles. The second evaluable lesion of patient 7 (4R) was measured as 170 % larger post-RT. This outlier is not shown in **b**, to enhance visibility, nevertheless was included in the statistical analyses.

RT response of individual patients is similarly plotted against baseline values in Fig. 3b. RT-related primary tumour volume changes ranged from −33.9 to +33.1 % (mean change +6 %, $p=0.84$). In most (9/12) cases, these changes did not exceed the RC (25 %). On the other hand, metastatic node volume changes ranged from −90.0 % to an outlier increase of +170.4 %, demonstrating a decrease exceeding the RC (44 %) in 5/18 lesions from 3/12 patients. RT-induced changes of lesion SUVs ranged from −54.9 to +7.6 % for SUV_{mean} and from −62.0 to +1.6 % for SUV_{max}. Examined separately, nodes demonstrated a 40±15 % decrease in SUV_{mean} that on average was 1.6 times higher than the 24±14 % decrease of primary tumours (1.9-fold for SUV_{max}). SUV_{mean} response correlated strongly with SUV_{max} response (rho 0.89, $p<0.0001$).

Malignant lesion SUV_{max} during RT (normalized to single/latest baseline value) is plotted against calendar days on RT in Fig. 4, as previously presented by Everitt et al. [21]. During the course of our response assessment window, no significant dose-response relationship was found between SUV_{max} response in primary tumours and days since start of RT (rho=0.27, $p=0.39$), nor with RT dose delivered or BED.

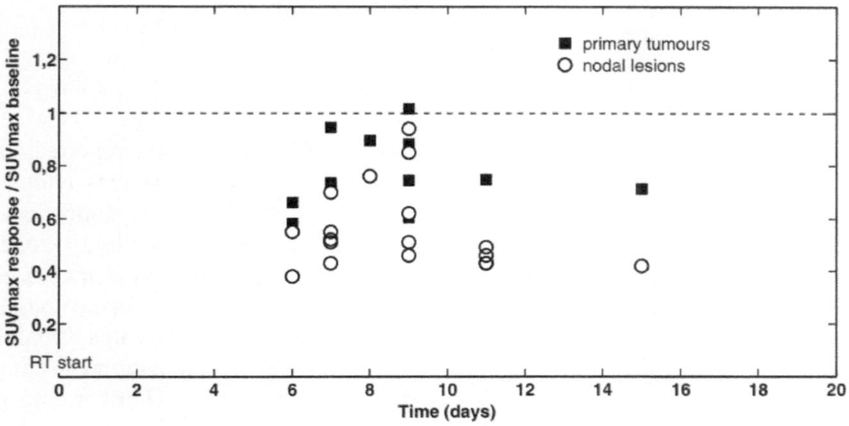

Figure 4. Lack of dose-response relationship between SUV_{max} response (expressed as ratio of SUV_{max} during RT to single/latest baseline value) and calendar days on RT. Primary tumours represented by squares and metastatic nodes by circles.

The results of the ANCOVA are outlined in Table 3. The mixed-effects model implemented on the reproducibility data set (model A) did not provide any evidence of a systematic effect (progression/decline) of the retest values in relation to the test values for any of the parameters SUV_{max}, SUV_{mean} or volume for either primaries or nodes. The fit of the response data to model B did not improve by adding BED as a covariate for any of the parameters SUV_{max}, SUV_{mean} or volume. Therefore, BED was not included in the final implementation of model B. On average, the model estimated a significant decrease in SUV_{mean} of 25 % [confidence interval (CI) −15 to −34 %] in the primary lesions post-RT. Furthermore, the treatment effect for nodes was significantly different to primaries ($p=0.004$), with a larger 40 % (CI −33 to −46 %) decrease. Similarly, the model estimated a significant RT-related decrease of primary tumour SUV_{max} by an average of 24 % (CI −13 to −34 %), which was significantly lower ($p=0.0006$) compared to the average 46 % (CI −39 to −52 %) decrease in SUV_{max} for nodes.

Table 3. Tabulated results of ANCOVA performed separately for lesion SUV_{mean}, SUV_{max} and volume at duplicate baseline scans (model A) and in response to RT (model B). The linear mixed-effects model was generally formulated as $\log10(y_{1ij})=\log10(y_{0ij})+(\beta_0+b_i)+\beta_1 x_{1ij}+\varepsilon_{ij}$. In model A, y_{0ij} is the initial baseline and y_{1ij} is the second baseline value for patient i and lesion j, whereas in model B, y_{0ij} is the pre-RT value and y_{1ij} is the post-RT value for patient i and lesion j. In both models, x_1 indicates the type of lesion (set to 0 if primary or 1 if node) such that β_0 is the 'intercept' for primaries and $\beta_0+\beta_1$ is the intercept for nodes. In both models, $b_i \sim N(0, \sigma_b^2)$ represents the cross-patient heterogeneity random term (σ_b^2 is the variance across patients) and $\varepsilon_{ij} \sim N(0, \sigma^2)$ represents the model error that is due to variability across lesions and 'pure' model error (σ^2 is the residual error variance). Note that parameter estimates are based on log-transformed data and hence need to be back-transformed to allow estimation of effect size. For example, the model-estimated mean RT-induced SUV_{mean} effect size ratio can be calculated from β_0, β_1 values from model $y_1/y_0-1=10^{(\beta_0+\beta_1)}-1$ for nodes. The proportion of the variation in the intercept that is accounted for by patient heterogeneity can be calculated as $\sigma_b^2/(\sigma^2+\sigma_b^2)$. The Akaike Information Criterion (AIC) provides a measure of the goodness of the fit to the four-parameter $\left(\beta_0,\beta_1,_{\sigma_b^2},_{\sigma^2}\right)$ models

Model A (reproducibility) parameters		SUV_{mean}	SUV_{max}	Volume
Fixed effects[a]	β_0[b]	−0.014±0.025 (0.60)	0.024±0.026 (0.37)	0.041±0.031 (0.11)
	β_1[c]	0.015±0.032 (0.65)	−0.025±0.027 (0.38)	−0.025±0.031 (0.43)
Random effects	σ_b^2	0.00000	0.00188	0.00300
	σ^2	0.00448	0.00291	0.00374

AIC		−28.78	−30.20	−25.42
Model B (response) parameters		SUV_{mean}	SUV_{max}	Volume
Fixed effects[a]	β_0[b]	−0.127±0.025 (0.0001)	−0.119±0.029 (0.0007)	0.018±0.073 (0.81)
	β_1[c]	−0.095±0.029 (0.004)	−0.147±0.035 (0.0006)	−0.177±0.089 (0.06)
Random effects	σ_b^2	0.00224	0.00154	0.00858
	σ^2	0.00556	0.00839	0.05579
AIC		−45.24	−37.02	15.46

[a]Model parameters for fixed effects presented as estimate ±standard error (p value)

[b]p values from statistical comparison against 0

[c]p values from statistical comparison against primary tumours

With regard to lesion volume, primary tumours demonstrated no significant change (4 %, CI −27 to +48 %, p=0.81) in response to treatment. In contrast, the model estimated an average decrease of 31 % (CI −6 to −49 %) in node volume that was significant (p=0.020) and significantly different to primary tumours (p=0.060).

For all three parameters, the random variation across patients estimated by model B was small compared to the variation across lesions. For SUV_{mean}, the cross-patient (nested) effect accounted for about 28.7 % of the total variance. The contribution of cross-patient variance to the total variance was even smaller for SUV_{max} and volume at 15.5 and 13.3 %, respectively. One year after recruiting the last patient (September 2013), the median follow-up time was 15.4 months after RT initiation (range 3–33 months). At that time point, 9 patients had documented local primary tumour progression, 5 had developed metastatic disease and 11 had died of which 1 (patient 2) before treatment completion. Median LRC and OS times were 12.2 (CI 6–18) and 19.5 (CI 9–30) months, respectively. Cox regression analysis identified no significant association between OS and baseline, on-RT or response values of primary tumour SUV_{mean} and SUV_{max} (p>0.08). However, LRC was found to be associated with primary tumour SUV_{max} on-RT (hazard ratio 2.31, CI 1.06–5.00, p=0.034) but not with SUV_{max} at baseline (hazard ratio 1.46, CI 0.97–2.18, p=0.068) or SUV_{mean} on RT (hazard ratio 5.80, CI 0.66–50.6, p=0.112).

DISCUSSION

We have confirmed previous studies on FLT parameter reproducibility and demonstrated that, in patients with NSCLC, RT induces an early, significant decrease in tumour FLT uptake which is lower than previously reported for concurrent chemo-RT at a similar time point [21]. After 1–2 weeks of RT, the magnitude of this response was found not to be driven by variations in the RT dose delivered but to vary between primary tumours and metastatic nodal lesions, possibly indicating distinct intrinsic radiosensitivities. This contrasts with the previously reported findings that FLT response did not to differ between lesion types after 5–6 weeks of chemo-RT and depended on the RT dose received [22].

Establishing the effect of treatment on a potential imaging biomarker is best performed in the context of validating its precision. Therefore, we performed a combined assessment of tumour FLT PET parameter reproducibility and response. To date, three groups have reported on the reproducibility of tumour FLT SUVs in patients with lung and other cancers [28–30], while two further publications addressed the issue of metabolic volume reproducibility [26, 27]. In all cases, tumour VOIs were delineated on PET images, either manually or using semi-automatic segmentation methods. In contrast, in our study, tumour VOIs were delineated primarily on anatomical CT images, aiming to capture the mean uptake across both avid and less avid tumour regions. Furthermore, previous studies largely included treatment-naive subjects, whereas most patients enrolled in our study had received induction chemotherapy before acquisition of the baseline scans. Consequently, average lesion SUV_{mean} in our subjects was substantially lower than in previous studies (SUV_{mean} ~2 compared to more than 3). Despite such differences, SUV_{mean} reproducibility results across studies were comparable: Reproducibility in our study was 14.9 % (primaries 8.9 %, nodes 18.0 %) compared to 10.5 % [28], 7.0 % [29] and 4.5 % [30] in previous reports exclusively or predominantly including primary lesions. Despite the use of image smoothing and absence of variability associated with VOI delineation, primary tumour SUV_{max} was less reproducible (SD 12.6 %) than SUV_{mean}. These results are in agreement with the main conclusion of a recent meta-analysis of FDG studies demonstrating SUV_{mean} as the most reproducible SUV parameter [31]. This superiority was lost in nodal lesions for which SUV_{max} was marginally more reproducible than SUV_{mean}.

In terms of volume reproducibility, we found that manual delineation of malignant NSCLC lesions by a single imaging expert yielded VOIs with volumetric precision at least equivalent to semi-automatic segmentation methods including fixed threshold, adaptive threshold or cluster-based methods implemented in two previous publications in patients with lung and breast cancer [26, 27]. However, it is expected that manual tumour delineation, unlike semi-automatic methods, will suffer from additional inter-observer variability [32]. In accordance with previous reports, we found that the volume reproducibility of manually delineated lesions correlated negatively with their size [26, 27]. Therefore, using the same confidence intervals across a wide spectrum of volumes is inappropriate. Optimal volumetric response assessment would require one or more cut-off values defined through analysis of a large reproducibility data set and/or simulation studies.

Taken together, this and other recent reports indicate that, in lung cancer, FLT SUV parameters are similarly robust to respective FDG parameters, with only a modest impact from the segmentation approach used. Changes of primary tumour SUV_{mean} exceeding 17 % and SUV_{max} exceeding 25 % are likely to be significant. Lesion volume, delineated manually on PET/CT images or with semi-automatic PET-based segmentation methods is generally a less precise parameter, especially for small lesions.

When we designed this study, we considered the choice of potential time points to assess response. Based on preclinical reports [17–20] and the first pilot clinical study [21], we elected an early assessment point aiming to obtain an early read-out of intrinsic radiosensitivity and minimize the confounding effect of volumetric changes and potential RT-related inflammatory changes on tumour uptake. Furthermore, to limit the variability of RT dose delivered at the time of on-treatment scans, while maintaining study feasibility, we restricted the response assessment window to 1 week.

We found that in the absence of significant changes in average primary tumour size, RT induced a significant decrease of about 25 % in FLT uptake after a week of treatment, as measured by both SUV_{mean} and SUV_{max}. In contrast, metastatic nodes sustained a significant decrease in mean volume associated with a decrease in FLT uptake significantly exceeding that observed in primary tumours. Considering that primary tumours routinely receive RT doses at least equivalent to metastatic nodes, the observed difference in uptake response may be attributed to genuine differences in biological behaviour between primary and metastatic nodal lesions in terms of perfusion, FLT-specific transport and/or phosphorylation in response to treatment. These processes cannot be separated by simple SUV measurements. Alternatively, the RT dose delivered to the metastatic nodes may differ from that to the primary tumour. Finally, considering the potential interaction of size and uptake, which may be enhanced in small/shrinking lesions, it is possible that the observed decreases of the size of some nodal lesions may have contributed to an artefactual decrease of measured uptake. On a different but relevant note, response results will differ on whether absolute or percentage differences are calculated. Considering that in most response-evaluable patients baseline primary tumour uptake exceeded that of metastatic nodes, an absolute difference response assessment would attenuate differences in response between primaries and nodes.

In addition to differences between primaries and nodes, we observed variable changes in FLT uptake across all lesions and across primaries and nodes separately. This is complicated further by the fact that different patients had variable numbers of evaluable lesions. To disentangle these interactions, we used a mixed-effects linear model. The statistical outcome suggests that the response variability across patients (i.e. a nested effect) had a limited contribution to the overall variability, which was mainly driven by lesion-to-lesion differences. In other words, response heterogeneity was most prominent across lesions rather than across patients. Variations in the RT dose delivered over the course of a week did not explain the variability in FLT responses in the early phase of treatment. Considering the spectrum of baseline variability and treatment-related changes illustrated in Fig. 3, this point in the course of RT SUV analysis may support early response stratification of lesions into responding and not responding.

Two previous studies have reported treatment-related FLT SUV_{max} changes, each in five patients each receiving concurrent chemo-RT. Everitt et al. were first to assess patients with NSCLC at variable time points ranging from 2 to 29 days of treatment [21]. After 10 Gy, primary tumour SUV_{max} reduced by 40 % in two cases, while in two subjects 20 Gy induced decreases exceeding 60 %, as compared to an average decrease of 24 % after 12–30 Gy in our study. These differences may to some extent reflect the added effect of concurrent chemotherapy. Vera et al. studied NSCLC patients using FLT, FDG and [^{18}F]fluoromisonidazole (FMISO for hypoxia) PET at baseline and after 4–5 weeks of radical concurrent/sequential chemo-RT [22]. The decrease in FLT SUV_{max} at this later time point was 46 ± 21 % in primary tumours, comparable to that previously reported by Everitt et al. [21] and appeared lower and more variable (29 ± 60 %) in mediastinal lymph nodes; nevertheless, no significant differences between primaries and nodes were found. In contrast to our results, and despite a narrower response assessment window (44–58 vs 12–30 Gy), they interestingly found that one third of the variations in FLT responses could be accounted by the dose-response relationship when considering tumours and nodes together and adjusting for inter-patient heterogeneity, possibly indicating that during the latter phase of treatment tumour uptake may be undergoing more dynamic changes. Neither lesion volumes nor changes in volume which could have confounded the changes in FLT uptake, especially in the later phase of treatment, were reported in this study.

Similarly to previous investigators [21], we observed a dramatic reduction in FLT uptake of normal bone marrow within the RT field. In this study, at least half of evaluable primary tumours and/or metastatic nodal lesions were adjacent or proximal to proliferating bone. It is worth noting that in such cases there is a risk for incorrect response assessment, which is exacerbated for RT compared to chemotherapy. For example, erroneous inclusion of a segment of proliferating bone marrow within the tumour VOI at baseline may lead to response overestimation. Such a risk may be higher in the absence of co-registered CT, or in cases of PET/CT mis-registration, and can have major effect on study results, in particular when SUV_{max} is used to assess response. We tried to minimize this risk by comprehensive co-registration assessment and exclusion of any overlap of the skeleton with tumour VOIs.

Compared to the concurrent approach, sequential chemo-RT lends itself to the separate study of systemic and local treatment on tumour response. Nevertheless, recent chemotherapy could still have influenced the changes observed on-RT by either affecting the baseline tumour proliferative status or through a persistent pharmacodynamic effect especially in the early course of RT. Although the interval between chemotherapy completion and baseline imaging in response-evaluable subjects was at least 2 weeks and duplicate baseline scans up to a week apart did not detect significant changes in tumour size or proliferative activity, induction chemotherapy could have confounded changes in tumour FLT uptake attributed to RT to a degree not quantifiable in this data set.

Although survival analysis was not a primary objective of this study, we explored potential relationships of primary tumour SUV parameters, at baseline, during treatment and their relative change, with tumour control and patient outcome.

Instead of defining arbitrary cut-off point(s) that would split the small sample size into smaller subgroups sensitive to the cut-off point(s) selected, we followed a univariate regression approach. Our results indicate a possible association of primary tumour SUV_{max}, but not SUV_{mean}, after 1–2 weeks of RT and eventual LRC. On the other hand, OS, potentially influenced by multiple variables in addition to local control, was not significantly associated with any local tumour imaging parameter. This interesting finding should be interpreted with caution because of the lack of detection power and the risk of type I error associated with multiple testing on a small sample size, which was further reduced by censoring. However, it could serve as an a priori hypothesis to be formally tested by a larger subsequent study, ideally with pre-planned multivariate analysis to account for additional clinical and imaging parameters.

Despite a larger number of patients compared to earlier work, our study was still limited in size. In our experience, patient recruitment in this setting can be challenging. Lung cancer patients are often symptomatic, frail or elderly and participation in a molecular imaging study is associated with the burden of additional scans without a potential therapeutic benefit. Comprehensive evaluation of FLT PET in this setting would require recruitment of large numbers of patients to be evaluated at various time points, in order to elucidate both the time course and heterogeneity of responses and repopulation. The logistic limitations related to accomplishing such a project in a single centre raise the importance of standardizing methodology and multi-centre collaborations, more easily achieved using SUV than kinetic analysis. A further limitation of our work arises from the lack of some form of respiratory motion correction. Respiratory motion and to a lesser extent partial volume effects are expected to induce an interaction between size and SUV, resulting in bias especially in small peripheral lesions [33, 34].

In summary, this is the first study demonstrating that RT, as single treatment modality, induces in a subgroup of patients an early, significant decrease of primary lung tumour FLT uptake in the absence of significant mean volumetric changes. Metastatic nodes follow a discrete pattern of change with some early volumetric regression and a larger decrease in FLT uptake. These results confirm the potential for FLT PET to report early on radiation response and to enhance the clinical development of novel drug-radiation combinations by providing an interpretable, early pharmacodynamic end point. The variability of responses observed indicates some potential for patient stratification in future clinical trials evaluating RT.

ACKNOWLEDGMENTS

This is a contribution from the Cambridge—Manchester Cancer Imaging Centre, which is funded by the EPSRC and Cancer Research UK and from the Manchester-UCL Lung Cancer Centre of Excellence, which is funded by CRUK. The authors gratefully acknowledge the financial support from AstraZeneca Pharmaceuticals, the Oglesby Charitable Trust and Cancer Research UK. We also thank Pamela Hindmarsh for her help with patient recruitment and the technical staff at the WMIC for PET scanning. We are also grateful to all participants for volunteering in the study.

REFERENCES

1. Parkin DM. Global cancer statistics in the year 2000. Lancet Oncol 2001; 2:533–43.
2. Price A. Lung cancer 5: state of the art radiotherapy for lung cancer. Thorax 2003; 58:447–52.
3. Bayman NA, Blackhall F, Jain P, Lee L, Thatcher N, Faivre-Finn C. Management of unresectable stage III non-small-cell lung cancer with combined-modality therapy: a review of the current literature and recommendations for treatment. Clin Lung Cancer 2008; 9:92–101.
4. Aupérin A, Le Péchoux C, Rolland E, Curran WJ, Furuse K, Fournel P, Belderbos J, Clamon G, Ulutin HC, Paulus R, et al. Meta-analysis of concomitant versus sequential radiochemotherapy in locally advanced non-small-cell lung cancer. J Clin Oncol 2010; 28:2181–90.
5. Tan DS, Thomas GV, Garrett MD, Banerji U, de Bono JS, Kaye SB, et al. Biomarker-driven early clinical trials in oncology: a paradigm shift in drug development. Cancer J 2009; 15:406–20.
6. Seddon BM, Workman P. The role of functional and molecular imaging in cancer drug discovery and development. Br J Radiol 2003; 76(76 Spec No 2):S128–38.
7. Weber WA, Wieder H. Monitoring chemotherapy and radiotherapy of solid tumors. Eur J Nucl Med Mol Imaging 2006; 33 Suppl 1:27–37.
8. Riesterer O, Milas L, Ang KK. Use of molecular biomarkers for predicting the response to radiotherapy with or without chemotherapy. J Clin Oncol 2007; 25:4075–83.
9. Chau CH, Rixe O, McLeod H, Figg WD. Validation of analytic methods for biomarkers used in drug development. Clin Cancer Res 2008; 14:5967–76.
10. Begg AC, Stewart FA, Vens C. Strategies to improve radiotherapy with targeted drugs. Nat Rev Cancer 2011; 11:239–53.
11. Bading JR, Shields AF. Imaging of cell proliferation: status and prospects. J Nucl Med 2008; 49 Suppl 2:64S–80.
12. Vesselle H, Grierson J, Muzi M, Pugsley JM, Schmidt RA, Rabinowitz P, et al. In vivo validation of 3′deoxy-3′-[(18)F]fluorothymidine ([(18)F]FLT) as a proliferation imaging tracer in humans: correlation of [(18)F]FLT uptake by positron emission tomography with Ki-67 immunohistochemistry and flow cytometry in human lung tumors. Clin Cancer Res 2002; 8:3315–23.
13. Muzi M, Vesselle H, Grierson JR, Mankoff DA, Schmidt RA, Peterson L, et al. Kinetic analysis of 3′-deoxy-3′-fluorothymidine PET studies: validation studies in patients with lung cancer. J Nucl Med 2005; 46:274–82.
14. Buck AK, Halter G, Schirrmeister H, Kotzerke J, Wurziger I, Glatting G, et al. Imaging proliferation in lung tumors with PET: 18F-FLT versus 18F-FDG. J Nucl Med 2003; 44:1426–31.
15. Yamamoto Y, Nishiyama Y, Ishikawa S, Nakano J, Chang SS, Bandoh S, et al. Correlation of 18F-FLT and 18F-FDG uptake on PET with Ki-67 immunohistochemistry in

non-small cell lung cancer. Eur J Nucl Med Mol Imaging 2007; 34:1610–6.

16. Brockenbrough JS, Souquet T, Morihara JK, Stern JE, Hawes SE, Rasey JS, et al. Tumor 3′-deoxy-3′-(18) F-fluorothymidine ((18)F-FLT) uptake by PET correlates with thymidine kinase 1 expression: static and kinetic analysis of (18)F-FLT PET studies in lung tumors. J Nucl Med 2011; 52:1181–8.
17. Sugiyama M, Sakahara H, Sato K, Harada N, Fukumoto D, Kakiuchi T, et al. Evaluation of 3′-deoxy-3′-18F-fluorothymidine for monitoring tumor response to radiotherapy and photodynamic therapy in mice. J Nucl Med 2004; 45:1754–8.
18. Yang YJ, Ryu JS, Kim SY, Oh SJ, Im KC, Lee H, et al. Use of 3′-deoxy-3′-[18F]fluorothymidine PET to monitor early responses to radiation therapy in murine SCCVII tumors. Eur J Nucl Med Mol Imaging 2006; 33:412–9.
19. Pan MH, Huang SC, Liao YP, Schaue D, Wang CC, Stout DB, et al. FLT-PET imaging of radiation responses in murine tumors. Mol Imaging Biol 2008; 10:325–34.
20. Murayama C, Harada N, Kakiuchi T, Fukumoto D, Kamijo A, Kawaguchi AT, et al. Evaluation of D-18F-FMT, 18F-FDG, L-11C-MET, and 18F-FLT for monitoring the response of tumors to radiotherapy in mice. J Nucl Med 2009; 50:290–5.
21. Everitt S, Hicks RJ, Ball D, Kron T, Schneider-Kolsky M, Walter T, et al. Imaging cellular proliferation during chemo-radiotherapy: a pilot study of serial 18F-FLT positron emission tomography/computed tomography imaging for non-small-cell lung cancer. Int J Radiat Oncol Biol Phys 2009; 75:1098–104.
22. Vera P, Bohn P, Edet-Sanson A, Salles A, Hapdey S, Gardin I, et al. Simultaneous positron emission tomography (PET) assessment of metabolism with (18)F-fluoro-2-deoxy-d-glucose (FDG), proliferation with (18)F-fluoro-thymidine (FLT), and hypoxia with (18)fluoro-misonidazole (F-miso) before and during radiotherapy in patients with non-small-cell lung cancer (NSCLC): a pilot study. Radiother Oncol 2011; 98:109–16.
23. Eisenhauer EA, Therasse P, Bogaerts J, Schwartz LH, Sargent D, Ford R, et al. New response evaluation criteria in solid tumours: revised RECIST guideline (version 1.1). Eur J Cancer 2009; 45:228–47.
24. Machulla HJ, Blocher A, Kuntzsch M, Piert M, Wei R, Grierson JR. Simplified labeling approach for synthesizing 3′-deoxy-3′-[18F]fluorothymidine ([18F] FLT). J Radioanal Nucl Chem 2000; 243:843–6.
25. Levitt SH. Technical basis of radiation therapy: practical clinical applications. 4th rev. ed. Berlin: Springer; 2006.
26. Hatt M, Cheze-Le Rest C, Aboagye EO, Kenny LM, Rosso L, Turkheimer FE, et al. Reproducibility of 18F-FDG and 3′-deoxy-3′-18F-fluorothymidine PET tumor volume measurements. J Nucl Med 2010; 51:1368–76.
27. Frings V, de Langen AJ, Smit EF, van Velden FH, Hoekstra OS, van Tinteren H, Boellaard R. Repeatability of metabolically active volume measurements with 18F-FDG and 18F-FLT PET in non-small cell lung cancer. J Nucl Med 2010; 51:1870–77.
28. Kenny L, Coombes RC, Vigushin DM, Al-Nahhas A, Shousha S, Aboagye EO. Imaging early changes in proliferation at 1 week post chemotherapy: a pilot study in breast cancer patients with 3′-deoxy-3′-[18F] fluorothymidine positron emission tomography. Eur J Nucl Med Mol Imaging 2007; 34:1339–47.
29. de Langen AJ, Klabbers B, Lubberink M, Boellaard R, Spreeuwenberg MD, Slotman BJ, et al. Reproducibility of quantitative 18F-3′-deoxy-3′-fluorothymidine measurements using positron emission tomography. Eur J Nucl Med Mol Imaging 2009; 36:389–95.
30. Shields AF, Lawhorn-Crews JM, Briston DA, Zalzala S, Gadgeel S, Douglas KA, et al. Analysis and reproducibility of 3′-deoxy-3′-[18F]fluorothymidine positron emission tomography imaging in patients with non-small cell lung cancer. Clin Cancer Res 2008; 14:4463–8.
31. de Langen AJ, Vincent A, Velasquez LM, van Tinteren H, Boellaard R, Shankar LK, et al. Repeatability of 18F-FDG uptake measurements in tumors: a metaanalysis. J Nucl Med 2012; 53:701–8.
32. Dewalle-Vignion AS, Yeni N, Petyt G, Verscheure L, Huglo D, Béron A, et al. Evaluation of PET volume segmentation methods: comparisons with expert manual delineations. Nucl Med Commun 2012; 33:34–42.
33. Hamill JJ, Bosmans G, Dekker A. Respiratory-gated CT as a tool for the simulation of breathing artifacts in PET and PET/CT. Med Phys 2008; 35:576–85.
34. El Naqa I, Low DA, Bradley JD, Vicic M, Deasy JO. Deblurring of breathing motion artifacts in thoracic PET images by deconvolution methods. Med Phys 2006; 33:3587–600.

SECTION III - SOLAR RADIATION

CHAPTER 15

MEASUREMENT BIASES EXPLAIN DISCREPANCIES BETWEEN THE OBSERVED AND SIMULATED DECADAL VARIABILITY OF SURFACE INCIDENT SOLAR RADIATION

Kaicun Wang

INTRODUCTION

Solar radiation is the ultimate energy source of the earth's climate system, which drives weather and climate change and vegetation growth[1]. Due to its importance, surface incident solar radiation (R_s) has been widely measured since the late 1950s. These observations have been archived by the Global Energy Balance Archive (GEBA)[2]. They have suggested a widespread decrease between the 1950s and 1980s ("global dimming")[2] with the subsequent brightening[3,4].

Recent studies[5,6] have compared the Coupled Model Intercomparison Project phase 3 (CMIP3) and phase 5 (CMIP5)[7] decadal variability of simulated R_s with observations collected by GEBA over land for the last half century and have reported large discrepancies. In particular, it was found that all of the 42 models of CMIP5 underestimated the trend of the observed R_s and none of the simulations of the CMIP5 models could reproduce the magnitude of the observed dimming trend over China and India[5]. From these comparisons, it could be inferred that the models are seriously flawed in their determination of the decadal variability of R_s. If this is so, their reported good ability to reproduce twentieth century climate could be called into question because R_s has an important contribution to decadal variability of surface air temperature[8,9,10].

In this study, we examine the decadal variability of observed R_s in China and find that the observed R_s may have overestimated the dimming rate due to the degradation problem of instruments before 1990 and overestimated the brightening rate due to instrument replacement from 1990 to 1993. When these sources of error are accounted for, the inference that there is serious disagreement between models and observations becomes much weaker.

RESULTS

Here, we evaluate the decadal variability of the observed R_s with an independent measurement of sunshine duration (SunDu). SunDu is a conventional meteorological observation that records the time duration during a day when the direct solar beam is greater than 120 W m^{-2}, which is defined by the world meteorological organization. The light-sensitive paper of a SunDu recorder is burned when the direct solar beam is higher than a threshold, i.e., 120 W m^{-2}. SunDu is measured through reading the length of the burned mark during a day.

R_s can be calculated from SunDu, i.e., with the method (Eq. (1)) proposed by Yang et al.[11], which has been regarded as having the capability of reflecting the impacts of clouds and aerosols on R_s accurately[12,13,14,15,16,17]. To apply the method globally or regionally, existing studies[12,13] tried to derive a suite of parameters by calibrating the equations with the observed R_s.

However, the burning threshold depends on the types of SunDu recorders and the sitting environment, i.e., its geographical location[16]. To address this issue, we calibrate the Eq. (1) to estimate R_s from SunDu at each station. We find 122

Citation: Kaicun Wang. Measurement biases explain discrepancies between the observed and simulated decadal variability of surface incident solar radiation, Scientific Reports 4, Article number: 6144 (2014). DOI:10.1038/srep06144 stations where both R_s and SunDu were measured for more than 10 years from 1958 to 2012 (Fig. 1), from which a reliable relationship between R_s and SunDu can be established at each station (Eq. (1) of Method Section). The relationship between R_s and SunDu may vary with geo-location and types of SunDu recorders. However, this relationship is expected to be stable for a station given the same SunDu recorder has been used. Under the assumption that the relationship between R_s and SunDu is stable for a station, the calibrated equation can be used to calculate R_s from SunDu for a longer time period, as SunDu has a longer observation history than R_s[16].

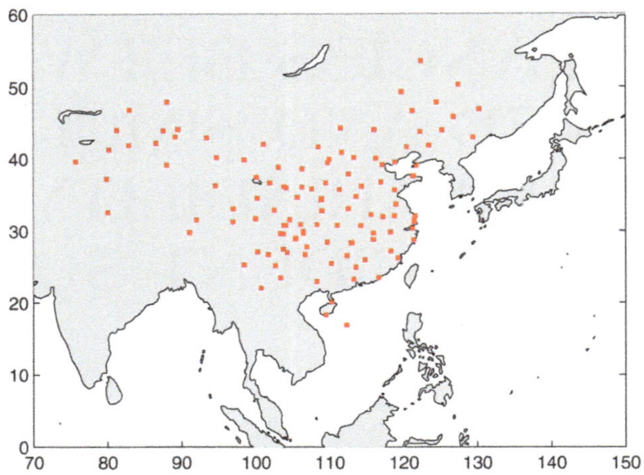

Figure 1: A map of the stations (red square) where data durations of both surface incident solar radiation (R_s) and Sunshine Duration (SunDu) were longer than 120 months from 1958 to 2012. There are 122 stations in total. The figure was produced using MATLAB.

Fig. 2 shows scatterplots of SunDu-derived R_s as a function of the observed R_s at four stations. The biases are near zero because Eq. (1) used to estimate R_s from SunDu was calibrated with the observed R_s at each station. The statistical results of the standard deviation and correlation coefficients of all the stations are shown in Fig. 3, which shows R_s can be accurately estimated from SunDu at daily and monthly time scales. SunDu has difficulty in estimating R_s at time scales shorter than one day, as only daily SunDu was documented.

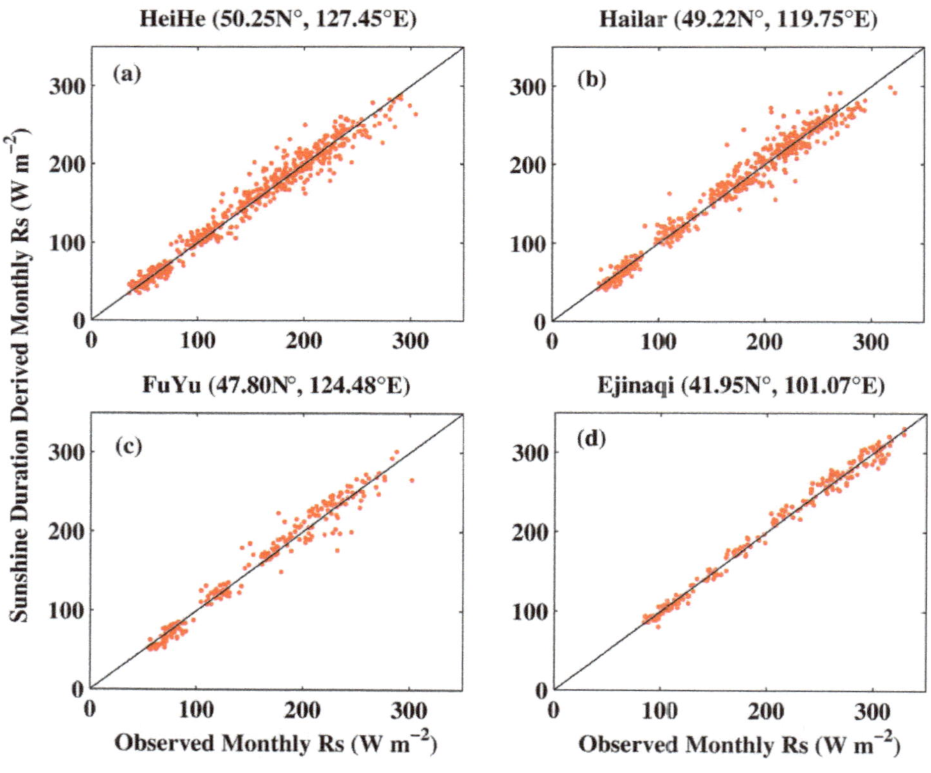

Figure 2: Scatterplots of monthly averages of Sunshine Duration (SunDu) derived surface incident solar radiation (R_s) as a function of the observed R_s at four stations. The biases, standard deviations, and correlation coefficients of the comparisons between SunDu-derived R_s and observed R_s at the four stations are: (a): −0.3 W m^{-2}, 12.0 W m^{-2}, 0.99, (b) −0.6 W m^{-2}, 12.9 W m^{-2}, 0.98, (c) −0.8 W m^{-2}, 12.5 W m^{-2}, 0.98, and (d) −0.4 W m^{-2}, 7.9 W m^{-2}, 0.99. The biases are near zero because Eq. (1) used to calculate R_s from SunDu was calibrated at each station with the observed R_s. Four examples are shown here and the statistical results of all the stations are shown in Fig. 3. The figure was produced using MATLAB.

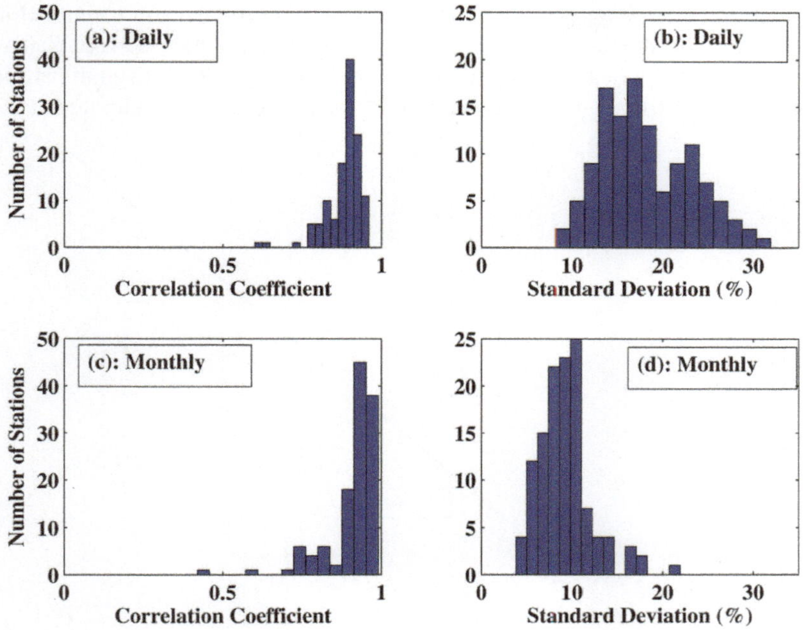

Figure 3: Histograms of the statistical parameters of the comparisons between daily and monthly observed surface incident solar radiation (R_s) and R_s derived from Sunshine Duration (SunDu). The correlation coefficients and relative standard deviations (normalized by multi-year averages at each station) calculated from daily data are shown in panels (a) and (b), and those calculated from monthly data are shown in panels (c) and (d). As the Eq. (1) used to calculate R_s from SunDu was calibrated at each station, the biases of the comparisons are near zero and are not shown here. The medians of the correlation coefficients and the relative standard deviations between observed and calculated daily R_s are 0.89 and 17.32%, respectively, and the values are 0.94 and 9.11% for monthly R_s. The figure was produced using MATLAB.

To provide accurate decadal variability of R_s, it is necessary to regularly and properly calibrate the instruments (i.e., the pyranometers) to measure R_s. However, a world-wide radiometric reference for such a calibration was not established until the year 1979[18,19]. Without an accurate and regular calibration, the instruments would lose their sensitivity and introduce a false dimming trend of the observed R_s[3]. SunDu recorders do not have this issue[20] as their recording material, the light-sensitive paper, is replaced every day. Fig. 4 shows that there were obvious instrument degradation problems for the observed R_s at the four stations in the Tibetan Plateau, while the SunDu-derived R_s were more stable and more homogeneous.

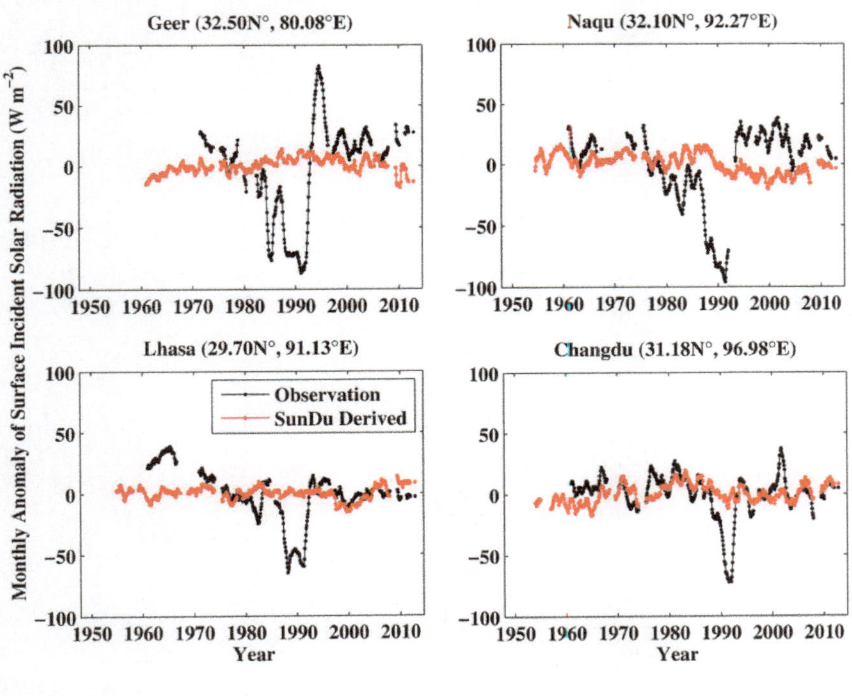

Figure 4: Time series of 12-month smoothed monthly anomalies of observed surface incident solar radiation (R_s) and R_s calculated from Sunshine Duration (SunDu) at four stations in the Tibetan Plateau. Observations of R_s are impacted by the performance of instruments (pyrheliometer and pyranometers). These instruments should be accurately and regularly calibrated. Otherwise, they would lose their sensitivity and produce a spurious dimming trend of R_s. On the contrary, the measurements of SunDu are much less sensitive to instrument calibration, as its recording material is replaced each day. There is significant evidence that the instruments used to measure R_s at these four stations had important calibration problems before 1992 when the new instruments were deployed. The figure was produced using MATLAB.

These instrument degradation issues were very common for the R_s measurements in China before 1990. Fig. 5 shows that trends of R_s from observations are substantially more negative than those of the SunDu-derived R_s from 1960 to 1989. There are four stations where the observed R_s had a near-zero trend while SunDu-derived R_s had significant positive or negative trends. Fig. 6 shows that this is because the instruments used to measure R_s were inaccurately calibrated at the stations at certain years.

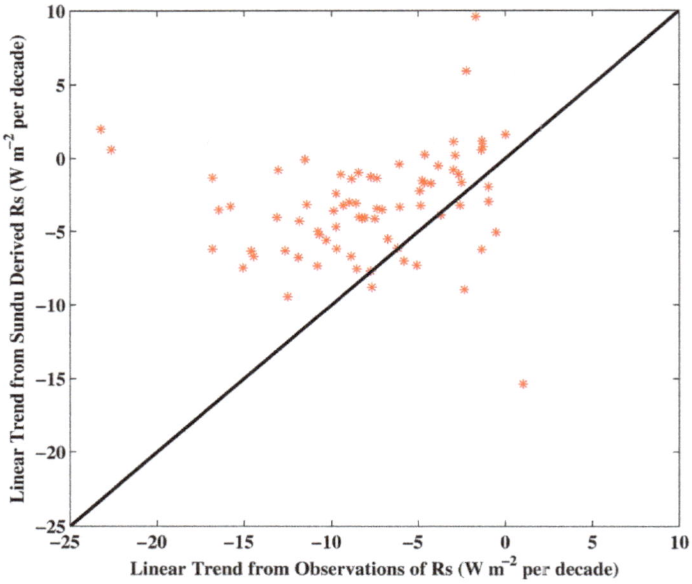

Figure 5: Scatterplot of the linear trends of observed R_s as a function of trends of SunDu-derived R_s. Each red star represents a station in China where the data duration of both the observed and calculated R_s were longer than 120 months during 1960 to 1989. There are 76 stations in total. Linear trends of observed surface incident solar radiation (R_s) are significantly more negative than those from sunshine duration (SunDu) derived R_s. The figure was produced using MATLAB.

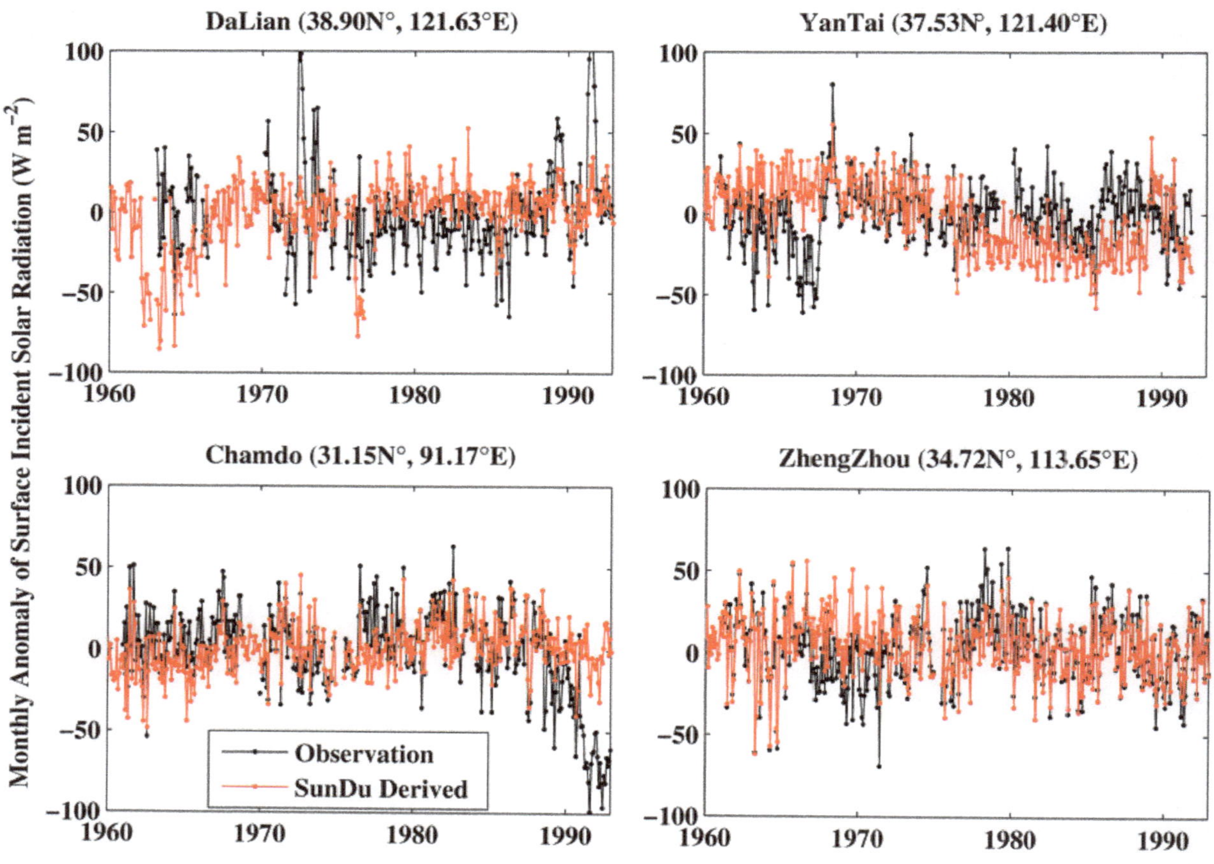

Figure 6: Time series of observed surface incident solar radiation (R_s) and R_s calculated from Sunshine Duration (SunDu) at four stations where the observed R_s showed a near-zero trend while SunDu-derived R_s had significant positive or negative trends (see Fig. 5). It is obvious that the instruments used to measure R_s were inaccurately calibrated at the DaLian station in the early 1970s and the early 1990s, YanTai station in the late 1960s, and ChamDo station in the late 1980s to the early 1990s. At these stations, the trends of SunDu-derived R_s are more reliable than those of observed R_s. The figure was produced using MATLAB.

Figs. 4–6 indicate that the lack of calibration or inaccurate calibration made the observed R_s values highly uncertain. Fig. 7 further shows that measurement biases may explain the discrepancies between the observed and simulated decadal variability of R_s. The linear trend of the observed R_s averaged over China from 1960 to 1989 was −8.5 W m^{-2} per decade, with a 95% confidence interval from −9.8 W m^{-2} per decade to −7.3 W m^{-2} per decade. None of the 48 Earth System Models of CMIP5 (CMIP5 ESM)[7,21] reproduced the observed trend (Fig. 7).

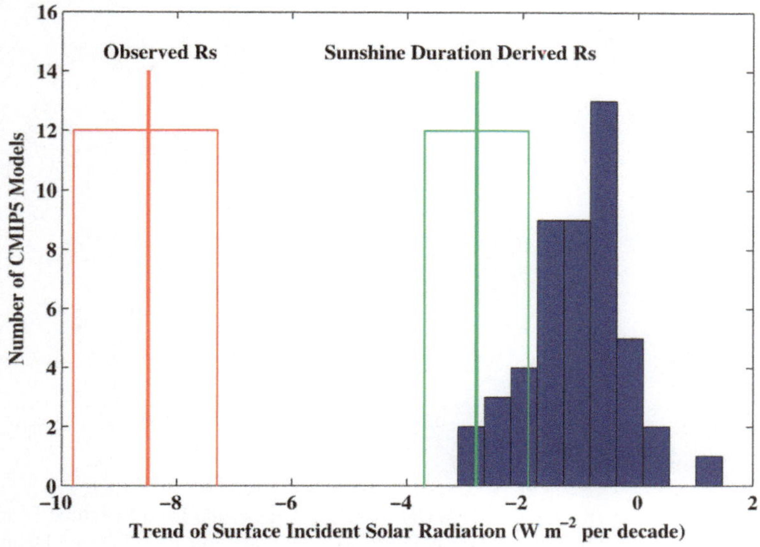

Figure 7: Histogram of the linear trends of surface incident solar radiation (R_s, blue bars) over China from 1960 to 1989 simulated by 48 CMIP5 models (see Ma et al.[21] for details of these models). None of the models reproduced the observed trend of −8.5 W m^{-2} per decade (thick red line, with the red box showing its 95% confidence interval) based on the raw data of R_s observations. However, some CMIP5 models, including NASA Goddard Institute for Space Studies (GISS) models, National Center for Atmospheric Research (NCAR) Community Earth System Models (CESM-CAM5), and Centre National de Recherches Meteorologiques Climate Model 5 (CNRM-CM5), reproduced our new estimates of the trend based on Sunshine Duration (SunDu) derived R_s, −2.8 W m^{-2} per decade (thick green line, with the green box showing its 95% confidence interval). The figure was produced using MATLAB.

However, many high-quality CMIP5 ESMs reproduced the trend of SunDu-derived R_s very well. The linear trend of the SunDu-derived R_s averaged over China during the same period was −2.8 W m^{-2} per decade, with a 95% confidence interval from −3.7 W m^{-2} per decade to −1.9 W m^{-2} per decade (Fig. 7). The R_s from NASA Goddard Institute for Space Studies (GISS) models show the best agreement with the SunDu-derived values. The four versions of GISS ESM simulated an average trend of R_s by −2.8 W m^{-2} per decade. Other CMIP5 ESMs, including the Centre National de Recherches Meteorologiques Climate Model 5 (CNRM-CM5-2, −2.9 W m^{-2} per decade) and National Center for Atmospheric Research (NCAR) Community Earth System Models (CESM1-CAM5-1-FV2, −2.4 W m^{-2} per decade and CESM1-CAM5, −2.0 W m^{-2} per decade), also had consistent simulations of R_s trend with SunDu-derived R_s. However, the interannual variability of R_s of CMIP5 is much less than those from the observed R_s and SunDu derived R_s because the models have difficulty in simulating variability of clouds[22].

It has been shown that aerosol is the dominating factor for the dimming of R_s in China from 1960 to 1990[23,24] although cloud has been believed to be the key factor for the decadal variability of R_s in the U.S.[25,26] and India[27] during recent decades. A recent study has shown that the CMIP5 models perform significantly different in simulating atmospheric aerosols over India[28]. This is because the atmospheric aerosol loading was interactively calculated by each individual model[10], although the same emission inventory[29,30,31,32] was used for all of the CMIP5 models[7]. Our results show that the GISS models perform best, which is partly because the GISS model team has made great effort in simulating aerosols[33,34,35,36].

Fig. 8 shows that the agreement of the long-term trends between SunDu-derived R_s and CMIP5 simulations is significantly better than those between observations and CMIP5 simulations over China from 1960 to 1989. The brightening rate of the measured R_s was impaired by instrument replacement between 1990 and 1993[13], as shown in Fig. 4. The observations of diurnal temperature range[8,37] confirmed that the observed brightening from 1990 to 1993 was not real. The observed increase in R_s is inconsistent with the observed increase in stratospheric aerosols because of Pinatubo volcano eruption in 1991[38]either. After 1995, variability of the three estimates of R_s from the observations, the SunDu and the CMIP5 model simulations agreed well because issues of the instruments used to measure R_s had been eliminated. During this period, the impact of increased aerosols on R_s[39] has been offset by the decreasing cloud cover fraction[13], and in turn R_s kept near constant.

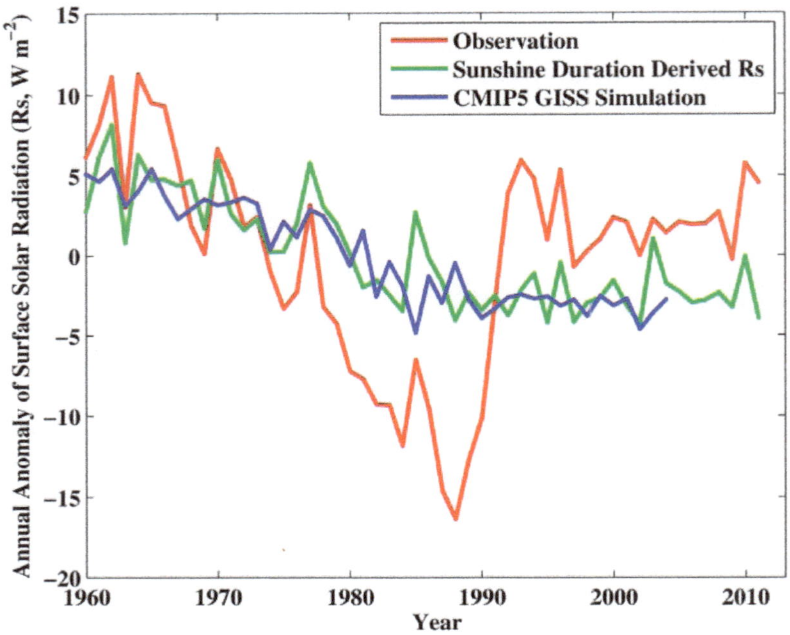

Figure 8: Time series of observed surface incident solar radiation (R_s, in red), R_s calculated from Sunshine Duration (SunDu, in green) and R_s simulated by CMIP5 GISS (in blue) averaged over China. The observed R_s overestimated the dimming trend from 1960 to 1989. The instrument replacement in China from 1990 to 1993 resulted in an abrupt increase to the observed R_s. The agreement of the long-term trends of R_s between sunshine duration (SunDu) derived R_s and CMIP5 NASA Goddard Institute for Space Studies (GISS) model simulations (averaged from four different model versions) is much better than those between observations and CMIP5 simulations. After 1995, variability of the three estimates of R_s from the observations, the SunDu and the CMIP5 model simulations agreed well because issues of the instruments used to measure R_s had been eliminated. The figure was produced using MATLAB.

DISCUSSION

The overestimation of the dimming trend of the observed R_s over China has been corroborated by independent studies on clouds and aerosols. Observed R_s was reported to have decreased by 21 W m^{-2} in eastern China from 1961 to 1990[40], with changes in aerosols regarded as the primary reason for this dimming trend[13,41]. Changes in cloud cover showed a decreasing trend[41], implying an increasing trend of R_s. The aerosol optical depth (AOD, vertical integration of optical extinction) over the same region during the same time has increased by 0.16[42]. Analyses have shown that R_s under clear sky conditions decreases by 8 Wm^{-2} in the winter seasons or 9 Wm^{-2} in the summer seasons for an AOD increase of 0.1 over China[43]. The change in AOD can explain at most a reduction of 1.6 × 9 = 14.4 Wm^{-2} of R_s, which is approximately two-thirds of the observed value, but probably considerably less because of masking by clouds. This is confirmed by the SunDu-derivedR_s, which showed a decrease of 8.4 W m^{-2} during the period.

Globally distributed *DTR* observations show that since 1985, brightening was only significant over Europe and there was a lack of brightening over other continents[8]. Furthermore, AOD derived from visibility observations has increased globally since 1973 except for Europe[39]. This explains why the CMIP5 ESM could only reproduce the observed brightening over Europe[5].

The inhomogeneity of observed R_s caused by inaccurate instrument calibration also impacted the observed R_s over Europe before 1990. A homogeneity test was applied to R_s measurements at 56 stations over Europe where at least 30 years of data of R_s were available at each station[44]. Sixteen of the 56 series (28.6% of the total) were found to be inhomogeneous[44]. After these datasets were appropriately adjusted, the dimming trend over Europe from 1961 to 1984 became −2.0 W m^{-2} per decade, substantially less than the −3.1 W m^{-2} per decade derived from raw data of the observed R_s[45].

METHODS

Sunshine Duration (SunDu) records the time during a day that the direct solar beam irradiance exceeds 120 Wm^{-2}. It was initiated 150 years ago and is one of the oldest and most robust measurements related to radiation[3]. Measurement of SunDu is insensitive to instrument calibration as its recording material is replaced each day.

SunDu has long been used to estimate R_s, and the earliest and most popular methods are those developed by Ångström[46] and subsequently modified by Prescott[47], which assumed a linear relationship between relative R_s and SunDu. Yang et al. proposed a revised Ångström-Prescott to estimate daily mean R_s from SunDu[11]:

$$R_s/R_c = a_0 + a_1 \cdot n/N + a_2 \cdot (n/N)^2 \quad (1)$$

where n is the measured SunDu; N is the theoretical values of SunDu, and R_c is the daily solar radiation at the surface under clear-sky conditions:

$$R_c = R_{cb} + R_{cd} = \int I_0 \cdot \overline{\tau_b} \cdot \sin(h) \cdot dt + \int I_0 \cdot \overline{\tau_d} \cdot \sin(h) \cdot dt \quad (2)$$

where R_{cb} is the daily mean direct solar radiation at the surface, R_{cd} is the daily mean diffuse solar radiation at the surface, I_0 is the solar radiation at the extraterrestrial level, $\overline{\tau_b}$ is the atmospheric transmittance for direct solar radiation, $\overline{\tau_d}$ is the atmospheric transmittance for diffuse solar radiation, h(rad) is the altitude angle of sun, and t(s) is the time. The atmospheric transmittances $\overline{\tau_b}$ and $\overline{\tau_d}$ depend on Rayleigh scattering, aerosol extinction, ozone absorption, water vapor absorption and permanent gas absorption. Rayleigh scattering and water vapor absorption can be calculated from surface meteorological observations, and ozone and permanent gas absorption can be calculated using their climatological values. In the calculation of aerosol extinction, winter- and summer-averaged aerosols based on Hess et al.[48] were included but the inter-annual variation of aerosols was not incorporated. Please refer to reference 11 for detailed information of the calculations.

The calculation of R_c does not include time varying aerosols because SunDu is impacted by changes in both clouds and aerosols. Direct solar radiation is generally lower than 120 W m^{-2} for scattered clouds (cumulus, stratocumulus)[20]. High and thin cirrus, as well as aerosols can reduce SunDu at low solar elevations, i.e., at times when the incident clear sky solar radiation is not much larger than 120 W m^{-2}. Recent studies confirmed such an inference and have shown that SunDu can accurately reflect the impact of change of aerosols and clouds on R_s[12,13,14,15,16,17] at time scales ranging from daily to decadal.

The parameters of Eq. (1), namely a_0, a_1, and a_2, can be obtained by tuning this equation with measurements of R_s and SunDu. In the existing studies, a suite of parameters are derived by calibrating Eq. (1) and then the method is applied regionally or globally[12,13]. This may limit the accuracy of the R_s estimates. In contrast, in this study, we calibrate Eq. (1) at each station in China where both R_s and SunDu observations were available at more than 10 years. We then apply Eq. (1) to calculate R_s from 1958 to 2012 at each station when observations of SunDu were available. Figs. 2–3 show that R_s can be calculated accurately from SunDu data at daily and monthly time scales. These two estimates of R_s allow us to investigate the homogeneity of these two estimates, which are shown in Figs. 4–8. In this study, we show that the R_s decreased at a rate of −2.8 W m^{-2} per decade from 1960 to 1989 over the 76 stations where both the observed R_s and SunDu were available at more than 120 months during the study period. In a previous study, Tang et al.[12] calculated R_s from SunDu with a suite of parameters of Eq. (1) for 716 weather stations in China and estimated an averaged trend of −2.3 W m^{-2} per decade from 1961 to 2000, which is a little weaker than our current estimate because R_s stopped decreasing after 1990 (Fig. 8).

In this study, we propose to combine the advantages of the observations of R_s and SunDu. The observed R_s can accurately quantify the variation of R_s in higher temporal resolution, i.e., hourly, and daily. However, it is impaired by the sensitivity drift of its measurement instruments. This limits its usage in climatic study. The SunDu is nearly free from the sensitivity drift problem. We use the observed R_s to calibrate Eq. (1) used to estimate R_s from SunDu at each station. This makes up the disadvantages of SunDu: (1) SunDu does not directly provide an estimate of R_s, (2) threshold of a SunDu recorder changes with recorder types and their sitting environment. In this paper, we show that the SunDu-derived R_s has an advantage of long-term stability and can be used to climatic studies, i.e., to evaluate climate model simulations, which only require estimates of R_s at coarse time resolution (monthly or annually). However, SunDu has difficulty in estimating R_s at time scales shorter than daily.

ACKNOWLEDGEMENTS

This study was funded by the National Basic Research Program of China (2012CB955302), the National Natural Science Foundation of China (41175126 and 91337111) and the New Century Excellent Talents Program. Robert E. Dickinson provided helpful comments on preparing the manuscript and Qian Ma processed some data for this study.

REFERENCES

1. Mercado, L. M. *et al.* Impact of changes in diffuse radiation on the global land carbon sink. *Nature* 458, 1014–U1087, 10.1038/nature07949 (2009).
2. Gilgen, H., Wild, M. & Ohmura, A. Means and trends of shortwave irradiance at the surface estimated from global energy balance archive data. *J. Clim.* 11, 2042–2061, 10.1175/1520-0442-11.8.2042 (1998).
3. Wild, M. Global dimming and brightening: A review. *J. Geophys. Res.* 114, D00D16, 10.1029/2008JD011470 (2009).
4. Wild, M. *et al.* From dimming to brightening: Decadal changes in solar radiation at Earth's surface. *Science* 308, 847–850, 10.1126/science.1103215 (2005).
5. Allen, R. J., Norris, J. R. & Wild, M. Evaluation of multidecadal variability in CMIP5 surface solar radiation and inferred underestimation of aerosol direct effects over Europe, China, Japan and India. *J. Geophy. Res.* 118, 6311–6336, 10.1002/jgrd.50426 (2013).
6. Wild, M. & Schmucki, E. Assessment of global dimming and brightening in IPCC-AR4/CMIP3 models and ERA40. *Clim. Dyn.*37, 1671–1688, 10.1007/s00382-010-0939-3 (2011).
7. Taylor, K. E., Stouffer, R. J. & Meehl, G. A. An overview of CMIP5 and the experiment design. *Bull. Amer. Meteorol. Soc.* 93, 485–498, 10.1175/bams-d-11-00094.1 (2012).
8. Wang, K. C. & Dickinson, R. E. Contribution of solar radiation to decadal temperature variability over land. *Proc Natl Acad Sci USA*110, 14877–14882, 10.1073/pnas.1311433110 (2013).
9. Padma Kumari, B., Londhe, A. L., Daniel, S. & Jadhav, D. B.Observational evidence of solar dimming: Offsetting surface warming over India. *Geophys. Res. Lett.* 34, L21810, 10.1029/2007gl031133 (2007).
10. Ghan, S. J. & Schwartz, S. E. Aerosol properties and processes: a path from field and laboratory measurements to global climate models. *Bull. Amer. Meteorol. Soc.* 88, 1059–1083, 10.1175/bams-88-7-1059 (2007).
11. Yang, K., Koike, T. & Ye, B. S. Improving estimation of hourly, daily, and monthly solar radiation by importing global data sets. *Agric. For. Meteorol.* 137, 43–55, 10.1016/j.agrformet.2006.02.001 (2006).
12. Tang, W. J., Yang, K., Qin, J., Cheng, C. C. K. & He, J. Solar radiation trend across China in recent decades: a revisit with quality-controlled data. *Atmos. Chem. Phys.* 11, 393–406, 10.5194/acp-11-393-2011 (2011).

13. Wang, K. C., Dickinson, R. E., Wild, M. & Liang, S. Atmospheric impacts on climatic variability of surface incident solar radiation.*Atmos. Chem. Phys.* 12, 9581–9592, 10.5194/acp-12-9581-2012 (2012).

14. Sanchez-Lorenzo, A., Calb, J., Brunetti, M. & Deser, C.Dimming/brightening over the Iberian Peninsula: Trends in sunshine duration and cloud cover and their relations with atmospheric circulation. *J. Geophys. Res.* 114, D00D09, 10.1029/2008JD011394 (2009).

15. Sanchez-Lorenzo, A. & Wild, M. Decadal variations in estimated surface solar radiation over Switzerland since the late 19th century. *Atmos. Chem. Phys.* 12, 8635–8644, 10.5194/acp-12-8635-2012 (2012).

16. Sanchez-Romero, A., Sanchez-Lorenzo, A., Calbó, J., González, J. A. & Azorin-Molina, C. The signal of aerosol-induced changes in sunshine duration records: A review of the evidence. *J. Geophy. Res.* 119, 2013JD021393, 10.1002/2013jd021393 (2014).

17. Soni, V. K., Pandithurai, G. & Pai, D. S. Evaluation of long-term changes of solar radiation in India. *Int. J. Climatol.* 32, 540–551, 10.1002/joc.2294 (2012).

18. Gueymard, C. A. & Myers, D. R. [Solar radiation measurement: progress in radiometry for improved modeling solar radiation at the Earth's surface]. *Modeling Solar Radiation at the Earth Surface*[Badescu, V. (ed.)] [1–28] (Springer-Verlag Berlin Heidelberg, 2008).

19. Fröhlich, C. in *WMO/CIMO Final Report, WMO No. 490, 97–110*. (PMOD/WRC intern: 545a, 1977).

20. Stanhill, G. & Cohen, S. Solar radiation changes in the United States during the Twentieth Century: Evidence from sunshine measurements. *J. Clim.* 18, 1503–1512, http://dx.doi.org/10.1175/JCLI3354.1 (2005).

21. Ma, Q., Wang, K. C. & Wild, M. Evaluations of atmospheric downward longwave radiation from 44 coupled general circulation models of CMIP5. *J. Geophy. Res.* 119, 4486–4497, 10.1002/2013JD021427 (2014).

22. Zhang, M. H. *et al.* Comparing clouds and their seasonal variations in 10 atmospheric general circulation models with satellite measurements. *J. Geophys. Res.* 110, D15s02, 10.1029/2004jd005021 (2005).

23. Qian, Y., Wang, W. G., Leung, L. R. & Kaiser, D. P. Variability of solar radiation under cloud-free skies in China: The role of aerosols. *Geophys. Res. Lett.* 34, 10.1029/2006GL028800 (2007).

24. Xia, X. A closer looking at dimming and brightening in China during 1961–2005. *Ann. Geophys.* 28, 1121–1132, 10.5194/angeo-28-1121-2010 (2010).

25. Augustine, J. A. & Dutton, E. G. Variability of the surface radiation budget over the United States from 1996 through 2011 from high-quality measurements. *J. Geophy. Res.* 118, 43–53, 10.1029/2012jd018551 (2013).

26. Long, C. N. *et al.* Significant decadal brightening of downwelling shortwave in the continental United States. *J. Geophys. Res.* 114, D00D06, 10.1029/2008JD011263 (2009).

27. Padma Kumari, B. & Goswami, B. N. Seminal role of clouds on solar dimming over the Indian monsoon region. *Geophys. Res. Lett*37, L06703, 10.1029/2009gl042133 (2010).

28. Sanap, S. D., Ayantika, D. C., Pandithurai, G. & Niranjan, K.Assessment of the aerosol distribution over Indian subcontinent in CMIP5 models. *Atmos. Environ.* 87, 123–137, http://dx.doi.org/10.1016/j.atmosenv.2014.01.017 (2014).

29. Lamarque, J. F. *et al.* Historical (1850–2000) gridded anthropogenic and biomass burning emissions of reactive gases and aerosols: methodology and application. *Atmos. Chem. Phys.*10, 7017–7039, 10.5194/acp-10-7017-2010 (2010).

30. Smith, S. J. *et al.* Anthropogenic sulfur dioxide emissions: 1850–2005. *Atmos. Chem. Phys.* 11, 1101–1116, 10.5194/acp-11-1101-2011 (2011).

31. Bond, T. C. *et al.* Historical emissions of black and organic carbon aerosol from energy-related combustion, 1850–2000. *Global Biogeochem. Cycles* 21, GB2018, 10.1029/2006gb002840 (2007).

32. Junker, C. & Liousse, C. A global emission inventory of carbonaceous aerosol from historic records of fossil fuel and biofuel consumption for the period 1860–1997. *Atmos. Chem. Phys.*8, 1195–1207, 10.5194/acp-8-1195-2008 (2008).

33. de Boer, G., Bauer, S. E., Toto, T., Menon, S. & Vogelmann, A. M.Evaluation of aerosol-cloud interaction in the GISS ModelE using ARM observations. *J. Geophy. Res.* 118, 6383–6395, 10.1002/jgrd.50460 (2013).

34. Lee, Y. H. & Adams, P. J. Evaluation of aerosol distributions in the GISS-TOMAS global aerosol microphysics model with remote sensing observations. *Atmos. Chem. Phys.* 10, 2129–2144, 10.5194/acp-10-2129-2010 (2010).

35. Li, J., Liu, L., Lacis, A. A. & Carlson, B. E. An optimal fitting approach to improve the GISS ModelE aerosol optical property parameterization using AERONET data. *J. Geophy. Res.* 115, D16211, 10.1029/2010jd013909 (2010).

36. Menon, S. *et al.* Analyzing signatures of aerosol-cloud interactions from satellite retrievals and the GISS GCM to constrain the aerosol indirect effect. *J. Geophy. Res.* 113, D14S22, 10.1029/2007jd009442 (2008).

37. Wang, K., Ye, H., Chen, F., Xiong, Y. & Wang, C. Urbanization effect on the diurnal temperature range: different roles under solar dimming and brightening. *J. Clim.* 25, 1022–1027, 10.1175/jcli-d-10-05030.1 (2012).

38. Stevermer, A. J., Petropavlovskikh, I. V., Rosen, J. M. & DeLuisi, J. J.Development of a global stratospheric aerosol climatology: Optical properties and applications for UV. *J. Geophys. Res.* 105, 22763–22776, 10.1029/2000jd900368 (2000).

39. Wang, K. C., Dickinson, R. E. & Liang, S. Clear sky visibility has decreased over land globally from 1973 to 2007. *Science* 323, 1468–1470, 10.1126/science.1167549 (2009).

40. Li, X., Li, W. & Zhou, X. Analysis of the solar radiation variation of the China in recent 30 years. *Quart. J. Appl. Meteorol.* 9, 24–31 (1998).

41. Xia, X. Significant decreasing cloud cover during 1954–2005 due to more clear-sky days and less overcast days in China and its relation to aerosol. *Ann. Geophys.* 30, 573–582, 10.5194/angeo-30-573-2012 (2012).

42. Luo, Y., Lu, D., Zhou, X., Li, W. & He, Q. Characteristics of the spatial distribution and yearly variation of aerosol optical depth over China in last 30 years. *J. Geophy. Res.* 106, 14501–14513, 10.1029/2001jd900030 (2001).

43. Xia, X. *et al.* A compilation of aerosol optical properties and calculation of direct radiative forcing over an urban region in northern China. *J. Geophy. Res.* 112, D12203, 10.1029/2006jd008119 (2007).

44. Sanchez-Lorenzo, A., Wild, M. & Trentmann, J. Validation and stability assessment of the monthly mean CM SAF surface solar radiation dataset over Europe against a homogenized surface dataset (1983–2005). *Remote Sens. Environ.* 134, 355–366, http://dx.doi.org/10.1016/j.rse.2013.03.012 (2013).

45. Norris, J. R. & Wild, M. Trends in aerosol radiative effects over Europe inferred from observed cloud cover, solar "dimming" and solar "brightening". *J. Geophys. Res.* 112, D08214, 10.1029/2006JD007794 (2007).

46. Angström, A. Solar and terrestrial radiation. Report to the international commission for solar research on actinometric investigations of solar and atmospheric radiation. *Q. J. R. Meteorol. Soc.* 50, 121–126, 10.1002/qj.49705021008 (1924).

47. Prescott, J. A. Evaporation from water surface in relation to solar radiation. *Trans R Soc Sci Austr* 64, 114–118 (1940).

48. Hess, M., Koepke, P. & Schult, I. Optical properties of aerosols and clouds: The software package OPAC. *Bull. Amer. Meteorol. Soc.* 79, 831–844, 10.1175/1520-0477(1998)0790831:opoaac>2.0.co;2 (1998).

CHAPTER 16

MONTHLY-AVERAGED HOURLY SOLAR DIFFUSE RADIATION MODELS FOR WORLD-WIDE LOCATIONS

T. Muneer, EJ Gago, and S. Etxebarria

Keywords: Solar radiation, Averaged-hourly solar diffuse fraction, Insolation, Solar diffuse radiation

INTRODUCTION

Solar radiation data are essential for the design of very many energy systems. These data are needed for obtaining solar energy resource assessment, its transmission and also to obtain the efficiency of energy delivery. A few examples are solar water heating, and space PV systems, daylighting, building air conditioning load and solar-driven ventilation. The starting point for the above computational chain is almost always global and diffuse horizontal radiation. Usually, the computations are carried out using hourly or sub-hourly data.

Note that not always it is possible to obtain a long-term series of hourly or sub-hourly data for the above parameters.

The most commonly measured solar data are global irradiation and these are available for a limited number of stations within any given country at an hourly, daily or monthly frequency. For example within the UK and Spain a historical records of hourly data are available for 71 and 31 stations, respectively.

Of these stations due to higher operational costs associated with diffuse radiation measurements the respective meteorological offices tend to record the latter variable at much fewer locations. For example, since the year 2002 within the UK the diffuse radiation is recorded at only two locations, at North latitudes of Camborne (50.21°) and Lerwick (60.80°).

On the contrary, through the work of NASA (http://eosweb.larc.nasa.gov/cgi-bin/sse/retscreen.cgi?email=rets@nrcan.gc.ca) it is now possible to obtain daily-averaged irradiation data for virtually any location in the world. A sample table of climatic data for Easthampstead (Bracknell) is provided in Table 1.

Citation: T. Muneer, EJ Gago and S. Etxebarria. Monthly-averaged hourly solar diffuse radiation models for world-wide locations, Future Cities and Environment, (2015); 1: 5. DOI:10.1186/s40984-015-0008-5.

Table 1. Climatic data for Easthampstead (Bracknell) with the NASA reported irradiation data and averaged measured data for the period 1981-1983

	Unit	**Climate data location**							
Latitude	°N	51,42							
Longitude	°E	–0,75							
Elevation	m	58,00							
Heating design temperature	°C	–1,74							
Cooling design temperature	°C	22,96							
Earth temperature amplitude	°C	14,35							
Frost days at site	day	37,00							
Month	Air temperature	Relative humidity	Daily solar radiation-horizontal	Atmospheric pressure	Wind speed	Earth temperature	Heating degree-days	Cooling degree-days	Average measured radiation
	°C	%	kWh/m²/day	kPa	m/s	°C	°C-d	°C-d	kWh/m²/day
January	4,2	83,90	0,77	100,8	6,3	3,1	426	1	0,71
February	4,3	80,20	1,39	101,0	5,8	3,6	380	1	1,28
March	6,4	76,80	2,34	100,9	6,0	6,2	353	4	2,18
April	8,6	69,80	3,59	100,7	5,1	9,1	279	21	3,55
May	12,7	64,00	4,57	100,9	4,7	13,8	168	92	4,11
June	16,1	60,80	4,84	100,9	4,4	17,7	75	177	4,86
July	18,6	60,20	4,80	100,9	4,4	20,4	25	261	4,77
August	18,6	61,20	4,23	100,9	4,3	20,3	26	264	4,23
September	15,5	66,30	2,86	100,9	5,0	16,5	83	164	2,85
October	11,7	74,10	1,73	100,7	5,5	11,5	191	73	1,57
November	7,3	83,20	0,96	100,7	5,9	6,4	318	11	0,80
December	4,9	85,00	0,60	100,8	6,1	3,8	404	3	0,60
Annual									
	10,7	72,10	2,72	100,8	5,3	11,0	2728	1072	
Measured at (m)					10,0	0,0			

Website: http://eosweb.larc.nasa.gov/cgi-bin/sse/retscreen.cgi?email=rets@nrcan.gc.ca

This information was downloaded from the above-mentioned NASA website. The NASA reported irradiation data were compared by the present research team against averaged measured data for one UK location for the period 1981–1983 (three complete years) (see Fig. 1). The statistics within the latter figure shows that there is a close concordance between the satellite-based NASA irradiation and the UK Meteorological Office measured data set.

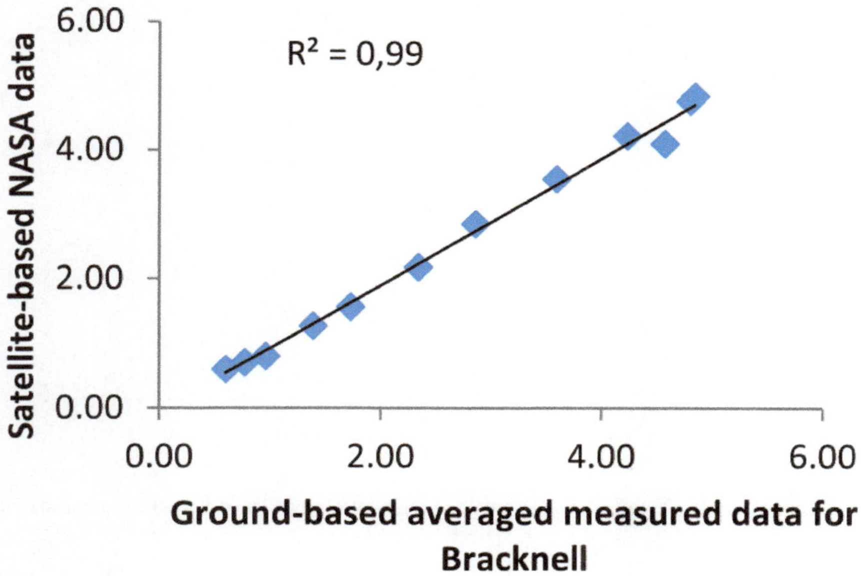

Figure 1. Comparison between NASA reported irradiation data and ground-based averaged measured data for Bracknell, kWh/m²-day.

Following the original work of Liu and Jordan (Liu & Jordan 1960) a great many number of research teams from around the world have produced regressions relating diffuse ratio (k) and clearness index (kt) regressions at an hourly, daily, monthly and annual frequency. Each of the above four category of regression is unique and statistically different as shown in the work of Muneer (Muneer 2004) and Saluja et al. (Saluja et al. 1988).

The present article was pooled from 14 world-wide locations to obtain a regression model to complete the above missing link. It was presently shown that the averaged–data based regressions are distinctly different from previously available hour-by-hour regressions.

The Unique Nature of Solar Radiation Regressions

Historically speaking, a large number of research teams from around the world have produces k-kt regressions that were based on an hour-by-hour, daily, monthly or annual data. Examples that may be cited here, are Liu and Jordan (daily, and monthly-averaged daily) (Liu & Jordan1960), Erbs et al. (hourly, daily and monthly-averaged daily) (Erbs et al. 1982), Hawas and Muneer (hour-by-hour, daily, monthly- and annual-averaged daily) (Hawas & Muneer 1984; Muneer & Hawas 1984; Muneer et al. 1984) and Stanhill (monthly- and annual-averaged daily) (Stanhill 1966).

Presently, Figs. 2 and 3 show the unique nature of hour-by-hour (Fig. 2: $k-k_t$ plot) and monthly-averaged hourly regressions (Fig. 3: $\bar{k}-\bar{k}_t$). An important point to note is that while Fig. 2 shows a convex profile, Fig. 3 demonstrates a concave behaviour. The latter two figures are based on data from common UK locations.

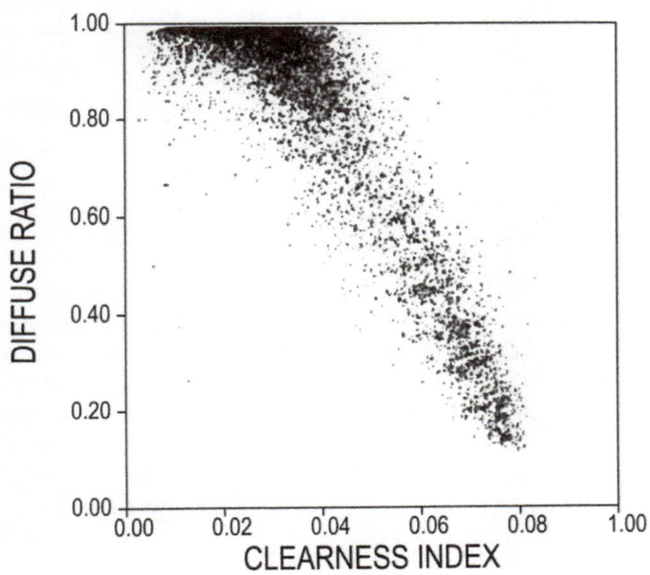

Figure 2. Hourly diffuse ratio versus clearness index for UK locations.

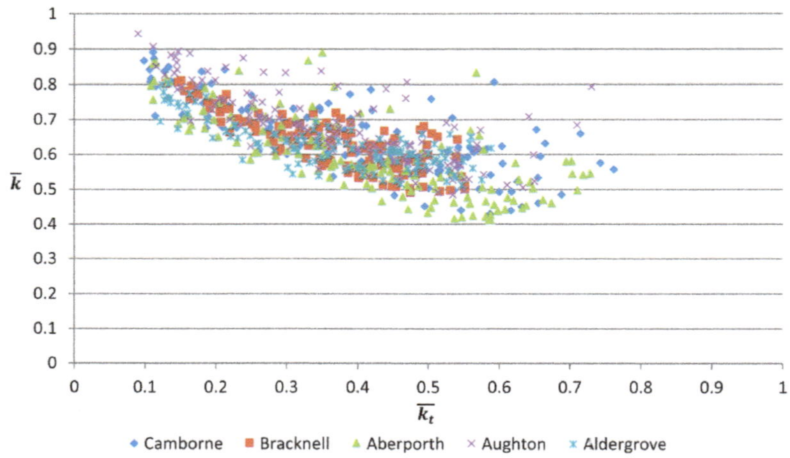

Figure 3. Monthly-averaged hourly plot for UK locations (arranged in an increasing order of latitude: Camborne 50.21° N, Aldergrove 54.65° N).

While there are established models for data of Fig. 2 there are no regressions available in literature for averaged-hourly data such as those shown in Fig. 3. The object of this article is to present the latter type of regressions.

Presently Developed Monthly-averaged Hourly $\bar{k}$-$\bar{k}_t$ Regressions

Fourteen worldwide locations were chosen for this study, details of which are shown in Table 2.

Table 2. The 14 worldwide locations that were presently investigated

Country	Location	Latitude	Longitude	Period of observation
India	Chennai	13.08	80.18	1990–1994
	Pune	18.32	73.85	1990–1994
Kingdom of Bahrain	Bahrain	26.03	50.61	2000–2002
State of Kuwait	Kuwait	29.22	47.98	1996–2000
Spain	Almeria	36.83	−2.38	1993–1998
Portugal	Faro	37.02	−7.96	1982–1986
	Lisbon	38.71	−9.15	1982–1990
Spain	Madrid	40.40	−3.55	1999–2001
	Girona	41.97	2.76	1995–2001
United Kingdom	Camborne	50.21	5.30	1981–1995
	Bracknell	51.42	0.75	1992–1994
	Aberporth	52.13	4.55	1975–1995
	Finningley	53.48	0.98	1982–1995
	Stornoway	58.22	6.39	1982–1995

Data consisted of hourly global and diffuse irradiation values for several years for each location, covering most of the range of latitude for the country. The location names have been arranged in an increasing order of latitude.

Monthly-averaged hourly values were calculated for the global and diffuse radiation considering the data period for each location. For each of them, the monthly-averaged hourly diffuse ratio ($\bar{k}$) and the corresponding clearness index ($\bar{k}_t$) were calculated from sunrise to sunset. The following conditions were used in each case to remove erroneously recorded data.

$$k_T = \frac{I_G}{I_E} \rightarrow I_G < I_E \quad (1)$$

$$k = \frac{I_D}{I_G} \rightarrow I_D \leq I_G \quad (2)$$

The monthly-averaged clearness index was then regressed against the monthly-averaged diffuse ratio for each location. Figure 4 shows one such scatter plot for Chennai and Lisbon. Furthermore, for each increment at bandwidth of clearness index of 0.05 width, the corresponding values of averaged diffuse ratio shown in Fig. 5 were obtained, shown here for pooled data from two Indian locations.

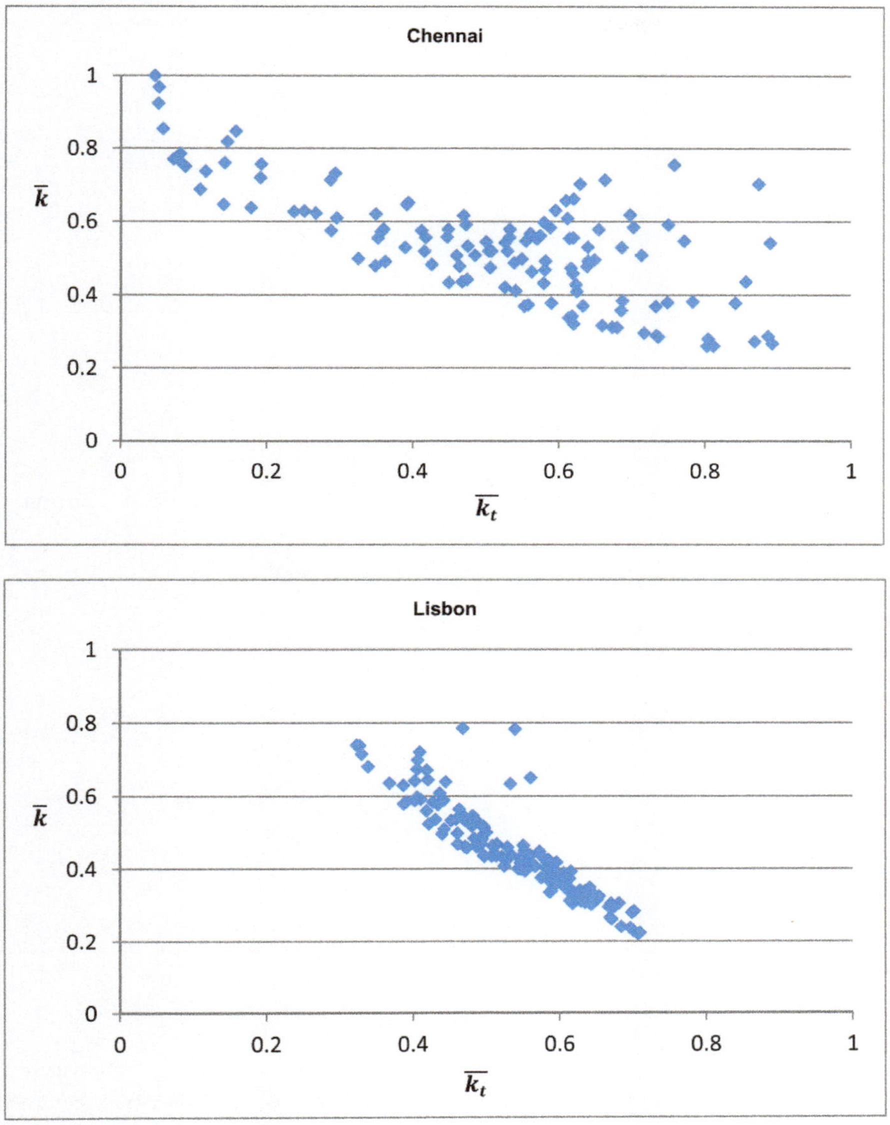

Figure 4. Monthly-averaged hourly diffuse ratio (y-axis) versus clearness index (x-axis) fot two locations. One Indian and other a South European.

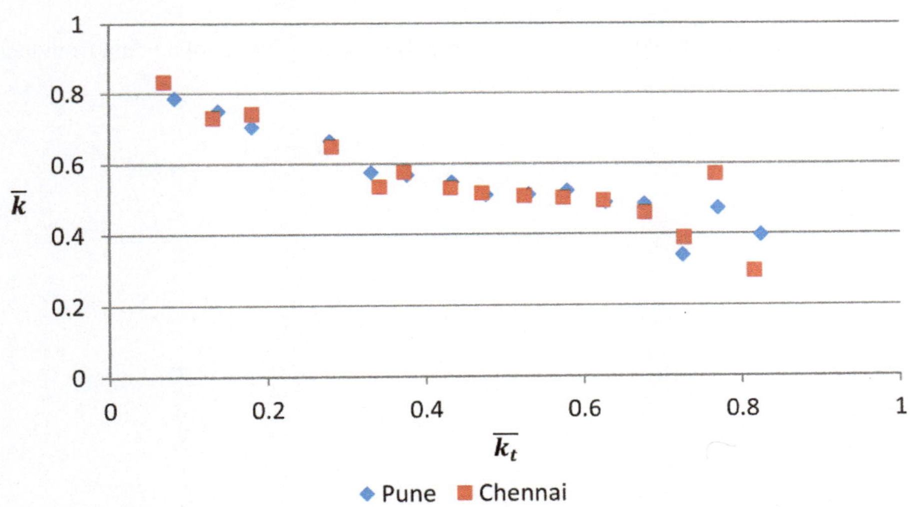

Figure 5. Averaged values of diffuse ratio for the locations between latitude 13-20° North.

Figures 6 and 7 respectively show the regressions for locations in a narrower range of latitudes (20-42° N) and worldwide sites with a more diverse range of latitudes (13-58°N).

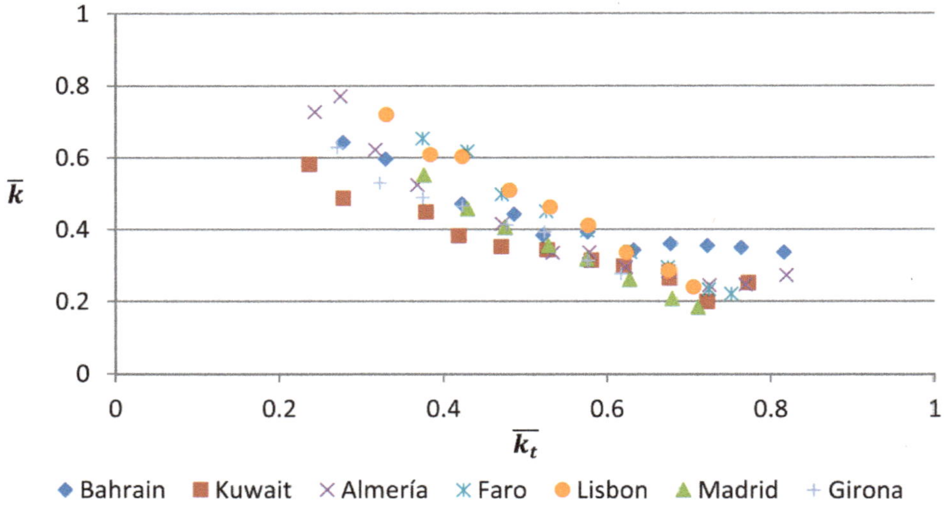

Figure 6. Averaged values of diffuse ratio for the locations between latitude 20-42° North.

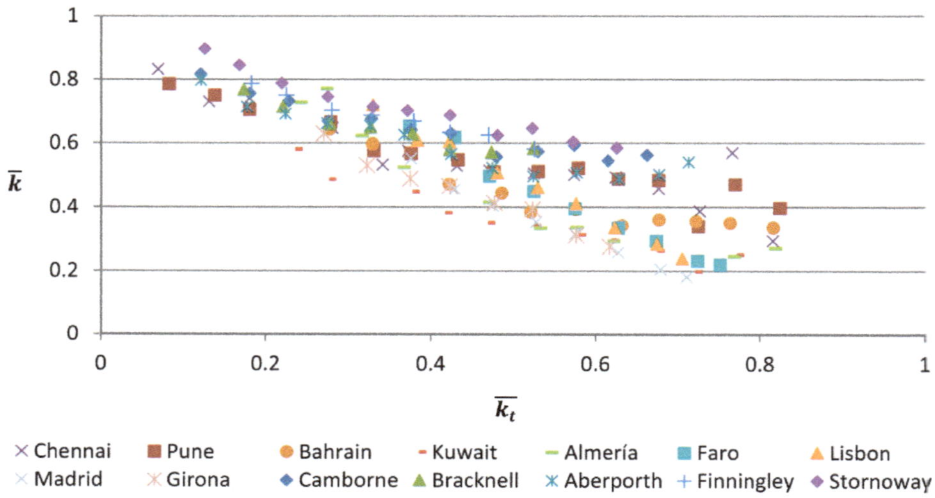

Figure 7. Averaged values of diffuse ratio for the all locations.

Note that Fig. 6 shows the potential for a single regression model. Figure 7 on the other hand indicates the existence of different sub-models and these shall now be explored further.

Figures 8, 9 and 10 respectively present regressions models that were obtained by pooling data from locations with a latitude range of 13-20° N, 20-42° N and 50-58° N.

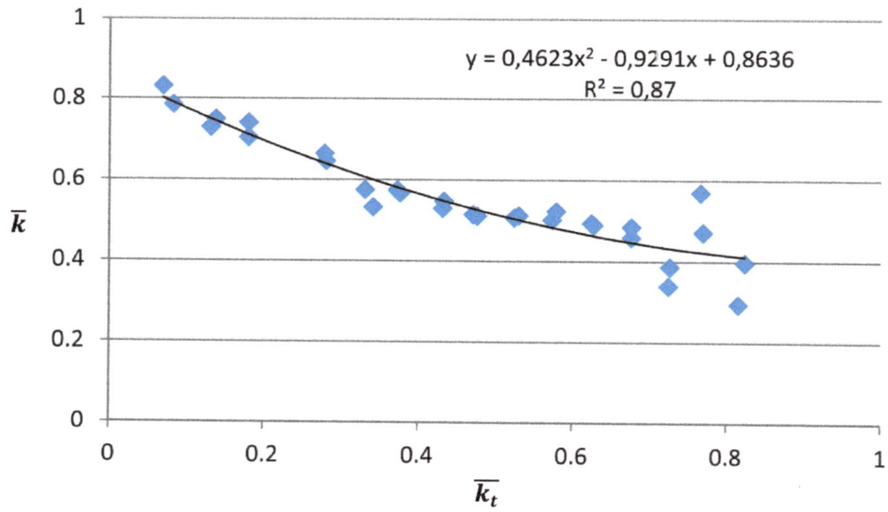

Figure 8. Averaged values of diffuse ratio for the locations between latitude 13-20° North (Chennai and Pune).

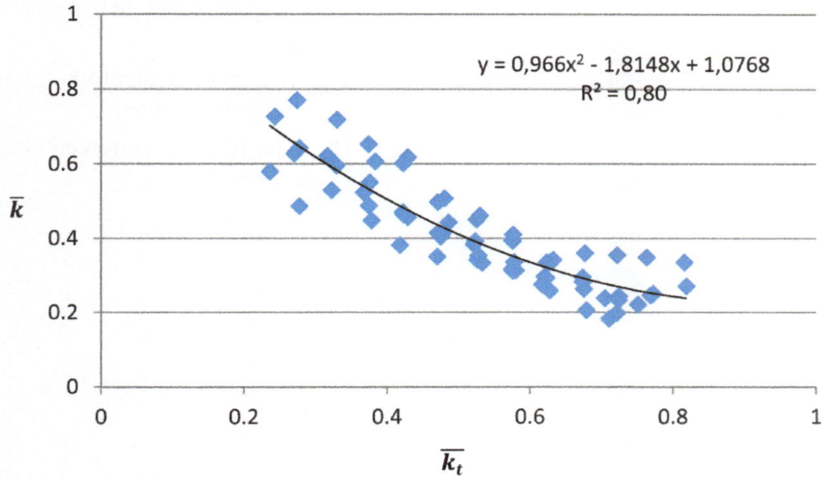

Figure 9. Averaged values of diffuse ratio for the locations between latitude 20-42° North (Bahrain, Kuwait, Almeria, Faro, Lisbon, Madrid and Girona).

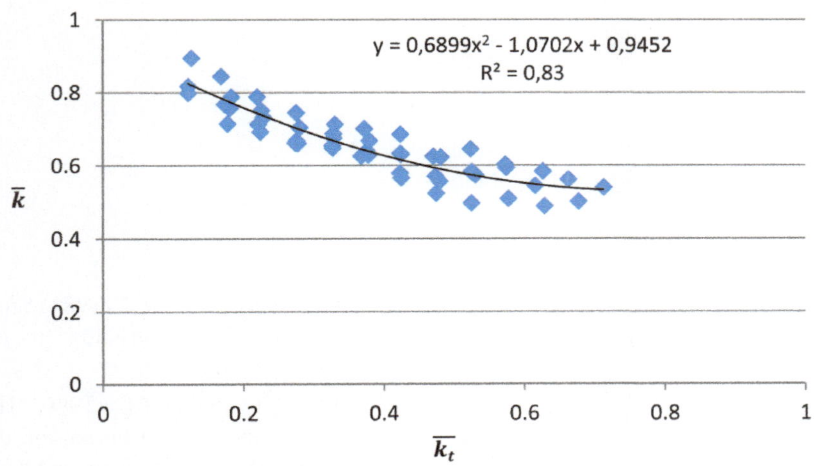

Figure 10. Averaged values of diffuse ratio for the locations between latitude 50-58° North (Camborne, Bracknell, Aberporth, Finningley and Stornoway).

Table 3 presents regressions equations and coefficient of determination (R^2) for each location.

Table 3. The regressions equations and coefficient of determination (R^2) for each location

Country	Location	Regression equations	R^2
India	Chennai	$y=0.5124x^2-0.9809x+0.8733$	0.83
	Pune	$y=0.4083x^2-0.873x+0.853$	0.92
Kingdom of Bahrain	Bahrain	$y=1.4455x^2-2.113x+1.1262$	0.98
State of Kuwait	Kuwait	$y=0.7088x^2-1.3237x+0.8299$	0.96
Spain	Almeria	$y=1.9414x^2-2.9329x+1.3637$	0.98
Portugal	Faro	$y=0.9184x^2-2.2173x+1.3654$	0.99
	Lisbon	$y=0.0721x^2-1.3001x+1.1246$	0.99
Spain	Madrid	$y=0.9087x^2-2.0465x+1.1808$	0.99
	Girona	$y=0.1781x^2-1.0867x+0.887$	0.98
United Kingdom	Camborne	$y=0.8188x^2-1.1127x+0.9365$	0.96
	Bracknell	$y=1.4394x^2-1.5414x+0.9878$	0.97
	Aberporth	$y=0.9797x^2-1.3032x+0.9403$	0.95
	Finningley	$y=0.451x^2-0.876x+0.9267$	0.99
	Stornoway	$y=7441x^2-1.1382x+1.0147$	0.98

Three points are worthy of note from Figs. 8, 9 and 10:

i. A strong correlation is observed between $\bar{k}$ and $\bar{k}_t$ with the respective coefficient of determination of 0.87, 0.80 and 0.83 (corresponding values of coefficient of correlation are 0.93, 0.89 and 0.91),

ii. In each case the shape of the regressed curve is concave, contrary to the convex profile for hour-by-hour regressions reported by research teams from around the world, and

iii. it is not possible to produce a single regressed curve for worldwide locations.

The latter point is reinforced via Fig. 11.

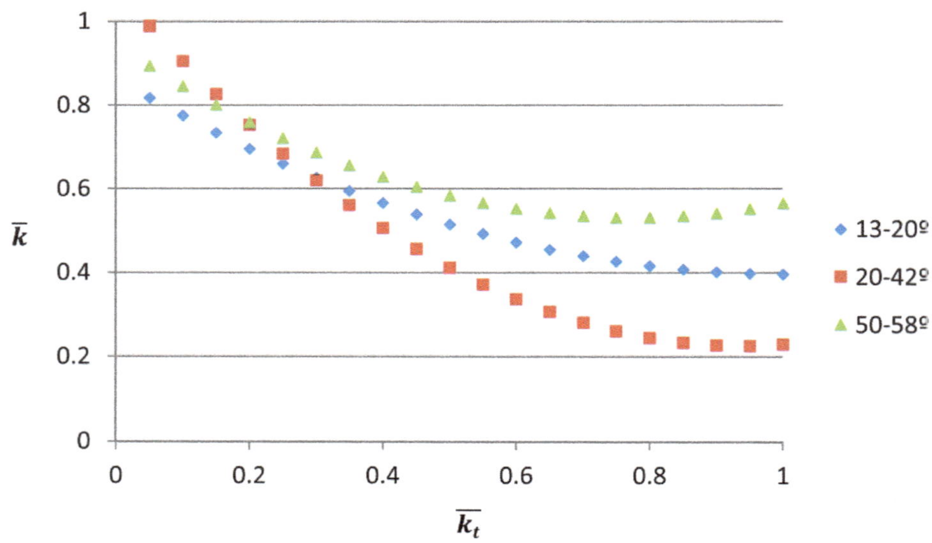

Figure 11. Monthly-averaged hourly regressions for three ranges of latitudes.

CONCLUSIONS

Monthly-averaged daily global irradiation data are now easily available from NASA website for any terrestrial location. Using established models such as those presented by Liu and Jordan (Liu & Jordan 1960), Collares-Pereira and Rabl (Collares-Pereira & Rabl 1979), Mani and Rangarajan (Mani & Rangarajan 1983), Muneer and Saluja (Muneer & Saluja 1996) and Lloyd (Lloyd 1982) it is then possible to decompose the daily–to averaged-hourly global irradiation. The missing link so far has been hourly averaged diffuse irradiation. The authors report a regression model to complete the above missing link for 14 world locations and show that the averaged–data regressions are distinctly different from previously available hour-by-hour regressions.

AUTHORS' CONTRIBUTIONS

Authors made substantial contributions to conception and design, and acquisition of data, and analysis and interpretation of data. Authors participated in drafting the article and revising it critically for important intellectual content. Authors give final approval of the version to be submitted and any revised version.

REFERENCES

1. Collares-Pereira M, Rabl A (1979) The average distribution of solar radiation correlations between diffuse and hemispherical and between daily and hourly insolation values. Solar Energy 22:155
2. Erbs DG, Klein SA, Duffie JA (1982) Estimation of the diffuse fraction of hourly, daily and monthly-averaged global radiation. Solar Energy 28:293
3. Hawas M, Muneer T (1984) Study of diffuse and global radiation characteristics in India. Energy Convers Manage 24:143
4. Liu YH, Jordan RC (1960) The interrelationship and characteristic distribution of direct, diffuse and total solar radiation. Sol Energy 4:1–19
5. Lloyd PB (1982) A Study of Some Empirical Relations Described by Liu and Jordan. Report no. 333, Solar Energy Unit, University College, Cardiff
6. Mani A, Rangarajan S (1983) Techniques for the precise estimation of hourly values of global, diffuse and direct solar radiation. Solar Energy 31:577
7. Muneer T (2004) Solar Radiation and Daylight Models, 2nd edn., Elsevier
8. Muneer T, Hawas M (1984) Correlation between daily diffuse and global radiation for India. En Conv Mgmt 24:151
9. Muneer T, Saluja GS (1996) Correlation between hourly diffuse and global solar irradiation for the UK. Building Services Engineering Research & Technology 7, 1
10. Muneer T, Hawas MM, Sahili K (1984) Correlation between hourly diffuse and global radiation for New Delhi. Energy Conv Mgmt 24:265
11. Saluja GS, Muneer T, Smith ME (1988) Methods for estimating solar radiation on a horizontal surface. Ambient Energy 9:59
12. Stanhill G (1966) Diffuse sky and cloud radiation in Israel. Solar Energy 10:96

CHAPTER 17

EVALUATION OF RADIOMETRIC AND ATMOSPHERIC CORRECTION ALGORITHMS FOR ABOVEGROUND FOREST BIOMASS ESTIMATION USING LANDSAT 5 TM DATA

Pablito M. López-Serrano, José J. Corral-Rivas, Ramón A. Díaz-Varela, Juan G. Álvarez-González, and Carlos A. López-Sánchez

Keywords: Multivariate adaptive regression splines, remote sensing, radiometric correction algorithms, terrain features

INTRODUCTION

Apart from sensor gains/offsets, solar irradiance and Sun-Earth geometry, the characteristics of electromagnetic energy detected by remote sensing optical sensors is affected by particles and other components present in the atmosphere. Hence, as solar radiation passes through the atmosphere (Sun-surface-sensor), it is affected by absorption or scattering by particles in suspension (aerosols) and other atmospheric elements, thus creating a hazy effect that distorts the radiometric properties of satellite images [1,2,3,4]. Various algorithms have been developed to correct such effects in the image. These include calibrations based on sensor parameters, solar-Earth geometry, dark object subtraction and radiative transfer [5,6,7,8]. Correction of atmospheric effects is important in relation to improving data quality [9,10]. However, the use of correction algorithms to minimize atmospheric effects, especially the scattering and absorption caused by aerosols, remains challenging [11]. This particularly applies to the parameterization of algorithms for calculating the surface reflectance for its eventual use in estimating aerial or aboveground forest biomass (AGB) [12].

AGB is an important parameter that provides information about the current status of forests and therefore facilitates forest management decisions [13,14]. The use of optical remote sensors of medium spatial resolution, such as the Landsat Thematic Mapper (TM), has become increasingly common in the last few decades. The use of these sensors for large-scale monitoring of AGB dynamics, particularly in the case of multi-temporal/multi-scene analyses or unevenly-distributed atmospheric effects in single-image analyses, frequently involves the application of different atmospheric correction algorithms. Such algorithms correct distortions between or within images other than those related to real land cover differences [15,16,17,18,19].

The aim of the present study was to evaluate four different atmospheric correction algorithms (surface reflectance)—COST (Cosine of the Solar Zenith Angle), a modification of the dark object subtraction method [20] with the addition of a multiplicative correction for atmospheric transmittance [21], ATCOR2 (Atmospheric Correction for Flat Terrain), [22]), FLAASH (Fast Line-of-sight Atmospheric Analysis of Spectral Hypercubes, [23,24]) and 6S (Second Simulation of Satellite Signal in the Solar Spectrum, [25]), and one radiometric correction algorithm (apparent reflectance at sensor), ToA

Citation: Pablito M. López-Serrano, José J. Corral-Rivas, Ramón A. Díaz-Varela, Juan G. Álvarez-González, and Carlos A. López-Sánchez. Evaluation of Radiometric and Atmospheric Correction Algorithms for Aboveground Forest Biomass Estimation Using Landsat 5 TM Data, Remote Sensing, 2016, 8(5), 369; DOI:10.3390/rs8050369.

(Top of Atmosphere), for estimating AGB from spectral data captured by the Landsat 5 TM sensor and topographic variables derived from a digital elevation model (DEM) generated using data collected by sampling of the permanent forest growth and soil research sites (SPIFyS) established in a temperate forest in the northwest of the state of Durango, Mexico.

Different methods could be used for remote AGB estimation in forests, including parametric and nonparametric approaches. However, since forest structure and biomass often entail nonlinear variability, variable interaction across scales and autocorrelation, nonparametric approaches often markedly outperform parametric methods [26].

In this study, we investigate remote AGB estimation of mixed and uneven-aged forests using the multivariate adaptive regression splines (MARS). To the best of our knowledge, MARS have rarely been used for remote estimation of AGB [27,28,29], but in these cases, the method has performed best for prediction than other parametric and non-parametric approaches, such us linear models, classification, regression trees and artificial neural networks [27] or hybrid tree-based algorithms [28,29].

MATERIALS AND METHODS

Study Area

The study area is located in the northwest of the state of Durango (Figure 1). The forest vegetation comprises pine (Pinusspp.), oak (Quercus spp.), fir (Abies spp.) and plurispecific stands with different proportions of species of the genera Pinusand Quercus, in accordance with the Land and Vegetation Use Map, scale 1:250,000, Series V [30]. The weather is cold in the canyons (with temperatures ranging from −20 °C in winter to 20 °C in summer) and mild or warm in the valleys (with temperatures ranging from 10 °C in winter to 40 °C in summer).

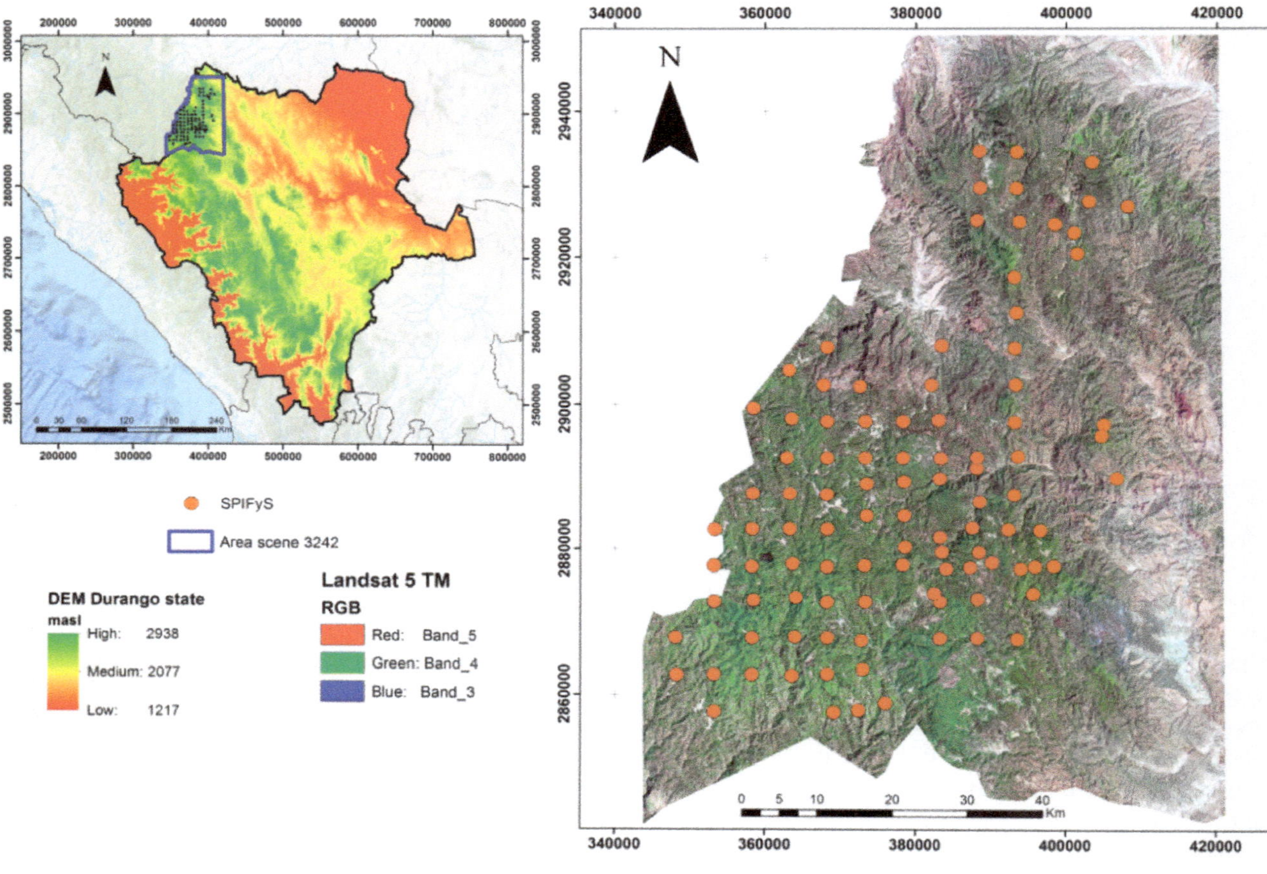

Figure 1. Location of the study area and of the permanent forest growth and soil research sites (SPIFyS).

Field Data

The field data were AGB values taken from a database of stand variables measured in 99 permanent forest growth and soil research sitesSPIFyS established during the winter of 2011 in accordance with the method developed by Corral-Rivas et al.[31]. The SPIFyS are square plots of a size of 50 × 50 m (surface area, 2500 m^2). The location of the sites was carried out by systematic sampling at the regional level using a squared grid of five kilometers, although a small squared grid (3 km) was used on very steep areas to include their variability.

In each sample plot, the tree species were recorded, and the diameter at breast height (cm) and total height (m) of all standing trees were measured. Species-specific models developed for the study area were used to estimate individual tree aboveground biomass [32]. The goodness of fit for such statistical models ranged from 0.87–0.99 (R^2), and the root mean square error (RMSE) varied from 22.8–95.2 kg. Once the tree aboveground biomass was estimated, all values from each sampling plot were summed and expressed on a per hectare basis. Table 1 shows the descriptive statistics of the main stand variables.

Table 1. Descriptive statistics of the main stand variables estimated from the 99 permanent sample plots. The dominant stand height was calculated as an average value from the 100 thickest trees per hectare.

Variable	Mean	Standard Deviation	Minimum Value	Maximum Value
Number of stems per ha	655.47	322.25	224	2264
Diameter at breast height (cm)	18.44	3.46	11.69	31.12
Dominant height (m)	14.62	3.72	6.87	24.81
Stand biomass ($Mg{\cdot}ha^{-1}$)	89.03	43.45	2.70	234.03

Spectral Data from the Landsat 5 TM Sensor

The image used in the study, which was captured by the Landsat 5 TM sensor in April 2011, is available at the U.S. Geological Service (USGS) website [33]. The sensor operates in seven bands of the electromagnetic spectrum: Band 1 (blue, 450–520 nm), Band 2 (green, 520–600 nm), Band 3 (red, 630–690 nm), Band 4 (near-infrared, 760–900 nm), Bands 5 and 7 (mid-infrared region, 1550–2350 nm) and Band 6 (which provides information in the thermal infrared region and is not used in this type of study). Likewise, the spectral indices Normalized Difference Vegetation Index (NDVI, [34]) and Modified Soil Adjusted Index (MSAVI2, [35]) were used. Such indexes are potentially less sensitive than single band values to artefacts due to differences in light conditions, exposed soil or terrain slope and orientation, which might eventually affect AGB estimation.

Radiometric Correction Algorithms

A useful prior step to the interpretation of satellite images is converting the digital numbers (DNs) stored in the original image into biophysical variables of standard significance (reflectance). These variables are comparable in the same sensor over time and over scenes, as well as between different sensors and between remote sensing and other methods of detecting electromagnetic energy. The correction is also advisable in the case of unevenly-distributed atmospheric effects in the image and also when vegetation indexes based on band ratios are included in the analyses [36,37,38,39,40,41]. In order to calculate surface reflectance, the atmospheric effects must be removed. This involves estimating the atmospheric transmissivity (both up and down welling), diffuse irradiance and atmospheric radiance due to scattering [42]. In the present study, we evaluated five different radiometric correction methods: the first four methods (namely ATCOR2, COST, FLAASH and 6S) including atmospheric corrections (surface absolute reflectance), while the fifth (ToA) without considering atmospheric effects (apparent reflectance at the sensor) for the final estimation of AGB.

Atmospheric Correction for Flat Terrain (ATCOR2)

The aim of ATCOR2 correction [22] is to remove the atmospheric effects in order to recover the physical parameters of the Earth's surface, including the surface reflectance, soil visibility and the temperature. The correction is carried out with the ATCOR module [43] included in ERDAS IMAGINE software, Version 2013 [44].

Cosine of the Sun Zenith Angle (COST)

This is a radiometric calibration method that considers the atmospheric effect and is based entirely on the characteristics of the satellite image, in contrast with other methods of atmospheric correction, like ATCOR2, FLAASH or 6S, requiring some extra parameters, such as atmospheric profiles, the aerosol models or visibility [21,45]. COST applies Dark Object Subtraction (DOS, [20]) to compensate for the additive components of the atmosphere, which mainly affect the shortest wavelengths. DOS does not take into account the multiplicative effect on the longer wavelengths. For initial estimation of the multiplicative effect, the value of the atmospheric transmittance along the path from the ground to the sensor (TAUz) was computed from the cosine of the solar zenith angle [46]. This correction was carried out by implementing the algorithm in the Model Maker® module of ERDAS IMAGINE software, Version 2013 [44].

Fast Line-of-Sight Atmospheric Analysis of Spectral Hypercubes (FLAASH)

This is an advanced atmospheric correction module based on the MODTRAN4 algorithm of radiative transfer developed by Spectral Sciences Inc. (Burlington, MA, USA) under the sponsorship of the U.S. Air Force Research Laboratory [23,24]. The technique is initially based on the standard equation of spectral radiance for each pixel of the sensor, which applies to the range of wavelengths of solar radiation (thermal emission is omitted) and a Lambertian and flat surface or their equivalents. It considers the radiance reflected from the Earth's surface and scattered by the atmosphere towards the sensor. The difference between these two radiances is due to the adjacency effect (spatial mixture of radiance among nearby pixels) caused by atmospheric scattering. The correction was carried out with the FLAASH module in ENVI® software, Version 5.1 [47].

Second Simulation of Satellite Signal in the Solar Spectrum (6S)

This procedure eliminates atmospheric effects on the reflectance values in images captured by sensors on board satellite or aircraft platforms. It is based on an advanced code of radiative transfer, designed for simulating the interaction between solar radiation and an atmospheric-surface system, together with a wide range of atmospheric, spectral and geometric conditions [25]. The code acts on the basis of the successive order of scattering (SOS) method and explains the polarization of radiation in the atmosphere by calculating the different components. The scenes used to belong to the National Landsat Archive Processing System (NLAPS) and correspond to the product obtained by Landsat 4–5 Thematic Mapper Level 1 of surface reflectance processed by the Standard Landsat Product Generation System (LPGS) and using the Landsat Ecosystem Disturbance Adaptive Processing System (LEDAPS) algorithm (available at the U.S. Geological Service website [33]).

Apparent Reflectance at the Top of Atmosphere (ToA)

This technique enables calculation of the apparent reflectance in a satellite image and consists of converting the DNs to radiance values and then to reflectance values. The word "apparent" refers to the fact that the reflectance has not been corrected for atmospheric effects and represents an initial normalization of the image [48]. The correction was carried out with the "apparent reflectance" method implemented in the "landsat" package [49] in the R software [50].

Parameters Derived from the Digital Elevation Model (DEM)

The primary and secondary terrain parameters were calculated from the DEM (Table 2), after the application of a low bandpass filter with a moving window of 5 × 5, with the aim of reducing the banding effect present in the original archive [51]. These parameters are considered as predictor variables for estimating AGB, because they are directly related to the distribution and development of forest species and can subsequently be evaluated [52,53].

Table 2. Additional field variables used to model the aboveground forest biomass (AGB).

Table 2. Additional field variables used to model the aboveground forest biomass (AGB).

Variable	Formula	Reference
Elevation	Digital Elevation Model	
Slope (β)	$\beta = \arctan\left[(G^2 + H^2)^{1/2}\right]$	
Transformed aspect (Trasp)	$Trasp = \frac{1-\cos((\pi / 180)(\alpha-30))}{2}$	[53]
Terrain Shape Index (TSI)	$TSI = \overline{Z}/R$	[52]
Wetness Index (WI)	WI = ln (As/tanβ)	[54]
Profile curvature (Ø)	$Ø = -2\frac{DG^2+EH^2+FGH}{G^2+H^2}$	[55]
Plan curvature (ω)	$\omega = 2\frac{DH^2+EG^2+FGH}{G^2+H^2}$	
Curvature (x)	x = ω − Ø	

where: $\overline{Z}$, average elevation; R, point radio altitude units; As, drainage area specified; tanβ, local slope angle; D, F, G and H were derived according to the equation of [56].

Generation of a Database

The database used to estimate AGB was generated by extracting the mean values of the satellite image pixels after each of the radiometric correction techniques and of the different DEM parameters by considering a buffer of 25 m for the geolocalization of the SPIFyS plots. The values were extracted using the "raster" package [57], implemented in R statistical software [50].

Statistical Analysis

Analysis of Variance

In order to establish whether there were any significant differences between the radiometric correction algorithms considered, analysis of variance (ANOVA) was used to compare the values of each spectral band of the sensor obtained by processing the images of the SPIFyS and applying the different correction algorithms. The correction algorithm was used as a fixed factor:

$$y_i = \mu + CA_i + \varepsilon_i \quad (1)$$

where y_i are the values of each spectral band of the sensor corrected by the algorithm i; CA_i is the correction algorithm used (fixed factor) and ε_i are the associated errors.

Prior to the application of the ANOVA, the dependent variables normality and homogeneity of variance were checked using respectively Shapiro–Wilk's test [58] and Levene's test [59]. When the results of these tests indicated that the ANOVA assumptions were not satisfied, the dependent variables were transformed by a natural log transformation. When the ANOVA indicated significant differences between correction algorithms ($\alpha = 0.05$), Tukey's multiple comparison test was used to identify which algorithms were different. Likewise, box plots were elaborated for each variable (spectral band) with the aim of facilitating graphical interpretation of the results. All analyses were carried out with R statistical software [50].

Multivariate Adaptive Regression Spline (MARS)

The statistical analysis was carried out by the non-parametric multivariate adaptive regression splines (MARS) proposed by Friedman [60], using the "earth" package [61] implemented in the R software [50]. This method involves constructing a non-linear regression model based on a product of functions denominated "smoothed basis functions" (splines). The predictors are incorporated in their structure as part of a function generating a model for the dependent variable, which may be continuous or binary, and at the same time automatically selects the predictors in the final model. The general form of the MARS non-parametric regression model, formulated on the dependent "y" variable and the "x" predictors, is as follows:

$$y = f(x) + \varepsilon \quad (2)$$

where ε is the error and f (x) is the unknown regression function, derived as follows:

$$f(x) = \beta_0 + \sum_{m=1}^{M} \beta_m B_m(x) \quad (3)$$

where β_0 is the intercept of the model, B_m (x) is the m-th basis function, βm is the coefficient of the m-th basis function andM is the number of basis functions in the model. Each basis function B_m(x) takes one of the following two forms: (i) a hinge function of the form max (0, x-k) or max (0, k-x), where k is a constant value; (ii) a product of two or more hinge functions that, therefore, can model the interaction between two or more predictors (x).

The optimal model was selected using the backward procedure. An overfitted model was generated with all possible predictor variables, and the model was pruned by removing terms one by one, deleting the least effective term at each step until the best submodel was found. Model subsets were compared using the generalized crossed validation (GCV) criterion. GCV is an approximation to the error that would be determined by leave-one-out validation and considers both the residual error and the model complexity. Therefore, the optimal model will be that yielding the lowest GCV.

$$GCV(\mathrm{M}) = \frac{\sum_{i=1}^{n} (y_i - f_M(x_i))^2}{n\left(1 - \frac{p_M}{n}\right)^2} \quad (4)$$

where y_i are the observed values of the dependent variable, n is the number of observations, $f_M(x_i)$ is the MARS model with M basis functions, x_i are the observed values of the predictors included in the MARS model and p_M is the number of parameters of the MARS model.

To analyze the importance of the independent variables that contribute most to the final model, three different criteria were used: (i) nsubsets, i.e., the number of times that each variable is included in a subset (in the final model); (ii) sqr_rss, i.e., the decrease in the sum of square errors (RSS) for each subset relative to the previous subset; and (iii) sqr_gcv, i.e., the decrease in the GCV value for each subset relative to the previous subset. These criteria are normalized on a scale of 100, to facilitate the interpretation of the contribution of each predictive variable in the model.

With the aim of evaluating the performance of the fitted model for each of the radiometric correction algorithms, the following statistics were determined to compare the AGB reference data for the monitoring plots with the estimates based on the images subjected to different corrections: root mean squared error (RMSE), the coefficient of determination (R^2) and the generalized coefficient of determination (GR^2):

$$\mathrm{RMSE} = \sqrt{\frac{\sum_{i=1}^{n} (y_i - \hat{y}_i)^2}{n - p}} \quad (5)$$

$$R^2 = 1 - \frac{\sum_{i=1}^{n} (y_i - \hat{y}_i)^2}{\sum_{i=1}^{n} (y_i - \bar{y}_i)^2} \quad (6)$$

$$GR^2 = \frac{1 - GCV}{GCV_{null}} \quad (7)$$

where y_i, $\hat{y}_i$ and $\bar{y}$ are, respectively, the observed, estimated and mean values of the dependent variable; n is the total number of observations used to fit the model; p is the number of parameters to estimate; and GCV_{null} is the GCV of a model with a single independent term (β_0).

Because the quality of the fit does not necessarily reflect the quality of the prediction, assessment of the validity of the model with an independent dataset is desirable [62]. Therefore, cross-validation was carried out by splitting the dataset into different numbers of folds (2–10), and the goodness-of-fit statistics (Equations (5)–(7)) were calculated for each fold (test data) by using the models fitted to the other folds (training data).

Generation of Thematic Maps

The final stage of the overall process illustrated was the calculation of AGB maps. These maps were derived by implementing the basic functions resulting from the MARS model fit for each of the atmospheric correction algorithms by using the raster calculator in ArcGIS® software [63].

An overview of the workflow described in the previous sections is presented in Figure 2.

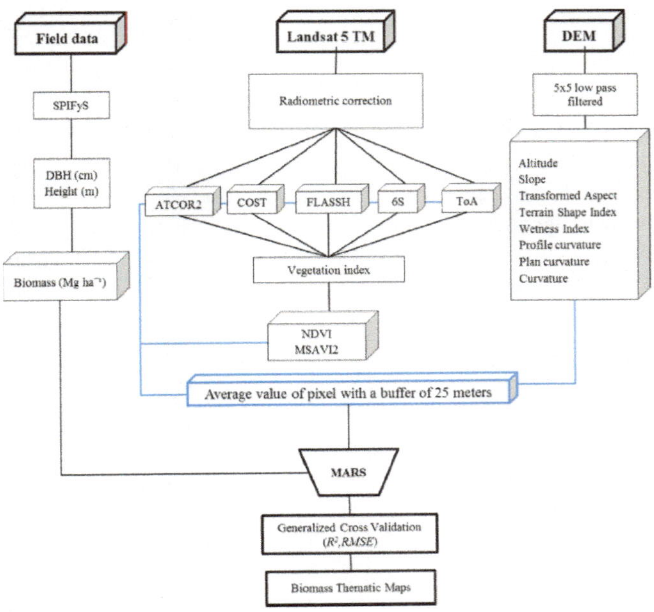

Figure 2. Flow diagram of the processes involved in estimating AGB.

RESULTS

In the first step, a visual comparison of the application of the different radiometric correction algorithms to the Landsat 5 TM image of the study area was done. All atmospheric correction algorithms were parameterized using the same type of "rural" aerosol, for zones not affected by urban or industrial sources and a visibility larger than 40 km. In comparison with the original image in DNs, the brightness of the other images differs due to the parameterization used in each algorithm to correct the radiometric and atmospheric effects (Figure 3).

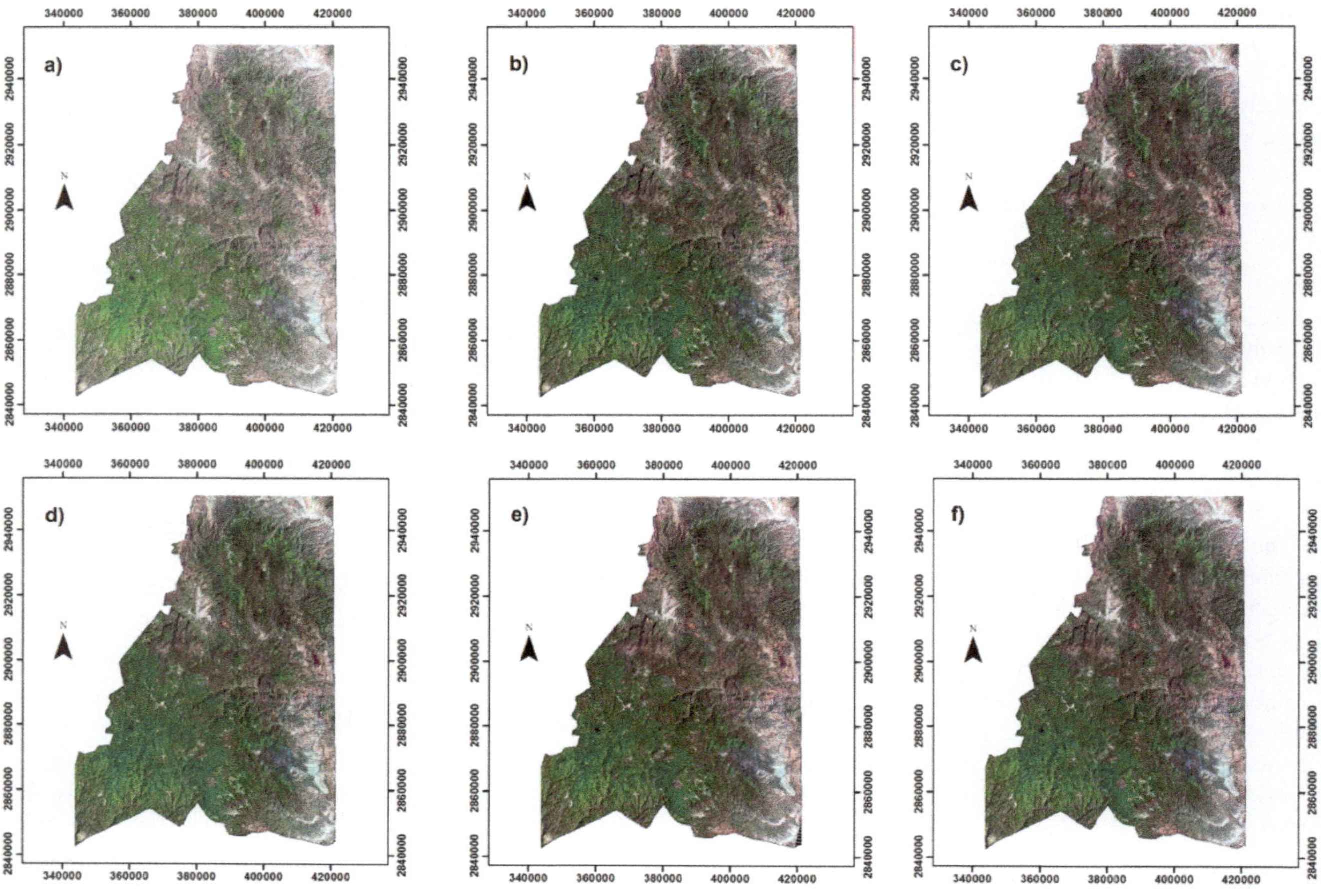

Figure 3. Comparison of the application of the different radiometric correction algorithms: (a) original image in DNs (multiband composition 5, 4 and 3); (b) ATCOR2; (c) COST; (d) FLAASH; (e) 6S; and (f) ToA.

The mean reflectances of the 99 SPIFyS plots obtained for each band of the Landsat 5 TM sensor and radiometric correction algorithm were graphically compared (Figure 4). The differences vary according to the atmospheric effects corrected by each particular algorithm. In general, the spectral signature of the vegetation showed in all cases typical behavior: low reflectance in the bands of the visible spectrum (450–690 nm) and high reflectance in the near- and mid-infrared bands (760–2350 nm). However, a clear difference appears depending on whether the radiometric correction algorithms were applied to variables with physical meaning (e.g., ground reflectance) rather than to DNs. In this respect, the ATCOR2 and FLAASH algorithms overcorrected the atmospheric effects (underestimation of transmissivity) in the short wavelength regions and underestimated them in the near- and mid-infrared regions, while COST and ToA produced the inverse spectral pattern. Finally, the performance of 6S was intermediate between that of the other algorithms evaluated.

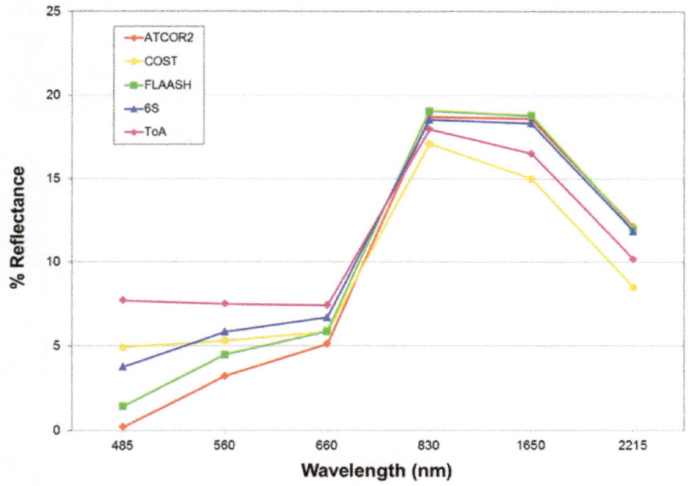

Figure 4. Spectral performance of each of the radiometric correction algorithms considered.

As the Shapiro–Wilk's test indicated that the corrected values of the spectral bands of the sensor were not normally distributed, therefore a log transformation was used. The ANOVA applied to the data from the 99 SPIFyS plots detected significant differences for all algorithms in the visible region (Figure 5), except for the COST and FLAASH algorithms inBand 3. Significant differences were observed in the near-infrared region for all algorithms tested, except ATCOR2 and 6S, which were included in the same population group (Tukey's test); they also shared characteristics with FLAASH and ToA. Finally, in the bands corresponding to mid-infrared regions, the algorithms ATCOR2, FLAASH and 6S did not provide significantly different results ($p > 0.05$).

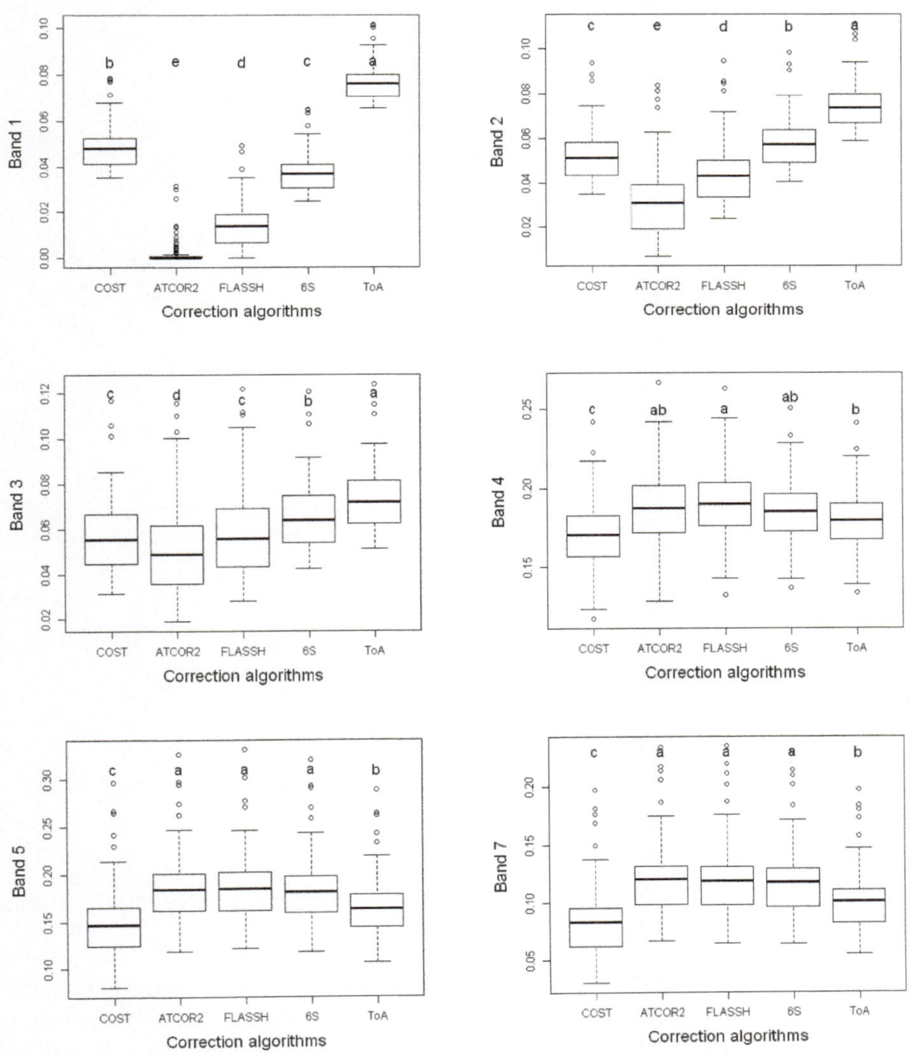

Figure 5. Box plots for each band of the Landsat 5 TM sensor and corresponding groupings of the radiometric correction algorithms (different letters indicate significant differences between algorithm performances, at $p < 0.05$).

The importance of the predictor variables (spectral bands and indices and topographic variables) for each of the MARS models fitted to the different radiometric correction algorithms was calculated (Figure 6). Results pointed out the near-infrared as the most relevant spectral region for AGB prediction. In fact, among the predictor variables, Band 7 made the greatest contribution to the capacity for predicting AGB for the different algorithms analyzed in almost all the cases except in algorithm 6S, where the variable Band 5 appeared as the most important in accordance with the number of times that each variable is included in a subset.

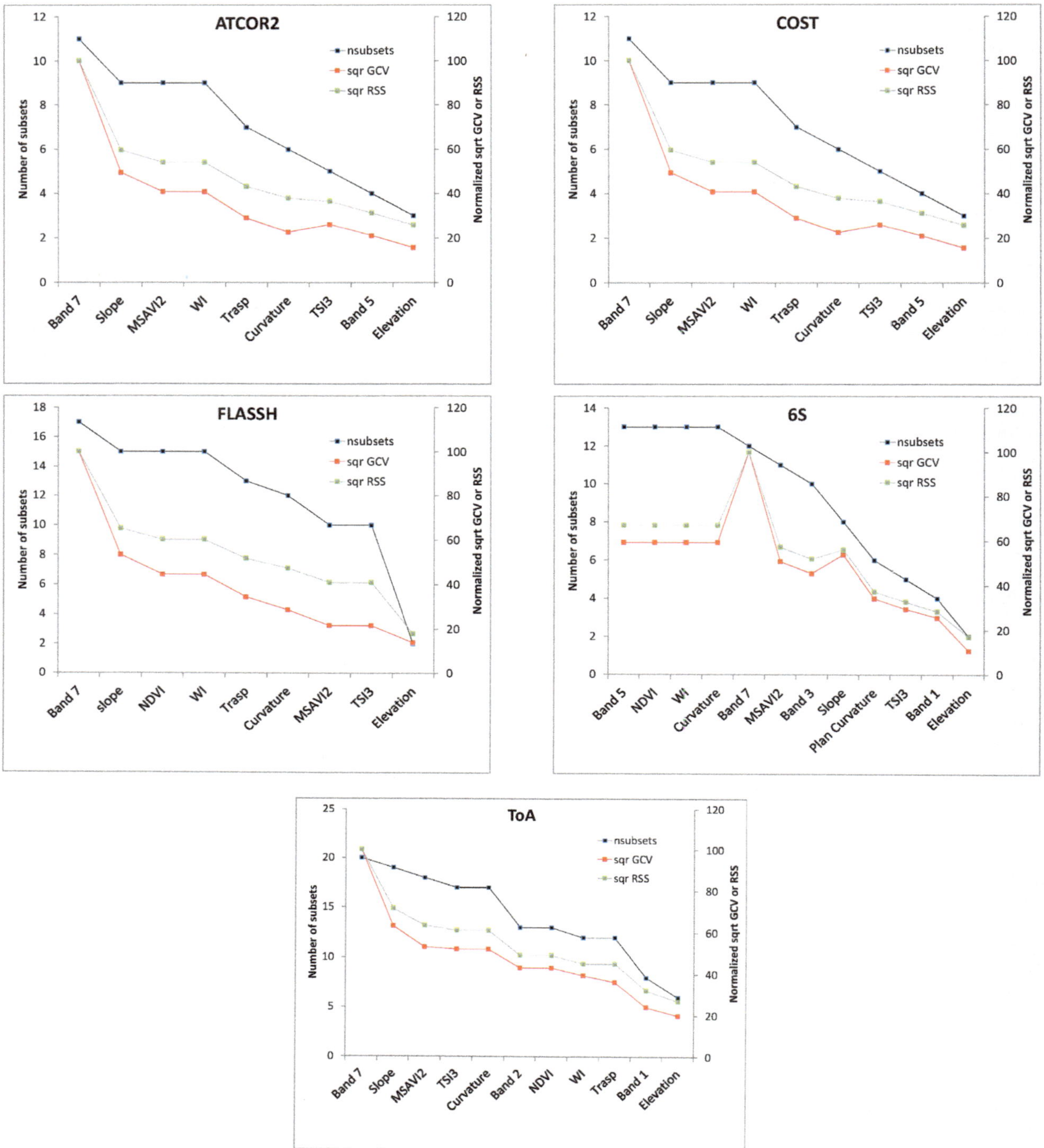

Figure 6. Importance and selection of predictor variables in the multivariate adaptive regression splines (MARS) models for each radiometric correction algorithm considered.

Table 3 shows the results of applying the MARS technique for estimating the AGB on the basis of different correction algorithms. The algorithm that yielded the best predictions was ToA (R^2 = 0.89, RMSE = 29.82 Mg·ha^{-1}; 33.49% of the average stand biomass). However, after the application of cross-validation, the generalized coefficient of determination (GCV) decreased to 0.68. By contrast, the algorithm with the lowest predictive power was ATCOR2 (R^2 = 0.75 and GR^2 = 0.59). The algorithm with the highest generalized coefficient of determination was 6S (GR^2 = 0.71).

Table 3. MARS model selection criteria for AGB estimation and the different radiometric correction algorithms considered.

Algorithm	Number of Terms	Number of Predictors	*GCV*	*RSS*	*GR²*	*R²*	RMSE	%RMSE
ATCOR2	12 of 31	9 of 17	780.84	45556.61	0.59	0.75	50.37	56.58
COST	16 of 29	9 of 17	572.13	26722.49	0.70	0.85	36.55	41.05
FLAASH	18 of 33	9 of 17	737.91	30530.20	0.61	0.83	36.43	40.92
6S	16 of 30	12 of 17	552.26	25794.27	0.71	0.86	33.48	37.61
ToA	21 of 30	11 of 17	601.91	20452.83	0.68	0.89	29.82	33.49

where: GCV, generalized cross-validation; RSS, residual sum of squares; GR^2, generalized coefficient of determination; R^2, coefficient of determination; RMSE, root mean squared error (Mg·ha^{-1}).

Figure 7 shows the variations in the goodness of fit statistics (R^2 and GR^2) obtained by application of the cross-validation technique (nfold = 2–10) to the MARS model fits to each of the algorithms considered. In this case, the COST algorithm produced the best results and the highest stability, followed by ToA and 6S.

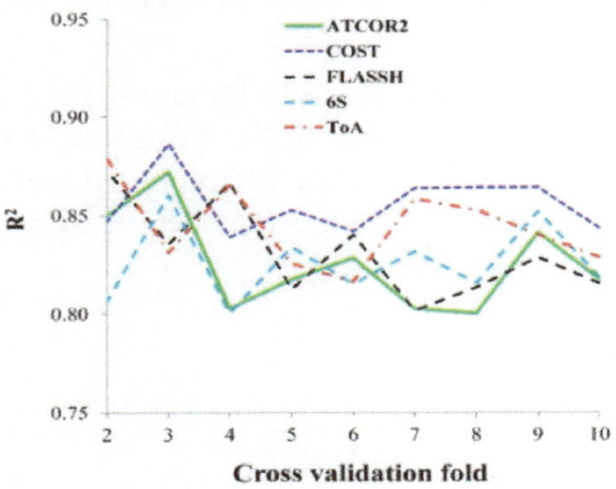

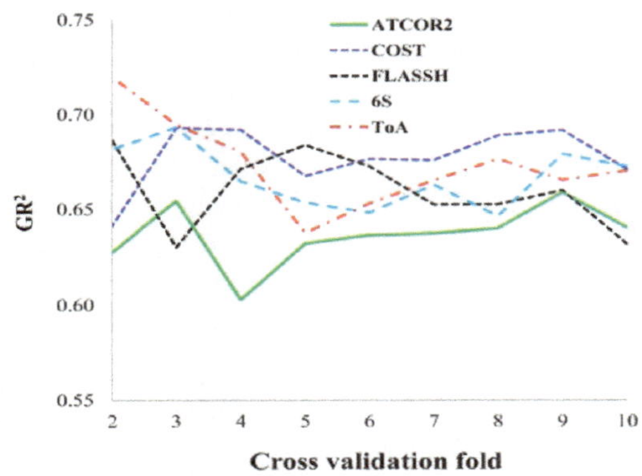

Figure 7. Variations in the goodness of fit statistics obtained by applying the cross-validation technique (nfolds = 2–10) to the MARS models.

Finally, AGB maps of the study area were generated by implementing the fitted MARS models for each radiometric correction algorithm on the satellite image using the raster calculator with ArcGIS® software [63] and then intersected with the vector layer of vegetation cover [30] (Figure 8).

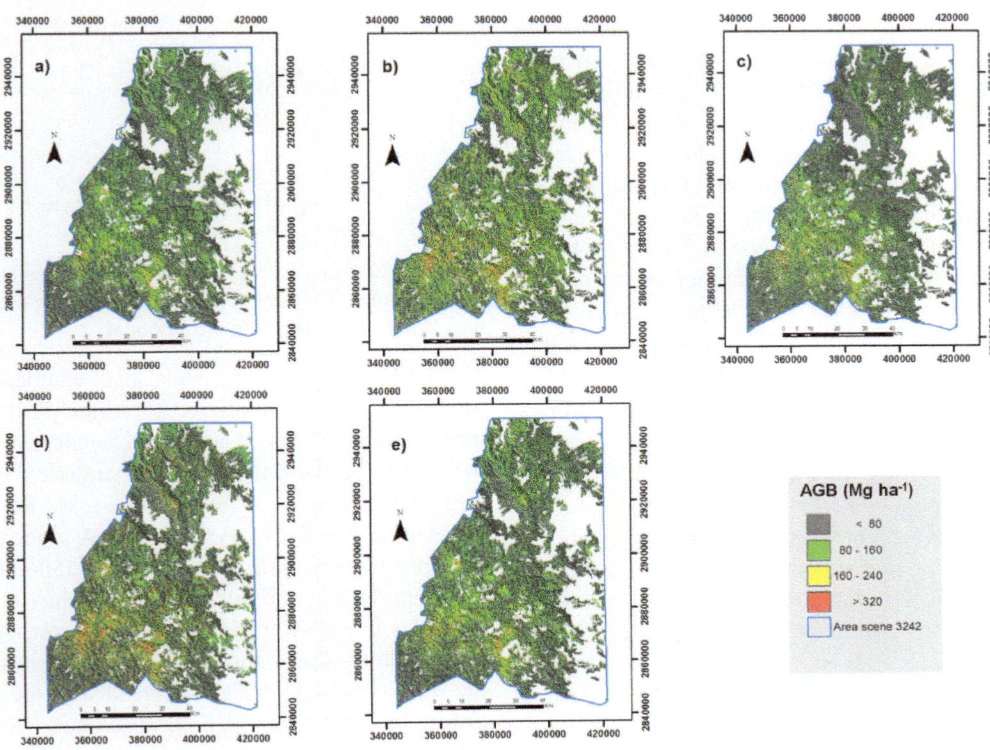

Figure 8. Maps of AGB in the study area generated from images corrected using the different radiometric correction algorithms considered. (a) ATCOR2; (b) COST; (c) FLAASH; (d) 6S; and (e) ToA.

DISCUSSION

The use of radiometric correction algorithms enabled the transformation of DNs to reflectance values (i.e., variables with biophysical meaning). The spectral reflectance of the forest cover in the study area was low (<0.10) in the visible region being typical of vegetated land (as chlorophyll absorbs most of the light received from the visible spectrum). Accordingly, the reflectance was higher (around 19%) in the near-infrared region, indicating the contrast between these regions of the electromagnetic spectrum [42,64] typical of green vegetation.

In accordance with [42], reflectance in the blue band (450–520 nm) was lower relative to the DNs and was distorted by the ToA algorithm, which assumes a transparent atmosphere over flat land and perfectly Lambertian surfaces. However, with the ATCOR2 algorithm, overcorrection at the shortest wavelengths in the visible region (i.e., green or red bands) is a consequence of scattering caused by particles of ozone and water vapor present in the atmosphere [65,66]. According to Broszeit and Ashraf [67], the images corrected using the COST algorithm are less accurate than those corrected with the ATCOR2 algorithm for vegetation cover, because COST automatically selects the lowest pixel values for each band to eliminate atmospheric haze from the data, whereas ATCOR2 uses specific parameters of atmospheric geometry and of the sensor for improved conversion of the reflectance data.

In the present study, the 6S algorithm performed more consistently than the other algorithms evaluated (ATCOR2, COST, FLAASH and ToA), because of the capacity of 6S to correct the effects of water vapor, high temperature and, therefore, high aerosol levels. This finding is similar to that reported by Nazeer et al. [68], who observed that, among five algorithms tested, 6S produced the smallest difference in field-measured surface reflectance and that obtained using the Landsat ETM sensor.

The analysis of variance applied to data from the 99 SPIFyS plots revealed similar behavior of the population means for the ATCOR2, FLAASH and 6S algorithms in the bands of the mid-infrared region. However, the bands in the visible and near-infrared regions indicated a statistically-significant difference in the configuration of the groups of algorithms. These findings are consistent with those reported by Mahiny and Turner [69], who compared the first four bands of the Landsat TM sensor under five radiometric correction methods (two relative approaches: pseudo invariant features (PIF) and radiometric control sets (RCS); and three absolute approaches: COST, 6S and ToA), showing that in most cases, the four bands produced significantly different results.

Regarding the use of the MARS technique for estimating AGB in the present study, the ToA algorithm initially showed the greatest predictive power (R^2 = 0.89, RMSE = 29.8 Mg·ha^{-1}; 33.49% of the mean biomass in the stand). This result showed a slightly better performance than that reported by Hamdan et al. [70] who estimated AGB by fitting regression models to reflectance data (corrected by ToA) from the SPOT-5 and ALOS PALSAR (R^2 = 0.803; RMSE = 32.6 Mg·ha^{-1}). Furthermore, in a study in southwest Colorado (USA), a lower correlation for biomass prediction (r = 0.86, RMSE = 45.6 Mg·ha^{-1}) with data corresponding to vegetation indices and texture analysis in Landsat TM images corrected by ToA radiometric correction was obtained [18]. However, further analyses in the present study, such as the use of the generalized error of cross-validation (GCV), indicated a GR^2 value of 0.68, pointing out a decrease in the predictive capacity of the model. Therefore, after application of GCV, the 6S algorithm proved to be optimal (GR^2 = 0.71) despite the potentially negative effect of considering a larger number of predictors (12 of 17) than in ToA correction. It should be taken into account that the GCV criterion considers both the residual error and also the model complexity, penalizing those models with a high number of parameters. The results are similar to those obtained by Nguyen et al. [71] in a study carried out in South Korea in which it was confirmed that the 6S algorithm fitted by the kNN technique (RMSE = 22.5 Mg·ha^{-1}) produced better results for estimating AGB than the other algorithms tested (DOS, FLAASH and ToA), especially for Landsat ETM bands in the infrared region. Furthermore, various studies have concluded that the MARS technique is a flexible method that yields robust predictions [72,73].

The scatterplot of observed versus predicted aboveground forest biomass obtained with the MARS model fitted to the spectral data corrected using the proposed algorithm (6S) is shown in Figure 9. No trends to under- or over-estimate were observed.

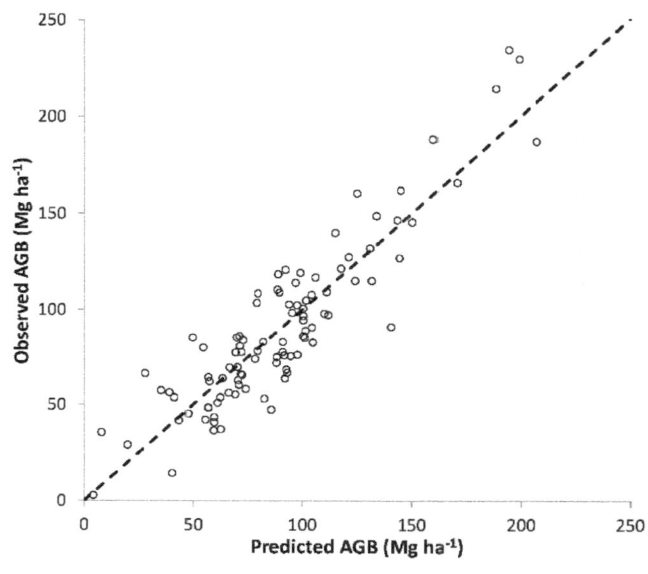

Figure 9. Observed versus predicted AGB obtained using the MARS model fitted to the spectral data corrected using the 6S algorithm. The broken line corresponds to the diagonal.

This statistical approach also enables identifying the importance of the predictive variables, in this case the near-infrared being the most important. Hence, in accordance with the nsubsets criterion, the spectral variable Band 7 (2080–2350 nm) contributed most to the fitted MARS models for the ATCOR2, COST, FLAASH and ToA algorithms, in contrast to algorithm 6S, in which Band 5 (1550–1750 nm) was the most important variable. However, the importance of the variables in algorithm 6S, under the criteria sqr_rss and sqr_gcv, indicates that Band 7 makes the greatest contribution to the MARS model, as also occurred with the other algorithms tested. In this respect, the variable Band 7 is associated with the moisture content of the forest stand, so that the greater the moisture content of the land cover, the greater absorption in this band of the electromagnetic spectrum; in other words, the surface reflectance captured by the sensor tends to decrease [74,75].

Among the topographical variables considered, the slope (β) and the wetness index (WI) contributed most to defining the MARS models and is also directly related to the moisture content in the field sites as a factor that controls run-off; the lower the value of β, the higher the moisture content and, therefore, the higher the AGB [18,76,77]. Hence, it is quite clear that radiometric and topographic variables related to water availability played a key role in the prediction of AGB in Durango's temperate forests.

Regarding the inclusion of vegetation indices, NDVI and MSAVI2 were the variables that contributed most to the MARS models, given their potential usefulness in estimating AGB. Inclusion of these indices improved the prediction of the biophysical variables in forest ecosystems: in the case of NDVI because of it high sensitivity to the chlorophyll content of the vegetation [78,79] and in the case of MSAVI2 because of its capacity to discriminate soil from vegetation, even in zones with scarce vegetation cover [80].

CONCLUSIONS

The study findings demonstrate the potential of the combined application of Landsat Thematic Mapper (TM) sensor satellite imagery and the consideration of topographical variables for estimating AGB, as well as the effects of different radiometric correction algorithms on the estimates obtained. The algorithm that showed the greatest spectral stability and that best estimated the AGB after application of the cross-validation technique was the 6S algorithm. However, each algorithm has advantages and disadvantages, and the user must parameterize each algorithm on the basis of the specific objectives. The MARS statistical method proved suitable for AGB estimation by using easy-to-obtain variables from remote sensing techniques. For all algorithms considered, the spectral band in the mid-infrared region (Band 7), the slope (β) and the wetness index (WI) of the land, both related to water availability, along with the vegetation indices MSAVI2 and NDVI were the most important predictor variables for estimating AGB. Generation of an AGB map from the fitted models may be used in local and regional forest management, thus facilitating the location and precise delimitation of zones with different levels of AGB. Further research could aim at testing the effects of radiometric corrections on biomass modelling on a multi-scene and/or multi-temporal basis.

ACKNOWLEDGMENTS

This research was supported by SEP-PROMEP (project: Seguimiento y Evaluación de Sitios Permanentes de Investigación Forestal y el Impacto Socio-económico del Manejo Forestal en el Norte de México) and by the research project EM2014-003 (Plan Galego de Investigación, Innovación e Crecemento 2011–2015; Consellería de Cultura, Educación e Ordenación Universitaria. Xunta de Galicia).

AUTHOR CONTRIBUTIONS

Pablito M. López-Serrano and Carlos A. López-Sánchez conceived of, designed and performed the experiments and wrote the manuscript. Jose J. Corral-Rivas, Ramón A. Díaz-Varela and Juan G. Álvarez-González analyzed the data and revised the manuscript.

REFERENCES

1. Jensen, J.R. A remote sensing perspective. In Introductory Digital Image Processing; Prentice Hall: Englewood Cliffs, NJ, USA, 1996.
2. Gao, B.C.; Montes, M.J.; Davis, C.O.; Goetz, A.F. Atmospheric correction algorithms for hyperspectral remote sensing data of land and ocean. Remote Sens. Environ. 2009, 113, S17–S24.
3. Tyagi, P.; Bhosle, U. Atmospheric correction of remotely sensed images in spatial and transform domain. Int. J. Image Process. 2011, 5, 564–579.
4. Tan, K.C.; Lim, H.S.; Matjafri, M.Z.; Adbullah, K. A comparison of radiometric correction techniques in the evaluation between LST and NDVI in Landsat imagery. Environ. Monit. Assess. 2012, 184, 3813–3829.
5. Hadjimitsis, D.G.; Papadavid, G.; Agapiou, A.; Themistocleous, K.; Hadjimitsis, M.G.; Retalis, A.; Michaelides, S.; Chrysoulakis, N.; Toulios, L.; Clayton, C.R.I. Atmospheric correction for satellite remotely sensed data intended for agricultural applications: Impact on vegetation indices. Nat. Hazards Earth Syst. Sci. 2010, 10, 89–95.
6. Li, F.; Jupp, D.L.; Thankappan, M.; Lymburner, L.; Mueller, N.; Lewis, A.; Held, A. A physics-based atmospheric and BRDF correction for Landsat data over mountainous terrain. Remote Sens. Environ. 2012, 124, 756–770.
7. Jaelani, L.M.; Matsushita, B.; Yang, W.; Fukushima, T. An improved atmospheric correction algorithm for applying MERIS data to very turbid inland waters. Int. J. Appl. Earth Obs. Geoinform. 2015, 39, 128–141.
8. Lee, C.S.; Yeom, J.M.; Lee, H.L.; Kim, J.J.; Han, K.S. Sensitivity analysis of 6S-based look-up table for surface reflectance retrieval. Asia Pac. J. Atmos. Sci. 2015, 51, 91–101.
9. Vanonckelen, S.; Lhermitte, S.; Van Rompaey, A. The effect of atmospheric and topographic correction methods on land cover classification accuracy. Int. J. Appl. Earth Obs. Geoinform. 2013, 24, 9–21.
10. Moreira, E.P.; Valeriano, M.M. Application and evaluation of topographic correction methods to improve land cover mapping using object-based classification. Int. J. Appl. Earth Obs. Geoinform. 2014, 32, 208–217.
11. Roy, D.; Wulder, M.; Loveland, T.; Woodcock, C.; Allen, R.; Anderson, M. LANDSAT-8: Science and product vision for terrestrial global change research. Remote Sens. Environ. 2014, 145, 154–172.
12. Ju, J.; Roy, D.; Vermote, E.; Masek, J.; Kovalsky, V. Continental-scale validation of MODIS-based and LEDAPS Landsat ETM+ atmospheric correction methods. Remote Sens. Environ. 2012, 122, 175–184.
13. Ediriweera, S.; Pathirana, S.; Danaher, T.; Nichols, D.; Moffiet, T. Evaluation of different topographic corrections for Landsat TM data by prediction of foliage

projective cover (FPC) in topographically complex landscapes. Remote Sens.2013, 5, 6767–6789.

14. Gagliasso, D.; Hummel, S.; Temesgen, H. A comparison of selected parametric and non-parametric imputation methods for estimating forest biomass and basal area. Open J. For. 2014, 4, 42–48.
15. Hantson, S.; Chuvieco, E. Evaluation of different topographic correction methods for Landsat imagery. Int. J. Appl. Earth Obs. Geoinform. 2011, 13, 691–700.
16. Balthazar, V.; Veerle, V.; Eric, F.L. Evaluation and parameterization of ATCOR3 topographic correction method for forest cover mapping in mountain areas. Int. J. Appl. Earth Obs. Geoinform. 2012, 18, 436–450.
17. Cortés, L.; Hernández, J.; Valencia, D.; Corvalán, P. Estimation of above-ground forest biomass using Landsat ETM+, Aster GDEM and Lidar. Forest Res. 2014.
18. Kelsey, K.C.; Neff, J.C. Estimates of aboveground biomass from texture analysis of landsat imagery. Remote Sens. 2014,6, 6407–6422.
19. Tian, X.; Li, Z.; Su, Z.; Chen, E.; Van der Tol, C.; Li, X.; Guo, Y.; Li, L.; Ling, F. Estimating montane forest above-ground biomass in the upper reaches of the Heihe River Basin using Landsat-TM data. Int. J. Remote Sens. 2014, 35, 7339–7362.
20. Vincent, R.K. An ERTS multispectral scanner experiment for mapping iron compounds. In Proceedings of the 8th International Symposium on Remote Sensing of Environment, Ann Arbor, MI, USA, 2–6 October 1972; pp. 1239–1247.
21. Chavez, P.S. Image-based atmospheric corrections-revisited and improved. Photogramm. Eng. Remote Sens. 1996, 62, 1025–1036.
22. Richter, R. A spatially adaptive fast atmospheric correction algorithm. Int. J. Remote Sens. 1996, 17, 1201–1214.
23. Adler-Golden, S.; Berk, A.; Bernstein, L.S.; Richtsmeier, S.; Acharya, P.K.; Matthew, M.W.; Anderson, G.P.; Allred, C.L.; Jeong, L.S.; Chetwynd, J.H. FLAASH, a MODTRAN4 atmospheric correction package for hyperspectral data retrievals and simulations. In Procedings of the 7th Annual JPL Airborne Earth Science Workshop, Pasadena, CA, USA, 12–16 January 1998; Green, R.O., Ed.; pp. 9–14.
24. Anderson, G.P.; Felde, G.W.; Hoke, M.L.; Ratkowski, A.J.; Cooley, T.W.; Chetwynd, J.H., Jr.; Gardner, J.A.; Adler-Golden, S.M.; Matthew, M.W.; Berk, A.; et al. MODTRAN4-based atmospheric correction algorithm: FLAASH (fast line-of-sight atmospheric analysis of spectral hypercubes). In Algorithms and Technologies for Multispectral, Hyperspectral, and Ultraspectral Imagery VIII (Proceedings of SPIE); Shen, S.S., Lewis, P.E., Eds.; Society of Photo Optics: Orlando, FL, USA, 2002; pp. 65–71.
25. Vermote, E.F.; Tanre, D.; Deuze, J.L.; Herman, M.; Morcette, J.J. Second simulation of the satellite signal in the solar spectrum, 6S: An overview. IEEE Trans. Geosci. Remote 1997, 35, 675–686.
26. Saatchi, S.S.; Harris, N.L.; Brown, S.; Lefsky, M.; Mitchard, E.T.A.; Salas, W.; Zutta, B.R.; Buermann, W.; Lewis, S.L.; Hagen, S.; et al. Benchmark map of forest carbon stocks in tropical regions across three continents. Proc. Natl. Acad. Sci. USA 2011, 108, 9899–9904.
27. Moisen, G.G.; Frescino, T.S. Comparing five modelling techniques for predict-ing forest characteristics. Ecol. Model.2002, 157, 209–225.
28. Güneralp, I.; Filippi, A.M.; Randall, J. Estimation of floodplain aboveground biomass using multispectralremote sensing and nonparametric modeling. Int. J. Appl. Earth Obs. Geoinform. 2014, 33, 119–126.
29. Filippi, A.M.; Güneralp, I.; Randall, J. Hyperspectral remote sensing of above-ground biomass on a river meander bend using multivariate adaptive regressionsplines and stochastic gradient boosting. Remote Sens. Lett. 2014, 5, 432–441.
30. Instituto Nacional de Estadística Geográfica e Informática (INEGI). Uso del Suelo y Vegetación Escala 1:250 000 Serie V, Información Vectorial; Instituto Nacional de Estadística Geográfica e Informática: Ciudad de Mexico, Mexico, 2012.
31. Corral-Rivas, J.J.; Vargas, B.; Wehenkel, C.; Aguirre, O.; Álvarez, J.G.; Rojo, A. Guía para el Establecimiento de Sitios de Inventario Periódico Forestal y de Suelos del Estado de Durango; Facultad de Ciencias Forestales: Universidad Juárez del Estado de Durango, Durango, México, 2009.
32. Vargas-Larreta, B. Estimación del Potencial de los Bosques de Durango Para la Mitigación del Cambio Climático. Modelización de la Biomasa Forestal. Proyecto FOMIX-DGO-2011-C01-165681; Comisión Nacional de Ciencia y Tecnología (CONACYT): Durango, Mexico, 2013.
33. United States Geological Survey. Available online: http://glovis.usgs.gov (accessed on 11 January 2011).
34. Rouse, J.W.; Haas, R.H.; Schell, J.A.; Deering, D.W.; Harlan, J.C. Monitoring the Vernal Advancements and Retrogradation (Greeen Wave Effect) of Natural Vegetation; NASA/GFSC: Greenbelt, MD, USA, 1974.
35. Baret, F.; Guyot, G. Potentials and limits of vegetation indices for LAI and APAR assessment. Remote Sens. Environ.1991, 35, 161–173.
36. Lavreau, J. De-hazing landsat thematic mapper images. Photogramm. Eng. Remote Ssens. 1991, 57, 1297–1302.
37. Guyot, G.; Gu, X.F. Effect of radiometric corrections on NDVI-determined from SPOT-HRV and Landsat-TM data.Remote Sens. Environ. 1994, 49, 169–180.
38. Richter, R. Atmospheric correction of satellite data with haze removal including a haze/clear transition region. Comput. Geosci. 1996, 22, 675–681.
39. Carlotto, M.J. Reducing the effects of space-varying, wavelength-dependent scattering in multispectral imagery. Int. J. Remote Sens. 1999, 20, 3333–3344.
40. Song, C.; Woodcock, C.E.; Seto, K.C.; Lenney, M.P.; Macomber, S.A. Classification and change detection using Landsat TM data: When and how to correct

atmospheric effects? Remote Sens. Environ. 2001, 75, 230–244.

41. Liang, S.; Fang, H.; Morisette, J.T.; Chen, M.; Shuey, C.J.; Walthall, C.L.; Daughtry, C.S.T. Atmospheric correction of Landsat ETM+ land surface imagery. II. Validation and applications. IEEE Trans. Geosci. Remote Sens. 2002, 40, 2736–2746.

42. Chuvieco, E. Teledetección Ambiental: La Observación de la Tierra, 1st ed.; Ariel Ciencia: Madrid, Spain, 2010.

43. Geosystems. Haze Reduction, Atmospheric and Topographic Correction. User Manual ATCOR2 and ATCOR3; Geosystems GmbH: Geneva, Switzerland, 2013.

44. ERDAS Inc. Erdas Imagine. Available online: http://www.hexagongeospatial.com/products/ERDAS-IMAGINE/details.aspx (accessed on 6 October 2014).

45. Chavez, P.S. An improved dark-object subtraction technique for atmospheric scattering correction of multispectral data. Remote Sens. Environ. 1988, 24, 459–479.

46. Moran, M.S.; Jackson, R.D.; Slater, P.N.; Teillet, P.M. Evaluation of simplified procedures for retrieval of land surface reflectance factors from satellite sensor output. Remote Sens. Environ. 1992, 41, 169–184.

47. EXELIS Inc. ENVI® 5.1 Fast Line-of-Sight Atmospheric Analysis of Hypercubes (FLAASH); EXELIS Inc.: Boulder, CO, USA, 2013.

48. Huang, C.; Yang, L.; Homer, C.; Wylie, B.; Vogelman, J.; DeFelice, T. At Satellite Reflectance: A First Order Normalization of LANDSAT 7 ETM+ Images. Available online: http://digitalcommons.unl.edu/usgspubs/109/ (accessed on 6 October 2014).

49. Goslee, S. Radiometric and Topographic Correction of Satellite Imagery. Package Landsat. Version 1.0.8. Available online: http://cran.r-project.org/web/packages/landsat/landsat.pdf (accessed on 18 May 2015).

50. R Core Team. R: A Language and Environment for Statistical Computing, R Foundation for Statistical Computing. Available online: http://www.R-project.org/ (accessed on 18 March 2014).

51. Instituto Nacional de Estadística Geográfica e Informática (INEGI). México Continuo de Elevaciones Mexicano 3.0 (CEM 3.0). Available online: http://www.inegi.org.mx/geo/contenidos/datosrelieve/continental/descarga.aspx(accessed on 6 May 2014).

52. McNab, W.H. Terrain shape index: quantifying effect of minor landforms on tree height. Forest Sci. 1989, 35, 91–104.

53. Roberts, D.W.; Cooper, S.V. Concepts and techniques of vegetation mapping. In Land Classifications Based on Vegetation: Applications for Resource Management; Ferguson, D., Morgan, P., Johnson, F.D., Eds.; General technical report INT-US Department of Agriculture, Forest Service, Intermountain Research Station (USA): Ogden, UT, USA, 1989; pp. 90–96.

54. Moore, I.D.; Nieber, J.L. Landscape assessment of soil erosion and non-point source pollution. J. Minn. Acad. Sci. 1989,55, 18–24.

55. Wilson, J.P.; Gallant, J.C. Digital terrain analysis. In Terrain Analysis: Principles and Applications; Wilson, J.P., Gallant, J.C., Eds.; John Wiley & Sons, Inc.: New York, NY, USA, 2000; pp. 1–28.

56. Zevenbergen, L.W.; Thorne, C.R. Quantitative analysis of land surface topography. Earth Surf. Proc. Landf. 1987, 12, 47–56.

57. Hijmans, R.J. Raster: Geographic Data Analysis and Modeling. R Package Version 2.4-20. Available online: http://CRAN.R-project.org/package=raster (accessed on 6 October 2015).

58. Shapiro, S.S.; Wilk, M.B. An analysis of variance test for normality (complete samples). Biometrika 1965, 52, 591–611.

59. Levene, H. Robust tests for equality of variances. In Contributions to Probability and Statistics: Essays in Honor of Harold Hotelling; Olkin, I., Ed.; Stanford University Press: Stanford, CA, USA, 1960; pp. 278–292.

60. Friedman, J.H. Multivariate adaptive regression spline. Ann. Stat. 1991, 19, 1–141.

61. Milborrow, S. Earth: Multivariate Adaptive Regression Splines. R Package Version 4.2.0. Available online: http://CRAN.R-project.org/package=earth (accessed on 6 October 2015).

62. Myers, R.H. Classical and Modern Regression with Applications; PWS-Kent Publishing Company: Belmont, CA, USA, 1990.

63. ESRI Inc. ArcGIS Desktop: Release 10; Environmental Systems Research Institute: Redlands, CA, USA, 2011.

64. Fernández, S.C.; Rodenas, A.Q. Teledetección: Avances y Aplicaciones; Diputación de Albacete: Albacete, Spain, 1999.

65. Buho, H.; Kaneko, M.; Ogawa, K. Correction of NDVI calculated from ASTER L1B and ASTER (AST07) data based on ground measurement. In Advances in Geoscience and Remote Sensing; Jedlovec, G., Ed.; In-Tech Press: Vienna, Austria, 2009.

66. Richter, R.; Schläpfer, D. Atmospheric/Topographic Correction for Satellite Imagery. ATCOR 2/3 User Guide, Version 9.0.0.; ReSe Applications Schläpfer: Langeggweg, Switzerland, 2015.

67. Broszeit, A.; Ashraf, S. Using different atmospheric correction methods to classify remotely sensed data to detect liquefaction of the February 2011 earthquake in Christchurch. In Proceedings of the SIRC NZ 2013—GIS and Remote Sensing Research Conference, Dunedin, New Zealand, 29–30 August 2013.

68. Nazeer, M.; Nichol, J.E.; Yung, Y.K. Evaluation of atmospheric correction models and Landsat surface reflectance product in an urban coastal environment. Int. J. Remote Sens. 2014, 35, 6271–6291.

69. Mahiny, A.S.; Turner, B.J. A comparison of four common atmospheric correction methods. Photogramm. Eng. Remote Sens. 2007, 73, 361–368.

70. Hamdan, O.; Hasmadi, I.M.; Aziz, H.K. Combination of SPOT-5 and ALOS PALSAR images in estimating aboveground biomass of lowland Dipterocarp forest. In

Proceedings of the IOP Conference Series: Earth and Environmental Science, Tomst, Russia, 7–11 April 2014.

71. Nguyen, H.C.; Jung, J.; Lee, J.; Choi, S.U.; Hong, S.Y.; Heo, J. Optimal atmospheric correction for above-ground forest biomass estimation with the ETM+ remote sensor. Sensors 2015, 15, 18865–18886.

72. Bilgili, A.V.; Van Es, H.M.; Akbas, F.; Durak, A.; Hively, W.D. Visible-near infrared, reflectance spectroscopy for assessment of soil properties in a semi-arid area of Turkey. J. Arid Environ. 2010, 74, 229–238.

73. Ghasemi, J.B.; Zolfonoun, E. Application of principal component analysis-multivariate adaptive regression splines for the simultaneous spectrofluorimetric determination of dialkyltins in micellar media. Spectrochim. Spectrochimi. Acta Part A Mol. Biomol. Spectrosc. 2013, 115, 357–363.

74. García, M.A.; Pérez, C.F.; De la Riva, J.; Fernández, J.; Pascual, P.E.; Herranz, A. Estimación de la biomasa residual forestal mediante técnicas de teledetección y SIG en masas puras de Pinus halepensis y P. sylvestris. In Proceedings of the IV Congreso Forestal Español, Zaragoza, Spain, 26–30 September 2005.

75. López-Serrano, P.M.; López-Sánchez, C.A.; Díaz-Varela, R.A.; Corral-Rivas, J.J.; Solís-Moreno, R.; Vargas-Larreta, B.; Álvarez-González, J.G. Estimating biomass of mixed and uneven-aged forests using spectral data and a hybrid model combining regression trees and linear models. iForest 2015.

76. Lam, C.S.Y. Comparison of Flow Routing Algorithms Used in Geographic Information Systems. Ph.D. Thesis, University of Southern California, Los Angeles, CA, USA, 2004.

77. Hoechstetter, S.; Walz, U.; Dang, L.H.; Thinh, N.X. Effects of topography and surface roughness in analyses of landscape structure–A proposal to modify the existing set of landscape metrics. Landsc. Online 2008, 3, 1–14.

78. Sesnie, S.E.; Dickson, B.D.; Rosenstock, S.S.; Rundall, J.M. A comparison of Landsat TM and MODIS vegetation indices for estimating forage phenology in desert bighorn sheep (Ovis canadensis nelsoni) habitat in the Sonoran Desert, USA. Int. J. Remote Sens. 2012, 33, 276–286.

79. Ali, M.; Montzka, C.; Stadler, A.; Menz, G.; Thonfeld, F.; Vereecken, H. Estimation and validation of rapideye-based time-series of leaf area index for winter wheat in the rur catchment (Germany). Remote Sens. 2015, 7, 2808–2831.

80. Yao, Z.; Liu, J.; Zhao, X.; Long, D.; Wang, L. Spatial dynamics of aboveground carbon stock in urban green space: A case study of Xi'an, China. J. Arid Land. 2015, 7, 350–360.

CHAPTER 18 A BAYESIAN METHOD FOR SHORT-TERM PROBABILISTIC FORECASTING OF PHOTOVOLTAIC GENERATION IN SMART GRID OPERATION AND CONTROL

Antonio Bracale, Pierluigi Caramia, Guido Carpinelli, Anna Rita Di Fazio, and Gabriella Ferruzzi

Keywords: Smart grid, photovoltaic generation, clearness index, forecasting, probability density functions, autoregressive models, Bayesian inference

INTRODUCTION

In recent years, power systems have been undergoing radical changes and in the near future their planning and operation will be undertaken according to the Smart Grid (SG) vision. The SG initiatives aim at introducing new technologies and services in power systems to make the electrical networks more reliable, efficient, secure and environmentally-friendly [1].

Increasing the exploitation of renewable energy sources (such as wind and solar energy) is certainly one of the most important goals of SGs. Indeed, the random behavior of such energy sources introduce challenging issues in the design of advanced tools and techniques for the optimal SG operation and control. In tackling these issues, forecasting is a fundamental task for an efficient utilization of the available distributed energy resources and for a secure and economic behaviour of the power system [2].

In general, the power system operator can use accurate forecast information about renewable power generation and load consumption to guarantee a balance between generation and demand at all the time with reduced capacity and costs of the operating reserves [3,4]. From the perspective of the producers, forecasting the renewable power output can be very useful for decision making on the energy market. In this way, not only the deviation between scheduled and actual generation can be minimized, but also the revenues are increased, thus reducing the penalties related to regulation costs and enhancing the competitiveness of renewable energies in comparison with dispatchable energy sources [5]. Finally, prosumers can use prediction models to plan their consumption patterns so as to match the power they generate on-site thus maximizing their benefits [6].

In the relevant literature, various forecasting methods have been proposed to estimate the expected power generated from a renewable energy source, which essentially differ in the type of the information characterizing the predicted output and in the time horizon of their application.

Concerning the type of information, two main forecasting methods can be adopted, referred to as deterministic and probabilistic forecasting. In the former one, a single value of the renewable power generation is provided and no uncertainty of the prediction is considered. In the latter one, the output value is accompanied with information on its intrinsic unpredictability and, then, it is more appropriate to solve problems of management and control in future SGs [3,5,7]. Probabilistic forecasting methods can be distinguished in two further categories according to the adopted approach: the prediction error or the direct approach. While the first one provides the uncertainty of the error deriving from the

Citation: Antonio Bracale, Pierluigi Caramia, Guido Carpinelli, Anna Rita Di Fazio, and Gabriella Ferruzzi, A Bayesian method for short-term probabilistic forecasting of photovoltaic generation in smart grid operation and control, Energies, 2013; 6, 733-747. DOI:10.3390/en6020733.

application of a deterministic forecasting method, the second one directly yields the statistic representation of the predicted output.

Concerning the time horizon, renewable generation forecasting can basically be divided into different time intervals, depending on the time frames corresponding to the tasks of grid operation and control and to the sessions of electricity markets. Short-term forecasting covers time intervals ranging from less than 1 hour to few hours ahead and is very useful for frequency regulation and load balancing. Medium term forecasting, up from several hours to few days ahead, is needed for unit commitment and energy trading. Finally, long-term forecasting can be required to support system planning and economic analyses in seasonal and annual horizons. However, recent renewable integration studies have shown that it is the short term forecasting that gains the most in a SG [3].

One of the most promising renewable energy conversion system to be integrated in SGs is the Photo Voltaic (PV) power generation, due to the expected cost reduction and the increased efficiency of both PV panels and converters [8]. The power generated by a PV power system varies according to the solar radiation on the earth's surface, which mainly depends on the installation site and the weather conditions. While the dependence on the specific location can be essentially predicted on a deterministic way, the atmospheric conditions (such as cloud cover, ambient temperature, relative humidity) are the main causes of the randomness of the solar radiation and it is very important to consider them when short-term forecasting is concerned [9,10].

Several methods have been proposed in the relevant literature for forecasting the PV power generated in a short time horizon. In [11] a recurrent neural network has been proposed to perform a short term forecasting of the PV power production using meteorological data of the last 16 days and has been compared with a feed-forward neural network. A method to predict PV power output has been presented in [12] by deriving hourly site-specific irradiance forecasts from data provided by a weather forecasts center. In [13] an advanced Grey-Markov chain model has been applied to predict the daily power production of grid-connected PV systems using operating data collected at 15 minute intervals. A two-stage method to predict hourly value of the PV power for time horizon up to 36 hours has been proposed in [14]. In [15] Kalman filters are applied to predict sub-hourly and hourly PV power production using solar irradiance as input. First studies on the application of Bayesian theory for PV power production forecasting are shown in [16,17].

In this paper, extending and improving the approach based on the Bayesian theory outlined in [16,17,18], a new method for short-term probabilistic forecasting is proposed, that directly yields to the statistic representation of the predicted PV power output. The proposed method forecasts at the generic hour h the probability density function (pdf) of the active power produced by a PV power system at the hour $h + k$ with k = 1,..., K, starting from the evaluation of samples of the pdf of the hourly clearness index at hour $h + k$. The forecast of the pdf of the hourly clearness index is obtained firstly selecting for the pdf an analytical expression and, then, evaluating the pdf parameters by applying the Bayesian Inference (BI). To this aim, an Auto Regressive (AR) time series model, representing the relationship between the pdf parameters, the clearness index and some explanatory meteorological variables, is used together with appropriate sets of historical measurements of the random variables involved in the AR model. Finally, a Monte Carlo (MC) simulation procedure is applied to generate the predicted pdf of the PV active power: a random sampling of the pdf of the hourly clearness index is performed and, using the PV system model, the PV power samples are obtained.

The key steps of the proposed method are: (i) the choice of the analytical expression of the pdf modeling the hourly clearness index; (ii) the definition of an adequate AR time series model so as to consider only the meteorological variables that most affect the hourly clearness index behaviour; and (iii) the selection of appropriate data vectors from historical measurements collected before the time of the forecast.

The peculiarity of the method is that it takes into account the dependence of the terrestrial solar radiation on some explanatory atmospheric variables and combines probabilistic techniques, such as BI and MC simulation, to provide a probabilistic forecasting of the PV power generation useful for optimal SG operation and control.

This paper is organized as follows: Section 2 briefly recalls the probabilistic forecasting method based on the Bayesian approach. In Section 3 the probabilistic method is applied to forecast the power production of a PV system. Finally, numerical simulations are reported in Section 4 to give evidence of the effectiveness of the proposed approach.

PROBABILISTIC FORECASTING METHOD BASED ON THE BAYESIAN APPROACH

The probabilistic forecasting method based on the Bayesian approach predicts at the generic hour $t = h$ the pdf of a random variable X_t at the hour $t = h + k$, with $k = 1,..., K$. For the sake of simplicity, in the following the analysis is referred to the case of $k = 1$.

In applying this method, the starting point is the knowledge of the analytical expression of the pdf $f_{X_t}(X_t)$ of the random variable to be forecasted. Usually, the analytical expression of the pdf is characterized by some distribution parameters and it is modeled as a conditional pdf. For the sake of conciseness, reference is made to only one distribution parameter (i.e., the mean value), generically referred to as ϑ_t, and the conditional pdf is indicated as $f_{X_t}(X_t|\vartheta_t)$.

Forecasting at $t = h$ the pdf $f_{X_{h+1}}\left(X_{h+1}|\vartheta_{h+1}\right)$ requires an estimation of ϑ_{h+1}. To this aim, a first order AR time series model can be used, representing the relationship between ϑ_{h+1} and both the measurements x_h and $(v_{1,h},\dots,v_{M,h})$collected at the hour h of, respectively, the random variable X_t to be forecasted and the M explanatory random variables $V_{1,t},\dots,_{VM,}t$ influencing X_t:

$$\vartheta_{h+1} = \alpha_1 x_h + \beta_1 v_{1,h} + \dots + \beta_M v_{M,h} + \alpha_0 \quad (1)$$

where α_0, α_1, β_1,... , β_M are the coefficients of the AR model. Explanatory variables are variables such that changes in their value are thought to cause changes in another variable.

In the classical statistics, α_0, α_1, β_1,... , β_M are assumed to be constant. Indeed, when Bayesian approach are adopted, such coefficients are modeled as random variables, known as prior random parameters, and the BI [19] allows to estimate the conditional pdf $p(\alpha_0, \alpha_1, \beta_1,\dots, \beta_M \mid S_{X_h})$ of the parameters $\alpha_0, \alpha_1, \beta_1,\dots, \beta_M$ given the set $S_{X_h} = (x_{s_1},\dots,x_{s_{N_h}})$ composed of N_h measurements of X_t observed before the hour h. The pdf $p(\alpha_0, \alpha_1, \beta_1,\dots, \beta_M \mid S_{X_h})$ is known as a posteriori distribution of the prior random parameters and it is very difficult to obtain its expression in closed form. Actually, only a simplified expression, known as unnormalized a posteriori distribution of the prior random parameters, and indicated as $q(\alpha_0, \alpha_1, \beta_1,\dots, \beta_M \mid S_{X_h})$, can be provided. Fortunately, the knowledge of the unnormalized a posteriori distribution of the prior random parameters is sufficient for developing algorithms that provide information about the normalised a posteriori distributions.

The unnormalized a posteriori distribution of the prior random parameters is derived from the application of the Bayes' rule assuming the independency of the prior random parameters so that:

$$q(\alpha_0,\alpha_1,\beta_1,\dots,\beta_M \mid \boldsymbol{S}_{X_h}) = p(\boldsymbol{S}_{X_h}|\alpha_0,\alpha_1,\beta_1,\dots,\beta_M)\prod_{i=0}^{1} p(\alpha_i)\prod_{j=1}^{M} p(\beta_j) \tag{2}$$

where $p(\boldsymbol{S}_{X_h}|\alpha_0,\alpha_1,\beta_1,\dots,\beta_M)$ is the likelihood function; and $p(\alpha_i)$ and $p(\beta_j)$ are the a priori distributions of the prior random parameters.

The a priori distributions are the initial pdfs of the prior random parameters which are not conditional on observed data. Their expressions can be vague or informative and reflects the knowledge that we have in advance about the pdfs that we are interested in.

The likelihood function is the conditional data distribution that is the pdf modeling X_t, whose realizations are contained in S_{X_h}, given the prior random parameters. Its expression can be derived making use of the $f_{X_t}(X_t|\vartheta_t)$ for the set S_{X_h} and assuming that $x_{s_1},\dots,x_{s_{N_h}}$ are independent realizations of X_t. Substituting for ϑ_t the AR time series model and using the vectors $\boldsymbol{S}_{V_{1,h}} = (v_{1,s_1},\dots,v_{1,s_{N_h}}),\ \dots\ ,\boldsymbol{S}_{V_{M,h}} = (v_{M,s_1},\dots,v_{M,s_{N_h}})$ of the N_h measurements of the explanatory variables $V_{1,t},\dots,V_{M,t}$ corresponding to S_{X_h}, it obtains:

$$p(\boldsymbol{S}_{X_h}|\alpha_0,\alpha_1,\beta_1,\dots,\beta_M) = \prod_{i=2}^{N_h} f_{X_t}(x_{s_i}|\vartheta_{s_i} = \alpha_1 x_{s_i-1} + \beta_1 v_{1,s_i-1} + \dots + \beta_M v_{M,s_i-1} + \alpha_0) \tag{3}$$

Once the unnormalized a posteriori distribution of the prior random parameters is known, it is trivial to evaluate the normalised a posteriori distributions of each parameter by applying the theory of the joint pdfs [20]. Then, the Monte Carlo Markov Chain (MCMC) simulation method based on the Metropolitan-Hasting algorithm [21] can be directly applied to the unnormalized distributions of every parameter to obtain samples of their a posteriori distributions. In the MCMC approach, a Markov chain is constructed, characterized by a transition probability matrix reflecting the a posteriori distributions of the prior random parameters. Then, the Markov chain is simulated until the samples are representative of the a posteriori distributions of every parameter.

Eventually, incorporating the AR time series model in this procedure, the samples derived from the a posteriori pdfs of $\alpha_0, \alpha_1, \beta_1,\dots, \beta_M$ can be used together with the measurements X_h and $v_{1,h},\dots,v_{M,h}$ collected at the hour h to obtain samples of ϑ_{h+1}. Finally, for each simulated sample of ϑ_{h+1}, the samples of the random variable X_t are drawn from the analytical expression of the pdf so as to provide the full predictive distribution

$$f_{X_{h\,h+1}}(X_{h+1}|\vartheta_{h+1}).$$

PROBABILISTIC FORECASTING OF THE PHOTOVOLTAIC GENERATION

In the following, the probabilistic forecasting method described in Section 2 is applied to predict at hour h the pdf of the PV power production at hour $h + 1$, starting from an estimation of the terrestrial hourly solar radiation, expressed in terms of the pdf of the hourly clearness index at hour $h + 1$. The next four subsections dealt with:

- The description of the adopted model for the PV system;
- The description of the pdf modeling the hourly clearness index;
- The definition of the AR time-series model including meteorological variables; and
- The probabilistic characterization of the prior random parameters.

PV System Model

The hourly active power produced by a PV system depends on the availability of the solar radiation at the installation site. The solar radiation in a given locality cannot be exactly predicted owing mainly to the irregular presence of clouds. The sky conditions are often taken into account by representing the terrestrial solar radiation in terms of clearness index that is defined as the ratio of the surface radiation to the extraterrestrial radiation for a given period [22].

When the PV system is equipped with a maximum power point tracker, an analytical relationship exists between the PV active power P_{PV_t} at the hour t and the corresponding hourly clearness index K_t, [22,23,24] that is defined as the ratio of the hourly total solar radiation on an horizontal plane I_t to the extra-terrestrial hourly total solar radiation I_0; it results:

$$P_{PV_t} = S_C \eta\,(TK_t - T'K_t^2) \tag{4}$$

where S_C is the array surface area; η is the efficiency of the PV system; and T and T′ are defined as:

$$T = \left[\left(R_b + \rho\frac{1-\cos\gamma}{2}\right) + \left(\frac{1+\cos\gamma}{2} - R_b\right)p\right] r_d \frac{H_0}{3600} \quad (5)$$

$$T' = \left(\frac{1+\cos\gamma}{2} - R_b\right) q r_d \frac{H_0}{3600} \quad (6)$$

where R_b is the ratio of beam radiation on a tilted surface to that on a horizontal surface at any time; ρ is the reflectance of the ground; γ is the inclination of the array surface to the horizontal plane; r_d is the ratio between diffuse radiation in hours and diffuse radiation in a day; H_o is the extra-terrestrial total solar radiation; and p, q are coefficients reported in [23], which link the diffuse fraction of the hourly total solar radiation on horizontal plane with the hourly clearness index.

The analysis of the relationship (4) clearly reveals that K_t is the only variable affecting P_{PV_t}, once the hour of the day, the installation site and the technical characteristics of the PV system are assigned. The hourly clearness index K_t is a random variable modelling the uncertain behaviour of the terrestrial solar radiation. The hourly PV active power P_{PV_t}, as function of K_t, is itself a random variable and its pdf can be determined by the pdf of the hourly clearness index.

In this paper, a MC simulation procedure is used to generate at the hour $t = h$ samples of the predictive pdf of the hourly PV active power $f_{P_{PV_{h+1}}}(P_{PV_{h+1}})$ by performing a random sampling of the pdf of the hourly clearness index $f_{K_{h+1}}(K_{h+1})$ estimated for the hour $t = h + 1$ and applying Equation (4).

Probability Density Function of the Hourly Clearness Index

The analytical expression of the pdf of the hourly clearness index can be experimentally obtained by a statistical analysis of historical solar measurements collected in the site in which the PV system is installed. In the literature, starting from the fitting of the hourly clearness index data collected in a specific location, the investigation has often resulted in the individuation of pdfs characterized by standard distributions. In [25] the hourly clearness index measurements recorded at various locations in Algeria are conveniently described by Beta distributions. In [26] bimodal distributions are considered more adequate to model clear and cloudy sky conditions of hourly clearness index measurements collected in different cities in the U.S.A. On the other hand, several attempts have been made to find universal standard pdfs that are independent of the location and the time period used to define the clearness index [27,28,29]. Following the latter approach, in this paper the model proposed in [29] has been adopted and the following modified Gamma distribution $f_{K_t}(K_t|C_t, \lambda_t)$ is used to model the pdf of the hourly clearness index K_t:

$$f_{K_t}(K_t|C_t, \lambda_t) = C_t \frac{\bar{k}_u - K_t}{\bar{k}_u} e^{\lambda_t K_t} \quad (7)$$

where $\bar{k}_u$ is the upper bound of the observed values of K_t; and Ct and λ_t are the distribution parameters, defined as:

$$C_t = \frac{\lambda_t^2 \bar{k}_u}{\left(e^{\lambda_t \bar{k}_u} - 1 - \lambda_t \bar{k}_u\right)} \quad (8)$$

$$\lambda_t = \frac{\left(2F_t - 17.519e^{-1.3118F_t} - 1062e^{-5.0426F_t}\right)}{\bar{k}_u} \quad (9)$$

with:

$$F_t = \frac{\bar{k}_u}{\bar{k}_u - \mu_{K_t}} \quad (10)$$

where μ_{K_t} is the mean value of the hourly clearness index K_t at hour t. Assuming the knowledge of $\bar{k}_u$, the distribution parameters C_t and λ_t only depend on the mean value μ_{K_t} and the pdf in Equation (7) can be rewritten as:

$$f_{K_t}\left(K_t \middle| \mu_{K_t}\right) = C_t(\mu_{K_t}) \frac{\bar{k}_u - K_t}{\bar{k}_u} e^{\lambda_t(\mu_{K_t})K_t} \quad (11)$$

AR Time-Series Model

To predict at the hour $t = h$ the pdf $f_{K_{h+1}}\left(K_{h+1}|\mu_{K_{h+1}}\right)$ at the hour $t = h + 1$ an estimation of the mean value $\mu_{K_{h+1}}$ is required, as shown in the Subsection 3.2. To this aim, an AR time series model can be used to define the relationship among such mean value and the measurements of the clearness index and of some meteorological variables influencing the solar radiation, such as the ambient temperature AT, the relative humidity RH, the wind speed WS and the cloud cover CC, where the cloud cover is defined as the ratio in % of the sky hidden by all visible cloud. In this paper, the following first order AR time series model is adopted:

$$\mu_{K_{h+1}} = \alpha_1 k_h + \beta_1 at_h + \beta_2 rh_h + \beta_3 ws_h + \beta_4 cc_h + \alpha_0 \quad (12)$$

where k_h, at_h, rh_h, ws_h, cc_h are the measurements of, respectively, the clearness index, the ambient temperature, the relative humidity, the wind speed and the cloud cover, which are collected at the hour $t = h$.

The inclusion of meteorological variables in the AR model significantly increases the computational efforts in the application of the proposed forecasting method. Despite of the highest complexity of the procedure, taking into account the dependence of the clearness index on the meteorological variables allows to perform a more accurate forecasting [10,30]. To reduce computational efforts, a correlation analysis can help to individuate the meteorological variables presenting the highest influence on the solar radiation. Such analysis is performed "off-line" and correlates historical measurements collected in the specific site in which the PV system is installed. In this way, only the meteorological variables presenting the highest correlation value with the clearness index are selected so as to found a good compromise between results' accuracy and computational efforts.

Probabilistic Characterization of the Prior Random Parameters

In this paper, the coefficients α_0, α_1, β_1, β_2, β_3, β_4 of the AR time series model in Equation (12) are assumed to be the prior random parameters of the BI. The a priori pdfs of the prior random parameters $p(\alpha_0)$, $p(\alpha_1)$, $p(\beta_1)$, $p(\beta_2)$, $p(\beta_3)$, $p(\beta_4)$ are usually chosen with a large variance so that the data, rather than the a priori distributions, determine the relevant parameters values in the a posteriori distributions [19,20,21]. In this paper the a priori pdfs are assumed to be Gaussian with a mean value $\mu = 0.5$ and a standard deviation $\sigma = 0.5$ so as:

$$p(\alpha_i) = \frac{1}{\sigma\sqrt{2\pi}} e^{\frac{(\mu-\alpha_i)^2}{2\sigma^2}} = \frac{1}{0.5\sqrt{2\pi}} e^{\frac{-\alpha_i^2}{2(0.5)^2}} \quad i = 0,1 \tag{13}$$

$$p(\beta_j) = \frac{1}{\sigma\sqrt{2\pi}} e^{\frac{(\mu-\beta_j)^2}{2\sigma^2}} = \frac{1}{0.5\sqrt{2\pi}} e^{\frac{-\beta_j^2}{2(0.5)^2}} \quad j = 1,\dots,4 \tag{14}$$

The likelihood function $p(\boldsymbol{S_{K_h}}|\alpha_0,\alpha_1,\beta_1,\beta_2,\beta_3,\beta_4)$ is the pdf in Equation (11) specified for the set $\boldsymbol{S_{K_h}} = (k_{s_1},\dots,k_{s_ih},\dots,k_{s_{N_h}})$ of N_h measurements of k_t observed before the hour h:

$$p(\boldsymbol{S_{K_h}}|\alpha_0,\alpha_1,\beta_1,\beta_2,\beta_3,\beta_4) = \prod_{i=2}^{N_h} f_{K_t}(k_{s_i}|\mu_{K_{si}}) = \prod_{i=2}^{N_h} C(\mu_{K_{s_i}}) \frac{\bar{k}_u - k_{s_i}}{\bar{k}_u} e^{\lambda(\mu_{K_{s_i}})k_{s_i}} \tag{15}$$

where:

$$\mu_{K_{s_i}} = \alpha_1 k_{s_{i-1}} + \beta_1 at_{s_{i-1}} + \beta_2 rh_{s_{i-1}} + \beta_3 ws_{s_{i-1}} + \beta_4 cc_{s_{i-1}} + \alpha_0 \tag{16}$$

Relationship (15) is obtained by substituting for $\mu_{K_{s_i}}$ the AR time series model in Equation (16). The generic measurements $k_{s_{i-1}}, at_{s_{i-1}}, rh_{s_{i-1}}, ws_{s_{i-1}}, cc_{s_{i-1}}$ are contained in the sets , $\boldsymbol{S_{K_h}} = (k_{s_1},\dots,k_{s_i},\dots,k_{s_{N_h}})$, $\boldsymbol{S_{AT_h}} = (at_{s_1},\dots,at_{s_i},\dots,at_{s_{N_h}})$, $\boldsymbol{S_{RH_h}} = (rh_{s_1},\dots,rh_{s_i},\dots,rh_{s_{N_h}})$, $\boldsymbol{S_{WS_h}} = (ws_{s_1},\dots,ws_{s_i},\dots,ws_{s_{N_h}})$, $\boldsymbol{S_{CC_h}} = (cc_{s_1},\dots,cc_{s_i},\dots,cc_{s_{N_h}})$, including N_h measurements collected before the hour h of, respectively, the clearness index and the meteorological variables.

According to Equation (2), the a posteriori unnormalized distribution $q(\alpha_0,\alpha_1,\beta_1,\beta_2,\beta_3,\beta_4,\boldsymbol{S_{K_h}})$ of the prior random parameters is equal to

$$q(\alpha_0,\alpha_1,\beta_1,\beta_2,\beta_3,\beta_4,\boldsymbol{S_{K_h}}) = \left[\prod_{i=2}^{N_h} C(\mu_{K_{s_i}}) \frac{\bar{k}_u - k_{s_i}}{\bar{k}_u} e^{\lambda(\mu_{K_{s_i}})k_{s_i}}\right] \prod_{i=0}^{1} \frac{1}{0.5\sqrt{2\pi}} e^{\frac{-\alpha_i^2}{2(0.5)^2}} \prod_{j=0}^{4} \frac{1}{0.5\sqrt{2\pi}} e^{\frac{-\beta_j^2}{2(0.5)^2}} \tag{17}$$

and the samples of the individual a posteriori distributions are evaluated by applying the MCMC simulation method based on the Metropolitan-Hasting algorithm. The samples of the a posteriori pdfs of $\alpha_0,\alpha_1,\beta_1,\beta_2,\beta_3,\beta_4$ are used in Equation (12) together with the measurements k_h, t_h, r_h, w_h, cc_h collected at the hour h to provide samples of the mean value $\mu_{K_{h+1}}$. Finally, for each samples of $\mu_{K_{h+1}}$, the samples of the hourly clearness index X_{h+1} are drawn from the analytical expression of the pdf in Equation (11). The simulated samples of X_{h+1} describes the predictive distribution $f_{K_{h+1}}(K_{h+1}|\mu_{K_{h+1}})$.

It should be noted that the choice of the measurements contained in the sets $\boldsymbol{S_{K_h}}, \boldsymbol{S_{AT_h}}, \boldsymbol{S_{RH_h}}, \boldsymbol{S_{WS_h}}, \boldsymbol{S_{CC_h}}$ represent a key issue in the BI, since they are used to make inference about the prior random parameters $\alpha_0,\alpha_1,\beta_1,\beta_2,\beta_3,\beta_4$. In general, these sets contain N_h measurements recorded before the hour h of the forecast. Actually, these data are not necessarily the ones collected from the hour $h-1$ to $h-N_h-1$, but can be selected with adequate criteria thus improving the accuracy of the proposed forecasting method. In [16] the homologue and the coded group criteria have been proposed. In the first one, the sets contain measurements at the hour h which are collected N_h days before the forecast (e.g., if the forecast has to be performed at h = 10:00, the sets include measurements recorded N_h days before at 10:00). In the second one, the sets contain a coded group of measurements around the hour h collected some days before the forecast (e.g. if the forecast has to be performed at h = 10:00, the sets include measurements from the 8:00 to 10:00 recorded N_h /3 days before). In addition, the measurements contained in $\boldsymbol{S_{K_h}}, \boldsymbol{S_{AT_h}}, \boldsymbol{S_{RH_h}}, \boldsymbol{S_{WS_h}}, \boldsymbol{S_{CC_h}}$ can be collected at time intervals different from an hour. In [17] the data of the clearness index and of the meteorological variables contained in the vectors are extracted from measurements registered at time intervals of 15 minutes. If this is the case, the application of the proposed forecasting method will provide at the hour h the predictive distribution of the clearness index at the first 15 minutes of the hour $h+1$. To estimate the pdf at the hour $h+1$ the following approach is adopted in this paper:

$$f_{K_{h+1}}\left(K_{h+1}\middle|\mu_{K_{h+1}}\right) = f_{K_{h+15'}}(K_{h+15'}\,|\mu_{K_{h+15'}}) \tag{18}$$

that is the pdf forecasted at $h + 1$ is assumed to be equal to the pdf forecasted at the first 15 minutes of the hour $h + 1$. Eventually, Figure 1 shows a block diagram describing the main steps applied in the proposed Bayesian approach.

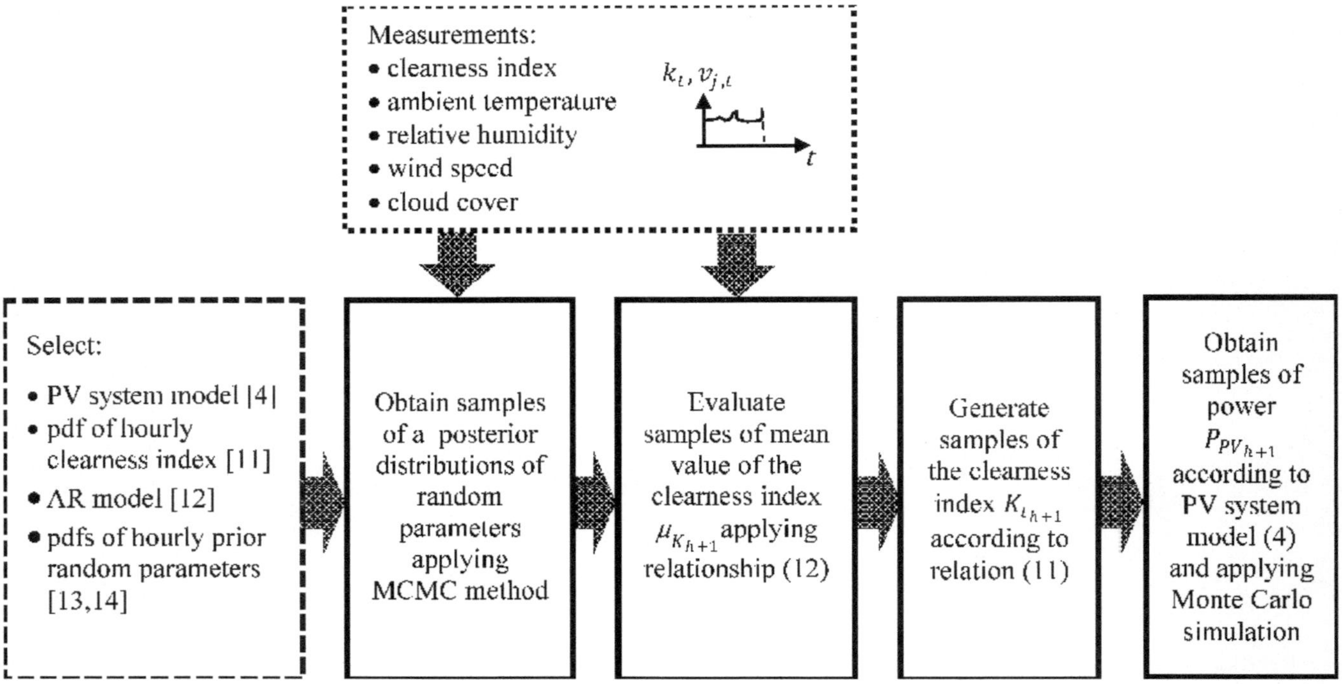

Figure 1. Block diagram describing the main steps applied in the proposed Bayesian approach.

EXPERIMENTAL SECTION

In this section, the proposed Bayesian forecasting method is applied to a 75-kWp PV system, presenting an array surface S_c = 600 m^2 and an efficiency η = 0.09. Measurements of the clearness index and of the meteorological variables cited in the Subsection 3.4 (air temperature, relative humidity, wind speed and total cloud cover) are available at the website of the National Renewable Energy Laboratory. In particular, a meteorological station in Colorado (39.742° N, 105.18° W) has been selected and measurements referred to the time interval [8 a.m., 8 p.m.] and collected every 15 minutes are chosen.

In the following, at first a correlation analysis is performed to individuate the meteorological variables to be included in the time series AR model; then, the proposed method is used to forecast the pdf of the hourly active power produced by the PV system.

To individuate the most suitable AR time series model, an "off-line" correlation analysis between the clearness index and the meteorological variables is carried out, on the basis of measurements recorded from January to December 2010. Figure 2reports the time evolution of the correlation coefficient between the clearness index and the meteorological variables. To avoid excessive computational efforts, only the meteorological variables furnishing the highest values of the correlation coefficient are taken into account. As such, the analysis of the Figure 2 clearly reveals that the total cloud cover and the relative humidity are the meteorological variables presenting the highest influence on the clearness index; consequently, the AR time-series model in Equation (12) reduces to:

$$\mu_{K_{h+1}} = \alpha_1 k_h + \beta_1 rh_h + \beta_2 cc_h + \alpha_0 \tag{19}$$

To make inference about the prior random parameters α_0,α_1, β_1 and β_2, the sets S_{K_h}, S_{CC_h}, S_{RH_h} (see Subsection 3.4) contain N_h = 144 measurements collected at time intervals of 15 minutes recorded before the hour h of the forecast.

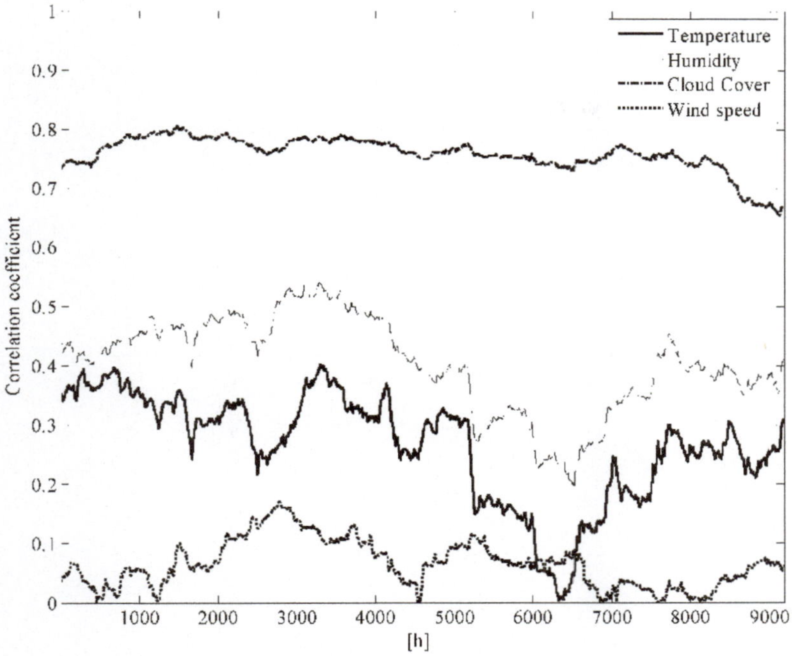

Figure 2. Time evolution of the correlation coefficient between the clearness index and the selected meteorological variables.

The application of the proposed approach to forecast the hourly PV active power is performed referring to the four seasons of the 2011. Figure 3, Figure 4, Figure 5 and Figure 6 show, respectively, the actual measured values of the PV active powers (red lines), the mean value (blue line) and the range between the 5th and 95th percentile values of the forecasted pdfs of hourly PV active power. In particular, the results refer to the Recommended Average days of winter (Figure 3), spring (Figure 4), summer (Figure 5) and autumn (Figure 6). In [22] Recommended Average Days are days which have the extraterrestrial radiation closest to the average value in the month. A similar behavior characterizes the vast majority of the considered days (in almost all considered days).

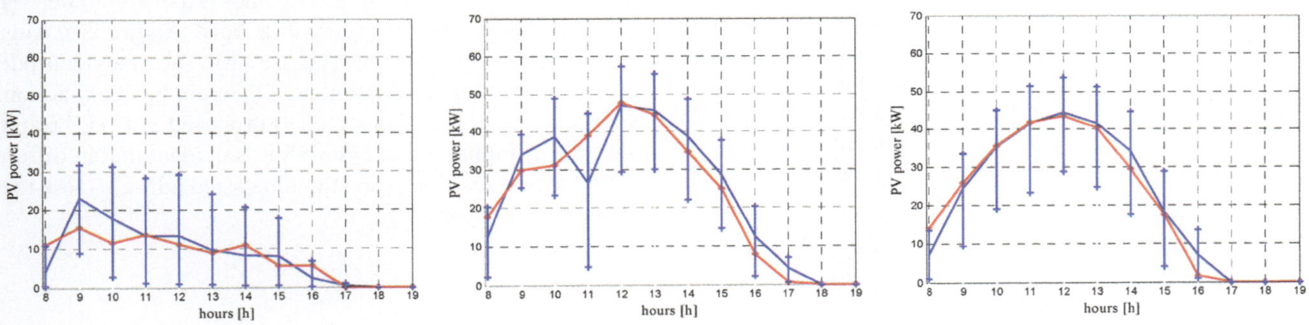

(a) (b) (c)

Figure 3. Actual measures of the hourly PV active power (red line); mean values (blue line) and range between 5th and 95th percentile values of the forecasted pdfs of the hourly PV active power. (a) 17 January; (b) 16 February; and (c) 10 December.

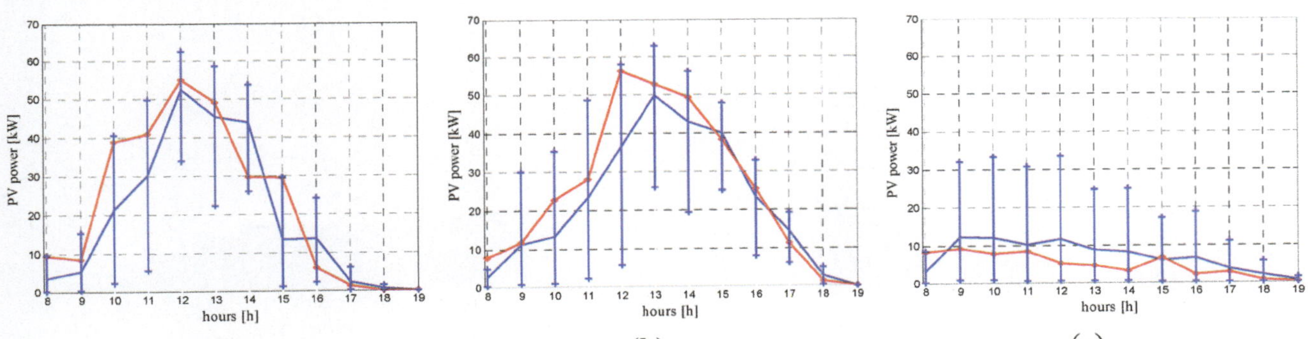

(a) (b) (c)

Figure 4. Actual measures of the hourly PV active power (red line); mean values (blue line) and range between 5th and 95th percentile values of the forecasted pdfs of the hourly PV active power. (a) 16 March; (b) 15 April; and (c) 15 May.

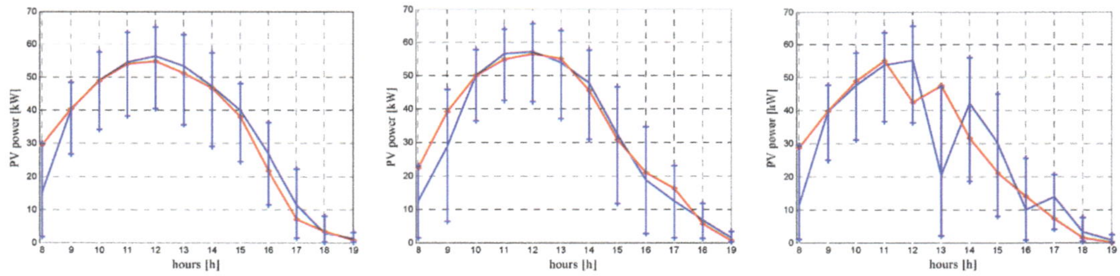

(a) (b) (c)

Figure 5. Actual measures of the hourly PV active power (red line); mean values (blue line) and range between 5th and 95th percentile values of the forecasted pdfs of the hourly PV active power. (a) 11 June; (b) 17 July and; (c) 16 August.

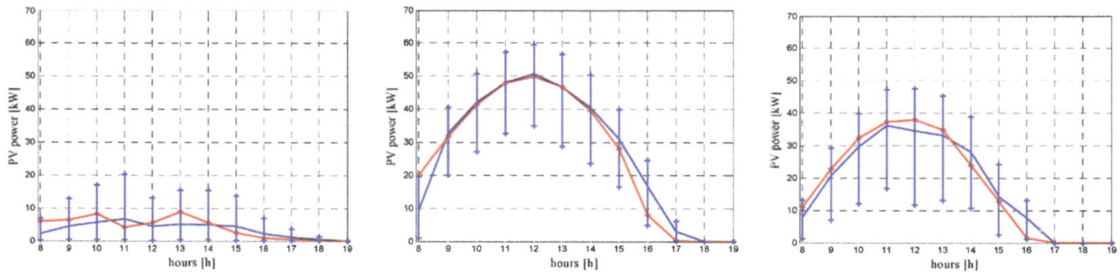

(a) (b) (c)

Figure 6. Actual measures of the hourly PV active power (red line); mean values (blue line) and range between 5th and 95th percentile values of the forecasted pdfs of the hourly PV active power. (a) 15 September; (b) 15 October and; (c) 14 November.

From the analysis of the figures, it appears that the actual values of the hourly PV active power are always comprised between the 5th and 95th percentile values. In addition, it should be noted that the mean value appears in most cases a good estimator for the forecasted pdfs, particularly in the range of hours between 11 a.m. and 3 p.m. At the beginning (end) of the period characterized by the presence of solar radiation, usually higher (lower) percentiles appear the most adequate estimators. Anyway, if the mean value of forecasted pdf would be used as the only estimator of the forecasted PV power, the Mean Absolute Relative Error (MARE), defined as:

$$MARE = \frac{1}{N}\sum_{h=1}^{N} \frac{\left|P_{PV_h} - P^*_{PV_h}\right|}{P_{PV_h}} \quad (20)$$

is estimated between 14.5% (winter season) and 18.0% (autumn season).

Finally, Figure 7 and Figure 8 show the forecasted (represented by a blue histogram) and the analytical (represented by a continuous red line) pdfs of the hourly PV active power in March (Figure 7a), April (Figure 7b), August (Figure 8a) and September (Figure 8b). The analytical pdf is obtained applying the fundamental theorem for the function of a random variable to Equation (9) proposed in [31]. From the analysis of Figure 7 and Figure 8 it is evident that in different conditions of solar radiation the forecasted pdfs are close to the analytical distributions.

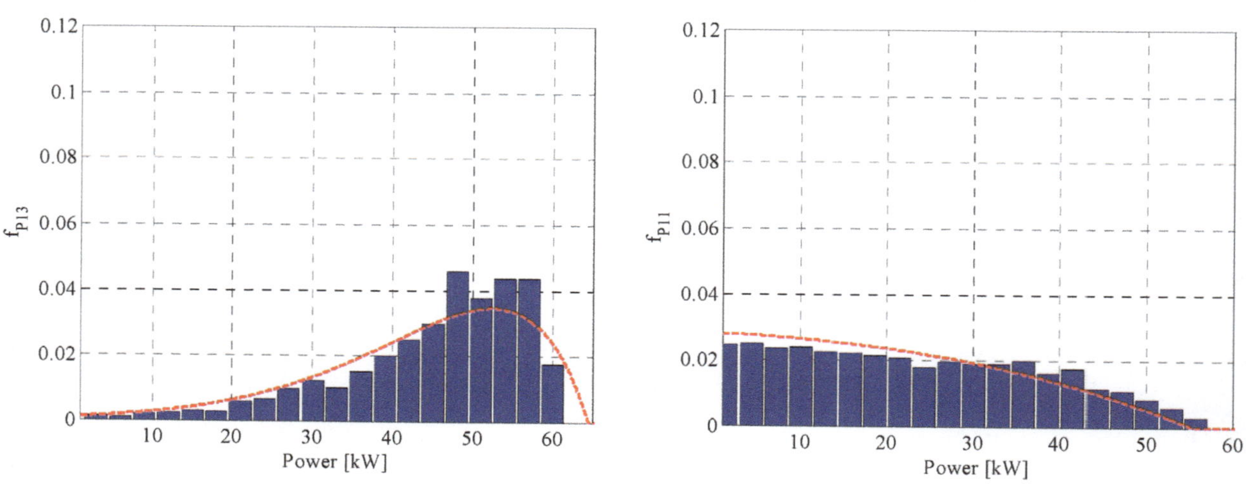

(a) (b)

Figure 7. Forecasted (histogram) and analytical (red line) pdfs of PV power. (a) h = 1 p.m. of 16 March; and (b) h = 11 a.m. of 15 April.

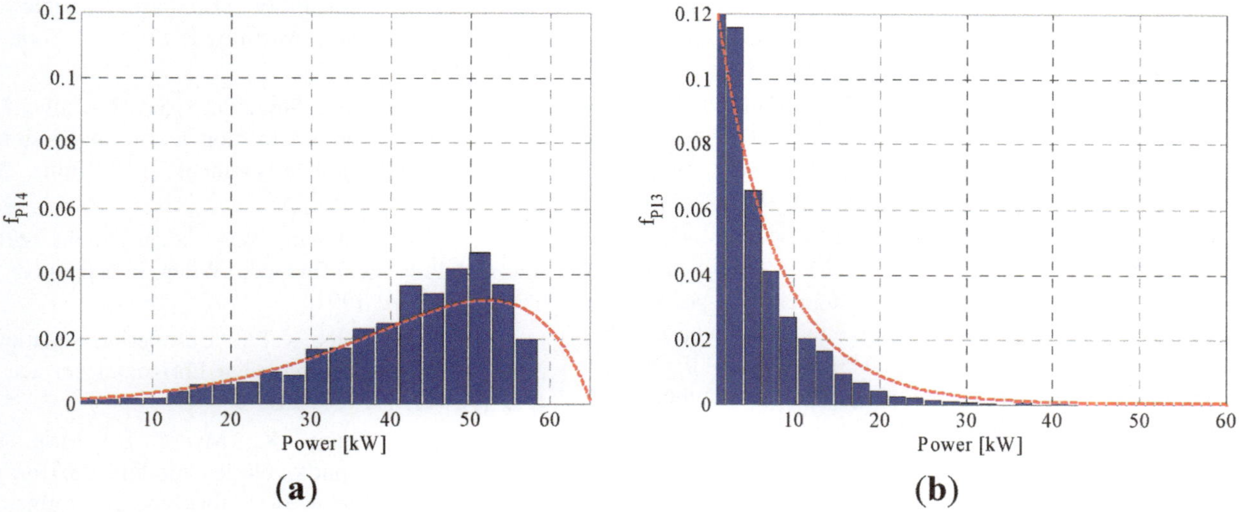

Figure 8. Forecasted (histogram) and analytical (red line) pdfs of PV power. (a) h = 2 p.m. of 16 August and; (b) h = 1 p.m. of 15 September.

CONCLUSIONS

A new method based on the Bayesian inference has been proposed to perform a short-term forecasting of the active power produced by a photovoltaic system starting from an estimation of the hourly clearness index. It takes into account the dependence of the terrestrial solar radiation on some explanatory atmospheric variables, including the cloud cover and humidity. The combination of probabilistic techniques, such as Bayesian inference and Monte Carlo simulation, allows to provide the predictive probability density function of the photovoltaic generated power, which is very useful for the optimal operation and control of the smart grids of the future.

However, if only a value is requested as estimator of the forecasted photovoltaic power, arises the problem of individuate which pdf parameter (mean value, percentiles ...) is the most representative for the distribution. Moreover, the non-linear relationship between the clearness index and the photovoltaic power output can reflect in not negligible errors in the forecasted distributions of the photovoltaic power. Then, future works will investigate the direct application of the proposed probabilistic forecasting method to the active power produced by the PV system, even if the application of the Bayesian inference in this case seems to be arduous. The research will also focus on the choice of the best parameter to be extracted from the predicted probability distribution so as to test the performance of the proposed method in terms of traditional measures of the forecasting accuracy; in this case comparison with ARIMA and neural networks methods will be affected.

ACKNOWLEDGEMENTS

This paper has been developed in the context of the Italian project PON Research and Competitiveness 2007–2013, Action II-PON 01_02864 "FC SMART GEN"—Fuel cell and smart hybrid generation from fossil and renewable sources.

REFERENCES

1. Bouhafs, F.; Mackay, M.; Merabti, M. Links to the future: Communication requirements and challenges in the smart grid. IEEE Power Energy Mag. 2012, 10, 24–28.
2. Pilo, F.; Pisano, G.; Soma, G.G. Optimal coordination of Energy resources with a two-stage online active management.IEEE Trans. Ind. Electron. 2011, 58, 4526–4537.
3. Potter, C.M.; Archambault, A.; Kenneth, W. Building a smarter smart grid to better renewable energy information. In Proceedings of Power Systems Conference and Exposition (PSCE 09), Seattle, WA, USA, 15–18 March 2009.
4. Smith, J.C.; Milligan, M.R.; De Meo, E.A.; Parson, B. Utility wind integration and operating impact state of art. IEEE Trans. Power Syst. 2007, 22, 900–907.
5. Pinson, P.; Chevallier, C.; Kariniotakis, G.N. Trading wind generation from short-term probabilistic forecasts of wind power. IEEE Trans. Power Syst. 2007, 22, 1148–1156.
6. Sharma, N.; Sharma, P.; Irwin, D.; Shenoy, P. Predicting solar generation from weather forecast using machine learning. In Proceedings of IEEE International Conference on Smart Grid Communications (SmartGridComm), Bruxelles, Belgium, 17–20 October 2011; pp. 528–533.
7. Watson, R. IEA Expert Meeting on Wind Forecasting Techniques; NREL Report. NREL (National Renewable Energy Laboratory): Golden, CO, USA, 2000.
8. Liserre, M.; Sauter, T.; Hung, J.Y. Future energy systems: Integrating renewable energy sources into the smart power grid through industrial electronics. IEEE Ind. Electron. Mag. 2010, 4, 18–37.
9. Mellit, A; Massi Pavan, A. A 24-h forecast of solar irradiance using artificial neural network: Application for performance prediction of a grid-connected PV plant at Trieste, Italy. Sol.Energy 2010, 84, 807–821.
10. Al Riza, D.F; Gilani, S.I.; Aris, M.S. Hourly solar radiation estimation using ambient temperature and relative humidity data. Int. J. Environ. Sci. Dev. 2011, 2, 188–193.

11. Yona, A.; Senjyu, T.; Funabashi, T. Application of recurrent neural network to short-term-ahead generating power forecasting for photovoltaic system. In Proceedings of IEEE Power Engineering Society General Meeting, Tampa, FL, USA, 24–28 June 2007.
12. Lorenz, E.; Hurka, J.; Heinemann, D.; Beyer, H.G. Irradiance forecasting for the power prediction of grid-connected photovoltaic systems. IEEE J. Sel. Top. Appl. Earth Obs. Remote Sens. 2009, 2, 2–10.
13. Li, Y.; He, L.; Nie, R. Short-term forecast of power generation for grid-connected photovoltaic system based on advanced Grey-Markov chain. In Proceedings of IEEE International Conference on Energy and Environment Technology (ICEET '09), Guilin, China, 16–18 October 2009; Volume 2, pp. 275–278.
14. Bacher, P.; Madsen, H.; Nielsen, P. Online short-term solar power forecasting. Sol. Energy 2009, 83, 1772–1783.
15. Hassanzadeh, M.; Etezadi-Amoli, M.; Fadali, M.S. Practical approach for sub-hourly and hourly prediction of PV power output. In Proceedings of IEEE Conferences North American Power Symposium, Arlington, TX, USA, 1–5 September 2010.
16. Bracale, A.; Caramia, P.; Fantauzzi, M.; Di Fazio, A.R. A Bayesian-based approach for photovoltaic power forecast. In Proceedings of Cigrè International Symposium on Smart Grid, Bologna, Italy, 13–15 September 2011.
17. Bracale, A.; Caramia, P.; De Martinis, U.; Di Fazio, A.R. An improved Bayesian-based approach for short term photovoltaic power forecasting in smart grids. In Proceedings of International Conference on Renewable Energies and Power Quality (ICREPQ 2012), Santiago De Compostela, Spain, 28–30 March 2012.
18. Bracale, A.; Caramia, P.; Carpinelli, G.; Di Fazio, A.R.; Varilone, P. A Bayesian-based approach for very short-term steady-state analysis of a smart grid. IEEE Trans. Smart Grids 2013. in press.
19. Gelman, A.; Carlin, J.B.; Stern, H.S.; Rubin, D.B. Bayesian Data Analysis; Chaoman & Hall: London, UK, 1995.
20. Papoulis, A. Probability, Random Variables and Stochastic Processes; McGraw-Hill: New York, NY, USA, 1991.
21. Zhang, J.; Pu, J.; McCalley, J.D.; Stern, H.; Gallus, W.A., Jr. A Bayesian approach to short term transmission line thermal overload risk assessment. IEEE Trans. Power Deliv. 2002, 17, 770–778.
22. Duffie, J.A.; Beckman, W.A. Solar Engineering of Thermal Processes, 2nd ed.; Wiley Interscience: New York, NY, USA, 1991.
23. Orgill, J.F; Hollands, K.T.G. Correlation equation for hourly diffuse radiation on a horizontal surface. Sol. Energy 1977, 19, 357–359.
24. Kroposki, B.; Emery, K.; Myers, D.; Mrig, L. A comparison of photovoltaic module performance evaluation methodologies for energy ratings. In Proceedings of First World Conference on Photovoltaic Energy Conversion (WPEC 1994), Hawaii, HI, USA, 5–9 December1994; pp. 858–862.
25. Ettoumi, F.Y.; Mefti, A.; Adane, A.; Bouroubi, M.Y. Statistical analysis of solar measurements in Algeria using beta distributions. Renew. Energy 2002, 124, 28–33.
26. Ibanez, M.; Beckman, W.A.; Sanford, A.K. Frequency distributions for hourly and daily clearness indices. J. Sol. Energy Eng. 2002, 26, 47–67.
27. Liu, B.Y.H.; Jordan, B.C. The interrelationship and characteristic distribution of direct, diffuse and total solar radiation. Sol. Energy 1960, 4, 1–19.
28. Bendt, P.; Collares-Pereira, M.; Rabl, A. The frequency distribution of daily insolation values. Sol. Energy 1981, 27, 1–19.
29. Hollands, K.T.G.; Huget, R.G. A probability density function for clearness index, with applications. Sol. Energy 1983, 30, 195–209.
30. Huang, Y.; Lu, J.; Liu, C.; Xu, X.; Wang, W.; Zhou, X. Comparative study of power forecasting methods for PV stations. In Proceedings of International Conference on Power System Technology (POWERCON 2010), Hangzhou, China, 24–28 October 2010; pp. 1–6.
31. Conti, S.; Raiti, S. Probabilistic load flow using Monte Carlo techniques for distribution networks with photovoltaic generators. Sol. Energy 2007, 81, 1473–1481.

INDEX

A

aboveground forest biomass (AGB) 227, 230
active infrared thermography (AIT) 153
adaptive radiation therapy (ART) 127, 137
analogue-to-digital converter (ADC) 26
Auto Regressive (AR) 242

B

Bayesian approach 242, 246, 250
Biological Concentration Factor (BCF) 35, 53
Biological Intake Value 35, 53
biophysics 165, 175, 176
Borehole measurements 72

C

cardiovascular disease (CVD) 112
Cell images 140
cholecystokinin 2 181
climate change 209
Concentration Factor (CF) 35, 53
Concentration ratios 35, 48, 53, 66
confidence intervals (CI) 111
Coupled Model Intercomparison Project phase 209

D

daylighting 219
Derived Consideration Reference Levels (DCRL) 93
digital elevation model (DEM) 228
double-strand breaks (DSB) 139

E

Eastern Cooperative Oncology Group (ECOG) 196
eddy current (EC) 153, 157
Effective Sample Size (ESS) 104
Electromagnetic thermography (EMT) 153
Evaluated Nuclear Structure Data File (ENSDF) 23
Extended Homogeneous source (EHS) 72

F

fetal bovine serum (FBS) 166

G

galactic cosmic rays (GCR) 111
Generalized Linear Mixed Models (GLMM) 87, 97
genome architecture 165, 175, 177
global irradiation 219, 226
green fluorescent protein (GFP) 166

H

high-energy and charge (HZE) 111
horizontal radiation 219
human umbilical vein endothelial cells (HUVEC) 139

I

infrared (IR) 153
intensity-modulated radiation therapy (IMRT) 127
International Atomic Energy Agency (IAEA) 35, 53
International Commission on Radiological Protection (ICRP) 99, 108
International Monitoring System (IMS) 19
International Space Station (ISS 111, 116
ischemic heart disease (IHD) 112
isochron method 5

L

linear energy transfer (LET) 95, 182
linear-quadratic (LQ) 182
low Earth orbit (LEO) 111

M

Markov chain Monte Carlo (MCMC) 100, 103
medullary thyroid cancer (MTC) 181
minigastrin analogue 181
Monte Carlo Markov Chain (MCMC) 243
Monte Carlo (MC) 242
Monte Carlo simulations (MCS) 73
multivariate adaptive regression splines (MARS) 228, 230, 234

N

National Center for Atmospheric Research (NCAR) 213
National Research Council (NRC) 111
Neural Network (NN) 74
never-smokers (NS) 112
non-small cell lung cancer (NSCLC) 195
nuclear chronometry 22
Nuclear chronometry 19
nuclear physics 3
nuclear power plant (NPP) 87

O

Overall survival (OS) 197

P

passive infrared thermography (PIT) 153
peptide receptor radionuclide therapy (PRRT) 181
Photo Voltaic (PV) 242
physics-mathematical pattern modeling and mining (PPMM) 154
positron emission tomography (PET) 195, 205
power systems 241
principal component analysis (PCA) 154
Principal Component Analysis (PCA) 74
probability mass function (PMF) 129
probability of causation (PC) 111
probability of detection (POD) 154
pulsed field gel electrophoresis 139

R

radiation measurements 219
radiation protection 102, 104
Radiometric dating methods 4
radionuclide metrology 3
radionuclides 3, 4, 8, 10, 13, 14, 15
Radiotherapy (RT) 195
Radium Contaminated Legacy Sites (RCLS) 71
relative biological effectiveness (RBE) 111
risk of exposure induced death (REID) 111
robust optimization model 128, 129
robust optimization (RO) 127
root mean square error (RMSE) 228
rubidium-strontium dating 5

S

Smart Grid (SG) 241
solar energy resource assessment 219
solar irradiance 227
solar particle events (SPEs) 111
Solar radiation 209, 215, 216
Solar radiation data 219
Standard deviations (SD) 144
Sun-Earth geometry 227
sunshine duration 209, 212, 214, 216

T

the Consultative Committee for Ionizing Radiation, CCRI 3
Thematic Mapper (TM) 227, 237
thermodynamic integration (TI) 103
thymidine kinase 1 (TK1) 195
total number of birds (TNB) 91
Transfer Factor (TF) 35, 53

V

volumes of interest (VOI) 197

W

Wildlife Transfer Database (WTD 35, 53

Y

yellow fluorescent protein (YFP) 166

Z

zirconium 99, 100, 101, 104, 105, 106, 107, 108, 109